The Physiology and Pharmacology of the Microcirculation
VOLUME 1

Physiologic and Pharmacologic Bases of Drug Therapy

Series Editors

Stanley Greenberg
and
Thomas M. Glenn

Department of Pharmacology
College of Medicine
University of South Alabama
Mobile, Alabama

Gene C. Palmer (Editor) Neuropharmacology of Central Nervous System and Behavioral Disorders, 1981

R. Douglas Wilkerson (Editor) Cardiac Pharmacology, 1982

Nicholas A. Mortillaro (Editor) The Physiology and Pharmacology of the Microcirculation, Volume 1, 1983

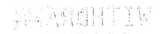

The Physiology and Pharmacology of the Microcirculation

VOLUME 1

EDITED BY

Nicholas A. Mortillaro

Department of Physiology
College of Medicine
University of South Alabama
Mobile, Alabama

1983

Academic Press

A Subsidiary of Harcourt Brace Jovanovich, Publishers
New York   London
Paris   San Diego   San Francisco   São Paulo   Sydney   Tokyo   Toronto

ACADEMIC PRESS, INC.
111 Fifth Avenue, New York, New York 10003

United Kingdom Edition published by
ACADEMIC PRESS, INC. (LONDON) LTD.
24/28 Oval Road, London NW1 7DX

Library of Congress Cataloging in Publication Data

Main entry under title:

The Physiology and pharmacology of the microcirculation.
    2 v, ';
    (Physiologic and pharmacologic bases of drug therapy)
    Includes index.
    1. Microcirculation. 2. Capillaries--Effect of
drugs on. I. Mortillaro, Nicholas A. II. Series.
QP106.6.P48 1982   612'.135   82-20562
ISBN 0-12-508301-7 (v.1)

To my wife Mildred, daughter Susan, and son Philip

Contents

8. Microcirculation of the Heart

Harvey V. Sparks, Jr., Jerry B. Scott, and Mark W. Gorman

9. Microcirculation of the Kidneys

L. Gabriel Navar, Andrew P. Evan, aŋd László Rosivall

Contributors

Numbers in parentheses indicate the pages on which the authors' contributions begin.

Albert Alm (299), Department of Ophthalmology, University Hospital, Uppsala 14, Sweden

George E. Barnes (209), Microcirculation Research Institute and Department of Medical Physiology, College of Medicine, Texas A & M University, College Station, Texas 77843

Jeffrey L. Borders (209), Microcirculation Research Institute and Department of Medical Physiology, College of Medicine, Texas A & M University, College Station, Texas 77843

Frederick A. Curro (39), Department of Pharmacology, College of Dentistry, Fairleigh Dickinson University, Hackensack, New Jersey 07601, and Department of Oral Surgery, New York University, New York, New York 10010

Andrew P. Evan (397), Department of Anatomy, School of Medicine, Indiana University, Indianapolis, Indiana 46226

Anthony H. Goodman (209), Microcirculation Research Institute and Department of Medical Physiology, College of Medicine, Texas A & M University, College Station, Texas 77843

Mark W. Gorman (361), Department of Physiology, Michigan State University, East Lansing, Michigan 48824

D. Neil Granger (157), Department of Physiology, College of Medicine, University of South Alabama, Mobile, Alabama 36688

Harris J. Granger (209), Microcirculation Research Institute and Department of Medical Physiology, College of Medicine, Texas A & M University, College Station, Texas 77843

Stan Greenberg (39), Department of Pharmacology, College of Medicine, University of South Alabama, Mobile, Alabama 36688

Gerald A. Meininger (209), Microcirculation Research Institute and Department of Medical Physiology, College of Medicine, Texas A & M University, College Station, Texas 77843

Nicholas A. Mortillaro (143), Department of Physiology, College of Medicine, University of South Alabama, Mobile, Alabama 36688

L. Gabriel Navar (397), Department of Physiology and Biophysics, Nephrology Research and Training Center, University of Alabama in Birmingham, Birmingham, Alabama 35294

Gene C. Palmer (1), Frist–Massey Neurological Institute, Nashville, Tennessee 37203

Michael A. Perry (157), Department of Physiology, College of Medicine, University of South Alabama, Mobile, Alabama 36688

*László Rosivall** (397), Department of Physiology and Biophysics, University of Alabama in Birmingham, Birmingham, Alabama 35294

Jerry B. Scott (361), Department of Physiology, Michigan State University, East Lansing, Michigan 48824

Harvey V. Sparks, Jr. (361), Department of Physiology, Michigan State University, East Lansing, Michigan 48824

Toshiki P. Tanaka (39), Kanagawa Dental College, Department of Pharmacology, 82 Inaoka, Yokosuka, Kanagawa, Japan

Aubrey E. Taylor (143), Department of Physiology, College of Medicine, University of South Alabama, Mobile, Alabama 36688

Richard J. Traystman (237), Department of Anesthesiology and Critical Care Medicine, Johns Hopkins Hospital, Baltimore, Maryland 21205

*Present address: Department of Pathophysiology, Semmelweis University Medical School, Budapest H-1445, Hungary.

Foreword

Since the early 1960s, an enormous amount of information has been generated with regard to the physiopharmacology of the microcirculation. The present volumes are compilations of microcirculatory phenomena by renowned experts, who have integrated present knowledge into concise overviews concerning *(1)* how oxygen delivery is regulated by the tissues, *(2)* the biochemistry of smooth muscle and endothelial cells, and *(3)* the mechanisms associated with movement of fluid and molecules across capillary wall barriers.

The two volumes are organized such that the first five chapters of Volume 1 cover the biochemistry, metabolism, pharmacology, and physiology of the general microcirculation. Then, the microcirculation of 14 different organs is presented, with special emphasis on the metabolic needs of each organ as it carries out its functions. The action of different physiological hormones such as the prostaglandins on microcirculatory phenomena is integrated into the overall functional aspects of each organ's biochemistry, fluid balance, transcapillary solute exchange, blood flow, etc. Each contributor approaches the microcirculatory function of each organ using precise modeling ideas, and, although computer models are not included in these chapters, the reader can easily follow the developments along the lines of input–output functions, which have been analyzed away from a black-box approach, because each organ system is discussed relative to its biochemistry, special metabolic needs, functional requirements, and its role in the overall organism's scheme of energy–function balance.

Dr. Mortillaro is to be congratulated for developing such a cohesive and informative set of chapters. The information contained in these volumes promises to serve as factual material for many years to come, because the chapters have sufficient depth to please the expert; they are also written in a style such that not only researchers but medical and graduate students will find the text most useful for learning the basic functional aspects of the microcirculation.

The *milieu internal* of Claude Bernard has not changed over the last century, yet our understanding of the regulatory phenomena associated with this milieu has expanded by orders of magnitude. A comparison of the effects of PCO_2 (or pH) on the cerebral circulation as compared to the peripheral vessels indicates how very differently organs can respond to the same stress, change of metabolic state, vascular pressure, etc. These volumes will give the reader a better appreciation and understanding of the complexities and interrelationships that exist within the body's vascular system as it works to provide nutrients to the many different types of functional cells. For the first time, the reader is treated to a physiological–pharmacological treatise on the microcirculation that focuses on the functional states and needs of each tissue as it relates to maintaining overall body hemostasis.

Aubrey E. Taylor

Preface

This work, the first of two volumes on *The Physiology and Pharmacology of the Microcirculation,* brings together the expertise of many active and eminent investigators in the field. The approach taken in presenting the latest information in this vast field differs from that of other publications on the same subject, and in this respect it is unique. Whereas previous publications have dealt with microcirculation along functional lines, each chapter covering a specific function of many tissue beds and organs, the initial five chapters of the present volume present introductory, overall views of basic concepts regarding the microcirculation, with each of the remaining chapters covering a specific organ system. Hence, the reader whose knowledge of the microcirculation is limited may find it advantageous to concentrate first on the introductory chapters before moving on, whereas the experienced reader may wish to go directly to the chapter(s) dealing with a specific organ system(s).

Chapter 1 treats the biochemistry of isolated elements of the microvasculature, with special emphasis on the central nervous system. Chapter 2 brings into focus that microvascular element, the vascular smooth muscle, discussing not only ultrastructural characteristics, innervation, and contraction–relaxation, but also the effects of both endogenous and pharmacological vasoactive substances on vascular smooth muscle. Chapters 3 and 4 are concerned with the exchange mode of the microcirculation, the former concentrating on an overview of the mechanisms involved in the regulation of transcapillary fluid exchange, the latter focusing on the permeability of capillaries to small and large molecules in a variety of tissues. Chapter 5 concludes the introductory section with a consideration of the control mechanisms modulating microcirculatory dynamics.

Beginning with Chapter 6, the emphasis shifts to a consideration of the micro-circulation in particular organs. Chapter 6 focuses on the cerebral circulation, considering not only the vascular anatomy, but also the regulation of cerebral blood flow in the adult, neonate, and fetus. In Chapter 7 the microcirculation of the eye is presented, with special emphasis on the part of its microcirculation responsible for providing the nutrition to the retina, that is, the retinal and choroidal circulation. Microcirculation of the heart is covered in Chapter 8, in which the functional anatomy, microcirculatory exchange, and the determinants of coronary blood flow are discussed. Finally, Chapter 9 concentrates on the microcirculation of the kidney, which is most directly related to the filtration of fluid into the tubular systems and the return of the tubular reabsorbate into the vascular system.

In Volume 2, the presentation of the microcirculation of particular organ continues with chapters on the lung, endocrine glands (with an emphasis on the salivary glands and exocrine pancreas), liver and spleen, stomach, small and large intestines, bone, skin, skeletal muscle, and the pathophysiology of the microcirculation.

I wish to thank the staff of Academic Press for their guidance and patience during the preparation of these volumes.

Nicholas A. Mortillaro

Contents of Volume 2
(in press)

1 Biochemical Mechanisms of the Microvasculature

Gene C. Palmer

I. Introduction

Since the late 1970s techniques have been developed to isolate and culture capillaries from both central and peripheral tissues. With the advent of these methods a host of biochemical and pharmacogic investigations has

1

helped to elucidate the physiologic and pathologic roles of the microcirculation. For various reasons the majority of the investigations have centered on the cerebral microvasculature, namely, capillaries, choroid plexus vessels, and pial vessels. The most obvious reason has been the enigma of the *blood–brain barrier*. Thus, capillaries have been considered to be the site of this perplexing structure. Capillaries in most regions of the brain have distinctive structural properties compared with capillaries in other organs. These special properties include overlapping endothelial cells jointed to one another by tight junctions, an absence of fenestrations in the endothelial cell wall, a paucity of pinocytotic vesicles, a high mitochondrial content, a lack of free permeability to water, a complete investiture of the capillary by astrocytic processes, the presence of monoamine nerve endings, a special complement of barrier enzymes, and carrier-mediated transport mechanisms. Regions of the brain not displaying evidence of a blood–brain barrier, that is, area postrema, pineal gland, and choroid plexus, contain capillaries that resemble those of peripheral organs. The choroid plexus, however, has tight junctions between the epithelial cells. In summation, the integrity of the capillary lining ensures that substances do not move in and out of the brain in an indiscriminate fashion but that, instead, their movement is a highly regulated process (see Raichle and Grubb, 1978; Hartman *et al.*, 1980; Cutler, 1980; Lindvall and Owman, 1980).

This chapter focuses principally on the biochemistry of isolated elements of the central microvasculature with reference made to isolated peripheral microvessels according to available data. These biochemical findings are correlated when possible to physiologic and/or pathologic conditions. The principal function of the capillary is to control the influx and efflux of substances into and out of the brain parenchyma. The choroid plexus is responsible for the formation and maintenance of the chemical composition of the cerebrospinal fluid. This structure also contains energy-dependent, saturable, and stereospecific processes to transport amino acids and metabolites. The pia-arachnoid likewise contains specialized mechanisms for transport but mainly removes substances from the brain by bulk flow mechanisms.

The movement of nonelectrolytes through cells of the blood–brain barrier and cerebrospinal fluid barriers may be regulated by passive diffusion, pinocytosis, or carrier transport. Passive diffusion occurs across a concentration gradient and depends on the lipid solubility and degree of ionization of the substance in question. Pinocytosis is not considered an important transport mechanism in cerebral capillaries; however, recent evidence indicates that neurohumoral transmission may control this system. The specialized carrier transport systems are the most important function of the central capillaries in controlling the entrance and egress of materials into and from the brain. Facilitated transport systems exist for the influx and efflux of glucose. The system maintains a higher brain parenchymal level of glucose, probably as a safety factor. Small amino acids are removed from the brain by a sodium-dependent carrier, whereas the entrance of neutral and large amino acids is controlled by a unidirectional equilibrium system. Carrier systems are also present for ketones (β-hydroxybutyrate). This mechanism is inducible during starvation and serves also as a safety margin for energy during neonatal development. The influx of ketones is linked to another safety condition, the efflux of lactate and pyruvate, thereby controlling the brain pH environment under hypoxic situations. Special carrier-mediated systems are located in the choroid plexus for ascorbic acid and in the capillaries for tetrahydrofolic acid (for review see Cutler, 1980).

II. Techniques for Isolation of Microvessels

Several methods have been developed to isolate relatively purified microvessels from a variety of tissues, especially from brain. When one is evaluating microvessels for biochemistry or pharmacology experiments, it is necessary to use preparations that are as pure as possible. For example, most capillary fractions contain red blood cells or mast cells, which possess unique metabolic characteristics. Preperfusion of the tissue with saline, balanced salt solutions, or appropriate buffers is one way of alleviating this problem. For brain tissues the pia must be removed, because it will isolate with the capillary fraction and in addition has different biochemical properties. Isolated cells should be monitored for purity by the use of phase-contrast microscopy and various enzyme markers; for example, alkaline phosphatase or γ-glutamyl transpeptidase can be determined either histochemically or biochemically. Some workers feel that isolation of cells with hyaluronidase, trypsin, or collagenase digestion adds further problems to biochemical analyses because of potential damage to the endothelium. The following discussion briefly outlines several popular methods, many of which are not difficult to perform.

A. Peripheral Endothelium

Endothelium from a variety of tissues has been successfully isolated either by perfusing the tissue with digestive enzymes and centrifuging down the isolated endothelium or by mincing the tissue in a buffered

balanced salt solution containing digestive enzymes. The freed endothelium and capillaries are isolated from the supernatant by centrifugation, washing, and recentrifugation and may be used directly or cultured
(Tomasi *et al.*, 1978; Folkman *et al.*, 1979; Spector *et al.*, 1980). One simple
process is to remove large vessels (aorta, human umbilical vessels), ligate
one end of a vessel, and fill it with a suitable medium (Earle's solution plus
buffers) containing 0.1% collagenase. After 10 min the suspension containing the endothelium is centrifuged at low speed; the cells are collected and
either placed in culture media or used directly for biochemical experimentation (Dembinska-Kiec *et al.*, 1980).

B. Central Microvessel Fractions

The first reported procedure by which viable capillary fractions were
removed from mammalian brain was carried out by Joō and Karnushina
(1973). The rodent cerebral cortex (freed of pia and external vessels) is
removed and chopped into fine pieces in cold 0.25 M sucrose. The tissue
is passed successively through nylon bolting cloth of 333- and 110-μm
pore size. The sucrose breaks up adherent astrocytic endfeet. The mixture is centrifuged at 1500 g for 10 min. The pellet is resuspended in sucrose, filtered through 110-μm nylon cloth, and recentrifuged (1500 g).
The second pellet is resuspended in 0.25 M sucrose, filtered, and layered
onto a sucrose gradient of 1.5, 1.3, and 1.0 M sucrose. The samples are
centrifuged in a swinging bucket rotor at 58,000 g for 30 min. The capillaries are collected from the final pellet.

An even more convenient capillary preparation was devised by Brendel
et al. (1974). Small pieces of bovine cortex are lightly homogenized in
Earle's balanced salt solution buffered with Hepes. The homogenate is
poured over a 153-μm nylon sieve and washed with buffer. The capillaries
are retained on the sieve, collected, rehomogenized, and washed two
more times. The capillaries thus removed have a high rate of metabolic
activity.

Goldstein and co-workers (1975) developed a popular method that readily yields a highly purified microvessel fraction. The brain region is
minced in an oxygenated salt solution (Ringer) containing glucose and bovine serum albumin. The mince is successively filtered through 670-, 335-,
and 116-μm nylon meshes and centrifuged at 1000 g for 10 min. The pellet
is suspended in 100 ml of buffer containing 25% bovine serum albumin
and recentrifuged at 1000 g for 15 min. The pellets containing capillaries

and free nuclei are resuspended in the original buffer and washed through a glass bead column (1.2 × 1.5 cm, bead size of 0.25 mm). The nuclei pass through, while the beads with adherent capillaries are placed in buffer and gently agitated. After the beads settle the capillaries are removed from the supernatant by centrifugation at 500 g for 5 min.

Variations of the three procedures described have been successfully employed by a variety of investigators (Mršulja et al., 1976; Maurer et al., 1980; Matheson et al., 1980; Head et al., 1980).

A technique using eight low-speed centrifugations for central capillary isolations was reported by Hwang et al. (1980). The cortex is first homogenized in a sucrose–Hepes–CaCl₂ buffer followed by centrifugations and resuspension of the pellets in Krebs–Ringer bicarbonate buffers. The speeds and times for the centrifugation steps are as follows: 1000 g, 10 min, twice; 100 g, 15 sec, twice; 200 g, 1 min, four times.

A variation of the density gradient technique for microvessel isolation was used by White et al. (1981). The tissue is first homogenized and centrifuged at low speed. The pellet is suspended into 2.13 M sucrose (in 1 mM MgCl₂), and gradients of 1.29 and 0.32 M sucrose are layered on top of the suspension. The samples are centrifuged for 30 min at 64,000 g, and the purified microvessels are collected at the 1.29–2.13 M sucrose interface.

For use in tissue culture studies, finely chopped sections of brain are suspended for 5 min in a balanced salt solution containing trypsin (0.5%). Fetal calf serum is added to stop the reaction, and the samples are centrifuged at 500 rpm for 10 min. The pellet is rewashed with a suitable growth medium and then cultured (Phillips et al., 1979).

Nathanson (1980b) separated vascular cells from epithelium in the cat choroid plexus. The tissue is cut in small pieces (phosphate-buffered saline) and placed into small conical centrifuge tubes containing Hepes buffer, Na⁺, K⁺, bicarbonate, glucose, and 0.1% trypsin. After 15 min incubation, the cells are allowed to settle and the supernatant containing free epithelial cells is added to a tube containing horse serum. The dissociation process on the pieces of choroid plexus is repeated and the combined supernatants are filtered through a 100-μm screen, sedimented, and washed twice in enzyme-free buffer. The final pellet is used for biochemical determinations. The remaining deepithelialized choroid vasculature is washed twice and the final pellet subsequently used.

These techniques for isolated microvessel preparations have contributed significantly to our understanding of the biochemical and pharmacologic processes associated with the blood–brain barrier.

III. Monoamine Mechanisms

A. *Innervation, Levels of Monoamines, and Regulatory Enzymes*

1. *Norepinephrine and Dopamine*

Direct biochemical measurements as well as improved methods of immunofluorescence and electron microscopy have localized norepinephrine (NE) and, to a lesser extent, dopamine (DA) nerve endings to the capillary endothelium, choroid plexus, and the pia-arachnoid of mammalian brain (Table I). The endothelia appear to receive their innervation via NE cell bodies localized in the locus coeruleus, whereas nerve endings to the choroid plexus and pia-arachnoid originate from the superior cervical ganglion. In this manner rats whose superior cervical ganglia were removed showed severe deficits in immunofluorescence of DA β-hydroxylase activity in the adrenergic fibers to the pia and choroid, whereas that to the cerebral capillaries was unaffected. Thus, the source of NE fibers to the capillaries was considered to be within the brain itself and was subsequently identified through physiologic, biochemical, histologic, and pharmacologic experimentation to be the locus coeruleus. There do not appear to be, however, specialized synaptic contacts on the endothelium. The adrenergic varicosity appears instead to contact directly the basal lamina of the capillary endothelium. In the choroid plexus two types of adrenergic endings make contact with either the stroma between the choroidal endothelium or on smooth muscle cells (Nielsen and Owman, 1967; Hartman *et al.*, 1972; Edvinsson and MacKenzie, 1977; Nakamura and Milhorat, 1978; Preskorn and Hartman, 1979; Hardebo and Owman, 1980; Hartman *et al.*, 1980; Suddith *et al.*, 1980; Marin *et al.*, 1980; Head *et al.*, 1980).

The enzymes for the synthesis and metabolism of NE and DA have been identified in the capillaries, pia-arachnoid, and choroid plexus of the brain (Table I). The activity of tyrosine hydroxylase in cerebral capillaries was sevenfold less than that in whole rat brain. On the other hand, the activities of dopa decarboxylase, dopamine β-hydroxylase, monoamine oxidase A and B, and especially catechol O-methyltransferase were considerably greater in the cerebral capillary, pial, or choroid plexus fractions (Lai *et al.*, 1975; Lai and Spector, 1978; Marin *et al.*, 1980; Lindvall and Owman, 1980; Kaplan *et al.*, 1981). These enzymes, especially the high activities of dopa decarboxylase, monoamine oxidase, and catechol O-methyltransferase, provide an additional blood–brain, enzymatic barrier to prevent the precursors of and circulating levels of catecholamines

TABLE I

Catecholamine Mechanisms in the Central Microvasculature

Mechanism	Cell type	Method used for identification	References[a]
Synthesizing enzymes			
Tyrosine hydroxylase	Capillaries	Biochemical	1
Dopa decarboxylase	Capillaries	Histochemical	2
	Pia-arachnoid	Fluorescence	3
	Choroid plexus	Biochemical	4
Dopamine β-hydroxylase	Capillaries	Immunofluorescence	5
	Pia	Biochemical	6
	Choroid plexus	Biochemical	6
Metabolizing enzymes			
Monoamine oxidase	Capillaries	Biochemical	1, 7
A and B	Pia	Biochemical	2
	Choroid epithelium	Biochemical	8
Catechol O-methyl-	Choroid endothelium	Immunofluorescence	2
transferase	Choroid epithelium	Immunofluorescence	9
	Pia-arachnoid	Immunofluorescence	9
Norepinephrine and dopamine levels	Pia and capillaries	Radioenzymatic assay	1, 6, 10
Norepinephrine uptake	Pia and capillaries	Biochemical	11, 12
Serotonin-induced release of norepi- nephrine	Pia	Biochemical	11
L-Dopa levels	Capillaries	Fluorescence	13
Norepinephrine endings	Choroid plexus	Electron microscope	14
	Pia	Electron microscope	15
	Capillaries	Electron microscope	16, 17

[a] References: 1, Lai *et al.* (1975); 2, Hardebo and Owman (1980); 3, Melamed *et al.* (1980); 4, Rebert (1977); 5, Hartman *et al.* (1972); 6, Marin *et al.* 1980); 7, Lai and Spector (1978); 8, Lindvall and Owman (1980); 9, Kaplan *et al.* (1981); 10, Head *et al.* (1980); 11, Marin *et al.* (1979); 12, Abe *et al.* (1980); 13, Spatz *et al.* (1980); 14, Nakamura and Milhorat (1978); 15, Swanson *et al.* (1977); 16, Nielsen and Owman (1967); 17, Suddith *et al.* (1980).

from entering the brain (for reviews see Edvinsson and MacKenzie, 1977; Hardebo and Owman, 1980).

2. Serotonin

This biogenic amine has received only limited study with regard to the central microcirculatory systems. With larger pial vessels topical application of serotonin induces a vasoconstriction, whereas the smaller vessels may vasodilate provided that they possess an active tone. The latter vasodilatory action is inhibited by the β-adrenergic blocking agent propranolol, suggesting an interaction of both serotonin and NE at receptor sites within these vessels (for discussion see Edvinsson and MacKenzie, 1977). In further work of this nature, Marin et al. (1979) showed that serotonin elicited a dose-related release of NE from cat pia. This efflux was reduced by prior superior cervical ganglionectomy or reserpine or cocaine treatment. However, some types of serotonin-containing nerve endings have been shown to terminate on rat cerebral microvessels. Lesions to the nucleus raphe dorsalis and medialis, as well as pretreatment with p-chlorophenylalanine (tryptophan hydroxylase inhibitor) or p-chloroamphetamine (toxic to the nucleus raphe), produce a decrease in serotonin content in the microvessels. Furthermore, injections of the precursor amino acid tryptophan elevate serotonin content in the vessels (Reinhard et al., 1979).

3. Histamine

Jarrott and co-workers (1979) demonstrated higher levels of histamine in bovine cerebral microvessels than in the cerebral gray matter, striatum, or hippocampus. Furthermore, Head et al. (1980) measured histamine levels in parenchymal microvessels from the rat, rabbit, and bovine brains. In further work endogenous levels of histamine and associated enzymes, L-histidine decarboxylase and histamine N-methyltransferase, were observed in guinea pig cerebral capillaries (Karnushina et al., 1980a). The absence of synaptosomes in the capillary fraction, as well as the low activity of histidine decarboxylase in the vessel preparations (also see Jarrott et al., 1979), indicated the source of histamine to be the mast cells rather than direct nerve endings. A functional role for histamine-elicited receptor activation will be subsequently discussed.

B. Functional Significance of Adrenergic Innervation on the Central Microvasculature

1. Capillaries

In the preceding section evidence was presented for direct adrenergic innervation on the basal lamina of brain capillaries. If capillaries are devoid of smooth muscle cells, then what physiologic role must these adrenergic nerves play with regard to capillary function? To address this question, Raichle and co-workers (Raichle et al., 1975, 1976; Raichle and Grubb, 1978; Grubb et al., 1978; Hartman et al., 1980) performed a series of experiments with monkeys that had undergone bilateral removal of the superior cervical ganglia. Water does not freely cross the cerebral capillary endothelium. Thus, by devising a complicated apparatus in which ^{15}O water is generated by a cyclotron and administered directly and rapidly into the carotid, it was possible to measure both cerebral blood flow (CBF) and the extraction of the diffusible tracer (^{15}O water) simultaneously during a single capillary transit through the brain. A prominent finding in these studies was that the rate of CBF and capillary permeability were not linked to one another. In the first experiments intraventricular administration of low doses of the α-adrenergic blocking agent phentolamine acted to increase CBF and decrease capillary permeability to water. With higher phentolamine doses CBF was depressed whereas capillary permeability was elevated. The low-dose effect was thought to be a result of adrenergic receptor blockade, which prevented the action of NE to increase water permeability across the capillary endothelium. The high-dose action could have been a direct drug stimulation of the vessel or a blockade of presynaptic, autoregulatory α receptors. In the latter case more NE would be released from the presynaptic nerve terminal. In further work, stimulation of the locus coeruleus (supplies the NE fibers to the capillaries) with the cholinergic agonist carbachol, or by direct, low-intensity electrical pulses, resulted in an increased capillary permeability to water and a decreased CBF. These actions of carbachol were inhibited by phentolamine. Central injections of antidiuretic hormone likewise increased capillary permeability to water without influencing CBF. These findings and those by Preskorn *et al.* (1980c; discussed in Section III,E,4,a) provide evidence that noradrenergic endings influence the permeability of small molecules across the blood–brain barrier and thus may act to maintain fluid fluxes in the brain under both normal and pathologic conditions.

2. Choroid Plexus

Both the secretory epithelium and blood vessels of the choroid plexus receive an abundant supply of adrenergic nerve endings from the superior sympathetic ganglia. When these nerves are denervated or electrically stimulated, the released NE exerts a marked inhibition on the bulk production of cerebrospinal fluid. When monoamine oxidase inhibitors were given to laboratory animals, the inhibitory action of intraventricularly administered NE was likewise enhanced with respect to cerebrospinal fluid formation. Both monoamine oxidase A and B are present in the choroid plexus. The B form, which is normally not found in sympathetic nerves, most likely deaminates excess plasma and extracellular levels of central dopamine. The A form may be similarly responsible in deaminating excess levels of NE, serotonin, and epinephrine, as well as maintaining the sympathetic tone to inhibit excess cerebrospinal fluid production (for discussion see Lindvall and Owman, 1980).

3. Pia

The pial vessels appear to function with either vasoconstriction or dilation in response to monoamines. In this regard they appear to function like peripheral or major central blood vessels. For example, when topically applied to brain, serotonin constricts larger pial vessels while dilating small vessels. Moreover, the existing tone of the vessel determines its response to monoamines. Acetylcholine also plays a dual role. At low doses it causes a dilatation, and at high doses pial constriction ensues. The vasodilatory response is associated with muscarinic receptors, whereas release of acetylcholine at axoaxonic interactions on NE nerves results in an inhibition of NE release via nicotinic receptors. Pial vessels are usually constricted in response to NE through mechanisms associated with α-adrenergic mechanisms. Stimulation of sympathetic nerves to the pia decreases blood flow via vasoconstriction. When the superior cervical ganglia are removed, the pial vessels dilate but tone returns when the adrenergic receptors develop sufficient supersensitivity to circulating monoamines. β-Adrenergic agonists will dilate pial vessels that are maintained in an active tonic state. When dopamine (low concentrations) was applied to pial vessels, a vasodilatation occurred. At higher doses dopamine induced a vasoconstriction; however, no such dopamine nerves have been identified with regard to pial innervation (Altura *et al.*, 1980). The interactions of various neurotransmitters with regard to pial function are therefore a complex issue (for review see Edvinsson and MacKenzie, 1977).

C. Catecholamine Receptors Identified by Ligand-Binding Techniques

In only two investigations have catecholamine receptors been identified in cerebral microvessels by the use of receptor ligand-binding techniques. Harik *et al.* (1980) examined ligand binding in rat and swine microvessels with the specific β-adrenergic antagonist dihydroalprenolol and the α-adrenergic ligand WB-4101. The microvessels from both species displayed binding to only the β ligand. The data for the rat are in keeping with the β-adrenergic stimulation of adenylate cyclase discussed in the following section. Microvessels from the bovine cerebrum show evidence of binding to α-adrenergic, β-adrenergic, and histamine$_1$ receptors (Peroutka *et al.*, 1980). Thus, anatomic evidence of adrenergic innervation of capillaries is supported by the capacity of released neurotransmitter agents to combine in a stereospecific manner to receptor sites within the innervated microvasculature.

D. Receptors Coupled to and Associated with Cyclic Nucleotide Systems

The enzyme adenylate cyclase is located at both pre- and postsynaptic locations within the central nervous system (CNS) and serves as a control point for intracellular metabolism. A neurotransmitter/neuromodulator or hormone is released presynaptically and is attracted to a receptor site. If the receptor is presynaptic, the activation thereof acts to slow down or limit the release of neurotransmitter. At postsynaptic sites receptor stimulation yields one of the following: fast inhibition, slow inhibition, fast excitation, or slow excitation. Any of these, including presynaptic actions, are coupled to metabolic events, namely, activation of adenylate cyclase, guanylate cyclase, ATPase, and phospholipase A or control of ionic channels. Receptor activation of adenylate cyclase occurs in at least three stages. (a) The neurohormone is recognized by a highly specific receptor; (b) the receptor action is magnified by GTP acting at a transducer or coupling site; (c) the catalytic site of adenylate cyclase in turn promotes the formation of adenosine cyclic 3',5'-monophosphate (cyclic AMP) from ATP; and (d) in some instances the stimulation of adenylate cyclase is associated with the release of the Ca^{2+}-activator protein (calmodulin) from the synaptic membrane into the cytosol. Apparently in these situations receptor activation cannot take place unless coupled to Ca^{2+} translocation and calmodulin release. This activated calmodulin assumes a more helical state and may, depending on the metabolic machinery of the particular cell, initiate one or more of the following: (a) activation of specific forms of either high- or low-K_m phosphodiesterases [cyclic AMP-dependent or guanosine 3',5'-monophosphate (cyclic GMP)-dependent types]; (b) activation of adenylate cyclase; (c) regulation of synaptic membrane phosphorylation via protein kinase; (d) regulation of (Ca^{2+},Mg^{2+})-ATPase, favoring extrusion of Ca^{2+}; (e) activation of phospholipase A, releasing arachidonic acid; (f) activation of phosphorylase kinase; (g) enhancement of neurotransmitter release; and (h) promotion of axoplasmic transport or disassembly of microtubules (Fig. 1).

Cyclic AMP exerts its intracellular action on metabolism primarily via an activation of a cyclic AMP-dependent protein kinase. The kinase consists of two subunits. The regulatory unit binds to cyclic AMP and effects a dissociation of the catalytic subunit, which in turn activates the protein

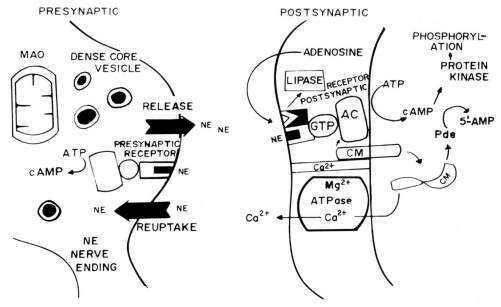

Fig. 1. Diagram of a postsynaptic monoamine receptor linked to the stimulation of cyclic AMP. CM, Calmodulin; Pde, phosphodiesterase; AC, adenylate cyclase; MAO, monoamine oxidase; NE, norepinephrine.

kinase. Protein kinase appears to be programmed into the rather specified metabolic processes depending on the cell in question. Actions attributed to protein kinase include control of synaptic permeability, neurotubular function, glycogen metabolism, induction of enzymes, and axoplasmic transport (for reviews see Daly, 1977; Nathanson, 1977; Palmer, 1981a).

1. Adenylate Cyclase–Cyclic AMP

The first indication that microvascular activation of adenylate cyclase was under hormonal regulation was observed in endothelial cells isolated from rat epididymal fat pad (Wagner *et al.*, 1972). The enzyme was located cytochemically on the luminal surface of intact capillaries, in micropinocytic invaginations, in free vesicles within the cytoplasm, and at the intracellular junctions. When intact capillaries were incubated with phosphodiesterase inhibitors, cyclic AMP accumulation was enhanced in response to NE, epinephrine, isoproterenol, prostaglandins E_1 and E_2, phenylephrine, and vasopressin. The sensitivity of the response to NE was attenuated in the presence of both α- and β-adrenergic blocking agents. Compared to the other types of microvasculature studied (Table II) these

TABLE II

Agents Eliciting Receptor Activation of Adenylate Cyclase
in the Microvasculature[a]

Species and tissue	Capillaries, endothelium	Pia-arachnoid	Choroid plexus	References[b]
Rat cerebrum	β_2, DA, GTP	β, GTP	—	1–6
Wistar rat cerebrum	H_1–H_2	—	—	7
Guinea pig cerebrum	Adenosine, NE, Isoproterenol, H_2, GTP, PGE_1, PGE_2, PGI_2	—	—	8, 9
Rabbit cerebrum	β, DA, H_1–H_2	β	β, DA, H_1–H_2, PGE_1	10, 11
Hypothalamus	NE, DA, H, GTP			12
Thalamus	NE, DA, H, GTP			12
Hippocampus	NE, DA, H, GTP			12
Brainstem	NE, DA, H, GTP			12
Cerebellum	NE, GTP			12
Cat brain	β_2, DA, GTP	β, DA, GTP	β, DA, H, GTP	13–16
Choroidal vascular	—	—	Isoproterenol	15
Choroidal epithelial	—	—	Isoproterenol	15
Bovine brain	—	—	Isoproterenol	16
Dog brain	—	—	Isoproterenol	16
Bovine aorta	PGI_2	—	—	17
Rabbit aorta	β	—	—	18
Rat epididymal fat	Vasopressin, α–β, PGE_1, PGE_2	—	—	19

[a] Abbreviations: β, β-adrenergic; α, α-adrenergic; H_1 or H_2, histamine$_1$ or histamine$_2$ receptors; NE, norepinephrine; PG, prostaglandin; DA, dopamine; GTP, GTP or 5′-guanylylimidodiphosphate.

[b] References: 1, Baca and Palmer (1978); 2, Palmer and Palmer (1978); 3, Palmer (1979); 4, Palmer (1980); 5, Herbst et al. (1979); 6, G. C. Palmer (unpublished); 7, Joó et al. (1975a); 8, Huang and Drummond (1979); 9, Karnushina et al. (1980a); 10, Palmer et al. (1980a,b); 11, Hammers et al. (1977); 12, Palmer (1981b); 13, Nathanson and Glasser (1979); 14, Nathanson (1980a); 15, Nathanson (1980b); 16, Nathanson (1979); 17, Dembinska-Kieç et al. (1980); 18, Buonassisi and Venter (1976); 19, Wagner et al. (1972).

endothelial cells from fat pads contain an adenylate cyclase that is activated by the widest variety of hormones including peptides.

　Further work by Joó and co-workers (Joó, 1972; Joó and Karnushina, 1973; Joó et al., 1975a,b) using histochemical methods (light and electron microscope) localized adenylate cyclase to rat brain capillaries. In the Wistar rat the enzyme was activated by histamine$_1$ and histamine$_2$ receptor agonists. Moreover, in keeping with the earlier observation (pinocytotic vesicles) by Wagner et al. (1972), they observed an enhanced rate of capillary pinocytotic activity as visualized histochemically with electron microscopy when dibutyryl cyclic AMP was injected into the mouse carotid (Joō, 1972). Thus, cyclic nucleotide systems may serve to enhance transport of substances across the blood–brain barrier. At about this time we began using the method of Joō and Karnushina (1973) to isolate and study neurohumoral activation of adenylate cyclase in rat cerebral capillaries. We found only an NE- and DA-activated system in the Sprague–Dawley strain of rats. This effect was magnified by the GTP analog 5′-guanylylimidodiphosphate [Gpp(NH)p]. Prostaglandins E_1, E_2, A_2, $F_{2\alpha}$, I_2, D_2, and 6-keto-$F_{1\alpha}$, octopamine, neurotensin, serotonin, and histamine analogs were ineffective. The action of NE was blocked by the mixed β blocker propranolol, but not by the α-adrenergic antagonist phentolamine or the DA antagonist haloperidol. The influence of DA was blocked only by haloperidol and highest concentrations of phentolamine. When detailed pharmacologic analyses were performed using a combination of β-adrenergic agonists–antagonists, the adrenergic stimulation was subtyped to be predominantly of a β_2 receptor (Baca and Palmer, 1978; Palmer and Palmer, 1978; Palmer, 1980; Palmer et al., 1980a,b). These data with β-adrenergic stimulation of adenylate cyclase were confirmed in incubated rat cerebral microvessels (Herbst et al., 1979; Table II).

In the cerebral cortex of another species, the guinea pig, adenylate cyclase in capillary fractions was stimulated by adenosine, β-adrenergic agonists, prostaglandins (E_1, E_2, I_2), GTP analogs, and histamine$_2$ receptors (Huang and Drummond, 1979; Karnushina et al., 1980a). In cat microvessels the enzyme was sensitive to β_2 agonists, GTP analogs, and DA (Nathanson and Glaser, 1979; Nathanson, 1980a). The capillary fractions from different brain regions (cerebrum, hypothalamus, hippocampus, thalamus, and brainstem) of the rabbit contain an enzyme system responsive to histamine, NE, DA, and Gpp(NH)p. The cerebellar enzyme from this tissue is sensitive only to NE and Gpp(NH)p (Palmer et al., 1980a,b; Palmer, 1981b). Adenylate cyclase in the endothelium from rabbit and bovine aorta is elicited by β-adrenergic agonists and prostaglandin I_2, respectively (Buonassisi and Venter, 1976; Dembinska-Kiec et al., 1980). These data indicate a difference in receptor-mediated responses for neurohumoral activation of adenylate cyclase among the different tissues from the same species, as well as variations in responses between species (Table II).

Only a few investigations have been carried out with respect to the receptors responsible for stimulation of adenylate cyclase in the pia-arachnoid. In the rabbit and rat only β-adrenergic agonists and Gpp(NH)p are active (Palmer et al., 1980a,b; G. C. Palmer, unpublished). Dopamine is effective in the cat pia, as are β-adrenergic compounds and GTP analogs (Nathanson and Glasser, 1979). In preliminary work pia from the gerbil was found to be sensitive to NE (G. C. Palmer and M. D. Taylor, unpublished).

Incubated preparations of rabbit choroid plexus were initially shown to accumulate cyclic AMP in response to added histamine and prostaglandin E_2, but not to NE (Hammers et al., 1977). With broken-cell preparations from the perfused brain the enzyme was shown to display a sensitivity to β_1- and β_2-adrenergic agonists, DA, and H_1-H_2 histamine agonists (Palmer et al., 1980a). In more detailed work with the cat choroid plexus, Nathanson (1979, 1980b) showed that activation of adenylate cyclase was mediated primarily by β_2 receptors; however, DA, GTP, and histamine were likewise effective. Moreover, when the epithelial cells of the choroid plexus were separated from the endothelium, the response was predominant in the epithelial secretory cells.

2. Guanylate Cyclase–Cyclic GMP

Until only recently it had been suggested that guanylate cyclase activity in the brain was confined to neuronal structures (Goridis et al., 1974; Kebabian et al., 1975; Nakane and Deguchi, 1978). A not surprising finding was that the enzyme is localized throughout all the cellular elements of the brain including glia, capillaries, pia, and choroid plexus (Ariano et al., 1980; Bloch-Tardy et al., 1980; Karnushina et al., 1980b; Palmer, 1981c). Karnushina and co-workers (1980b), using both histochemical and biochemical techniques, first localized guanylate cyclase to the luminal and basal membranes of capillaries. In biochemical analyses of capillary fractions guanylate cyclase was activated by Triton X-100 (Karnushina et al., 1980b) and by sodium azide, hydroxylamine, and Ca^{2+} (when the Mn^{2+} level was lowered). Agents that did not influence the enzyme included acetylcholine, histamine, enkephalin, and calmodulin (see also Palmer, 1981c).

When compared to other brain cells the pia-arachnoid contained the highest level of guanylate cyclase activity, followed by the total cerebral cortex and choroid plexus. The rate of basal activity was lowest in the capillaries. Moreover, the enzymes from the three tissues comprising the microvasculature plus the glia were scarcely sensitive to activation by azide and hydroxylamine. The latter compounds were more potent in fractions associated with neuronal endings, for example, neuronal perikarya, synaptosomes, and total cortex (Table III). There did not appear to be separate forms of guanylate cyclase (soluble and particulate) when homogenates of the pia-arachnoid and capillary fractions were centrifuged at 100,000 g for 1 h. In both preparations the enzymes were sensitive to stimulation by Ca^{2+} in the presence of low Mn^{2+} levels, and neither prepa-

TABLE III

Distribution of Guanylate Cyclase among Cellular Elements of the Rat Brain[a,b]

Conditions	Capillaries	Pia	Choroid plexus	Cortex glia	Cortex neurons	Cortex synaptosomes	Cortex
			Activity (pmol cyclic GMP/min × mg sample protein)				
0.5 mM Mn^{2+}	2 ± 0.8	17 ± 3	7 ± 2	8 ± 1	1.5 ± 0.6	6.5 ± 0.5	8.2 ± 1
0.5 mM Mn^{2+} + 2.5 mM Ca^{2+}	8 ± 0.9*	27 ± 2*	13 ± 1*	10 ± 1.5	6 ± 1.5*	13.1 ± 2*	20 ± 1*
3 mM Mn^{2+}	5 ± 0.7	35 ± 4	14 + 1	8 ± 0.5	6 ± 1	8.6 ± 0.6	19 ± 1
3 mM Mn + NaN$_3$[c]	10 ± 1.8*	33 ± 6	15 + 1	9 ± 0.4	9 ± 1*	39 ± 4*	66 ± 8*
3 mM Mn + NH$_2$OH[c]	8 ± 1.4*	38 ± 6	15 ± 1	15 ± 0.8*	8 ± 1*	100 ± 17*	57 ± 4*

[a] Values are the mean activity ±SEM of respective tissue homogenates (N = 5–8). An asterisk denotes significant difference from respective (Mn^{2+} concentration) control values.

[b] The method is described by Palmer (1981c).

[c] The values for NaN$_3$ and NH$_2$OH represent the maximal stimulation obtainable with these compounds. The concentration ranges were 0.5–1.0 mM.

ration displayed any degree of selectivity toward activation by azide or hydroxylamine (Palmer, 1981c).

The metabolic role of guanylate cyclase in the control of biochemical events within the microvasculature is unknown at this time. More work will be required in order to ascertain whether separate cyclic AMP- or cyclic GMP-dependent protein kinases even exist in these tissues. The histochemical visualization of the enzyme in the luminal and basal membranes of capillaries reveals a site where adenylate cyclase is localized (Joō et al., 1975b). Whether the enzyme serves to control the action of cyclic AMP, regulate the transendothelial transport of vesicles, or maintain the integrity of the basal lamina are topics for future discovery. The pia-arachnoid and choroid plexus possess the capability for a temperature-, oxygen-, and energy-dependent process for the uptake of both cyclic AMP and cyclic GMP. Hammers and co-workers (1977) believe that the exchange of cyclic nucleotides from the cerebrospinal fluid to the plasma takes place via this carrier-mediated, energy-dependent, ATPase-coupled system. However, the cells themselves within the choroid plexus and pia-arachnoid respond to environmental stimuli and synthesize the two cyclic nucleotides whose function is presently unknown.

3. Phosphodiesterases

In their initial report Hammers et al. (1977) mentioned the presence of a high specific activity of phosphodiesterase in homogenates of rabbit choroid plexus. Both cyclic AMP and cyclic GMP were hydrolyzed by this preparation. Microvessels isolated from bovine cerebral cortex exhibited significant cyclic AMP and cyclic GMP phosphodiesterase activities. The low-K_m form of the enzyme displayed a requirement for Mg^{2+} and Ca^{2+}. All enzyme forms were inhibited by methylxanthines, by low doses of imidazole, and in the presence of the opposite cyclic nucleotide (Stefanovich, 1979). I looked at the properties of cyclic AMP phosphodiesterase in capillary fractions isolated from perfused rat brain. The enzyme displayed a capacity for metabolism of cyclic AMP under conditions of high (0.4 mM) and low (1 μM) substrate concentration. Neither form of the enzyme was activated by Ca^{2+}. If calmodulin was added to homogenates or soluble forms (100,000 g supernatant) of the enzyme, no activation occurred, even though calmodulin was readily isolated from the capillaries. A kinetic analysis of the data suggested the presence of only one form of cyclic AMP-dependent phosphodiesterase in capillaries of the rat cerebral cortex (Palmer, 1980).

No investigations to date have dealt with the exact physiologic role of phosphodiesterase in the brain microcirculation. The enzyme may act to protect the brain from levels of cyclic nucleotides within the plasma, but these nucleotides would only penetrate the blood–brain barrier with difficulty. Most likely, the phosphodiesterases control in a precise manner the levels of cyclic AMP and cyclic GMP within the highly localized microenvironments of the cerebral microvasculature.

E. Biochemical Alterations or Regulation of Receptor Systems within the Microvasculature

1. Hypertension

When the cerebral capillaries were isolated from spontaneously hypertensive rats or the normotensive Wistar–Kyoto strain, the stimulation of adenylate cyclase by NE, DA, isoproterenol (mixed β-adrenergic agonist), salbutamol (β_2 agonist), and dobutamine (β_1 agonist) was significantly reduced in the hypertensive animals (Palmer, 1979). When the brains of the hypertensive rats were examined by histofluorescence microscopy, the degree of adrenergic staining around capillaries was considerably greater in these animals (Palmer *et al.*, 1980b). Other investigators had observed abnormally high levels of dopamine in the cerebral cortex of the spontaneously hypertensive rat (Versteeg *et al.*, 1976). This dopamine concentration is not due to enhanced metabolism by monoamine oxidase (Lai and Spector, 1977). Thus, the increased levels of catecholamines available for release during synaptic activity might induce a compensatory subsensitivity at postsynaptic receptor sites. This type of up-and-down regulation of receptor activity (Wagner *et al.*, 1979) was demonstrated in a study in which hypertensive rats were either chronically treated with the α-adrenergic agonist clonidine or the β antagonist propranolol to lower blood pressure. Stimulation of adenylate cyclase in the clonidine-treated animals by NE or DA was reduced. Alternatively, when the postsynaptic receptors were blocked with propranolol, the resultant adenylate cyclase was hyperresponsive to NE alone. In only the latter case was any specificity in receptor responses noted. In general, the receptor changes in the hypertensive rats appeared to be nonspecific (Palmer and Greenberg, 1978).

In chronic hypertension both blood–brain barrier lesions and edema are known to occur. Apparently the elevated blood pressure overextends the capillary wall, resulting in increased cerebrovascular permeability (Adachi *et al.*, 1966; Giacomelli *et al.*, 1970; Domer *et al.*, 1980). If adrenergically mediated cyclic AMP mechanisms are associated with microvascular permeability, as suggested by the work of Joó *et al.* (1975a) and Preskorn *et al.* (1980a,b,c), perhaps the reduced responsiveness of this

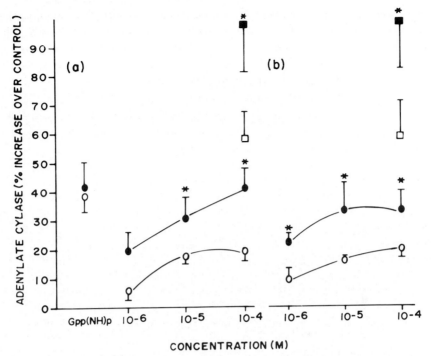

Fig. 2. Action of norepinephrine (a) or isoproterenol (b) on the stimulation of adenylate cyclase in homogenates of perfused pia-arachnoid isolated from either control or reserpine-treated rats (daily injections of 1 or 2 mg/kg for 7 days). The values are the mean ± SEM ($N = 4$) percent enzyme stimulation over respective basal activities (19.1 ± 1.1 pmol of cyclic AMP formed each minute per milligram protein. The concentration of 5′-guanylylimidodiphosphate [Gpp(NH)p] was $10^{-5} M$. Incubations consisted of 100 µg of enzyme protein incubated at 37°C for 8 min (see Palmer, 1979). *, Denotes significant difference from controls (Student's two-tailed t test); ○, control; ●, reserpine; □, Gpp(NH)p control; ■, Gpp(NH)p reserpine.

system to NE or amphetamine-induced permeability in hypertensive rats reveals a failure of a molecular mechanism to compensate (Domer *et al.,* 1980). It would be of interest to observe the action of centrally acting antihypertensive agents (propranolol, clonidine, and α-methyl-Dopa) to influence this system in hypertensive animals. One such agent, reserpine, which depletes central and peripheral monoamines and is occasionally used for hypertension, will in fact induce a greater sensitivity of catecholamine-elicited adenylate cyclase in pial vessels from normotensive rats. The cerebral capillaries were unaffected by reserpine (G. C. Palmer, preliminary observations; Fig. 2).

In another study with spontaneously hypertensive or diabetic rats the vessels in the chorid as viewed with electron microscopy contained an accumulation of basement membrane and proliferation of endothelium. These changes were thought to contribute to the narrowing of the vascular lumen (Hori *et al.*, 1980).

2. X Irradiation

If neonatal rats received a series of unilateral X-ray exposures (200 R at 2 and 3 days and 150 R at 5, 7, 9, 11, 13, and 15 postnatal days) and then were sacrificed at maturity (200 g weight), there was considerable histologic damage to the retina and hippocampus. The sensitivity of the hippocampal adenylate cyclase to stimulation by NE or DA was seriously impaired. Moreover, the overlying cortex and pial vessels displayed a similar reduced enzyme responsiveness to NE, whereas the cerebral capillary enzyme was not significantly altered. On the other hand, the retina displayed a supersensitivity of the DA-elicited adenylate cyclase (Chronister *et al.*, 1980; Palmer *et al.*, 1981). For capillary and pial data see Fig. 3. It was not known whether the X irradiation caused injury to the developing cells or inhibited DNA-dependent repair- and receptor-maintenance programs. However, histologic observations of the pia revealed a hyperplasia, which may indicate the elevation in basal enzyme activity so observed.

Radioactive yttrium (^{90}Y) was implanted into the parietal cortex of dogs and cats. A side effect of this neurosurgical procedure is severe brain edema. If animals were treated with the histamine$_2$ receptor antagonist metiamide, brain edema was prevented (Joō *et al.*, 1976). In view of the findings with certain species that histamine activates capillary adenylate cyclase, it is tempting to suggest an involvement of this histamine-coupled system in the molecular mechanisms of cerebral edema. In addition, a therapeutic rationale for treatment of cerebral edema is indicated by this study.

Microwave radiation, on the other hand, does not appear to alter drastically the permeability of parenterally administered fluorescein across the blood–brain barrier of rats. Increased fluorescein uptake was seen only when the rats were made hyperthermic in a warm-air environment. These investigations by Merritt *et al.* (1978) were in contrast to earlier work which showed that such administration of radiation did alter the rat brain permeability to saccharides (Frey *et al.*, 1975; Oscar and Hawkins, 1977).

3. Ischemia

Gerbils were subjected to bilateral common carotid occlusion for 6 min followed by isolation of brain capillaries. There was noted a decrease in the specific capillary uptake of 2-deoxy-D-glucose. At 3 h recirculation

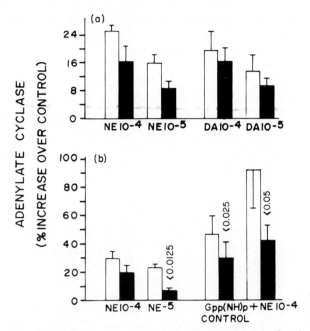

Fig. 3. Activation of adenylate cyclase in homogenates of isolated perfused cerebral capillaries (a) or pia (b) following a sequence of unilateral X irradiation (200 rads at postnatal days 2 and 3, plus 150 rads at days 5, 7, 9, 11, and 13). The animals were utilized at the adult stage (200 g weight). The mean values ± SEM (N = 5) are the percentage stimulation of enzyme activity over respective basal activity: capillaries—control (□), 21.4 ± 2; X ray (■), 19.1 ± 3; pia-arachnoid—control (□), 16 ± 3; X ray (■), 25 ± 2 (P < .05) (expressed as picomoles of cyclic AMP formed each minute per milligram protein); P values (Student's paired t test) show significant changes. DA, Dopamine; Gpp(NH)p, 5'-guanylylimidodiphosphate; NE, norepinephrine. Incubations consisted of 80–100 μg of enzyme protein incubated at 37°C for 8 min (see Palmer, 1979).

time, uptake of the sugar was enhanced. The return to normal uptake was seen in cerebral capillaries from animals whose cerebral circulation was reestablished for 5 h. Shorter time periods of carotid occlusion did not yield this depressed uptake of 2-deoxy-D-glucose (Spatz *et al.*, 1977).

In further work with bilateral carotid occlusion of gerbils the sensitivity of pial or cerebral capillary adenylate cyclase was unchanged following recirculation. However, the method for isolation of capillaries is itself carried out under ischemic conditions (G. C. Palmer and M. D. Taylor, unpublished; I. Karnushina, personal communication).

4. Drug-Induced Alterations

a. Tricyclic Antidepressants. These compounds have been used therapeutically for a number of years to treat psychiatric conditions of endogenous depression and have likewise been indicated for clinical use in migraine and sleep disturbances. The well-described biochemical action of these compounds has been their capacity to block the reuptake of released monoamines back into the presynaptic nerve terminal. In this vein, the tertiary tricyclic drugs imipramine and amitriptyline are thought to be more potent with respect to preventing the reuptake of serotonin, whereas their respective secondary amine metabolites, desipramine and nortriptyline, are more potent toward inhibiting the reuptake of released NE. Thus, on the basis of these findings and other evidence, two major types of depression, that is, noradrenergic and serotoninergic, are thought to occur as a result of functional deficits in the activity of one or the other of these two monoamines (Davis and Garver, 1978). On the other hand, several additional molecular mechanisms of these compounds have been presented: anticholinergic–antihistamine effects (Richelson and Divinetz-Romero, 1977; Palmer *et al.*, 1977), antagonism at adrenergic receptors (Palmer, 1976), and pre- or postsynaptic adrenergic receptor subsensitivity induced by chronic treatment of these agents (Frazer *et al.*, 1974; Vetulani *et al.*, 1976).

Raichle *et al.* (1975) had previously shown that capillaries in the monkey brain possessed a selective permeability to include simple passive diffusible compounds, namely, water and short-chain aliphatic alcohols. In a novel series of experiments conducted by Preskorn and co-workers (Preskorn and Hartman, 1979; Preskorn *et al.*, 1980a,b,c) all tricyclic antidepressants (doxepin > amitriptyline > imipramine > nortriptyline > desipramine > protriptyline) were shown to increase the capillary permeability of rat brain to labeled water and ethanol. This action was rapid in onset (5 min), was reversible (15 min), was dose dependent, was greatly enhanced after chronic treatment (2 weeks), and occurred at plasma concentrations demonstrating therapeutic efficacy in patients. Furthermore, this enhancement of capillary permeability was abolished by the α-adrenergic blocking agent phentolamine or by destruction of noradrenergic nerve endings with 6-hydroxydopamine. The injection of the anticholinergic drug atropine did not influence capillary permeability to the two substances, thus ruling out anticholinergic actions of the tricyclic antidepressants. These important findings revealed that capillary permeability in the brain was under adrenergic neuronal control. Moreover, the order of potency for tricyclic antidepressants to enhance capillary permeability to water and ethanol correlated with α-adrenergic receptor binding affinities within the brain (U'Prichard *et al.*, 1977). Thus, sustained elevations in central levels of NE by these drugs, in keeping with their postulated primary mechanism of action (blocking reuptake of NE), led to an enhanced exchange of compounds across the blood–brain barrier. Because the compounds were even more effective on a chronic basis, perhaps this action might be due to a subsensitivity of the presynaptic α-adrenergic receptor (autoreceptor). If this were the case, a diminished action of the autoreceptor would limit its capacity to slow down the release of NE from the presynaptic terminal and allow more NE to act at the postsynaptic capillary sites. One other aspect was noted: high levels of the tricyclic antidepressants inhibited capillary permeability. This could be due to the well-known adrenergic blocking actions of these drugs when given at high concentrations (Preskorn *et al.*, 1980c; Palmer, 1976). Nevertheless, these findings establish an important relationship between therapeutic drug use and associated changes in blood–brain barrier mechanisms.

b. d-Amphetamine and 6-Hydroxydopamine.   The compound ^{68}Ga-EDTA is used as a brain-scanning agent in nuclear medicine in order to localize pathologic failure in the blood–brain barrier. When either 6-hydroxydopamine or *d*-amphetamine was acutely given to rats before intraventricular injection of ^{68}Ga-EDTA, the rate of diffusion of this substance out of the brain was increased. Administration of either the antipsychotic drug pimozide or chronic (30 days) 6-hydroxydopamine did not produce this change. The major action of amphetamine in the brain is to release DA or NE and block their reuptake. Under certain conditions the drug may produce a psychosis indistinguishable from paranoid schizophrenia. In addition, despite destruction of NE and DA nerve endings, 6-hydroxydopamine may damage the central reward system and be linked to schizophrenia. The authors of this work (Braun *et al.*, 1980) suggested that the reduced capacity of the blood–brain barrier caused by these agents could result in a lowering of the brain barrier to circulating neurotoxins or DA, which in turn might induce behavioral changes including psychosis. Psychosis is postulated to occur as a result of excess functioning of the brain DA system. One other study was necessary, that being on the capacity of the antipsychotic pimozide to inhibit these actions of amphetamine and 6-hydroxydopamine.

c. Lysergic Acid Diethylamide.   The powerful hallucinogen lysergic acid diethylamide (*d*-LSD), when given to the conscious rat, increased blood flow to certain regions of the brain (cerebellum and frontal and parietal cortex) at a time when behavioral effects were prominent. The significance of these data is poorly understood but might correlate with increased functional demands placed on a particular brain region so influenced by psychotropic drug action (Goldman *et al.*, 1975).

IV. Other Receptor Mechanisms and Associated Biochemical Events

A. Prostaglandins

Prostaglandins (PG) are synthesized in vascular tissue and when released act to control blood vessel tone within the immediate environment. Recent evidence indicates that prostaglandins may be synthesized at several intracellular sites in the vascular wall including the endothelial cells. Stimuli such as thrombin, trypsin, or the calcium ionophore A-23187 can initiate a sequence of events starting with the activation of phospholipase A_2, which releases arachidonic acid. The enzyme cyclooxygenase then transforms the arachidonic acid to the short-lived prostaglandin precursor prostacyclin (PGI_2). Prostacyclin release from endothelium may also act as a local vasodilator and inhibitor of platelet aggregation (Spector et al., 1980; Maurer et al., 1980).

Isolated bovine cerebral microvessels incubated in glucose–bicarbonate buffer synthesized PGI_2, $PGF_{2\alpha}$, PGE_2, and thromboxane. However, addition of exogenous arachidonic acid was without effect on synthesis. Activation of lipase by the peptide melittin stimulated the synthesis of $PGF_{1\alpha}$ and $PGF_{2\alpha}$. Alternatively, when bovine artery endothelial cells were grown in tissue culture, arachidonic acid addition elicited the production of $PGF_{1\alpha}$ (Maurer et al., 1980). The prostaglandins of the endothelial system in the pial vessels may play a role in cerebral injury. Wei et al. (1980) investigated concussive brain injury in cats. Injured pial vessels as observed through a cranial window displayed sustained dilation, reduced responsiveness of the vasoconstrictive actions of hypocapnia, and a high density of endothelial lessions. When the animals were pretreated with cyclooxygenase inhibitors, these responses to concussion were absent. Likewise, when free-radical scavengers were applied topically to the cortex, the pial vessels again did not display the responses to concussion. Therefore, the immediate cause of cerebral arteriolar damage in concussive brain injury might be the generation of free radicals, which in turn initiate the synthesis of prostaglandins.

The endothelium from peripheral vessels has been more extensively studied. Linoleic acid may act as an inhibitor of the stimulation of PGI_2 synthesis in cultured liver endothelium, perhaps by competing with arachidonic acid for the cyclooxygenase (Spector et al., 1980). These cultured cells as well as cultured arterial endothelium readily produce PGI_2 in reply to an added arachidonic acid challenge (Moncada et al., 1977; Maurer et al., 1980). In addition, in rat liver endothelial cells, PGE_2 induces the formation of cyclic AMP, which in turn inhibits the synthesis of PGI_2 (Tomasi *et al.*, 1978), whereas in vascular endothelia PGI_2, PGH_2, and PGE_1 or PGE_2 elicit cyclic AMP formation (Dembinska-Kiec *et al.*, 1980; Hopkins and Gorman, 1981). What further role cyclic AMP performs with regard to endothelial metabolism is unknown. Despite the postulated direct actions of the cyclic nucleotide in the mediation of vascular relaxation (Namm and Leader, 1976), cyclic AMP in the endothelium appears to affect vascular reactivity through its influence on prostaglandin metabolism.

B. γ-Aminobutyric Acid

The powerful inhibitory transmitter γ-aminobutyric acid (GABA) was shown in a single study to bind rather specifically to receptor sites in isolated cerebral pial vessels. The vascular receptor for GABA appears to be limited to the cerebral circulation, as peripheral vessels were devoid of these GABA actions. These findings of Krause *et al.* (1980) correlated with earlier reports that glutamate decarboxylase (GABA synthesis) and GABA transaminase are also associated with cerebral blood vessels but not appreciably with peripheral blood vessels. The actions of GABA on the regulation of cerebral circulation are not clear, but the transmitter may cause vasodilation and increase local cortical blood flow (see Mršulja and Djuricic, 1980; Krause *et al.*, 1980). No studies have been conducted with GABA receptors on either cerebral microvessels or choroid plexus.

V. Transport Processes and Related Carrier Enzymes

A. ATPase or GTPase

The employment of two techniques, namely, cytochemistry following brain perfusion and electron microscopy, revealed the presence of a (K^+, Na^+)-ATPase at only the antiluminal surface of capillaries isolated from rat brain. When the plasma membranes were fractionated from isolated capillaries of bovine brain, the (K^+, Na^+)-ATPase was found only in the heavy membrane fraction. These and studies with other enzyme systems led Betz *et al.* (1980) to conclude that luminal and antiluminal membranes of brain capillaries are functionally and biochemically different. The antiluminal location of (K^+, Na^+)-ATPase is consistent with its proposed role in maintaining a constant CNS concentration of K^+ in the face of large variations in the plasma level of K^+. The ATPase might also permit the formation of cerebrospinal fluid by capillaries (Goldstein, 1979; Milhorat *et al.*, 1971). In addition, neutral amino acids were transported from the brain by an Na^+-dependent, ouabain-sensitive process, indicating a coupling of ATPase to egress of certain amino acids out of the brain (Betz and Goldstein, 1978).

Djuricic and co-workers (1980) likewise reported the presence of (K^+,Na^+)-ATPase in rat brain capillaries, as well as a distinct form of GTPase. The GTPase was postulated to act as a regulator of GTP levels that inhibit hexokinase, thereby limiting the transport of glucose. During periods of high energy demand, inhibitors of glucose transport such as GTP must be removed without interference of other transport mechanisms, that is, ATPase activity. The latter enzyme is also capable of degradation of GTP.

In contrast to the previous data Joō (1979) characterized the ATPase system of the rat cerebral capillaries. Because the enzyme was insensitive to ouabain inhibition he postulated that it must be a (Ca^{2+},Mg^{2+})-ATPase. In support of the findings of Betz *et al.* (1980), the enzyme was localized to the basal lamina (antiluminal surface). This enzyme was inhibited in a rapid and reversible manner by such divalent metals as $NiCl_2$ and $HgCl_2$. The two agents produced a leakage of the cerebral capillaries followed by the formation of collagen-like fibers within the basal lamina. Perhaps another role of the ATPase is to maintain the functional integrity of the basal lamina.

Potassium transport may be another function of ATPase in cerebral capillaries. The uptake of labeled rubidium-86, a K^+-like analog, was used to evaluate this system (Goldstein, 1978). The uptake in these studies and those of Eisenberg *et al.* (1980) was linear, blocked by ouabain, and 10-fold more active than in peripheral capillaries. Potassium in the interstitial fluid is maintained at a constant 2.8 mM concentration, and when the cerebrospinal fluid level of K^+ is elevated the pump functions to remove it from the brain to the plasma. Autoradiographic studies indicate a binding of ouabain to the surface of cerebral capillaries; presumably the carrier is located at the antiluminal surface. The pump is maintained by oxidative metabolism of both glucose and palmitate. Cerebral vessels also take up sodium by a mechanism inhibited by ouabain. This (K^+,Na^+)-ATPase responsible for the pump of K^+ was similar in both choroid plexus and capillaries. Goldstein (1978) postulated that deficits in this transport pathway could contribute to brain edema and that inhibition of the pump by steroids could be a therapeutic site of action (Chaplin *et al.*, 1981).

B. Amino Acids

Experimental evidence has indicated the presence of possibly 18 separate transport mechanisms for amino acids in the brain. This is most likely the result of different metabolic requirements among the various cell types comprising the nervous system (for discussion see Sershen and Lajtha, 1976). For example, the cerebrospinal fluid contains low levels of amino acids, which are thought to be cleared against a concentration gradient by an energy-dependent, saturable process found within the choroid plexus (Lorenzo and Cutler, 1969; Sessa *et al.*, 1976). The barrier for amino acids selectively excludes from the brain those that are nonessential. Thus, transmitter-like substances having the potential to alter the normal physiologic activity of specific brain cells are prevented from entering the brain, as indicated by their low capacity to cross the capillary endothelium. In this manner taurine, glutamate, glycine, and GABA enter the brain at only low rates (Sershen and Lajtha, 1976). Transport of essential amino acids into isolated capillaries of newborn rats is generally faster than in the adult. In addition, the uptake of neutral and basic amino acids in these preparations is not energy dependent in that inhibitors of (K^+,Na^+)-ATPase do not generally affect transport. However, the system is temperature and pH dependent, as well as saturable and stereospecific. Cross-competition between closely related compounds for uptake has likewise been shown to occur. It is suspected, but not conclusively proved, that this facilitated transport mechanism in the capillaries is bidirectional. This Na^+-independent carrier-mediated process for amino acid transport corresponds to the so-called L system (Christensen, 1969; Lorenzo and Cutler, 1969; Sershen and Lajtha, 1976; Sessa *et al.*, 1976; Hjelle *et al.*, 1978; Betz and Goldstein, 1978).

The so-called A system for amino acid transport described by Christensen (1969) is a Na^+-dependent, energy-requiring, ouabain-sensitive transport mechanism that possibly functions to translocate small neutral and nonessential amino acids. It was originally thought that the system did not function in the brain. However, Betz and Goldstein (1978) and Betz *et al.* (1980) discovered both the presence of (K^+,Na^+)-ATPase on the antiluminal membrane of capillaries and an energy-requiring, Na^+-dependent, ouabain-sensitive mechanism of amino acid transport in isolated cerebral capillaries. In a similar preparation Hwang *et al.* (1980) described a somewhat different two-step process for cystine. The first step was a binding process followed by energy-mediated transport. As postulated by Betz and Goldstein (1978) and Betz *et al.* (1980), it seems likely that this A system is a means whereby the brain can, by virtue of this specific efflux mechanism, maintain constant low levels of selected amino acids. This might prove also to be a process whereby excess levels of transmitter substances, that is glutamate, glycine, taurine, and GABA, are controlled. The cystine transport reported by Hwang *et al.* (1980) may, on the other hand, correspond to a separate ASC (alanine–serine–cysteine)-preferring system (Christensen, 1969). Whether this ASC system results in cystine entry into or egress from the brain is unknown.

White (1980) reported the existence of a vinblastine-sensitive protein transport system within the microvasculature of the rat brain. At least one species of protein above 71,000 molecular weight and one below 27,000 were transported. The physiologic significance of this process is, however, unknown.

C. Carrier Enzymes

γ-Glutamyl transpeptidase catalyzes the transfer of a γ-glutamyl residue of glutathione to amino acids. After the amino acid is converted to its γ-glutamyl derivative at or near the cell surface, a translocation step occurs, bringing the γ-glutamyl amino acid into the cell. The amino acid is then released through the action of another enzyme, γ-glutamylcyclotransferase, with concomitant formation of L-pyrrolidonecarboxylic acid, which is converted to glutamate and then to glutathione to complete the cycle. This physiologic process of degradation of glutathione appears to be involved in amino acid transport (Meister and Tate, 1976; Orlowski *et al.*, 1974). The enzyme γ-glutamyl transpeptidase has highest activities in cells associated with amino acid transport, that is, the brush border of the proximal convoluted tubules of the kidney, the apical portion of the intestinal epithelium, neuronal perikarya, the choroid plexus, glia, and brain capillaries (Albert *et al.*, 1966; Orlowski *et al.*, 1974; Sessa *et al.*, 1976; Reyes and Palmer, 1976). Isolated capillaries from the cerebrum contain the highest activities of γ-glutamyl transpeptidase, representing a 4- to 22-fold purification over the respective cortical homogenate (Orlowski *et al.*, 1974; Goldstein *et al.*, 1975; Reyes and Palmer, 1976; Sessa *et al.*, 1976; Hwang *et al.*, 1980). The enzyme is located histochemically throughout the capillary cell, and biochemical fractionation techniques show it to be heavily concentrated in both the light and heavy cell membrane fractions (Orlowski *et al.*, 1974; Mršulja *et al.*, 1976; DeBault and Cancilla, 1980; Betz *et al.*, 1980). The presence of glial cells appears to be necessary to induce the formation of γ-glutamyl transpeptidase in the capillaries (DeBault and Cancilla, 1980). As a clinical correlate, a mildly retarded patient with glutathionemia and marked glutathionuria was shown to have a drastic reduction of γ-glutamyl transpeptidase in cultured skin fibroblasts (Schulman *et al.*, 1975). It would be interesting to correlate such changes with central mechanisms.

D. Sugars

Isolated cerebral capillaries are highly metabolically active. With respect to oxygen consumption the rate of utilization may be 5–10 times higher than for other types of vascular tissue. Oxygen consumption is stimulated by succinate, indicating the function of the citric acid cycle. However, additional processes such as glycolysis and fatty acid oxidation are highly active (Brendel *et al.*, 1974).

D-Glucose enters the brain by a carrier-mediated (facilitated) transport system. Different brain cells have different carrier systems due to their individual metabolic requirements (Diamond and Fishman, 1973). Isolated cerebral capillaries have been evaluated for D-glucose transport mechanisms utilizing either the partially metabolized derivative 2-deoxy-D-glucose or the nonmetabolizable form, 3-*O*-methyl-D-glucose. In suspensions of capillaries from rat brain, labeled 2-deoxy-D-glucose or 3-*O*-methyl-D-glucose was accumulated by a linear, saturable, and temperature-dependent (maximum at 37°C) process. Uptake was competitively blocked by selected hexose isomers, namely, D-glucose, D-mannose, and 3-methyl-D-glucose, but not by D-ribose, D-galactose, D-xylose, or L-glucose. In addition, the postulated glucose-carrier antagonists phloretin, phlorizin, and cytochalasin B potently inhibited 2-deoxy-D-glucose uptake. The uptake process was neither rate limiting for the metabolism of 2-deoxy-D-glucose nor coupled to an Na^+-dependent ATPase energy-requiring mechanism. In this regard, ouabain or 2,4-dinitrophenol was minimally effective in preventing uptake (Betz *et al.*, 1979; Goldstein *et al.*, 1975, 1977). In less extensive studies these data were confirmed using 2-deoxy-D-glucose and 3-*O*-methyl-D-glucose uptake in isolated capillaries from the rabbit or gerbil. The 3-*O*-methyl analog also prevented uptake of 2-deoxy-D-glucose (Mršulja *et al.*, 1976; Spatz *et al.*, 1977). The enzyme glucose-6-phosphatase apparently is not coupled to glucose transport in the brain capillaries as suggested but may instead enhance the backward flow (efflux) of glucose from the brain during periods of rest (Anchors *et al.*, 1977).

Under conditions of cerebral ischemia in the gerbil there was an augmented uptake of 2-deoxy-D-glucose from the blood to the brain (Spatz *et al.*, 1974). Other investigators had observed a general depression of glucose transport across the blood–brain barrier during conditions of anoxia and hypoxia (Betz *et al.*, 1974; Berson *et al.*, 1975). Spatz and co-workers (1977) looked at the effect of 2-deoxy-D-glucose uptake in isolated cerebral capillaries of the gerbil following bilateral carotid occlusion. After a 6-min period of ischemia there was a decreased period of 2-deoxy-D-glucose uptake (1–5 min) followed by postischemic recovery to normal uptake (10 min) and then a transient increase (up to 1 h). The uptake could be inhibited by 3-*O*-methyl-D-glucose. In isolated capillaries from ischemic rabbit brain a deficit in 2-deoxy-D-glucose uptake was also observed. Spatz *et al.* (1977) thought that the depression in uptake following ischemia might indicate an impairment of an energy-dependent system, loss of functional integrity of the capillary endothelium, or saturation of the entry mechanism in the damaged tissue. The transient elevation of 2-deoxy-D-glucose uptake could have been due to leakage of the damaged capillary endothelium.

Lead exposure to rats resulted in an accumulation of the metal in brain capillaries. When rats were exposed to lead from 5 to 25 postnatal days, there was a block in facilitated transport and an increase in passive transport of 3-*O*-methyl-D-glucose in isolated capillaries of the rat brain. The younger animals were more susceptible to the effects of lead. Under *in vitro* conditions, when lead was added to incubated capillaries, facilitated transport was abolished (Kolber *et al.*, 1980).

A degradative product of heme, bilirubin, in an unconjugated-nonprotein bound form readily penetrates the neonatal brain, causing a cerebral encephalopathy. The compound was shown to bind to isolated 1-month-old rat capillaries in a concentration- and pH-dependent manner. Bilirubin inhibited in a noncompetitive manner the uptake of 2-deoxy-D-glucose in these preparations (Katoh-Semba and Kashiwamata, 1980).

VI. Other Enzyme Systems

A. General

As listed in Table IV the activity of a variety of other enzyme systems has been measured in brain capillaries and the choroid plexus. Alkaline phosphatase was determined by several investigators presumably as a marker enzyme to assess the purity of isolated capillary preparations. Likewise, 5'-nucleotidase and acid phsophatase were determined. Butyrylcholinesterase was highly evident in capillaries (Mršulja *et al.*, 1976; Spatz *et al.*, 1980). Perhaps this enzyme represents another barrier enzyme that prohibits excess intracerebral and plasma levels of acetylcholine from entering the brain parenchyma.

TABLE IV

Other Identified Enzymes in Brain Capillaries or Choroid Plexus

Enzyme	Tissue and species	References
Alkaline phosphatase	Rat cerebral capillaries	Joō and Karnushina (1973); Goldstein et al. (1975); Panula et al. (1978); Joō (1979); Phillips et al. (1979); Spatz et al. (1980)
	Bovine cerebral capillaries and choroid plexus	Orlowski et al. (1974); Sessa et al. (1976); Phillips et al. (1979); Betz et al. (1980)
Acid phosphatase	Bovine choroid plexus	Sessa et al. (1976)
5'-Nucleotidase	Bovine capillaries	Orlowski et al. (1974); Sessa et al. (1976); Betz et al. (1980)
Thiamine pyrophosphatase	Rabbit cerebral capillaries	Mršulja et al. (1976)
Glucose-6-phosphatase	Rat cerebral capillaries	Goldstein et al. (1975)
Butyrylcholinesterase	Rat and rabbit capillaries	Mršulja et al. (1976); Spatz et al. (1980)
Enzymes of glycolysis and gluconeogenesis	Gerbil and rat capillaries	Mršulja and Djuricic (1980)
Enzymes of pentose shunt	Gerbil and rat capillaries	Mršulja and Djuricic (1980)
Glycogen-metabolizing enzymes	Gerbil and rat capillaries	Mršulja and Djuricic (1980)

B. Sugar Metabolism

Mršulja and Djuricic (1980) measured the activities of 48 enzymes in isolated gerbil and rat cerebral capillaries. The activities of enzymes associated with glycolysis (glycero-P-dehydrogenase, pyruvate kinase, and lactate dehydrogenase), except hexokinase and phosphofructokinase, were found to be lower than in corresponding brain parenchyma. Hexokinase might have a capillary role in glucose transport because the K_m for glucose transport is close to that of hexokinase. Alternatively, in parenchyma the main function of hexokinase is energy production. Phosphofructokinase has a rate-limiting role in glycolysis. The activities of the gluconeogenetic rate-limiting enzymes, fructose-1,6-diphosphatase and glucose-6-phosphatase, were higher in the capillary fraction. Thus, gluconeogenesis occurs in these blood vessels. Enzymes of the pentose shunt were also determined in capillaries (glucose-6-P dehydrogenase, 6-P-gluconate dehydrogenase, transaldolase, ribose-5-P isomerase, ribulose-5-P epimerase, and transketolase). The last enzyme, transketolase, which links the shunt with the glycolytic pathway, had the lowest activity. The capillaries readily synthesize glycogen, as glycogen synthase activity was higher than in parenchyma. However, the activities of the glycogen-splitting enzymes phosphorylase a and b were lower in capillaries. Phosphorylase might prove to be a substrate for NE-receptor-coupled cyclic AMP activation of protein kinase.

C. Actin

Using isolated capillaries from adult brain, LeBeux and Willemot (1978) observed the presence of actin-like filaments in the cytoplasm. The fibers were smooth-surfaced, averaged 6 nm in diameter, were branched with anastomoses, were intertwined in loosely meshed networks, and were anchored to the plasma membrane. After exposure to heavy meromycin the filaments increased in width (18–20 nm) and were tightly packed. The heavy side arms coating the microfilaments disappeared after exposure to ATP. Owman et al. (1978) likewise observed actin and myosin in brain capillaries. Therefore, these microfilaments might represent a contractile property of the capillary. Perhaps a cyclic AMP-mediated event could trigger a contractile mechanism whereby the tight junctions between endothelia could be opened, allowing for a change in blood–brain barrier permeability. Moreover, the actin filaments may be involved in cyclic AMP-mediated transport of pinocytotic vesicles (Wagner et al., 1972; Joō, 1972) or may function as elements of a cytoskeletal system in the cytoplasmic matrix (LeBeux and Willemot, 1978).

VII. Conclusions

The isolation of microvessels from the brain and peripheral vasculature provides a readily available means of studying biochemical mechanisms associated with the function of these microorgans. Recent biochemical research has focused on two major areas, namely, the monoamine systems and the carrier-mediated transport processes. The monoamine systems appear to be unique because current opinion has confined their vascular function to one of constriction or dilation. With the exception of the pial vessels, the brain capillaries and choroid plexus are devoid of smooth muscle components. The data presented in this chapter indicate that noradrenergic transmission regulates permeability of the central capillaries to

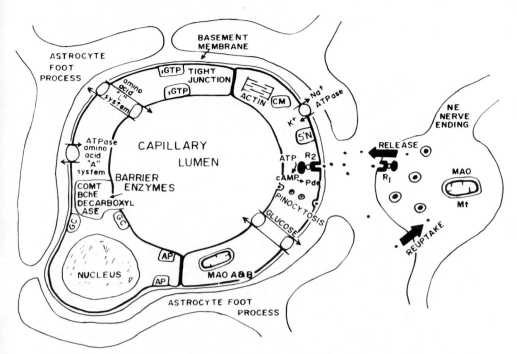

Fig. 4. Diagram of a brain capillary showing suggested biochemical mechanisms associated with the blood–brain barrier (see also Betz and Goldstein, 1980). AP, Alkaline phosphatase; BChE, butyrylcholinesterase; cAMP, cyclic AMP; CM, calmodulin; COMT, catechol O-methyltransferase; γGTP, γ-glutamyl transpeptidase; GC, guanylate cyclase; MAO, monoamine oxidase; Mt, mitochondria; NE, norepinephrine; 5′N, 5′-nucleotidase; Pde, phosphodiesterase; R_1, presynaptic NE receptor; R_2, postsynaptic NE receptor.

water and small molecules. Moreover, the enzymes associated with adrenergic metabolism serve an additional role as an enzyme barrier mechanism. The transport processes found in the microvasculature provide a key role in limiting the entrance of specified molecules into the brain and promoting their exit. Interesting findings have separated the intracellular sites of these molecules into the endothelial luminal and the antiluminal plasma membranes. Recent work suggests biochemical alterations of the central vasculature in the disease states of hypertension, ischemia, inborn errors of metabolism, damage by radiation, as well as functional alterations by pharmacologic agents. These basic research findings should provide a framework for more detailed investigation into these and many other pathologic processes, for example, seizures, edema, and diabetes. It is hoped that research of this nature will ultimately lead to a better design of therapeutic agents or medical approaches for the treatment of these conditions. For details and a summary of the functional biochemistry of central capillaries see Fig. 4.

Acknowledgments

I would like to thank S. Jo Palmer for technical help with the research reported herein. Additional appreciation is expressed to Judi Naylor for typing the manuscript. The work quoted was supported by NSF grant PCM 7911782 and the Frist–Massey Neurological Institute.

References

Abe, T., Abe, K., Rausch, W. D., Klatzo, I., and Spatz, M. (1980). *Adv. Exp. Med. Biol.* **131,** 45–55.

Adachi, M., Rosenblum, W. I., and Feigin, I. (1966). *J. Neurol. Neurosurg. Psychiatry* **29,** 451–455.

Albert, Z., Orlowski, M., Rzucidlo, Z., and Orlowska, J. (1966). *Acta Histochem.* **25,** 312–320.

Altura, B. M., Gebrewold, A., and Lassoff, S. (1980). *Br. J. Pharmacol.* **69,** 543–544.

Anchors, J. M., Haggerty, D. F., and Karnovsky, M. L. (1977). *J. Biol. Chem.* **252,** 7035–7041.

Ariano, M. A., Butcher, L. L., and Appleman, M. M. (1980). *Neuroscience* **5,** 1269–1276.

Baca, G. M., and Palmer, G. C. (1978). *Blood Vessels* **15,** 286–298.

Berson, F. G., Spatz, M., and Klatzo, I. (1975). *Stroke* **6,** 691–696.

Betz, A. L., and Goldstein, G. W. (1978). *Science (Washington, D.C.)* **202,** 225–227.

Betz, A. L., and Goldstein, G. W. (1980). *Adv. Exp. Med. Biol.* **131,** 5–16.

Betz, A. L., Gilboe, D. D., and Drewes, L. R. (1974). *Brain Res.* **67,** 307–316.

Betz, A. L., Csejtey, J., and Goldstein, G. W. (1979). *Am. J. Physiol.* **236,** C96–C102.

Betz, A. L., Firth, A. J., and Goldstein, G. W. (1980). *Brain Res.* **192,** 17–28.

Bloch-Tardy, M., Fages, C., and Gonnard, P. (1980). *J. Neurochem.* **35,** 612–615.

Braun, U., Braun, G., and Sargent, Th., III (1980). *Experientia* **36,** 207–209.

Brendel, K., Meezan, E., and Carlson, E. C. (1974). *Science (Washington, D.C.)* **185,** 953–955.

Buonassisi, V., and Venter, J. C. (1976). *Proc. Natl. Acad. Sci. USA* **73,** 1612–1616.

Chaplin, E. R., Free, R. G., and Goldstein, G. W. (1981). *Biochem. Pharmacol.* **30,** 241–245.

Christensen, H. N. (1969). *Adv. Enzymol. Relat. Areas Mol. Biol.* **1,** 1–20.

Chronister, R. B., Palmer, G. C., and Gerbrandt, L. (1980). *Brain Res. Bull.* **5,** 649–651.

Cutler, R. W. P. (1980). *In* "Neurobiology of Cerebrospinal Fluid" (J. H. Wood, ed), Vol. 1, pp. 41–51. Plenum, New York.

Daly, J. (1977). "Cyclic Nucleotides in the Nervous System." Plenum, New York.

Davis, J. M., and Garver, D. L. (1978). "Psychobiology of Affective Disorders." Upjohn, Kalamazoo, Michigan.

DeBault, L. E., and Cancilla, P. A. (1980). *Science (Washington, D.C.)* **207,** 653–655.

Dembinska-Kiec, A., Rucker, W., and Schonhofer, P. S. (1980). *Naunyn–Schmiedebergs Arch. Pharmacol.* **311,** 67–70.

Diamond, I., and Fishman, R. A. (1973). *J. Neurochem.* **20,** 1533–1542.

Djuricic, B. M., Stojanovic, T., and Mršulja, B. B. (1980). *Experientia* **36,** 40–42.

Domer, F. R., Sankar, R., Cole, S., and Wellmeyer, D. (1980). *Exp. Neurol.* **70,** 576–585.

Edvinsson, L., and MacKenzie, E. T. (1977). *Pharmacol. Rev.* **28,** 275–348.

Eisenberg, H. M., Suddith, R. L., and Crawford, J. S. (1980). *Adv. Exp. Med. Biol.* **131,** 57–67.

Folkman, J., Haudenschild, C. C., and Zetter, B. R. (1979). *Proc. Natl. Acad. Sci. USA* **76,** 5217–5221.

Frazer, A., Pandey, G., Mendels, J., Neeley, S., Kane, M., and Hess, M. E. (1974). *Neuropharmacology* **13,** 1131–1140.

Frey, A., Feld, S., and Frey, B. (1975). *Ann. N.Y. Acad. Sci.* **247,** 433–439.

Giacomelli, F., Wiener, J., and Spira, D. (1970). *Am. J. Pathol.* **59,** 133–159.

Goldman, H., Fischer, R., Nicolou, N., and Murphy, S. (1975). *Experientia* **31,** 328–329.

Goldstein, G. W. (1978). *Adv. Neurol.* **20,** 11–16.

Goldstein, G. W. (1979). *J. Physiol. (London)* **286,** 185–195.

Goldstein, G. W., Wolinsky, J. S., Csejtey, J., and Diamond, I. (1975). *J. Neurochem.* **25,** 715–717.

Goldstein, G. W., Csejtey, J., and Diamond, I. (1977). *J. Neurochem.* **28,** 725–728.

Goridis, C., Massarelli, R., Sensenbrenner, M., and Mandel, P. (1974). *J. Neurochem.* **23,** 135–138.

Grubb, R. L., Jr., Raichle, M. E., and Eichling, J. D. (1978). *Brain Res.* **144,** 204–207.

Hammers, R., Clarenbach, P., Lindl, T., and Cramer, H. (1977). *Neuropharmacology* **16,** 135–141.

Hardebo, J. E., and Owman, C. (1980). *Ann. Neurol.* **8,** 1–11.

Harik, S. I., Sharma, V. K., Wetherbee, J. R., Warren, R. H., and Banerjee, S. P. (1980). *Eur. J. Pharmacol.* **61,** 207–208.

Hartman, B. K., Zide, D., and Udenfriend, S. (1972). *Proc. Natl. Acad. Sci. USA* **69,** 2722–2766.

Hartman, B. K., Swanson, L. W., Raichle, M. E., Preskorn, S. H., and Clark, H. B. (1980). *Adv. Exp. Med. Biol.* **131,** 113–126.

Head, R. J., Hjelle, J. T., Jarrott, B., Berkowitz, B., Cardinale, G., and Spector, S. (1980). *Blood Vessels* **17,** 173–186.

Herbst, T. J., Raichle, M. E., and Ferrendelli, J. A. (1979). *Science (Washington, D.C.)* **204,** 330–332.

Hjelle, J. T., Baird-Lambert, J., Cardinale, G., Spector, S., and Udenfriend, S. (1978). *Proc. Natl. Acad. Sci. USA* **75,** 4544–4548.

Hopkins, N. K., and Gorman, R. R. (1981). *J. Clin. Invest.* **67,** 540–546.

Hori, S., Nishida, T., Mukai, Y., Pomeroy, M., and Mukai, N. (1980). *Res. Commun. Chem. Pathol. Pharmacol.* **29,** 211–228.

Huang, M., and Drummond, G. I. (1979). *Mol. Pharmacol.* **16,** 462–472.

Hwang, S. M., Weiss, S., and Segal, S. (1980). *J. Neurochem.* **35,** 417–424.

Jarrott, B., Hjelle, J. T., and Spector, S. (1979). *Brain Res.* **168,** 323–330.

Joō, F. (1972). *Experientia* **28,** 1470–1471.

Joō, F. (1979). *In* "Frontiers in Matrix Biology" (A. M. Robert, R. Boniface, and L. Robert, eds.), pp. 166–182. Karger, Basel and New York.

Joō, F., and Karnushina, I. (1973). *Cytobios* **8,** 41–48.

Joō, F., Rakonczay, Z., and Wollemann, M. (1975a). *Experientia* **31,** 582–583.

Joõ, F., Toth, I., and Jancsó, G. (1975b). *Naturwissenschaften* **8,** 397.

Joõ, F., Szucs, A., and Csanda, E. (1976). *J. Pharm. Pharmacol.* **28,** 162–163.

Kaplan, G. P., Hartman, B. K., and Creveling, C. R. (1981). *Brain Res.* **204,** 353–360.

Karnushina, I. L., Palacios, J. M., Barbin, G., Dux, E., Joõ, F., and Schwartz, J. C. (1980a). *J. Neurochem.* **34,** 1201–1208.

Karnushina, I., Toth, I., Dux, E., and Joõ, F. (1980b). *Brain Res.* **189,** 588–592.

Katoh–Semba, R., and Kashiwamata, S. (1980). *Biochim. Biophys. Acta* **632,** 290–297.

Kebabian, J. W., Bloom, F. E., Steiner, A. L., and Greengard, P. (1975). *Science (Washington, D.C.)* **190,** 157–159.

Kolber, A. R., Krigman, M. R., and Morell, P. (1980). *Brain Res.* **192,** 513–521.

Krause, D. N., Wong, E., Degener, P., and Roberts, E. (1980). *Brain Res.* **185,** 51–57.

Lai, F. M., and Spector, S. (1977). *Br. J. Pharmacol.* **59,** 393–395.

Lai, F. M., and Spector, S. (1978). *Arch. Int. Pharmacodyn. Ther.* **233,** 227–234.

Lai, F. M., Udenfriend, S., and Spector, S. (1975). *Proc. Natl. Acad. Sci. USA* **72,** 4622–4625.

LeBeux, Y. J., and Willemot, J. (1978). *Exp. Neurol.* **58,** 446–454.

Lindvall, M., and Owman, C. (1980). *J. Neurochem.* **34,** 518–522.

Lorenzo, A. V., and Cutler, R. W. P. (1969). *J. Neurochem.* **16,** 577–585.

Marin, J., Salaices, M., and Sanchez, C. F. (1979). *J. Pharm. Pharmacol.* **31,** 818–821.

Marin, J., Salaices, M., and Garcia, A. G. (1980). *J. Pharm. Pharmacol.* **32,** 64–65.

Matheson, D. F., Oei, R., and Roots, B. I. (1980). *Neurochem. Res.* **5,** 683–695.

Maurer, P., Moskowitz, M. A., Levine, L., and Melamed, E. (1980). *Prostaglandins Med.* **4,** 153–161.

Meister, A., and Tate, S. S. (1976). *Annu. Rev. Biochem.* **45,** 559–604.

Melamed, E., Hefti, F., and Wurtman, R. J. (1980). *Brain Res.* **198,** 244–248.

Merritt, J. H., Chamness, A. F., and Allen, S. J. (1978). *Radiat. Environ. Biophys.* **15,** 367–377.

Milhorat, T. H., Hammock, M. K., Fenstermacher, J. D., Rall, D. P., and Levin V. A. (1971). *Science (Washington, D.C.)* **173,** 330–332.

Moncada, S., Herman, A. G., Higgs, E. A., and Vane, J. R. (1977). *Thromb. Res.* **11,** 323–344.

Mršulja, B. B., and Djuricic, B. M. (1980). *Adv. Exp. Biol. Med.* **131,** 29–43.

Mršulja, B. B., Mršulja, B. J., Fujimoto, T., Klatzo, I., and Spatz, M. (1976). *Brain Res.* **110,** 361–365.

Nakamura, S., and Milhorat, T. H. (1978). *Brain Res.* **153,** 285–293.

Nakane, M., and Deguchi, T. (1978). *Biochim. Biophys. Acta* **25,** 275–285.

Namm, D. H., and Leader, J. P. (1976). *Blood Vessels* **13,** 24–47.

Nathanson, J. A. (1977). *Physiol. Rev.* **57,** 158–256.

Nathanson, J. A. (1979). *Science (Washington, D.C.)* **204,** 843–844.

Nathanson, J. A. (1980a). *Life Sci.* **26,** 1793–1799.

Nathanson, J. A. (1980b). *Mol. Pharmacol.* **18,** 199–209.

Nathanson, J. A., and Glaser, G. H. (1979). *Nature (London)* **278,** 567–569.

Nielsen, K. C., and Owman, C. (1967). *Brain Res.* **6,** 773–776.

Orlowski, M., Sessa, G., and Green, J. P. (1974). *Science (Washington, D.C.)* **184,** 66–68.

Oscar, K., and Hawkins, T. (1977). *Brain Res.* **126,** 281–293.

Owman, C., Edvinsson, L., Hardebo, J. E., Groschel-Stewart, U., Unsicker, K., and Walles, B. (1978). *Adv. Neurol.* **20,** 35–37.

Palmer, G. C. (1976). *Neuropharmacology* **15,** 1–7.

Palmer, G. C. (1979). *Biochem. Pharmacol.* **28,** 2847–2849.

Palmer, G. C. (1980). *Neuropharmacology* **19**, 17–23.
Palmer, G. C. (1981a). *In* "Neuropharmacology of Central Nervous System and Behavioral Disorders" (G. C. Palmer, ed.), pp. 571–623. Academic Press, New York.
Palmer, G. C. (1981b). *Neurosci. Lett.* **21**, 207–210.
Palmer, G. C. (1981c). *Neuroscience* **6**, 2547–2553.
Palmer, G. C., and Greenberg, S. (1978). *Prog. Neuro-Psychopharmacol.* **2**, 585–587.
Palmer, G. C., and Palmer, S. J. (1978). *Life Sci.* **23**, 207–216.
Palmer, G. C., Wagner, H. R., Palmer, S. J., and Manian, A. A. (1977). *Commun. Psychopharmacol.* **1**, 61–69.
Palmer, G. C., Chronister, R. B., and Palmer, S. J. (1980a). *J. Neurobiol.* **11**, 503–508.
Palmer, G. C., Palmer, S. J., and Chronister, R. B. (1980b). *Adv. Exp. Med. Biol.* **131**, 147–162.
Palmer, G. C., Christie, B. C., Chronister, R. B., and Gerbrandt, L. K. (1981). *Fed. Proc. Fed. Am. Soc. Exp. Biol.* **40**, 626.
Panula, P., Joó, F., and Rechardt, L. (1978). *Experientia* **34**, 95–96.
Peroutka, S. J., Moskowitz, M. A., Reinhard, J. F., Jr., and Snyder, S. H. (1980). *Science (Washington, D.C.)* **208**, 610–612.
Phillips, P., Kumar, P., Kumar, S., and Waghe, M. (1979). *J. Anat.* **129**, 261–272.
Preskorn, S. H., and Hartman, B. K. (1979). *Biol. Psychiatry* **14**, 235–247.
Preskorn, S. H., Hartman, B. K., and Clark, B. H. (1980a). *Psychopharmacology (N.Y.)* **70**, 1–4.
Preskorn, S. H., Hartman, B. K., Raichle, M. E., and Clark, B. (1980b). *J. Pharmacol. Exp. Ther.* **213**, 313–320.
Preskorn, S. H., Hartman, B. K., Raichle, M. E., Swanson, L. W., and Clark, H. B. (1980c). *Adv. Exp. Med. Biol.* **131**, 127–138.
Raichle, M. E., and Grubb, R. L., Jr., (1978). *Brain Res.* **143**, 191–194.
Raichle, M. E., Hartman, B. K., Eichling, J. O., and Sharp, L. G. (1975). *Proc. Natl. Acad. Sci. USA* **72**, 3726–3730.
Raichle, M. E., Eichling, J. O., Straatmann, M. G., Welch, M. J., Larson, K. B., and Ter-Pogussian, M. M. (1976). *Am. J. Physiol.* **230**, 543–552.
Rebert, R. R. (1977). *Pharmacologist* **19**, 201.
Reinhard, J. F., Jr., Liebmann, J. E., Schlosberg, A. J., and Moskonitz, M. A. (1979). *Science (Washington, D.C.)* **206**, 85–87.
Reyes, E., and Palmer, G. C. (1976). *Res. Commun. Chem. Pathol. Pharmacol.* **14**, 759–762.
Richelson, E., and Divinetz-Romero, S. (1977). *Biol. Psychiatry* **12**, 771–785.
Schulman, J. D., Goodman, S. I., Mace, J. W., Patrick, A. D., Tietze, F., and Butler, E. J. (1975). *Biochem. Biophys. Res. Commun.* **65**, 68–73.
Sershen, H., and Lajtha, A. (1976). *Exp. Neurol.* **53**, 465–474.
Sessa, G., Orlowski, M., and Green, J. P. (1976). *J. Neurobiol.* **7**, 51–61.
Spatz, M., Go, G. K., and Klatzo, I. (1974). *In* "Pathology of Cerebral Microcirculation" (J. Cervos-Navarro, ed.), pp. 361–366. de Gruyter, Berlin.
Spatz, M., Mršulja, B. B., Micic, D., Mušulja, B. J., and Klatzo, I. (1977). *Brain Res.* **120**, 141–145.
Spatz, M., Bembry, J., Dodson, R. F., Hervonen, H., and Murray, M. R. (1980). *Brain Res.* **191**, 577–582.
Spector, A. A., Hoak, J. C., Fry, G. L., Denning, G. M., Stoll, L. L., and Smith, J. B. (1980). *J. Clin. Invest.* **65**, 1003–1012.
Stefanovich, V. (1979). *Neurochem. Res.* **4**, 681–687.

Suddith, R. L., Savage, K. E., and Eisenberg, H. M. (1980). *Adv. Exp. Med. Biol.* **131,** 139–145.

Swanson, L. W., Connelly, M. A., and Hartman, B. K. (1977). *Brain Res.* **136,** 166–173.

Tomasi, V., Meringolo, C., Bartolini, G., and Orlandi, M. (1978). *Nature (London)* **273,** 670–671.

U'Prichard, D., Greenberg, D., Sheehan, P., and Snyder, S. (1977). *Science (Washington, D.C.)* **199,** 197–198.

Versteeg, D. H. G., Palkovits, M., van der Gugten, J., Wijnen, H. L. J. M., Smeets, G. W. M., and deJong, W. (1976). *Brain Res.* **112,** 429–434.

Vetulani, J., Stawarz, R. J., Dingell, J. V., and Sulser, F. (1976). *Naunyn–Schmiedebergs Arch. Pharmacol.* **293,** 109–114.

Wagner, H. R., Palmer, G. C., and Davis, J. N. (1979). *In* "Neuropharmacology of Cyclic Nucleotides" (G. C. Palmer, ed.), pp. 152–172. Urban & Schwarzenberg, Munich and Baltimore.

Wagner, R. C., Kreiner, P., Barrnett, R. J., and Bitensky, M. W. (1972). *Proc. Natl. Acad. Sci. USA* **69,** 3175–3179.

Wei, E. P., Kontos, H. A., Dietrich, W. D., Povlishock, J. T., and Ellis, E. F. (1980). *Circ. Res.* **48,** 95–103.

White, F. P. (1980). *J. Neurochem.* **35,** 88–94.

White, F. P., Dutton, G. R., and Norenberg, M. D. (1981). *J. Neurochem.* **36,** 328–332.

2 Regulation of Vascular Smooth Muscle of the Microcirculation

Stan Greenberg
Frederick A. Curro
Toshiki P. Tanaka

THE PHYSIOLOGY AND PHARMACOLOGY
OF THE MICROCIRCULATION, VOLUME 1

I. Introduction

The final common macromolecular factor regulating both arterial pressure and fluid homeostasis at the tissue level is the vascular smooth muscle (VSM) of the microcirculation. Although the VSM is modulated by the level of circulating humoral factors, the central and peripheral nervous systems, and endogenous local factors such as platelets, leukocytes, and mast cells, with their inherent vasoactive products, it is the ultimate capacity of the VSM to respond to these factors with either contraction or relaxation that determines the hemodynamic events resulting from these modulating factors. Despite the plethora of information on VSM function in large arteries and veins, little information is available on the pharmacologic and humoral responsiveness of the microcirculation (Mellander and Johansson, 1968; Vanhoutte, 1978; Kaley and Altura, 1978; Altura, 1978a,b, 1981; Bohr et al., 1978). Information on microvascular mechanisms of contraction and relaxation is almost nonexistent, although recent studies have attempted to investigate receptor mechanisms in microvessels from brain (Estrada and Krause, 1982; Gerritsen, 1982) and other organs. The specific aims of this chapter are to provide the reader interested in VSM and the microcirculation with the current knowledge relating to (a) the ultrastructural characteristics of the VSM, (b) the innervation of the VSM of the microcirculation, (c) the role of the endothelium as a modulator of VSM function, (d) the structural and functional basis of VSM contraction and relaxation, and (e) the effects of vasoactive endogenous and pharmacologic substances on the VSM and the mechanisms by which these substances alter vascular resistance.

Although this chapter cannot be encyclopedic either in providing definitive answers to each of the problems or in covering the entire pharmacologic armamentarium of therapeutic modalities, it is hoped that the information presented will serve as a base from which young investigators in the field will initiate questions and the experimental techniques from which the answers will arise.

II. Vascular Smooth Muscle in the Microcirculation

A. *Ultrastructural Characteristics of Vascular Smooth Muscle*

Rhodin (1974, 1980) and Majno (1965) stressed that "microcirculation" is the collective name for the smallest components of the cardiovascular channels, the arterioles, capillaries, and venules, each with its own characteristic structure and function. Because each organ has a unique microcirculation, knowledge of the macroanatomy of the microcirculation of one vascular bed does not imply knowledge of the macroarchitectural arrangement of others (Rhodin, 1981). Thus, the generalized discussion in this chapter tries to encompass the major characteristics of most vascular beds, with individualities delineated in the discussions of specific microcirculations within this volume. Figure 1 shows the general architecture of the systemic vascular tree of a mammalian organism.

Arterioles are essentially small arteries [<0.5 mm outer diameter (OD)] with at least two layers of smooth muscle cells. The smallest arterioles contain one layer of smooth muscle cells or several cells scattered widely apart within the vessel wall (Rhodin, 1980, 1981). Both arterioles and precapillary sphincters contain an inner lining of endothelial cells, which maintain the fluid integrity of the vessel by means of "tight junctions." Myoendothelial junctions penetrate the connective tissue basal lamina and separate the smooth muscle from the endothelial cells in arterioles from many organs (Williamson *et al.,* 1969). These myoendothelial junctions appear to serve as a site for circulating humoral factors to reach the smooth muscle from the vascular space. Within the connective tissue of the arteriolar wall nonmyelinated nerve terminals impinge on the VSM cells to form the myoneural or neuroeffector junction. It is from the nodular terminal varicosities that neurotransmitter is released, diffuses across the synaptic cleft, and interacts with the appropriate receptors on the VSM cell to produce vasoconstriction or vasodilation.

The capillaries (5 μm OD) are tubes joined by flat endothelial cells and by junctional areas, predominantly tight junctions (Rhodin, 1980, 1981). These are discussed elsewhere in this volume. However, some capillaries are surrounded by precapillary cells called pericytes (Weibel, 1974), which have their own basal lamina. These pericytes may have the capacity to contract and therefore could alter capillary blood flow. The endothelial cells of the capillaries contain actin and perhaps myosin filaments and may exhibit active contraction. Simionescu *et al.* (1982) showed that endothelial cells from large veins contracted in response to histamine.

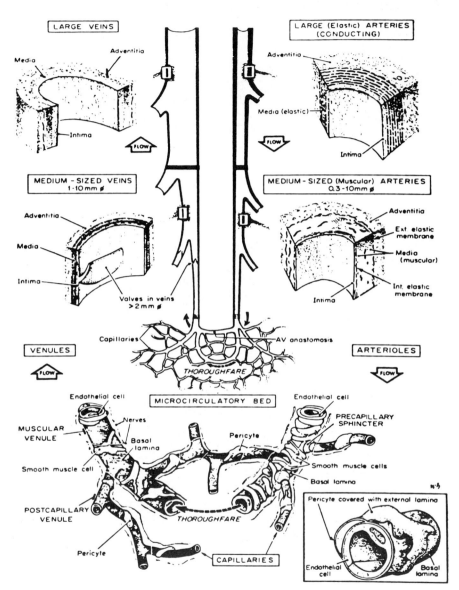

Fig. 1. Schematic drawing summarizing major characteristics of principal segments of blood vessels of mammals. (From Rhodin, 1980, with permission.)

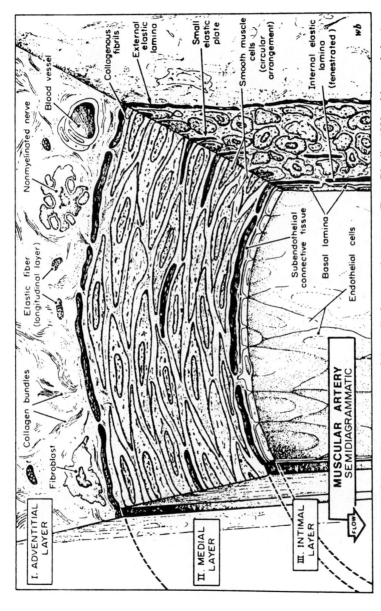

Fig. 2. Summary of the major components of the wall of a muscular artery. (From Rhodin, 1980, with permission.)

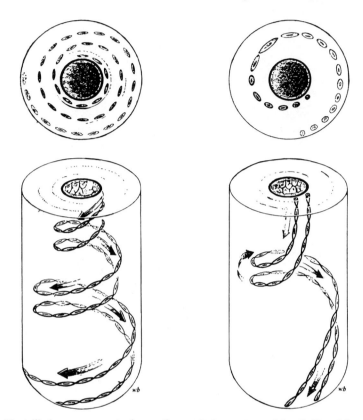

Fig. 3. Most likely arrangement of smooth muscle in most arterioles (left) and in some bovine vessels (right). (From Rhodin, 1980, with permission.)

These contractions, much slower than those of the VSM, may modulate microcirculatory VSM tone or, more likely, the opening and closing of "pores" in the endothelial spaces. According to Rhodin (1968) arterial capillaries lie closer to the arterioles than the venules and are endowed with a continuous endothelium. Venous capillaries are endowed with a fenestrated endothelium and lie closer to the venules than the arterioles. This arrangement would be consistent with a mechanism for hemodynamic mediation of fluid transfer.

Figures 4 and 5 show the five basic venules in the microcirculation. The endothelium of the venular capillaries is continuous with the endothelium of the venules up to the collecting veins. All endothelial cells have a continuous cytoplasm with a variable number of cytoplasmic vesicles (Rhodin, 1981). The tight junction of the venous endothelium is "looser" than that of the arteriolar and capillary endothelium, and the junctional regions

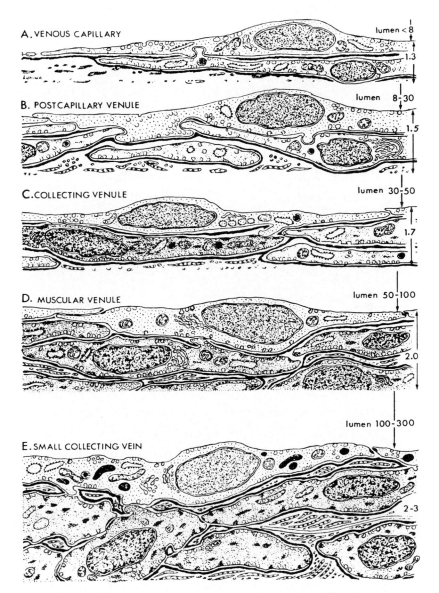

A. VENOUS CAPILLARY   lumen < 8

1.3

B. POSTCAPILLARY VENULE   lumen 8-30

1.5

C. COLLECTING VENULE   lumen 30-50

1.7

D. MUSCULAR VENULE   lumen 50-100

2.0

lumen 100-300

E. SMALL COLLECTING VEIN

2-3

Fig. 4. Summary of transition of venous segments in microcirculation. Lumen measurements in micrometers. (From Rhodin, 1968, with permission.)

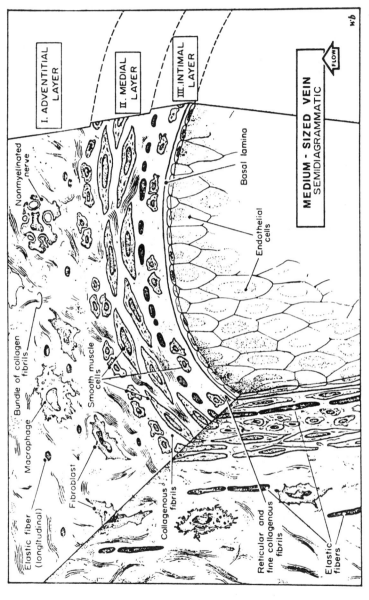

I. ADVENTITIAL LAYER

II. MEDIAL LAYER

III. INTIMAL LAYER

MEDIUM - SIZED VEIN
SEMIDIAGRAMMATIC

FLOW

Nonmyelinated nerve

Elastic fiber (longitudinal)

Bundle of collagen fibrils

Macrophage

Fibroblast

Smooth muscle cells

Collagenous fibrils

Reticular and fine collagenous fibrils

Elastic fibers

Basal lamina

Endothelial cells

wb

Fig. 5. Major components of wall of medium-sized vein. (From Rhodin, 1980, with permission.)

can open up the intercellular clefts when stimulated with histamine and 5-hydroxytryptamine (5-HT). According to Rhodin (1980, 1981) this precedes leukocyte migration into the portion of the vein in which the damage has occurred. A discontinuous layer of pericytes surrounds the postcapillary venules and then gives rise to layers of venous smooth muscle cells, which are of a lower number and density than those of the arterioles. The venules are also innervated primarily with an adrenergic innervation, and release of transmitter results in slower and less powerful contractions of the venules.

In small arterioles the muscle cells are elongated, fusiform with tapering ends, generally about 5 μm in diameter, and about 20 μm in length with an irregular profile, thus providing a high surface-to-volume ratio (Gabella, 1981). The cell membrane is trilaminar and of uniform thickness. Electron-dense bands of inpocketings, known as caveolae, surface vesicles, or plasmalemmal vesicles, are grouped in rows, two to four caveolae wide, parallel to the long axis of the cell. More than 33% of the plasma membrane at the cell surface forms caveolae, which are continuous with the extracellular space. Popescu (1974) suggested that these caveolae may be involved in the transmembrane transport of calcium ion across the plasma membrane. The cell membrane is coated by a basal lamina and is involved in the formation of cell-to-cell junctions (Gabella, 1981).

Bands of electron-dense material approximately 300–400 μm reinforce the cell membrane on the cytoplasmic side in VSM. These dense bands project into the cytoplasm in the form of wedge-shaped protrusions and are opposed to the fibrous material of VSM and the extracellular space. It has been suggested that these dense bands may serve as a mechanical link between the plasma membrane and the collagen fibrils of VSM. However, this remains questionable (Gabella, 1981). The sarcoplasmic reticulum of VSM is abundantly present beneath and parallel to the cell membrane, near the nuclear poles where Golgi and mitochondria are also present, and among the myofilaments. The function of the sarcoplasmic reticulum is still poorly understood. The granular endoplasmic reticulum is probably involved in protein synthesis, whereas the smooth sarcoplasmic reticulum is involved in the regulation of ion concentration, notably that of calcium. Mitochondria, the energy packets of the cell, are localized primarily in the regions of the cells near the poles of the nuclei, whereas some are scattered near the cellular membrane and sarcoplasmic reticulum. The Golgi apparatus is also usually situated in the region of the nuclear poles and is associated with the rough endoplasmic reticulum. The Golgi, as in all cells, is associated with protein synthesis in VSM. Although microtubules exist in VSM, no function has been assigned to them. Smooth muscle cells may be associated with phagocytitic activity, and it is not incidental that VSM contains lysosomes.

The VSM contains thick, thin, and intermediate-sized filaments. The thick filaments may be helically arranged, as in skeletal muscle, and are found in hexameric units arranged in a helical conformation with a 72-nm periodicity. The cells of VSM also contain thin filaments of actin, usually arranged in hexagonal packing, which normally extend for several micrometers along the cell length and then branch and divide. The thin filaments also appear to be tropomyosin. The native tropomyosin can be separated into tropomyosin and leiotonin, which may serve the same function as troponin, in VSM. The intermediate filaments are approximately 10 nm in diameter and are localized in the proximity of dense bodies, the cell surface, and dense bands. Although the intermediate filaments do not appear to penetrate the dense bodies, it has been suggested that these filaments form the cytoskeleton of the smooth muscle cell, which gives support to the myofilaments. In this regard, the dense bodies of VSM, which run parallel to the myofilaments and are at times continuous with the dense bands, have insertions with thin filaments (Gabella, 1981; Ashton *et al.*, 1975). It has also been suggested that these dense bodies and dense bands correspond to the Z bands of skeletal muscle, thus making the entire VSM cell the sarcomeric unit of contraction. According to Gabella (1981), "The distribution of myofilaments and the occurrence of dense bands—instead of Z lines—probably accounts for the remarkable amount of shortening a smooth muscle cell can undergo. It may also account for the wide changes in shape of the cell transverse profile."

Smooth muscle cells are usually separated from each other by 100-nm gaps containing collagen and elastin fibrils and extracellular matrix material. However, regions of opposition of smooth muscle cells occur (Fig. 6 and 7). Tight junctions appear to exist in some VSM in the circle of Willis (Tani *et al.*, 1977). Nexuses or gap junctions exist in most VSM and are characteristic of the gap junctions found in most cells (for review see Henderson, 1975). The nexuses appear to be the site of electrical activity propagated from one cell to another. A typical smooth muscle cell is presented in Fig. 8.

B. Innervation of the Microcirculation

Drugs and humoral substances may affect microvascular smooth muscle either directly by altering the level of VSM tone, or indirectly by interfering with neurotransmission to the microcirculation. Table I summarizes

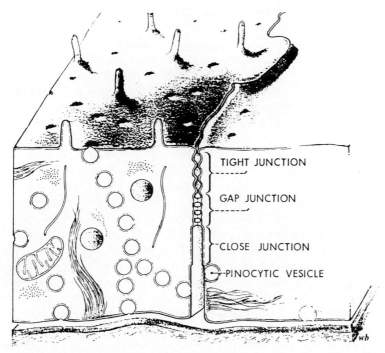

Fig. 6. Summary of general appearance of several types of cell junctions. Pinocytic vesicle: 500–600 Å. Junctions: tight (zonula occludens), punctate fusions; gap (macula communicans), gap = 20 Å, polygonal lattice of subunits; close, gap = 40 Å. Markers for molecules with ϕ (in Å) = 5 (ionic lanthanum); 20 (colloidal lanthanum); 17–20 (heme peptides); 25 × 34 × 42 (myoglobin); 50 (horseradish peroxidase); 45–200 (dextrans); 110 (ferritin). (From Rhodin, 1980, with permission.)

the density of innervation of the microcirculation as determined by histochemical fluorescence measurement of adrenergic nerve density and electron microscopic evidence of the presence of adrenergic nerves. The precapillary sphincters and collecting venules appear to be devoid of adrenergic innervation, whereas the small veins, arterioles, and terminal arterioles appear to be richly endowed with adrenergic varicosities. There is little evidence for a cholinergic innervation of the microcirculation, with the exception of the brain (D'Alecly and Rose, 1977; Heistad and Marcus, 1978) and the kidney. However, microvascular smooth muscle in the systemic and peripheral circulations appears to be endowed with both cholinergic and adrenergic receptors (Estrada and Krause, 1982; Altura, 1978a,b, 1981). Kadowitz and Hyman (1973) and Kadowitz *et al.* (1975a,b, 1976, 1981) have shown that the pulmonary circulation of many

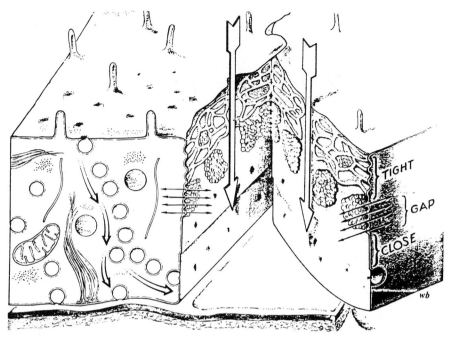

Fig. 7. Summary of general appearance of several types of cell junctions as seen from freeze-fracture segments. (From Rhodin, 1980, with permission.)

species responds to stimulation of both parasympathetic and adrenergic nerves and that the small blood vessels are innervated with both adrenergic and cholinergic varicosities. However, the size of the vessels at which the innervation disappears has not been determined. In contrast, Su *et al.* (1978) and Su and Bevan (1976) measured the contractile responses of small pulmonary arteries from rabbits to stimulation of adrenergic nerves and showed that the response to nerve stimulation disappears in vessels between 200 and 400 μm (OD). This would suggest that terminal arterioles of the pulmonary circulation may not be richly innervated with adrenergic nerve fibers.

Assuming the adrenergic innervation in the macrocirculation and that in the microcirculation are similar, then the factors that control the release of neurotransmitter should also be similar. Tables II and III summarize their purported mechanism of action. When such drugs as guanethidine, bretylium, and guanacline inhibit the release of norepinephrine (NE) from adrenergic nerves innervating the microcirculation, the more densely innervated microcirculatory components should exhibit the greatest decrease in VSM tone. Similar changes in the microcirculation should be ob-

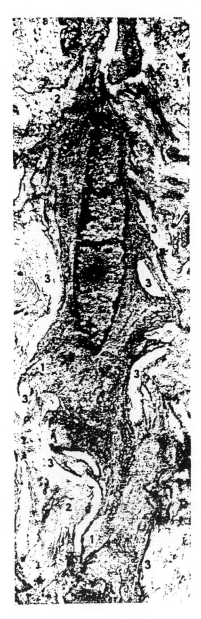

Fig. 8. Typical smooth muscle cell from abdominal aorta of squirrel monkey. (From Rhodin, 1980, with permission.)

TABLE I

Density of Adrenergic Innervation in Splanchnic and
Skeletal Muscle Microvessels[a]

	Evidence[b]	
Microvessel	Electron micrographic	Histochemical
Small muscular arteries	++++	++++
Arterioles	++++	+++
Terminal arterioles	++	++
Precapillary sphincters	±	−
Collecting venules	−	−
Muscular venules	±	±
Small veins	++	++

[a] From Altura (1978a,b) with permission.
[b] +, Degree of innervation; −, lack of innervation.

served with the α-adrenoceptor antagonists and agents such as reserpine, which prevents the retention of NE in the granular pool of NE, and 6-hydroxydopamine (6-OHDA), which causes degeneration of adrenergic nerves. When these compounds are administered, arterioles and terminal arterioles relax or dilate, whereas muscular venules do not exhibit an in-

TABLE II

Influence of Drugs that Affect Tissue Levels of Catecholamines on
Reactivity of Mesenteric Arterioles and Muscular Venules to Exogenously
Applied Constrictor Doses of Norepinephrine[a,b]

		Microvessel and response to NE	
Drug	Dose	Arterioles (20–28 μm)	Muscular venules (34–35 μm)
Procaine	10^{-4}–10^{-5} M^c	Potentiated	No effect[e]
Cocaine	10^{-4}–10^{-5} M	Potentiated	No effect[e]
Bretylium	5–10 mg/kg[d]	Potentiated	No effect[e]
Guanethidine	5–10 mg/kg	Potentiated	No effect[e]
Reserpine	3–5 mg/kg	Potentiated	No effect[e]

[a] From Altura (1978a,b) with permission.
[b] ED_{30} doses of norepinephrine (NE) were applied topically before and after administration of the drugs.
[c] Procaine and cocaine were superfused on the mesenteric vessels for 30–45 min.
[d] Bretylium, guanethidine, and reserpine were administered acutely intravenously 20–45 min before a challenge to control ED_{30} doses of NE.
[e] Signifies that the constrictor responses to NE were equivalent to those before drug administration.

TABLE III

Effects of Inhibitors of Catecholamine Degradation on Responsiveness of
Rat Mesenteric Arterioles and Venules to Exogenously
Applied Norepinephrine[a,b]

Inhibitor[c]	Dose[d] (mg/kg)	Arterioles (21–28 μm)	Venules (36–45 μm)
MAO inhibitor			
Tranylcypromine	5–15	Potentiated	No effect[e]
Iproniazid	150–300	Potentiated	No effect[e]
COMT inhibitor			
Pyrogallol	150–300	Potentiated	Potentiated

[a] From Altura (1978a,b) with permission.
[b] ED_{30} doses of norepinephrine (NE) were applied topically before and after administration of the inhibitors.
[c] MAO, Monoamine oxidase; COMT, catechol O-methyltransferase.
[d] Inhibitors were administered 30–60 min before challenge with control ED_{30} doses of NE.
[e] Signifies that the constrictor responses to NE were equivalent to those before administration of the MAO inhibitors.

crease in diameter (Altura and Hershey, 1967; Altura, 1971a, 1978a,b, 1981). These findings provide pharmacologic evidence supporting the lack of innervation of venules in the microcirculation.

This conclusion is also supported by studies evaluating the effects of drugs that release NE from adrenergic nerves (indirectly acting sympathomimetic amines) on microvascular reactivity. Norepinephrine, epinephrine, and the selective α_1-receptor agonist phenylephrine act directly on VSM to elicit contraction, whereas tyramine, ephedrine, and amphetamine are indirectly acting sympathomimetic amines. The directly acting receptor antagonists contract intact rat venules, whereas the indirectly acting sympathomimetic amines are devoid of this activity (Altura, 1978b). All these findings support the conclusion that small venules (30–60 μm OD) probably receive little or no adrenergic innervation.

Substances other than NE may be released from adrenergic nerves innervating the microvascular smooth muscle. There is sufficient evidence that purines may be coreleased with other transmitters from nerves or sites innervating VSM. Thus, adenosine triphosphate (ATP) and other purines may function as modulators of neurotransmission in VSM (Su, 1977; DeMey *et al.*, 1979; Moylan and Westfall, 1979; Levitt and Westfall, 1982). The purines may function as inhibitors of neurotransmission (Su, 1977), are released upon stimulation of adrenergic nerves (Su, 1975; Burnstock, 1976), have their release facilitated by NE and inhibited by α_1-receptor antagonists, α_2-receptor antagonists, α_2-receptor agonists, and 6-

OHDA (Levitt and Westfall, 1982), and cause relaxation of blood vessels with high tone. The purines may be derived from the NE storage vesicle, which releases its content of ATP, binding protein, and neurotransmitter by exocytosis (Smith and Winkler, 1972). However, experiments of Levitt and Westfall (1982) in which they destroyed the adrenergic varicosities with 6-OHDA and inhibited NE release by approximately 80% and purine release by approximately 60% suggest that the purine may be released from sites other than the NE-containing vesicle of adrenergic nerves or from nonadrenergic nerves. Further studies are necessary to evaluate the site and mechanism of purine nucleotide release and the significance of purinergic nerves in the microcirculation.

C. Mechanisms of Inactivation of Norepinephrine

Five potential mechanisms are involved in the termination of action of NE released from adrenergic nerves. Interference with these mechanisms can alter the microvascular effects of NE. Diffusion of NE from its receptor site and transport across the vascular wall to the vascular space accounts for one mechanism. Blood flow to the microvasculature is an important determinant of the elimination of NE by this mechanism. The NE released from adrenergic nerves may be taken back up into the nerve terminal by a sodium-dependent, ouabain-inhibitable, energy-dependent, cocaine-inhibitable, saturable, stereospecific transport mechanism (uptake$_1$). Once taken back into the nerve terminal, the NE is primarily deaminated by monoamine oxidase (MAO) and subsequently methylated by catechol O-methyltransferase (COMT), the lesser neuronal metabolic mechanism. In contrast, in the event of inhibition of uptake$_1$ or when the concentration of NE is exceedingly high, NE is taken up into the VSM by a sodium-dependent, saturable, stereospecific, hydrocortisone- and cholesterol-inhibitable mechanism (uptake$_2$). Once taken up into the VSM, NE is primarily subjected to the action of COMT with some metabolism via MAO. Finally, the binding of NE to collagen, elastin, and the extracellular matrix may play a role in terminating the action of NE in VSM (for references see reviews by Bevan, 1982; Langer et al., 1981; Smith and Winkler, 1972).

The importance of each of these pathways in the microcirculation has been indirectly assessed by the administration of inhibitors of some of these systems and the evaluation of their effects on the responses to exogenous administration of NE. As summarized in Table III, inhibition of uptake$_1$ and MAO enhances the responses of both arterioles and venules to NE. These data also support the conclusion that the arterioles, but not the venules, are innervated with adrenergic nerves and that MAO is the primary mechanism of NE inactivation. In the venules, uptake$_2$ and COMT are primarily involved in terminating the action of NE.

D. Endothelium as a Site of Humoral Factor Inactivation and Production

The endothelium is no longer thought to be a simple barrier to diffusion of substances across the vascular wall but a site for the synthesis and degradation of hormones and the transport of drugs, an active mediator of antithrombotic activity, and an obligatory factor in active vasodilation. This discussion focuses on the role of the endothelium in metabolism and generation of vasoactive agents and its obligatory role in vasodilation.

Norepinephrine, 5-HT (serotonin), and other biogenic amines are taken up into endothelial cells by carrier-mediated, saturable transport mechanisms apparently distinct for each amine (Hughes et al., 1969; Strum and Junod, 1972; Ryan and Ryan, 1981). Histamine and epinephrine appear to be refractory to endothelial-mediated uptake. Once taken up into the endothelial cells, NE and 5-HT are metabolized and some of the metabolites are released into the vascular space (Junod, 1972a,b; Shepro et al., 1975). Thus, drugs that compete for these transport processes may enhance the concentration of 5-HT and NE available to interact with the smooth muscle, whereas drugs that stimulate the uptake of these substances into the endothelium may decrease the action of 5-HT and NE on the microvasculature. Because imipramine, iproniazide, hydrocortisone, cholesterol, chlorpromazine, and amphetamine inhibit the endothelial uptake of 5-HT and NE into endothelial cells, some of the adverse effects attributed to these drugs may result from their capacity to compete with these biogenic amines for binding sites along the endothelial cell surface (Junod, 1972a,b; Orton et al., 1975; Ryan and Ryan, 1981).

Adenosine is taken up by endothelial cells. This action is inhibited by dipyridamole, a coronary and peripheral vasodilator. Pearson et al. (1978) and Ryan and Ryan (1981) have suggested that some of the effects of dipyridamole may be related to its capacity to inhibit the endothelial uptake of adenosine. The enzyme involved in the degradation of adenine nucleotides, 5'-nucleotidase, is abundant along the luminal surface of endothelial cells, primarily in association with caveolae and/or pinocytotic vesicles (Smith and Ryan, 1970, 1971; Ryan and Smith, 1971a,b). Adenosine diphosphate is degraded to AMP, which in turn is metabolized to adenosine and inosine. The adenosine is taken up into the endothelial cell and resynthesized to ADP and ATP. The significance of this endothelial nucleo-

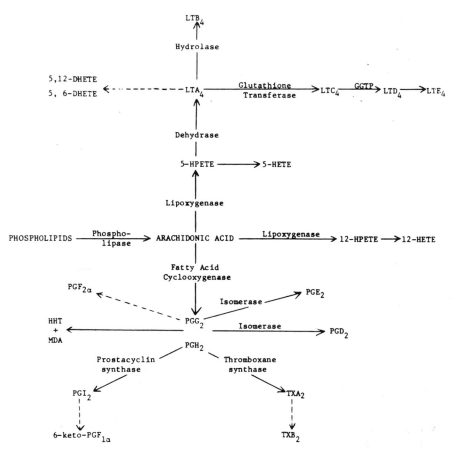

Fig. 9. Scheme of the major metabolic transformations of arachidonic acid. The enzymes responsible for the conversions are shown in between the arrows. The dashed arrows indicate nonenzymatic transformations. GGTP, γ-Glutamyl transpeptidase; HETE, hydroxy-5,-8,10,14-eicosatraenoic acid; HHT, hydroxyheptadecatetraenoic acid; HPETE, hydroperoxyeicosatetraenoic acid; LT, leukotriene; MDA, malonyldialdehyde; TX, thromboxane. (From Salmon, 1982. *In* Cardiovascular Pharmacology of the Prostaglandins. Copyright 1982, Raven Press, New York.)

tide metabolic mechanism is still hypothetical. However, circulating ADP is a stimulator of platelet aggregation. Endothelial inactivation of ADP and its production of the vasodilator antiaggregating agent adenosine may be a mechanism designed to prevent platelet aggregation. Moreover, inosine is believed to be protective of VSM under conditions of hypoxia (Bloom *et al.*, 1979). The significance of adenosine as a mediator of reactive hyperemia, at the level of the microcirculation, also becomes important in view of the capacity of adenosine to release a subsequent vasodila-

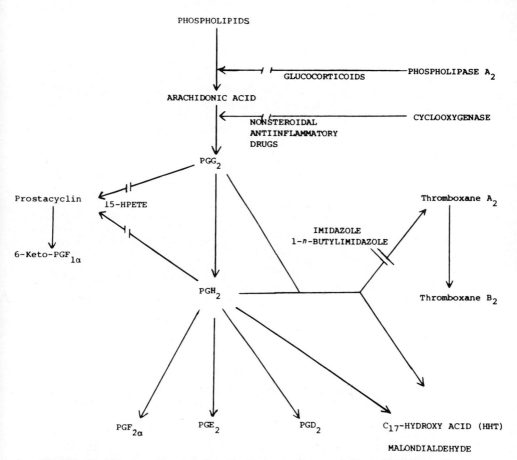

Fig. 10. Arachidonic acid metabolism by cyclooxygenase and sites of inhibitors. (From Salmon, 1982. *In* Cardiovascular Pharmacology of the Prostaglandins. Copyright 1982, Raven Press, New York.)

tor metabolite from the endothelium itself (see Section II,E). Thus, endothelial uptake of ADP may protect the VSM against platelet aggregation and aid in promoting VSM relaxation. Further studies are needed to define the significance of this system in the microcirculation.

Figures 9–12 summarize the synthetic and degradative mechanisms for prostaglandins (PG). The endothelium is a site of selective PGE_2 and prostacyclin (PGI) production. It appears that the larger arteries synthesize PGI, whereas the endothelium of the smaller arteries synthesizes PGE (Gerritsen, 1982). The endothelium is also a site for inactivation of PGE and PGF. Prostaglandins of this series are taken up by a probenecid-inhib-

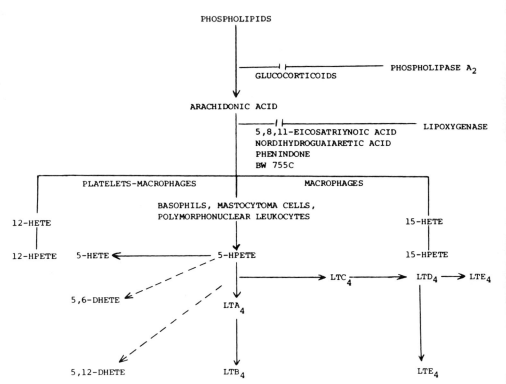

Fig. 11. Arachidonic acid metabolism by lipoxygenase. (From Salmon, 1982. *In* Cardiovascular Pharmacology of the Prostaglandins. Copyright 1982, Raven Press, New York.)

itable active uptake process (Bito and Baroody, 1975; Eling and Anderson, 1976) and metabolized primarily to the dihydro-15-ketoprostanoid derivative. Prostaglandins of the A, B, and I series, and perhaps thromboxanes, may not be taken up by the endothelium (Ryan and Ryan, 1980, 1981). The prostaglandin synthase appears to be a membrane-bound enzyme localized to the plasma membrane, whereas the enzymes responsible for degradation appear to be cytoplasmic (soluble). Endogenous prostanoids may be synthesized at the surface of the cell membrane and diffuse down a concentration gradient to the outside of the cell, where they act. The prostanoids that accumulate within the cell may be degraded within the cell of synthesis by the metabolizing enzyme system, accounting for the lack of preformed storage sites for prostanoids.

The functions of the endothelial cells are many. Although PGI and adenosine formed by the endothelium are vasodilator metabolites, the function of endothelial-derived PGI appears to be modulation of aggregation rather than vasodilation. Figure 13 is a model derived from Gorman

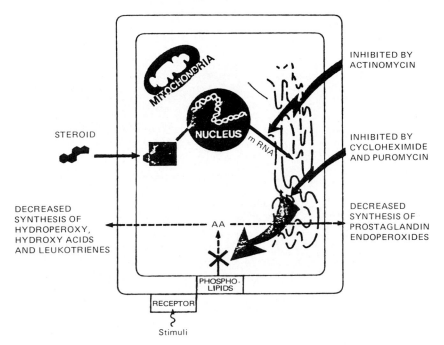

STEROID

INHIBITED BY
ACTINOMYCIN

INHIBITED BY
CYCLOHEXIMIDE
AND PUROMYCIN

DECREASED
SYNTHESIS OF
HYDROPEROXY,
HYDROXY ACIDS
AND LEUKOTRIENES

DECREASED
SYNTHESIS OF
PROSTAGLANDIN
ENDOPEROXIDES

AA

PHOSPHO-
LIPIDS

RECEPTOR

Stimuli

Fig. 12. Mechanism of inhibition of arachidonate metabolism. (From Salmon, 1982. *In* Cardiovascular Pharmacology of the Prostaglandins. Copyright 1982, Raven Press, New York.)

(1982) summarizing the interaction between the platelet and the vascular endothelium. It is believed that the interaction of the aggregating platelets with the endothelial wall and/or the release of lipid peroxides from the aggregating platelets results in action of prostacyclin synthase and elaboration of PGI. The PGI then acts on the platelet to stimulate an increase in cyclic AMP, which results in a decline in free calcium, inhibition of release of 5-HT and ADP, granule stabilization, and decreased release of thromboxane A_2 from the platelet. All of this decreases platelet adhesiveness and prevents aggregation and thrombus formation, if not platelet deposition on the endothelium. Indirectly, this action of the endothelium prevents the release of a potent coronary and cerebral vasoconstrictor, thromboxane A_2, and in this manner does protect the VSM from the deleterious constrictor influences of the circulating humoral factors.

In addition to the antithrombogenic effect of PGI, endothelial cells of veins and capillaries possess plasminogen activator (Todd, 1959, 1964). Moreover, endothelial cells bind thrombin, which rapidly suppresses the fibrinolytic activity of the endothelial cells (for references see Ryan and Ryan, 1981). Thrombin has also been reported to contract VSM (White, 1982). Thus, the endothelium of the microcirculation is both antithrombo-

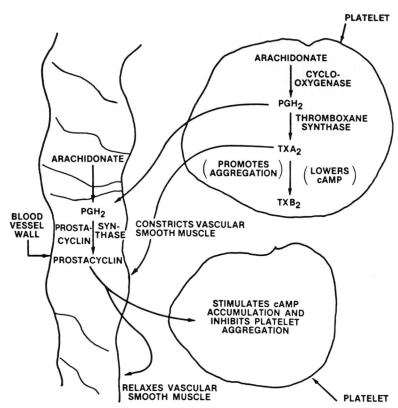

Fig. 13. Model for interaction of PGI₂ with platelets and endothelium. (From Gorman, 1982, with permission.)

genic and hemostatic. The significance of these activities and their relationship to the VSM remain to be explored.

The endothelium also modulates VSM function by acting on polypeptide hormones. The two most important of these act in Yin–Yang fashion to produce vasoconstriction and vasodilation, respectively. They are angiotensin and bradykinin. Endothelial cells contain peptidases, the most important of which is dipeptidyl carboxypeptidase [angiotensin-converting enzyme (ACE) or kinase II], which activates the vasoconstrictor decapeptide angiotensin I to the potent pressor octapeptide hormone angiotensin II and inactivates the nonapeptide vasodilator bradykinin to the pepta- and heptapeptides, which are relatively inactive (see Ryan and Ryan, 1977a,b, 1980). Thus, ACE can convert an active vasodepressor agent to a potent inactive metabolite and convert a prohormone to one of the most potent pressor agents in the circulation.

The ACE is localized along the external surface of the endothelial cells and some smooth muscles (e.g., uterus) and VSM (for references see Ryan and Ryan, 1977a,b, 1980), thus allowing conversion of these substances in the vascular space. The enzyme hydrolyzes the histidine–phenylalanine bond of angiotensin I and forms angiotensin II. The ACE both inactivates and degrades bradykinin by first hydrolyzing the proline–phenylalanine bond of the nonapeptide (inactivation) and then the serine–phenylalanine bond of the heptapeptide (degradation). The angiotensin II formed can then be acted on by endothelial aminopeptidase A to form the potent adrenal cortical stimulating hormone deaspartylangiotensin II (angiotensin III).

The rates of inactivation of bradykinin and activation of angiotensin II by the endothelium may play an important role in determining the microvascular pressures in such diverse diseases as hypertension and diabetes and in pregnancy, in which renin substrate is tremendously increased, providing a potential high concentration of angiotensin I, shock, and other conditions associated with altered endothelial activity. In view of this the finding of Stalcup *et al.* (1979a,b) and Stalcup (1982) that hypoxia inhibits ACE activity suggests that increased levels of vasodilator substances such as bradykinin may compromise the circulation, in the face of a decreased angiotensin II and III pressor influence, in neonatal and adult respiratory distress syndromes, not because of altered VSM function but rather because of endothelial mechanisms. The significance of the Stalcup experiments must await confirmation by independent investigations.

The brief summary provided herein shows that the endothelium of VSM has the potential for synthesizing and degrading humoral factors important in microvascular function. Disease-induced or drug-induced alterations of the vascular endothelium may modify microcirculatory VSM function as effectively as those interventions that alter the VSM directly. Evaluation of drug effects on the microcirculation must be interpreted in terms of the effects of the drugs or interventions on both the VSM and the endothelium. Whether there are therapeutic goals that can be achieved by interfering with or promoting the endothelial mechanisms involved in prostanoid, NE, 5-HT, and adenosine metabolism remains to be shown by future investigation.

E. Endothelium as a Mediator of Vascular Relaxation and Contraction

It is well known among physiologists and pharmacologists studying VSM that humoral substances such as bradykinin and acetylcholine (ACh) contract VSM *in vitro,* despite the inherent vasodilator properties in the microcirculation (McGiff *et al.,* 1972; Needleman *et al.,* 1974; Furchgott, 1955; Bohr *et al.,* 1978; Vanhoutte, 1978; Somlyo and Somlyo, 1968). Vanhoutte *et al.* (1973) suggested that the vasodilator response of ACh may result from an inhibitory effect on adrenergic neurotransmitter release, whereas ACh directly contracts VSM. However, some investigators reported ACh-mediated relaxation of VSM *in vitro* (Jeliffe, 1962; Kuriyama and Suzuki, 1978; Lee *et al.,* 1978).

Serendipitously, Furchgott and Zawadski (1979, 1980a,b,c) and Furchgott *et al.* (1981) found that if the endothelial surface of the blood vessel were not in contact with the glass or wax surface of the material used to prepare helical strips of blood vessels, or if care were taken to avoid contact of the skin with the endothelial surface of vessels, or if rings, rather than helical strips, of VSM were prepared, these blood vessels relaxed in response to ACh and a whole series of vasodilator compounds that had previously been shown to contract VSM *in vitro.* Subsequent analyses demonstrated that rubbing the endothelial surface with wet filter paper or wooden dowels obliterated the endothelium and VSM relaxation *in vitro.* These observations have been confirmed by several investigators (Altura and Chand, 1981; DeMey and Vanhoutte, 1978, 1980a,b,c,d, 1981; Greenberg *et al.,* 1982a,b; Tanaka *et al.,* 1982a).

Although the characteristics of ACh-dependent relaxation appear to be mediated by distinct endothelial cholinergic muscarinic receptors that differ from those on the smooth muscle (see Section III,H) the responses to ATP, adenosine, bradykinin, the calcium ionophore A-23187, ADP, and substance P appear to be dependent on the presence of an intact endothelium for either full or partial expression of their relaxant action (Furchgott *et al.,* 1981; Greenberg *et al.,* 1982a,b; Altura and Chand, 1981). Utilizing a sandwich technique in which endothelial-incompetent VSM was mounted as a sandwich with endothelial-competent VSM oriented so that it could neither relax nor contract to vasoactive substances, administration of ACh and other substances produced relaxation in the endothelial-deficient VSM. This suggested to Furchgott and Zawadski (1980a,b,c,d) that ACh and other substances released a vasoactive substance from the endothelium that acted on the smooth muscle to promote relaxation of VSM.

To prostaglandinologists the most likely candidate for a mediator of endothelial-dependent relaxation of VSM is prostacyclin (Needleman *et al.,* 1976; Moncada *et al.,* 1976a,b). Furchgott *et al.* (1981) tested prostacyclin, cyclic GMP, bradykinin, and cyclic AMP as potential mediators of endothelial-induced relaxation of VSM *in vitro.* Each of these were ruled out as possible candidates because the magnitude of relaxation produced

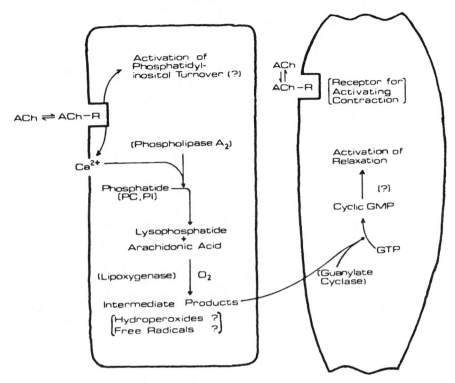

Fig. 14. Hypothetical scheme for ACh endothelial-dependent relaxation in endothelial (left) and smooth muscle (right) cells. PC, Phosphatidylcholine; PI, phosphatidylinositol. (From Furchgott *et al.*, 1981. *In* Vasodilation. Copyright 1981, Raven Press, New York.)

did not approach that of the stimulating substance. However, anoxia inhibited ACh-mediated relaxation, as did 5,8,11,14-eicosatetraynoic acid (ETYA), a lipoxygenase inhibitor. The inhibition of relaxation was selective for endothelial-mediated relaxation and not antagonistic for isoproterenol, nitroglycerin, AMP, or adenosine. The possibility that ACh increased intracellular calcium ion in the endothelium was considered. This resulted in an increased phospholipase A_2 activity and the activation of a lipoxygenase with the formation of either relaxant hydroperoxides or free radicals (Fig. 14). The intermediate lipoxygenase products then acted on the VSM cell to stimulate the accumulation of cyclic GMP (Hidaka and Asano, 1977; Hidaka *et al.*, 1979; Goldberg *et al.*, 1978; Schultz *et al.*, 1979; Spies *et al.*, 1980), which in some undefined manner relaxed the VSM. Although a more specific inhibitor of lipoxygenase BW-755-C, 3-amino-1-[*m*-(trifluoromethyl)phenyl]-2-pyrazoline, did not inhibit endothelial-mediated relaxation by ACh, the free-radical scavengers hydro-

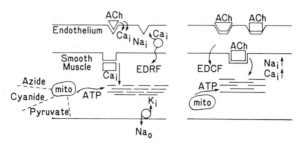

Fig. 15. Alternate mechanism for ACh-mediated relaxation (left) and contraction (right). EDCF, Endothelial-derived contractile factor; EDRF, endothelial-derived relaxation factor.

quinone and the antimalarial agent quinacrine inhibited endothelial-dependent ACh-mediated relaxation of VSM. Quinacrine inhibits phospholipase A_2 activity but may also inhibit the ACh receptor or the actions of ACh on calcium ion in the endothelium.

Although the hypothesis proposed by Furchgott et al. (1981) is attractive, there is some difficulty in reconciling the data and the interpretation. A finite time is required to inhibit lipoxygenase and phospholipase A_2 by these inhibitors. Their actions on VSM occur within 1 min. The concentration of inhibitor required to inhibit endothelial-dependent relaxation is 10–100 times that required for inhibition of lipoxygenase. The effects of the inhibitors are acutely reversible. ETYA acetylenates the lipoxygenase and irreversibly inhibits the enzyme. Finally, Greenberg et al. (1982b) showed that ETYA, hydroquinone, and other inhibitors, in low concentrations sufficient to inhibit lipoxygenase, did not inhibit bradykinin- or ACh-mediated relaxation of canine mesenteric arteries, but in high concentrations inhibited both ACh and NE responses in mesenteric arteries and veins even in the absence of endothelium (Greenberg et al., 1982b; Greenberg and Kadowitz, 1982). The experiments of Greenberg et al. (1982b) showed that ACh endothelial-dependent relaxation was inhibited by ouabain in concentrations that did not affect the responses to NE or ACh responses in endothelial-deficient preparations. An alternative hypothesis is summarized in Fig. 15. The interaction of ACh, bradykinin, and other endothelial-dependent substances releases an unknown mediator from the endothelium. This substance acts on the VSM to stimulate an influx of potassium ion and hyperpolarizes the cell by stimulating an electrogenic sodium pump within the VSM cell membrane. As the membrane potential moves mostly toward the potassium equilibrium potential, the permeability of calcium ion is decreased. This results in a decreased calcium–calmodulin interaction and a decreased phosphorylation of the p-myosin light chain (see Section II,J) and relaxation of VSM. Alternatively, several distinct mediators may exist in the endothelium, and the effects of the mediator on the VSM may be dependent on the type of mediator released from the endothelium, which is dependent in turn on the vasoactive relaxant substance. The nature of the endothelial mediator of VSM relaxation and the significance of endothelial-mediated relaxation to *in vivo* microcirculatory function remain to be defined.

The endothelium may be involved not only in VSM relaxation, but in contraction of the VSM as well. Endothelial destruction inhibits the contractile responses of porcine VSM to transmural nerve stimulation (Greenberg *et al.*, 1980) and ACh (Greenberg *et al.*, 1982a,b; Tanaka *et al.*, 1982b) in canine mesenteric and pulmonary veins. The magnitude of the change is only 20% of the maximal contractile response to ACh and approximately 50% of the response to nerve stimulation. This, at least for nerve stimulation, may have a pathophysiologic correlate in shock, in that pulmonary and systemic blood vessels obtained from shocked swine and dogs exhibit endothelial destruction and depression of the response to nerve stimulation (Greenberg *et al.*, 1980). It is possible that the effects of the endothelial mediator differ on arterial and venous smooth muscle or that the endothelial mediator differs when obtained from artery and vein. The nature of the factors obligatory for both endothelial-mediated relaxation and contraction remains to be elucidated.

F. Smooth Muscle as a Site of Production of Humoral Factors

Agonist-mediated contraction of VSM is attended by an increased release of prostaglandins, prostacyclin, and thromboxanes derived from the VSM (Salmon *et al.*, 1978; McGiff *et al.*, 1976; Needleman *et al.*, 1976; Hagen and White, 1978; Greenberg *et al.*, 1981; Greenberg and Kadowitz, 1982) as well as the endothelium. The mechanisms of synthesis and degradation are shown in Figs. 9–12. Local production of these prostanoids appears to be involved in VSM function and modulation of adrenergic neuroeffector transmission (see reviews by Kadowitz *et al.*, 1982a,b; Kadowitz and Hyman, 1982; Armstrong, 1982; Hedquist, 1977) because Marcus *et al.* (1982) showed that endothelial denudation of VSM resulted in smooth muscle production of PGI without any effect on platelet aggregation or thrombus formation.

The release of prostanoids from the VSM and the endothelium as well appears to be modified and/or regulated by many factors that affect either the biosynthesis or degradation of the prostanoids. Bradykinin, angiotensin II, and thrombin may activate phopholipase A_2 activity, thereby in-

creasing the release of arachidonic acid from phospholipid, or may promote the activity of phosphatidyl-inositol phosphodiesterase (Bell and
Majerius, 1980; Bell *et al.*, 1980), increasing the synthesis of prostaglandins. β-Thromboglobulin and its precursor γ-thromboglobulin appear to
inhibit PGE and PGI synthesis in aortic smooth muscle in culture (see
Pearson, 1982). Low-density lipoproteins (LDL), if present for 60 min or
more, inhibit PGI production whereas high-density lipoproteins counteract the effect of LDL but do not exert any effect on their own. The mechanism, although speculative, may be related to the capacity of LDL to bind
to specific cell receptors, be taken up into the endothelium and perhaps
smooth muscle, and destroy the cells (Brown and Goldstein, 1979; Evensen, 1979). Albumin can increase the transport of free fatty acids into the
cell, thereby increasing substrate for PG cyclooxygenase and increasing
or decreasing prostanoid synthesis.

Macrocortin, a 15,000-dalton protein, may be induced by nonsteroidal
antiinflammatory agents acting on the cell. This protein may inhibit phospholipase A_2 activity, thereby decreasing prostanoid synthesis (Blackwell
et al., 1978, 1980). A plasma factor that may be a phospholipid bound to
albumin has been found to contract the perfused coronary arteries of
hearts *in situ* and stimulate $PGF_{2\alpha}$ synthesis. The action of this phospholipid is antagonized by indomethacin. This substance, which acts only
when in free phospholipid form, stimulates both lipoxygenase and cyclooxygenase activity and promotes platelet aggregation as well as VSM
contraction. The mechanism of this inhibitor remains obscure (Moretti *et
al.*, 1976; Moretti and Abraham, 1978a,b; Moretti and Lin, 1980).

Normal human plasma appears to contain a substance, designated re-
ciprocal coupling factor, that both enhances $PGF_{2\alpha}$ breakdown and inhibits $PGF_{2\alpha}$ synthesis. This factor, enhanced by sufinpyrazone, increases in
diabetes and decreases in thyrotoxicosis and may be a natural antithrombotic substance (Hoult and Moore, 1982). Several factors exist in human
plasma that stimulate PGI synthesis and possibly inhibit thromboxane
synthase activity (see Pearson, 1982). These have not yet been characterized but may play a role in protecting the endothelium and VSM against
thrombosis or vasoconstriction in such disease states as renal failure, in
which their activity increases, and may play an adversary role in disease
states in which they are diminished, such as hemolytic uremic failure and
thrombocytopenic purpura (Pearson, 1982; Tables IV and V).

Thus, the VSM as well as the endothelium can synthesize prostanoids.
The synthesis of these factors is not controlled solely by the VSM but is
also subject to modulation by plasma factors of a diverse nature. Drug effects on the microvasculature, rather than being simply endothelial or
VSM dependent, may also modify VSM function by altering the synthesis

TABLE IV
Some Biological Effects of Leukotrienes

Vasodilation: PGE_2/PGI_2
Edema: PGE_2/PGI_2; leukotrienes C_4, D_4, and E_4
Leukocyte migration (adhesion, chemotaxis): Leukotriene B_4
Contraction: Leukotrienes C_4, D_4, E_4

---

and/or activation of these plasma factors, which subsequently affects the synthesis and degradation of these prostanoids and, secondarily, VSM tone. The prudent investigator will now be wise to consider the hematologic effects of pharmacologic antagonists when evaluating microcirculatory function.

G. Mechanisms of Vascular Smooth Muscle Excitation

The poor longitudinal transmission of electrical activity and the large amount of connective tissue in blood vessels make the recording of electrical activity in VSM more difficult than in any other smooth muscle preparation. However, for the sake of completeness, the electrical activation of VSM is discussed here briefly. The electrical activation of VSM plays a role in mediating VSM contraction, although both the nature of this activity and the importance differ in different vessels and with different modes of contraction within the same VSM (Keatinge, 1979).

The resting membrane potential of VSM is mediated by the permeability of the cell membrane to potassium ion. The relatively greater permeability to sodium ion results in a higher resting membrane potential in VSM and other smooth muscles than in skeletal muscle or nerve. A coupled sodium–potassium transport exchange mechanism is responsible for maintaining the gradient of sodium and potassium ion across the VSM cell. The smooth muscle of the arterioles is generally electrically quiescent except at times of release of neurotransmitter from the adrenergic nerves innervating the VSM. Upon release of NE, the VSM becomes partially depolarized and fires bursts of action potentials. The rate of firing of these action potentials appears to be related to the magnitude of increase in mechanical tension (Speden, 1964; von Loh and Bohr, 1973). Several discharges of the nerves in succession are required to initiate or fire an action potential (Hirst, 1977; Holman and Suprenant, 1979). The action potential is followed by a brisk contraction. Both the action potentials and the subsequent contractions are conducted for only a limited distance and seldom involve more than one arteriole (Hirst, 1977).

TABLE V

Interactions between Blood Components and Prostaglandin Synthesis[a,b]

Blood component	Tissue or system tested	Outcome
Plasma, serum, Cohn fractions IV and V, especially IV-4, haptoglobin, and albumin	Seminal vesicle microsomes	PG synthesis ↓
	Isolated rat fundus strip preparation contracted with arachidonic acid	Prevents increase in tone
Plasma or albumin	Soybean lipoxygenase	Oxygen uptake ↓
	Platelet lipoxygenase	↓PG, TXB_2, HETE synthesis
Plasma or serum (labile, nondialyzable factor)	Cultured bovine endothelial cells	↑PGI_2, synthesis (bioassay or RIA)
Platelet-derived β-thromboglobulin	Cultured bovine endothelial cells	↓PGI_2, synthesis (bioassay)
Plasma	"Exhausted" rat aorta rings	↑PGI_2, release (bioassay)
Plasma or lipid extract of albumin	Perfused rabbit heart	PG-Dependent vasoconstriction ↑
	Cardiac or renal microsomes (rabbit)	↑PG synthesis
	Platelets and platelet microsomes	↑PG, TXB_2, HETE synthesis
Plasma or albumin	Platelet aggregation to arachidonate	Biphasic effect
	Platelet aggregation to arachidonate	↓Aggregation and ↑release of arachidonate metabolites
Plasma or factor bound to albumin from adult, but not fetus	Human thyroid adenoma/mononuclear cell coculture	↓PGE yield
Serum, probably platelet-derived growth factor	Cultured 3T3 mouse fibroblasts	↑Phospholipase A_2 activity and PGE_2, $PGF_{2\alpha}$ release
Serum (plasma less effective)	Cultured MC5-5 mouse fibroblasts	↑PGE_2 release by RIA
Serum	Phagocytosing rat leukocytes	↓PGE_2 release by bioassay
Haptoglobin and acute-phase sera	Arachidonate hypotension in rabbit	Agents protect (via ↓PG synthesis?)
Albumin	Spontaneous decomposition of endoperoxide PHG_2	↑PGD_2 formation at expense of PGE_2
Plasma, platelet rich or platelet poor	Spontaneous decomposition of prostacyclin	Plasma ↓rate; platelets may convert PGI_2 to 6-keto-PGE_1

[a] From Hoult and Moore (1982). *In* Cardiovascular Pharmacology of the Prostaglandins. Copyright 1982, Raven Press, New York.

[b] Abbreviations: PG, prostaglandin; TXB_2, thromboxane B_2; HETE, 12L-hydroxy-5,8,10,14-eicosatetraenoic acid; PGI_2, prostacyclin; RIA, radioimmunoassay.

Sodium ion and, to a limited extent, calcium ion appear to carry the current in the smooth muscle cells of VSM (Keatinge, 1968a,b). The action potentials can be obtained in calcium-free solution, indicating that they are due primarily to the sodium current. However, unlike the sodium channels of nerve and skeletal muscle, tetrodotoxin cannot block the action potential or the entry of sodium into VSM. The action potentials of VSM can be blocked by verapamil, the calcium-channel-blocking agent, which also blocks these tetrodotoxin-resistant sodium channels in other smooth muscles (Golenhofen and Lammel, 1972). However, the action of verapamil is neither uniformly consistent nor specific. Specific, independent calcium channels also appear to exist in VSM, and these appear to be involved in the resting permeability of VSM to calcium ion. These channels seem to be distinct from those of the voltage-dependent calcium channel, in that they are not blocked by verapamil or D-600 (Weiss, 1981a,b; Vanhoutte, 1980).

Under special circumstances, such as anoxia, blood vessels exhibit widely conducted action potentials preceded by rhythmic changes in mechanical tension or pressure. This type of activity is also present under naturally occurring physiologic conditions in portal veins and some venules (Axelsson *et al.,* 1967; Funaki, 1961; Funaki and Bohr, 1964). Such contractions have a propulsive action, which is inefficient but of value in the dual circulation of the liver (Keatinge, 1979). Under normal conditions the high resting potassium permeability of most VSM, which increases on depolarization, prevents and opposes the development of regenerative action potentials (Mekata, 1971; Keatinge, 1978). Unlike the normal action potentials of VSM, these repetitive spike discharges of rhythmically active VSM appear to be mediated by a slowly inactivating calcium and magnesium current, which is independent of sodium ion (Keatinge, 1978). The significance of this unique magnesium channel remains speculative. However, Keatinge (1978, 1979) suggests that an increase in intracellular magnesium between spike discharges may aid in promoting VSM relaxation, thus contributing to the rhythmic fluctuations in VSM tone.

H. Sources of Activator Calcium in Vascular Smooth Muscle

The manner in which excitation of VSM by vasoactive agents initiates an increase or decrease in tension development remains an unresolved matter. Three major mechanisms exist to explain the sources of activator calcium in VSM. Humoral factors and agonists that either increase spike discharge or promote a maintained depolarization are believed to stimulate the opening of voltage-dependent channels, which increase the entry of both sodium ion and calcium ion. Both the number of channels that are open and the time during which they remain open determine the relative increase of extracellular calcium ion into the cell. Entry of calcium ion in response to electrical activation of VSM seems to be an integral component of the response because the electrical activity fails in calcium-free media at a time when the intracellular concentration of calcium ion falls to a threshold level for contraction (Hinke, 1965; Keatinge, 1979). It has been suggested that this process of calcium entry triggers the release of intracellular calcium ion from sequestered sites and thereby raises the ionized concentration of calcium ion above 10^{-7} M to initiate the contractile process (Sigurdsson et al., 1975), similar to a process that occurs in striated muscle. However, little evidence exists to support this hypothesis. The calcium ion that enters from extracellular or membrane-bound sites may be sufficient to interact with calmodulin, thereby activating the contractile proteins (Section II,J). The entry of activator calcium ion linked to changes in the membrane potential of VSM has been designated electrical–mechanical coupling (Somlyo and Somlyo, 1968, 1970; Bohr, 1973) or spike activation mechanisms (SAM) (Golenhofen et al., 1973; Fig. 16).

Norepinephrine can contract VSM either with or without a concomitant change in membrane potential (Bohr et al., 1978; Somlyo and Somlyo, 1968, 1970; Altura and Altura, 1977a,b; Altura, 1978a,b, 1981; Vanhoutte, 1978, 1980, 1981a,b; Weiss, 1981a,b). The contractile responses of VSM to low concentrations of NE are inhibited rapidly by withdrawal of extracellular calcium ion, whereas those to high concentrations are not inhibited (Weiss, 1977). Moreover, the responses to NE, some prostanoids, thromboxanes (Greenberg et al., 1973a,b; Bevan et al., 1973; Hudgins and Weiss, 1968; Greenberg, 1981a; McNamara et al., 1980; Altura and Altura, 1977b), and other vasoactive substances are not antagonized by inhibitors of calcium influx into the cell, such as nifedipine, D-600, or verapamil (for references see Vanhoutte, 1980; Weiss, 1981a,b). However, the responses to these agonists are inhibited by metabolic inhibitors, anoxia, or a reduction in temperature. It is thought that these agonists increase membrane permeability to calcium ion by opening up receptor-linkage voltage-independent channels in the cell membrane, as well as by causing a release of intracellular calcium ion from sequestered sites within the VSM cell (Bohr et al., 1978; Weiss, 1981a,b). Keatinge (1979) has suggested that the increase in membrane permeability of calcium ion and/or the release of intracellular sequestered calcium ion brought about by vasoactive agents acting through pharmacomechanical coupling (Somlyo and Somlyo, 1968) or spike-free activation mechanisms (SFAM) (Golenhofen et

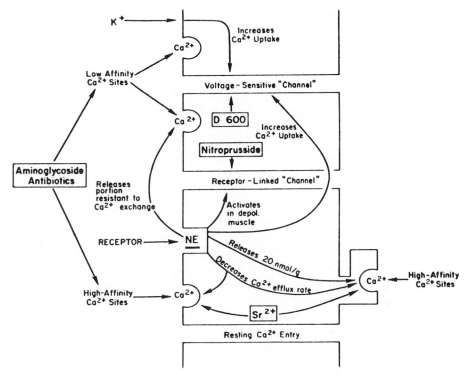

Fig. 16. Model for sites of action of different inhibitory agents on calcium uptake pathways and associated calcium-binding sites in vascular smooth muscle. (From Weiss, 1981, with permission.)

al., 1973) must do so by releasing or stimulating the synthesis of a chemical mediator or event, since the temperature sensitivity of the process indicates a chemical rather than a physical process. It is unlikely that the mediator is a prostanoid, despite the suggestion of Horrobin *et al.* (1976). These investigators showed that indomethacin inhibited the contractile responses of NE in rat VSM. In most preparations, indomethacin enhances the responses to NE (see Greenberg and Kadowitz, 1982). The chemical mediator, if one exists, remains unknown.

Vasodilators may bring about a decrease in VSM tone by (*a*) antagonizing or opposing the electrical changes produced by vasoconstrictor agonists, thereby decreasing the entry of extracellular calcium ion into the cell; (*b*) directly reducing calcium influx into the cell by promoting electrical changes opposite to, but independent of, those produced by vasoconstrictor agents; (*c*) directly increasing the efflux of calcium ion from the cell; or (*d*) promoting the sequestration of intracellular calcium ion by sarcoplasmic reticulum, mitochondria, or other subcellular organelles (Vanhoutte and Leusen, 1981; Vanhoutte, 1978, 1981a,b). Other evidence also suggests that vasodilators may promote VSM relaxation either by decreasing the binding of calcium ion to the regulatory protein calmodulin (Stull and Sanford, 1981) or by increasing the rate of dephosphorylation of myosin light chains (Small and Sobieszek, 1977, 1980; Perry and Grand, 1979). In the latter instances, relaxation is promoted in the absence of a change in free ionized calcium ion.

In summary, extracellular, intracellular, and membrane-bound calcium ions may serve as sources of activator calcium ion in VSM. Whereas SAM or electrical–mechanical coupling mechanisms may be associated with the entry of calcium from the outside of the cell through voltage-dependent channels, SFAM or pharmacomechanical coupling appears to be related to the entry of calcium into the cell via voltage-independent channels and release of sequestered calcium ion from within the cell. Relaxation of VSM is associated with decreases in the entry and release of calcium from these sources but may also be associated with direct effects of vasodilator compounds on the contractile proteins or calmodulin. Although graded depolarization appears to be evident in the microcirculation smooth muscle cells (Chernukh and Timkina, 1976; Funaki and Bohr, 1964; Kumamoto, 1977), the pools of activator calcium involved in VSM contraction and relaxation remain to be defined.

I. Energy and Vascular Smooth Muscle Contraction

The VSM is unique in that it utilizes a large amount of energy for a long period of time to maintain arterial pressure, without undergoing fatigue. The VSM maintains the integrity of the arterial pressure with approximately 4% of the basal metabolic rate of energy production, whereas equivalent energy utilization by skeletal muscle would require twice the energy output provided by the total basal metabolic rate of the organism (Paul, 1980). This efficient utilization of energy occurs with VSM in which the basal pool of high-energy phosphates is 2–5 μmol per gram of blood vessel, a value of 10–20 times lower than that found in skeletal muscle. Since the basal rate of high-energy phosphate utilization in VSM is 1–3 μmol/g per minute preformed ATP cannot serve as a source of energy for the maintenance of VSM tone. Rather, newly synthesized ATP from oxidative metabolism and phosphocreatine via the Lohman reaction

$$\text{Phosphocreatine} + \text{ADP} \rightleftharpoons \text{ATP} + \text{creatine}$$

must subserve VSM tension development. Thus, in VSM intermediary metabolism is more important than in skeletal muscle, where brief contractions are supported from preformed high-energy phosphate pools and the energy debt is repaid after the contraction is completed.

Steady-state oxygen consumption is coupled to isometric force development in VSM. Thus, the energy production by mitochondria should be limited by the amount of available ADP. It has been suggested that the limiting source of ADP in the VSM is derived from the hydrolysis of ATP via actomyosin ATPase activity (Nishiki *et al.*, 1978). However, because of the relatively low concentration of ADP in VSM this has not yet been verified experimentally. The major sources of substrate for energy production in VSM appear to be both exogenous glucose and preformed glycogen. However, VSM can utilize lipid substrates in both the presence and absence of glucose (Furchgott, 1966; Paul, 1980), because the enzymes for the conversion of lipids, proteins, and carbohydrates into ATP appear to exist in VSM and the respective substrates can support VSM contraction. The preferred substrate under physiologic conditions remains to be elucidated.

The VSM is unique among tissues in that approximately 90% of its glucose metabolism results in lactate formation (aerobic glycolysis) with approximately 30% of its ATP produced by this mechanism. Peterson and Paul (1974) and Gluck and Paul (1977) provided convincing evidence that the formation of lactate was increased by vasoconstrictor agents where the (K,Na)-ATPase was functional but that ouabain-induced contracture was associated with a decreased lactate production. It has been suggested that aerobic glycolysis provides the energy to support the sodium–potassium pump mechanism (Paul, 1980; Hellstrand and Paul, 1980, 1982) involved in maintaining the normal intracellular concentration of sodium and potassium ion (Table VIII, p. 108).

Although ATP is essential for both contraction and relaxation, relaxation appears to be more sensitive to inhibition by blockade of oxidative metabolism than contraction. DeMey and Vanhoutte (1978), Furchgott *et al.* (1981), and Greenberg *et al.* (1982b) have shown that hypoxia, azide, and cyanide abolish ACh-, adenosine-, and bradykinin-mediated relaxation of VSM in concentrations that do not inhibit contraction by NE. Although the metabolic bases for these events remain undefined, the data suggest that the increase in vascular resistance with hypoxia or hypoxic-induced vasoconstriction *in vitro* may result from abolition of vasodilator mechanisms, which then allow vasoconstrictor mechanisms to proceed unopposed. Further studies are necessary to elucidate the metabolic factors regulating VSM functions.

A discussion of the metabolic factors affecting VSM would be incomplete without an examination of the role of the cyclic nucleotides in VSM. The present state of knowledge concerning the role of cyclic AMP and cyclic GMP in VSM is, at best, controversial. Drugs that stimulate the

TABLE VI

Alterations in Activities of Enzymes of the Prostaglandin System in Pathophysiologic States[a,b]

Species, organ	Treatment	Prostaglandin synthesis (microsomes)	Prostaglandin metabolism (cytosol)
Rat kidney	Adrenalectomy	—	↑
	Renal hypertrophy	↓	—
	New Zealand hypertension	N/C	↓
	Renal artery clamp hypertension	↑	—
	Wistar–Okamoto hypertension	—	↓[c]
	Wistar–Okamoto hypertension	↑[d]	—
	Wistar–Okamoto hypertension	?[e]	↓
Rat lung	Pregnant	—	↑
	Parturition	—	↓
Guinea pig lung	Exposure to 100% O_2, 2 days	N/C	↓
Rabbit kidney	Ureter-obstructed hydronephrotic	↑[d]	—
	Renal vein constricted	↑[d]	—
Rabbit lung	Late pregnant/progesterone-treated	—	↑
	Parturition	—	↓

[a] From Hoult and Moore (1982). *In* Cardiovascular Pharmacology of the Prostaglandins. Copyright 1982, Raven Press, New York.

[b] Key: ↑, activity increased; ↓, activity decreased; N/C, no change in activity; —, not tested.

[c] Refers to the enzyme 9-hydroxyprostaglandin dehydrogenase. 15-Hydroxyprostaglandin dehydrogenase activity was normal.

[d] Synthesis from perfused organ.

[e] Assay was in crude homogenate: degradation interferes.

accumulation of cyclic AMP as well as cyclic GMP produce relaxation of VSM. However, increases in these nucleotides within the VSM cell may also be associated with contraction of the smooth muscle or no change in smooth muscle tone. The evidence leading to the hypothesis proposed for the action of cyclic nucleotides in VSM will be summarized here. For a detailed discussion of this topic the reader is referred to excellent reviews (Amer, 1977; Andersson *et al.*, 1972; Bar, 1974; Berridge, 1975; Diamond, 1978; Crain and Appleman, 1978; Goldberg *et al.*, 1973; Kukovetz *et al.*, 1981).

The original concept to emerge was that if cyclic AMP was associated with relaxation then cyclic GMP would oppose relaxation or initiate contraction. This concept was experimentally verified when it was shown that some vasoconstrictors, such as phenylephrine and $PGF_{2\alpha}$, increased cyclic GMP levels in bovine and canine arteries and veins (Dunham *et al.*, 1974; Kadowitz *et al.*, 1973, 1975a; Joiner *et al.*, 1975). This stimulation of cyclic GMP formation was indirect and not due to agonist-mediated ef-

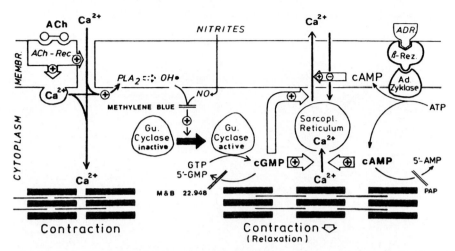

Fig. 17. Schematic representation of role of cyclic GMP and AMP in smooth muscle relaxation. Ad. Zyklase, Adenylate cyclase; ADR, adrenalin; β-Rez., β-receptor; Gu. cyclase, guanylate cyclase; PAP, papaverine; Sarcopl. Reticulum, sarcoplasmic reticulum. (From Kukovetz *et al.*, 1981. *In* Vasodilation. Copyright 1981, Raven Press, New York.)

fects on guanylate cyclase, but rather was a calcium-dependent event associated with an inhibition of phosphodiesterase activity. However, this concept was shattered when it was shown that nitrites produced relaxation in VSM, which was associated with an increase in cyclic GMP (Katsuki *et al.*, 1977). This effect was independent of calcium ion and occurred in broken-cell preparations. Methylene blue inhibited nitrate- and nitroprusside-induced relaxation and the accumulation of cyclic GMP (Kadowitz *et al.*, 1981; Gruetter *et al.*, 1979). Moreover, drugs that inhibited phosphodiesterase potentiated the relaxant effects of these vasodilators (Kukovetz *et al.*, 1979a,b). The reported effects of the nitroso compounds were not secondary to an increase in cellular calcium ion because (*a*) these compounds increased calcium efflux from VSM without increasing calcium influx (Zsoster *et al.*, 1977); (*b*) in the absence of extracellular calcium ion, nitrates and nitroprusside decreased calcium efflux from rabbit renal arteries and inhibited KCl-induced contraction, indicating that calcium sequestration was enhanced (Hester *et al.*, 1979); and (*c*) nitrites and nitroprusside do not directly inhibit calcium sequestration by sarcoplasmic reticulum from rabbit aorta (Thorens and Hausler, 1979). Thus, although the evidence is at best circuitous and circumstantial, it is possible that cyclic GMP could regulate VSM relaxation by stimulating calcium sequestration by sarcoplasmic reticulum or enhancing calcium extrusion from the VSM cell (Fig. 17).

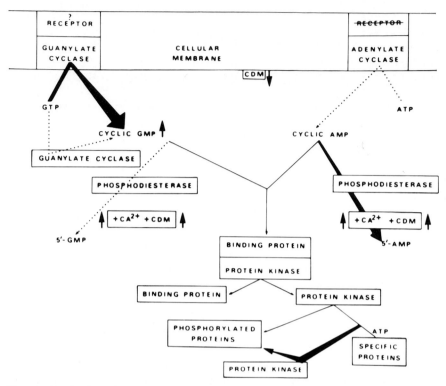

Fig. 18. Mechanism of cyclic nucleotide action. Specific proteins include histones, nonhistone chromosomal proteins, ribosomes, membrane proteins, and certain enzymes. CDM, Calmodulin. (From Criss and Kakiuchi, 1982, with permission.)

The evidence supporting a role and mechanism for cyclic AMP in VSM is firmer. Cyclic AMP stimulates calcium sequestration by subcellular organelles involved in reducing the free concentration of calcium ion, such as sarcoplasmic reticulum and mitochondria. Cyclic AMP accumulates in most VSM when β-receptor-mediated vasodilation occurs and when vasodilator phosphodiesterase inhibitors are employed. Cyclic AMP levels are decreased in conditions associated with increased tension development, such as hypertension (Amer, 1973, 1977; Amer et al., 1974), whereas cyclic AMP-dependent protein kinase (Fig. 18) appears to be involved in the regulation of the relaxation component of contractile protein regulation (see below). Thus, it is possible that stimulation of adenylate kinase, via β-receptor-linked or independent mechanisms, or inhibition of phosphodiesterase results in an increase in cyclic AMP, enhanced calcium extrusion from the cell or sequestration within the subcellular organelles involved in calcium regulation, or both, and subsequent relaxation. Alternatively, the influx of calcium ion may be inhibited by cyclic AMP, which could result in a decrease in calcium binding to calmodulin and relaxation. Finally, cyclic AMP-dependent protein kinase appears to be involved in the inactivation of myosin light-chain kinase, which can promote relaxation even in the absence of changes in calcium ion.

The available data support the hypothesis that both cyclic AMP and cyclic GMP mediate relaxation of VSM, probably by decreasing the concentration of ionized calcium that can interact with calmodulin and possibly by phosphorylating myosin light-chain kinase or dephosphorylating myosin. P. J. Kadowitz (personal communication) has suggested that cyclic GMP may be involved in the action of pharmacologic agents, whereas cyclic AMP mediates the responses to physiologic mediators and modulators of VSM tone. Further studies are necessary to resolve this question.

J. Biochemical Mechanisms Regulating Vascular Smooth Muscle Contraction and Relaxation

The major contractile proteins in VSM are actin, myosin, tropomyosin, and leiotonin A and C (Adelstein and Klee, 1980; Stull and Sanford, 1981; Small and Sobieszek, 1980; Ebashi *et al.*, 1978). Leiotonin C, a calcium-binding protein, differing from both calmodulin and troponin C, may be involved in the regulation of the thin contractile filament, actin, whereas calmodulin appears to be involved in the phosphorylation of the thick filament, myosin. Troponin, present in cardiac and skeletal muscle, may not exist in VSM. Calcium regulation of VSM contraction differs from that for skeletal and cardiac muscles. In the latter muscle, calcium ion removes an inhibitory effect of troponin C on the interaction between actin and myosin. In VSM, calcium ion activates the inactive state of myosin (Fig. 19).

Actin is a globular protein (MW 43,000) that polymerizes at physiologic ionic strength into a double-helical filament. In addition to its structural role in muscle, actin activates ATP hydrolysis by myosin. Tropomyosin (MW 66,000) sits in the groove created by the two strands of actin. The actual function of tropomyosin in VSM is unknown, but tropomyosin enhances the capacity of actin to activate myosin ATPase activity (Small and Sobieszek, 1977, 1980). Leiotonin A and C may, but this is questionable (Ebashi *et al.*, 1978), take the place of troponin and interact with both tropomyosin and actin. Myosin is a hexameric protein consisting of two heavy chains (MW 200,000) and two pairs of light chains (MW 20,000 and 15,000). The 20,000-dalton light chain (hereafter referred to as *p*-myosin light chain) can undergo reversible, covalent phosphorylation and de-

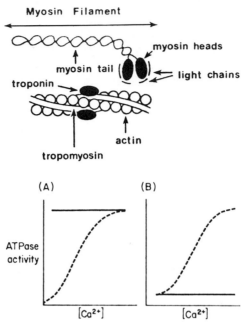

Fig. 19. Regulatory proteins and contractile elements of vascular smooth muscle. Lower panel: ATPase activity of calcium-independent (A) and calcium-regulated (B) actomyosin. Note the lower level of calcium-dependent activity in the absence of calcium (heavy black line). (From Triggle, 1981, with permission.)

phosphorylation, which is believed to be responsible for the velocity of shortening of smooth muscle. The enzymes responsible for myosin phosphorylation (protein kinases) are made up of two proteins: a calcium-binding small protein, known as calmodulin, and a larger protein, which contains most, if not all, of the catalytic activity (Dabrowksa *et al.*, 1978). The catalytic enzyme appears to be regulated by calmodulin.

When an agonist interacts with the cell membrane or intracellular organelles to increase the concentration of free, ionized calcium ion above 10^{-7} M, it is believed that four molecules of calcium bind to calmodulin (calcium–calmodulin). The calcium–calmodulin complex then binds to the inactive form of the myosin light-chain kinase to form the active complex calcium–calmodulin–myosin kinase (active). This active complex of calcium–calmodulin–myosin kinase catalyzes the phosphorylation of the p-myosin light chains, resulting in an active form of myosin susceptible to activation by actin. Myosin light-chain phosphatase, a calcium-independent enzyme, dephosphorylates p-myosin light chain, allowing the cycle to begin anew. It is the phosphorylation and dephosphorylation of the myosin light chains that results in the interaction between actin and myosin and thereby the cyclic attachment and detachment of the myosin heads to the actin filament. The attachment of the myosin heads to the actin results in a change in the angle of the orientation of the actin–myosin, which allows the filaments to slide past each other, similar to the mechanism in skeletal and cardiac muscle. Adenosine triphosphate provides the energy for this process, and actin activation of myosin ATPase activity releases this energy (Adelstein and Klee, 1980).

Conti and Adelstein (1980) suggested that relaxation by agonists (e.g., epinephrine) results from stimulation of adenylate cyclase, which stimulates the formation of cyclic AMP from ATP. The increased cyclic AMP binds to the regulatory subunit of inactive protein kinase to expose the catalytic subunit of protein kinase. This catalytic subunit of protein kinase phosphorylates myosin light-chain kinase. Because the phosphorylated form of the myosin light-chain kinase is less capable of binding with calmodulin, the myosin light-chain kinase is, in effect, inactivated. A decreased myosin kinase activity results in a decreased phosphorylation of myosin. Since dephosphorylated or unphosphorylated myosin cannot interact with actin, VSM tension declines.

Thus, it appears that changes in the level of ionized calcium may regulate the binding of calmodulin to myosin kinase and the degree of activity of the myosin light-chain kinase through cyclic AMP-dependent protein kinase activity. Moreover, drugs that affect the interaction between calcium and calmodulin greatly affect VSM tone and thereby arterial pressure and resistance. It must be stated that the mechanism of contraction and relaxation summarized above is still speculative. Many questions relating to the concentrations and affinity of the kinases and the calcium–calmodulin interaction have not been answered. Moreover, the role of leiotonin A and C in VSM contraction and relaxation is unknown. Further studies are necessary to validate the proposed concept. However, at present, on the basis of the available evidence, it appears that the phosphorylation and dephosphorylation of myosin may be the most important factor regulating VSM contraction and relaxation (for further discussion see Adelstein, 1978; Adelstein and Eisenberg, 1980; Small and Sobieszek, 1980; Ebashi et al., 1978).

K. Mechanisms of Vascular Smooth Muscle Contraction and Relaxation

The evidence presented above suggests that contraction of VSM may occur by four distinct mechanisms. Ions, such as potassium, and low concentrations of NE may induce changes in sodium permeability across the cell membrane, decreasing the membrane potential and causing an influx of sodium and calcium ions through voltage-dependent calcium channels. The increased influx of calcium ion results in the binding of calcium to calmodulin, with the subsequent binding to and activation of p-myosin light-chain kinase. The complex of calcium–calmodulin and activated p-myosin light-chain kinase results in the phosphorylation of the light chain of myosin and the subsequent events that mediate contraction. The contractile response may be regulated or modulated by the simultaneous production of vasodilator substances such as prostacyclin or PGE_2. These modulators may act by increasing adenylate cyclase activity, with its increased production of cyclic AMP and cyclic AMP-dependent protein kinase, which then acts by affecting the dephosphorylation of myosin light-chain kinase. Similarly, high concentrations of NE or 5-HT may induce discreet changes in the voltage-independent calcium channels, increasing the concentration of intracellular calcium ion with its attendant effects on the biochemical events mediating contraction.

In contrast, vasoactive agents, such as thromboxane A_2 and the endoperoxide analog 9a,11a-epoxymethanoprostaglandin H_2, vasopressin, oxytocin, and other agents may act to promote an intracellular release of sequestered calcium ion from within the cell. This process may also involve the presence of a second mediator other than the cyclic nucleotide system, in that some of these agonists would appear to be impermeable to the cell (Ryan and Ryan, 1981). The biochemical processes subserving this mode of activation may differ from that of NE, in that (a) the responses to agonists that appear to release intracellular calcium ion are susceptible to inhibition by anoxia and metabolic inhibitors and (b) the responses are highly magnesium dependent (see discussion of individual agents, Section III). Drugs such as ouabain may contract VSM by inhibiting the transport (K,Na)-ATPase. Inhibition of this enzyme results in an accumulation of sodium ion in the cell, partially depolarizing the membrane and increasing calcium entry via voltage-dependent calcium and sodium channels, whereas intracellular sodium ion may inhibit calcium binding and the loss of potassium may cause a loss of magnesium ion and subsequent inhibition of relaxation. Finally, the possibility exists that drugs, or perhaps humoral agents, may contract VSM by (a) inhibiting the dephosphorylation of myosin light-chain kinase, (b) enhancing the binding of calcium to calmodulin, or (c) promoting the phosphorylation of the 20,000-dalton myosin light chain. Although these three mechanisms have not yet been demonstrated, they serve as potential models for drug-induced contraction of VSM.

The process of contraction is subserved by energy derived from the Embden–Myerhoff pathway. However, when this cycle is inhibited, energy (ATP) derived from the pentose phosphate shunt and anaerobic metabolism appears to be sufficient to maintain the integrity of the contractile process for many humoral agonists. The exceptions to this seem to be prostanoids, 5-HT, vasopressin, and oxytocin, as well as the contractile responses to ACh.

Relaxation of VSM may be mediated by several distinct and independent mechanisms. Calcium-blocking agents are believed to promote relaxation of VSM by inhibiting voltage-dependent and voltage-independent entry of calcium ion into the intracellular compartment of VSM, thereby decreasing the availability of ionized calcium to the calmodulin–leiotonin–actomyosin system of contractile and regulatory proteins (for references see Stull and Sanford, 1981). In addition, several calcium-channel-blocking agents also appear to decrease or prevent the mobilization of tightly bound or sequestered intracellular calcium ion, thereby contributing to the relaxant action of such drugs as dilitazem and nifedipine on VSM (Weiss, 1981a,b).

Nitroprusside, nitrites, and other drugs are believed to stimulate the conversion of GTP to cyclic GMP, which inhibits contraction of VSM by an as yet unknown mechanism (Goldberg *et al.*, 1978; Hidaka and Asano, 1977; Kadowitz *et al.*, 1982a,b). Acetylcholine, ATP, adenosine, and bradykinin may stimulate the formation of a hydroperoxide vasodilator material within the vascular endothelium (Furchgott and Zawadski, 1979, 1980a,b,c), which may then act on the smooth muscle to stimulate guanylate cyclase and promote relaxation (Furchgott *et al.*, 1981). The (sodium–potassium)-activated, magnesium-dependent ATPase pumping mechanism located in the cell membrane may also play a role in vasodilation (Haddy, 1978; Webb *et al.*, 1981; Bonaccorsi *et al.*, 1977; Anderson, 1976). Drugs that promote relaxation by this mechanism may stimulate the activity of the pumping mechanism, thereby promoting an accumulation of potassium ion within the cell, decreasing the sodium ion concentration, and promoting a hyperpolarization of the VSM cell (Bonaccorsi *et al.*, 1977; Jones, 1980; Limas and Cohn, 1974). Finally, as stated above, vasodilators may directly affect the binding of calcium ion to calmodulin, thereby decreasing the capacity of myosin kinase to phosphorylate myosin. Alternatively, vasodilators may directly affect the dephosphorylation of myosin light-chain kinase. Although the mechanisms of action of some humoral factors and pharmacologic modalities have been elucidated, it is unknown whether these mechanisms persist in the VSM of the microcirculation.

Energy is required for relaxation as well as contraction, and relaxation is therefore an active process. In many types of VSM, the vasodilator response to ACh, adenosine, or bradykinin is inhibited in solutions with low

pO_2 values (DeMey and Vanhoutte, 1978). Similarly, metabolic inhibitors such as azide and cyanide, in concentrations that do not affect VSM contraction, abolish relaxation of VSM in response to ACh and prostanoids (Greenberg *et al.*, 1973a,b, 1974a,b, 1982b). The mechanism may be related to the fact that relaxation is more dependent on ATP than contraction or that the inability of ATP-dependent calcium sequestration mechanisms to function overrides the signal provided by dephosphorylation of myosin (see Section II,I).

III. Humoral Factors Affecting Vascular Smooth Muscle

A. Catecholamines

The microcirculation of most species is endowed with receptors on the VSM for catecholamines. Adrenergic receptors have been classified into α- and β-adrenergic receptors (Alquist, 1948) and subclassified into α_1 and α_2 receptors as well as β_1 and β_2 adrenoceptors (see reviews by Bertelsen and Pettinger, 1977; Wikberg, 1979; Vanhoutte, 1982). The α_1 adrenoceptors may be presynaptic or postsynaptic. Primarily the latter are activated by epinephrine > norepinephrine > phenylephrine > clonidine and are inhibited by prazosin > phentolamine > yohimbine > tolazoline > clonidine. α_2-Adrenergic receptors appear to be found both on presynaptic and on postsynaptic sites of the adrenergic neuroeffector complex (primarily the former), are extrasynaptic in location on the postsynaptic side, are activated by clonidine > α-methylnorepinephrine > norepinephrine > epinephrine > phenylephrine, and are inhibited by yohimbine > phentolamine > tolazoline >>> prazosin. The β_2 receptors are located primarily on VSM and other smooth muscles as well as presynaptically, are activated by isoproterenol and terbutaline, and are inhibited by propranolol, pindolol, and other nonselective β-receptor blocking agents. So-called selective β_1 blocking agents inhibit VSM responses mediated by β_2 receptors if the concentration of blocking agent is high enough.

A gradient of sensitivity to the α sympathomimetic actions of the catecholamines exists in the microcirculation, that is, metarterioles > precapillary sphincters > terminal arterioles > muscular venules > collecting venules. The capacity of metarterioles and venules to respond to both NE and α-methylnorepinephrine suggests that the microcirculation is endowed with both α_1 and α_2 postsynaptic receptors, but the former are the dominant species (Altura and Hershey, 1967; Altura, 1971a, 1978a,b, 1981; Baez, 1977b; Furness and Marshall, 1974). The microcirculatory VSM, including the precapillary sphincters, responds in graded fashion to catecholamines (Altura, 1981) and, with the exception of the muscular venules, responds to circulating levels of NE and epinephrine (Chin and Evonuk, 1971). Antagonists of α adrenoceptors block the microvascular responses to NE and other α-adrenoceptor stimulants, confirming the thesis that the contractile responses to these agents are mediated by α-receptor stimulation (Altura, 1978a,b, 1981; Miller and Harris, 1975).

A controversy exists concerning the *in vivo* and *in vitro* sensitivity of the venules of the microcirculation to catecholamines, in which the veins appear to be as sensitive or more so than the arteries to catecholamines, whereas with topical administration the venules appear to be less responsive than the arteries (Shepherd and Vanhoutte, 1975; Vanhoutte, 1978; Miller and Weigman, 1977; Greenberg *et al.*, 1973b, 1981; Greenberg and Kadowitz, 1982; Kadowitz *et al.*, 1982a,b; Altura, 1978a,b, 1981). Altura (1981) argues that mesenteric and cremaster arterioles close more and exhibit a greater sensitivity than venules to NE. However, the smallest microscopic venules, endowed with pericytes, are more sensitive to NE than larger venules without pericytes. Therefore, pericytes may contribute to the overall venous response to catecholamines. Although the argument explains the differences in sensitivity of cremaster and mesenteric venules and microscopic venules, it does not answer the question of why differences exist in the *in situ* and *in vitro* studies with topical application. It is possible, but speculative, that differences in rates of diffusion of NE, topography of receptors, or other modulating influences *in vivo* can override the differences in sensitivity of the VSM itself to NE. Moreover, species differences cannot be ruled out. Finally, it is difficult to expect total venous closure in the face of an adequate distending pressure. It is possible that if tension could be measured in these microvessels, or pressure with microtechniques, then the order of sensitivity of the venules might be found to increase more so than the arteries. Further studies must resolve this conflict.

The VSM of the microcirculation appears to be endowed with β adrenoceptors, which mediate vasodilation, suppression of the responses to adrenergic nerve stimulation, and inhibition of the responses to NE and 5-HT (Shepherd and Vanhoutte, 1975; Vanhoutte, 1978). Microvascular β receptors have been found in the mesenteric, hepatic, pancreatic, cerebral, renal, skeletal, and adipose tissue microvascular beds in numerous rodent species (for references see Altura, 1978a,b, 1981). Miller and Harris (1975) failed to find evidence of isoproterenol-induced vasodilation of the bat microcirculation. β-Receptor-mediated vasodilation of arterioles, but not venules, is exquisitely sensitive to inhibition of aging animals (Fleisch and Hooker, 1976; Altura and Altura, 1977b). The absence of responses in the experiments of Miller and Harris (1975) cannot be due to aging since neither artery nor vein responded to isoproterenol. It is possible that β adrenoceptors may not be present in the microcirculation of all strains and species. Whereas the rat arterioles and venules are endowed with β receptors, as are those of man, the bat may be devoid of this mechanism for vasodilation.

Mechanism of Action of Catecholamines

α-Adrenoceptor-mediated vasoconstriction produces many events within the VSM cell. Some of these events are primary in the process of excitation and contraction, and some merely subserve the contractile process, whereas one mechanism may tend to limit the magnitude of contraction or vasoconstriction.

In VSM in which spontaneous electrical activity is coupled to mechanical activity, NE increases the rate of firing of the action potential and increases mechanical activity (Johansson *et al.*, 1967; Nakajima and Horn, 1967; Keatinge, 1976, 1979). In normally electrically quiescent VSM, NE appears to depolarize the VSM partially and elicit contraction, whereas high concentrations of NE produce an even greater depolarization, equivalent to that of removing calcium from the physiologic salt solution bathing the VSM (Haeusler, 1972, 1973; Mekata and Niu, 1972; Keatinge, 1979; von Loh and Bohr, 1973; Haeusler and Thorens, 1980a,b). Associated with the electrical and mechanical activity of the VSM cell in response to NE is an increase in sodium and calcium influx or, in some VSM, an increase in the release of calcium from sequestered intracellular sites and an increase in potassium efflux from the cell (Guignard and Friedman, 1970; Jones, 1973; Haeusler and Thorens, 1980a,b). The increased influx of calcium ion is believed to occur via both voltage-dependent and voltage-independent calcium channels (Weiss, 1977, 1981a,b) and may also be associated with an increase in magnesium ion into the cell (Greenberg, 1981c). It is now believed that the increased calcium ion interacts with and binds to calmodulin. The calcium–calmodulin complex binds to the dephosphorylated form of myosin light-chain kinase, which is inactive, to form the activated complex calcium–calmodulin–MLCK, which then phosphorylates the higher molecular weight myosin light chain (*p*-myosin). *p*-Myosin is activated by actin and further activated as actomyosin by tropomyosin, with subsequent hydrolysis of ATP, liberation of the energy, and promotion of the sliding-filament mechanism (see Section II,J). Subserving this contraction are the concomitant biochemical changes produced by NE via α-adrenergic receptor activation, namely, stimulation of glycogenolysis and phosphorylase, and oxygen consumption, which generates ATP from both ADP and breakdown of preformed glycogen and lipid stores (Weston, 1972; Namm, 1971; Diamond, 1978; Paul, 1980). In addition, the aerobic glycolytic pathway, stimulated by NE, may aid in preventing the dissipation of the sodium–potassium gradient by providing energy for the sodium–potassium pump mechanism (Paul, 1980; Hellstrand and Paul, 1980, 1982). The increase in cyclic AMP observed with NE in VSM is not found with phenylephrine and so may be mediated via β adrenoceptors in the VSM (Dunham et al., 1974).

Along with the contractile response to NE is an associated increase in the efflux of prostaglandins from the VSM cell (McGiff et al., 1972; Needleman et al., 1973a,b; Needleman, 1976; Needleman and Isakson, 1980; Greenberg and Kadowitz, 1982). It has been suggested that the prostanoids may limit the magnitude of the contractile response to NE, thus protecting the VSM against excessive contraction. Evidence supporting this thesis is that many inhibitors of prostanoid synthesis enhance the magnitude of NE-induced contraction and enhance the sensitivity of the VSM to this amine (for references see Needleman, 1980; Greenberg, 1982a,b). However, more specific inhibitors such as ETYA do not affect the contractile response of VSM to NE (Goldberg et al., 1975a,b, 1976; Greenberg and Kadowitz, 1982). It is possible that nonspecific perturbations of the membrane produced by vasoconstriction result in the release of prostanoids or that the release of prostanoids from the VSM in vitro may reflect the terminal events of a tissue undergoing degeneration and death (Vanhoutte, 1980). Further studies are necessary to evaluate the significance of prostanoid release by NE in VSM.

It has been suggested that the interaction of epinephrine or isoproterenol with β receptors of the VSM may result in an increase in adenylate cyclase activity and cyclic AMP, which both stimulates calcium sequestration by subcellular organelles, such as sarcoplasmic reticulum and mitochondria, and stimulates calcium efflux from the cell. Both of these events decrease the free, ionized calcium concentration, decrease the interaction of calcium with calmodulin, and reverse the contractile events outlined above. In addition, cyclic AMP is synthesized from ATP and may decrease the ATP available for myosin phosphorylation. Finally, cyclic AMP binds to the regulatory subunit of inactive protein kinase to expose the catalytic subunit of protein kinase. This catalytic unit of protein kinase phosphorylates myosin light-chain kinase. Because the phosphorylated form of the myosin light-chain kinase is less capable of binding with calmodulin the myosin light-chain kinase is, in effect, inactivated. A decreased myosin kinase activity results in a decreased phosphorylation of myosin. Since dephosphorylated or unphosphorylated myosin cannot interact with actin, VSM tension declines.

B. Serotonin

Serotonin released from the vascular wall or the platelets may act as a local modulator of microcirculatory tone (Page, 1968; Jarrott *et al.*, 1975; McGrath, 1977, 1978). Serotonin can directly affect the VSM or act indirectly through adrenergic nerves to increase or decrease neurogenically mediated tone (Haddy *et al.*, 1959; Page, 1968). Serotonin accumulates in adrenergic nerve terminals and dense granules believed to be the intraneuronal storage sites for NE (Nishino *et al.*, 1970; Snipes *et al.*, 1968). Densely innervated blood vessels accumulate both 5-HT and NE in neuronal and extraneuronal storage sites within the VSM (Berkowitz *et al.*, 1975; Curro and Greenberg, 1982a,b; Thoa *et al.*, 1969; Weiss and Rosecrans, 1971a,b).

Serotonin also directly activates the VSM. The contractile responses of VSM to 5-HT are believed to result from an interaction between 5-HT and structurally specific protein moieties (receptors) on the VSM membrane (Freyburger *et al.*, 1952; Innes, 1962; Innes and Kohli, 1970; Page, 1968). McGrath (1978) suggested that the contractile responses of VSM and non-VSM preparations to 5-HT are, in part, mediated by an indirect sympathomimetic effect of 5-HT. 5-Hydroxytryptamine also interacts with the postsynaptic α receptors of VSM. Receptors for 5-HT exist in VSM but cross-reactivity between 5-HT and α receptors exists in some 5-HT and α-receptor agonists and antagonists (Apperley *et al.*, 1976, 1977, 1980; Clement *et al.*, 1969; Curro *et al.*, 1978; Edvinsson and Owman, 1977; Edvinsson *et al.*, 1978; Gyermek, 1966; Offermeier and Ariens, 1966a,b; Wakade *et al.*, 1970). Clement *et al.* (1969) suggested that the parallelism between 5-HT- and NE-induced contractions of VSM indicates that 5-HT and NE may interact with a single population of α receptors or a population of receptors that are very similar. The same conclusions were reached by many investigators utilizing a diverse group of VSM and other smooth muscle preparations (Apperley *et al.*, 1976, 1977, 1980; Clement *et al.*, 1969; Curro *et al.*, 1978; Edvinsson and Owman, 1977; Edvinsson *et al.*, 1978; Gyermek, 1966; Offermeier and Ariens, 1966a,b; Wakade *et al.*, 1970).

Studies indicate that two classes of 5-HT receptors exist in VSM (Curro *et al.*, 1978; Apperley *et al.*, 1980; Black *et al.*, 1981). 5-HT$_1$ receptors are activated by 5-HT and inhibited by methysergide (MSG), and 5-HT$_2$ receptors are activated by 5-HT and MSG, inhibited by α-receptor antagonists, and refractory to inhibition by MSG. Removal of extracellular magnesium ion (Mg_o) from physiologic salt solutions (PSS) bathing VSM also inhibits contractile responses to 5-HT (Goldstein and Zsoster, 1978), but it is uncertain whether this is an effect on 5-HT_1 or 5-HT_2 receptors.

Curro *et al.* (1978) and Curro and Greenberg (1982a,b) examined the interaction of adrenergic nerves, calcium and magnesium ion, pH, and sulfhydryl group reagents on the receptors for 5-HT in rodent and canine arteries and veins. In the rat mesenteric arteries (RMA), inhibition of neuronal reuptake and extraneuronal reuptake of NE with cocaine and hydrocortisone, respectively, enhanced the responses of the RMA to 5-HT. Depletion of NE with reserpine (1.5 mg/kg daily for 6 days) and inhibition of NE release with guanethidine did not inhibit the responses of RMA to 5-HT. These data support the conclusion that 5-HT is sequestered and/or inactivated by neuronal and extraneuronal mechanisms similar to that of NE but that the contractile responses of the RMA to 5-HT are not mediated by an indirect sympathomimetic effect of 5-HT. The responses of the RMA to 5-HT were inhibited by methysergide, a 5-HT receptor antagonist, and by the α-adrenergic receptor antagonists phentolamine and yohimbine. Tolazoline and prazosin did not affect the responses of RMA to 5-HT. These data support the conclusion that the 5-HT receptor of RMA is a 5-HT_1 receptor but that α_2 antagonists exert cross-reactivity with the 5-HT_1 receptor. An increase in the concentration of extracellular calcium ion (Ca_o) from 0.4 to 3.2 mM did not affect the sensitivity of RMA to 5-HT but decreased the antagonistic potency of phentolamine and methysergide. Reductions in the concentration of extracellular magnesium ion (Mg_o) depressed the responses of the RMA to 5-HT and decreased the blocking potency of methysergide and phentolamine. These data support the conclusion that Ca_o and Mg_o are involved in the interaction of 5-HT with 5-HT_1 receptors in RMA and that the 5-HT receptor contains a labile, sulfhydryl, or disulfide bond.

The contractile response of the canine dorsal metatarsal vein (DMV) to 5-HT differed in some aspects from that of the RMA. Agonist–antagonist interactions and ion–agonist and antagonist interactions were evaluated against the contractile responses to 5-HT and phenylephrine and the specific binding of $5\text{-}[2\text{-}^{14}\text{C}]\text{HT}$ to intact DMV. Decreases and increases in pH from pH 7.4 selectively reduce or abolish the responses to 5-HT and MSG. Reduction of disulfide bonds with dithiothreitol also selectively inhibits 5-HT- and MSG-induced contractions of DMV. These changes were associated with concomitant alterations in $5\text{-}[2\text{-}^{14}\text{C}]\text{HT}$ binding and decreases in the affinity for the 5-HT receptor. Reductions in extracellular sodium ion enhanced the contractile responses to 5-HT and MSG, whereas alterations in extracellular potassium ion did not affect the contractile responses of DMW to 5-HT or MSG. Similarly, reductions in extracellular sodium resulted in an increase in 5-[2-^{14}C]HT binding followed by a decrease in this parameter. Alterations in extracellular potassium ion did not affect 5-[2-^{14}C]HT binding at physiologic concentrations of potassium ion. Increases in extracellular calcium ion from 0.8 to 3.2 mM did not affect the sensitivity (ED$_{50}$) of the DMV to 5-HT or MSG but decreased the blocking potency of the antagonists against 5-HT. Reductions in concentration of extracellular magnesium ion from 2.4 to 0 mM lowered the ED$_{50}$ for 5-HT but decreased the blocking potency of the antagonists against 5-HT. Increases in extracellular calcium ion concentration did not affect the specific binding of 5-[2-^{14}C]HT to DMV, whereas increases in extracellular magnesium ion concentration from 0 to 2.4 mM increased the affinity and maximum binding capacity of 5-[2-^{14}C]HT in DMV. The data support the conclusion that the 5-HT$_2$ receptor of DMV contains a pH-sensitive, labile, ionizable binding site either containing a reducible disulfide group or maintained in a specific conformation by a disulfide group which is an integral moiety of the 5-HT$_2$ receptor complex. This receptor complex is not modulated by physiologic concentrations of monovalent cations but is subject to modulation by divalent cations. Since extracellular calcium ion modulates the sensitivity of the antagonists for 5-HT but not 5-HT itself, the data support the conclusion that extracellular calcium ion may allosterically modify the 5-HT$_2$ receptor complex of DMV. Extracellular magnesium ion alters the sensitivity of the DMV to 5-HT, MSG, and 5-HT receptor antagonists and alters both the affinity and maximum binding capacity of the 5-HT$_2$ receptors of DMV. These data support the conclusion that magnesium ion is an integral component of the 5-HT$_2$ receptor complex in DMV.

Kier (1968) and Korolkovas (1970) postulated that a three-point attachment of 5-HT at its receptor site involves the terminal and indole nitrogen atoms and the hydroxyphenyl ring of the indole moiety as absolute requirements for the binding of 5-HT with its receptors in smooth muscle. The minimal steric requirement for α-adrenergic receptor activity appears to be the interatomic distance between the phenyl ring and the terminal amino group on the α-carbon atom (Belleau, 1967). Phentolamine could interact with both postulated receptors because it possesses a hydroxyl group on the 3 position of the phenyl ring, a tertiary amine group, and a second nitrogen atom on the imidazole ring. Similarly, yohimbine possesses a complex ring structure, which also allows it to have three-point attachment to a 5-HT receptor. In contrast, prazosin and tolazoline do not possess a third ring structure allowing for this three-point attachment. Thus, the presence of the third ring or nitrogen atom may enable α-adrenergic receptor blocking agents to interact with 5-HT receptors.

The serotonergic receptor is composed of anionic and cationic binding sites for the complementary attachment of cationic and anionic sites of the serotonergic receptor agonists (Kier, 1968; Korolkovas, 1970). Changes in pH should affect the ionization of the charged amino acid moieties within the peptide chain of the receptor complex. This should result in a decreased number of active binding sites available for interaction with the complementry charged moieties of the 5-HT receptor agonists (Kier, 1968; Korolkovas, 1970). It is clear from the data presented that alkalosis and acidosis resulted in a preferential inhibition of the contractile responses of DMV to 5-HT and MSG, and not to phenylephrine. Moreover, alterations in pH depressed the maximum specific 5-[2-^{14}C]HT binding and increased the K_D (decreased the affinity) of the 5-HT receptor for its substrate. Therefore, the data support the conclusion that the 5-HT$_2$ receptors of DMV contain pH-sensitive peptide linkages or ionizable groups that either directly, or indirectly at an allosteric site, modulate the binding of 5-HT to its receptor. Moreover, the data add further support for the concept that the 5-HT and α-adrenoceptors differ within both RMA and DMV, as well as other VSM.

It may be argued that alkalosis and acidosis depress VSM contractility by affecting the release of calcium ion from the sarcoplasmic reticulum or by changing the plasticity of the contractile proteins (Alexander, 1968). The decrease in specific 5-HT binding with changes in pH could then be related to degradation of the 5-HT from the pH changes itself. Since the contractile responses of DMV to phenylephrine were not inhibited by the alkalotic or acidotic solution, it is unlikely that pH-induced alterations in the plasticity of DMV or changes in the release of calcium ion from the sarcoplasmic reticulum can explain the preferential inhibition of 5-HT-induced contraction of DMV.

DTT reduces disulfide bonds to form reduced sulfhydryl groups within the VSM (Freidman, 1973; Greenberg et al., 1976). The formation of disulfide bonds between the oxidized form of DTT and the reduced sulfhydryl groups of the DMV should be minimal since the redox potential of this type of reaction would be against an electrochemical potential gradient. Thus, the selective inhibition of MSG- and 5-HT-induced contractions of DMV by DTT and DTNB as well as their inhibitory effects on 5-[2-^{14}C]HT binding supports the conclusion that a disulfide bridge(s) is an integral component of the 5-HT$_2$ receptor of DMV. The reversal experiments with DTNB also support this conclusion.

DTNB alkylates both sulfhydryl and disulfide groups and inhibits the contractile responses of DMV to each of the agonists tested. However, when added to DMV in which the disulfide groups have been reduced with DTT, DTNB reverses the inhibitory effect of DTT on 5-HT- and

MSG-induced contractions of DMV. This effect is probably related to the formation of a redox potential chain among the VSM sulfhydryl groups, oxidized DTT, and DTNB (Freidman, 1973). With other reactions, such as the formation of a nitrobenzoate–sulfhydryl complex, the effect would be equivalent to alkylation of the reduced sulfhydryl groups with a resultant abolition of the responses to 5-HT and MSG (Freidman, 1973). Therefore, the data with DTT and DTNB support the conclusion that a disulfide bridge is an integral moiety of the 5-HT$_2$ receptor complex in DMV.

Alterations in [Na$_o$] from 120 to 160 mM and changes in [K$_o$] from 2 to 10 mM did not affect the contractile responses of the DMV to 5-HT or MSG and did not affect the binding of 5-[2-^{14}C]HT in any significant manner. The small changes in the contractile responses of the DMV to 5-HT and MSG could be related to alterations in calcium permeability produced by the changes in [Na$_o$] since they also affected the contractile responses to phenylephrine in a similar manner (van Breeman et al., 1979). Moreover, the changes in contractile responses of the DMV to 5-HT were not accompanied by changes in either the maximum binding capacity or affinity of the 5-HT receptors within DMV. In addition, alterations in [Na$_o$] and [K$_o$] did not affect the antagonist–agonist interaction between 5-HT and phentolamine or cyproheptadine. Thus, it is unlikely that physiologic concentrations of monovalent ions such as Na$_o$ or K$_o$ modulate the 5-HT$_2$ receptors of DMV.

The roles of Ca$_o$ and Mg$_o$ as modulators of the 5-HT receptors in VSM remain poorly defined. Although a wide variety of calcium-channel-blocking agents inhibit NE- and 5-HT-induced contraction (Triggle, 1976; van Nueten et al., 1978, 1980, 1981; Weiss, 1978, 1981a,b), these experiments do not delineate a direct association between the divalent ions and the 5-HT or NE receptors of VSM. Removal of calcium from PSS inhibits the protective effect of NE against dibenamine blockade of α receptors in rabbit thoracic aorta. This suggests that the NE–receptor interaction is a calcium-dependent process. The pA$_2$ for the NE–phentolamine interaction in rat thoracic aorta is decreased by calcium-displacing local anesthetics. This suggested that these local anesthetics did not inhibit agonist binding to the receptor but acted allosterically to decrease the affinity of both agonist and antagonist to their receptor (Triggle, 1976; Curro and Greenberg, 1982a,b).

Increases in [Ca$_o$] from 0.8 to 3.2 mM decreased the responses of DMV to phenylephrine but not to 5-HT and MSG. Alterations in [Ca$_o$] did not affect the maximum binding capacity of affinity of 5-HT for its receptors within DMV. Yet the inhibitory effect of α-adrenoceptor antagonists on 5-Ht and MSG was diminished to a far greater extent than was the inhibitory effect against phenylephrine. Although we did not measure the binding of the antagonist to DMV, since alterations in [Ca$_o$] did not affect the agonist–5-HT interaction within DMV yet diminished the antagonist–agonist interaction for these 5-HT$_2$ receptors, the data support the conclusion that Ca$_o$ appears to modify allosterically the binding of the 5-HT$_2$ receptor antagonists to sites within the receptor complex. These sites do not appear to be essential for the interaction of 5-HT with its receptor in DMV.

Magnesium ion exerts diverse and complex actions on VSM tone and contractile responses to vasoactive agents. Magnesium ion is essential for the activity of many enzyme systems and exerts both a complementary and opposing action with calcium ion in many biological systems (Altura and Altura, 1974a,b, 1976, 1981). Elevations in [Mg$_o$] result in competition with Ca$_o$ for binding sites on the sarcolemmal membrane of VSM (Weiner et al., 1980), thereby regulating myogenic tone (Altura and Altura, 1981; Weiner et al., 1980). Removal of Mg$_o$ enhances spontaneous contractions of VSM by increasing passive inward calcium permeability (Weiner et al., 1980), yet relatively selectively decreases the contractile responses of VSM to prostanoids (Altura et al., 1976; Greenberg, 1981c) and 5-HT (Curro and Greenberg, 1982a,b; Greenberg and Curro, 1982a,b; Goldstein and Zsoster, 1978). Moreover, increases in [Mg$_o$] above 4.8–7.2 mM depress the contractile responses of DMV to many agonists in a nonequivalent manner, probably by suppressing membrane excitation and inward calcium permeability and diminishing a pool of activator calcium ion derived from the membrane-bound or extracellular compartment of VSM (Weiner et al., 1980). The relationship of [Mg$_o$] to the 5-HT receptors of VSM has not been established. Decreases in [Mg_o] depress the contractile responses of rabbit and canine VSM to 5-HT and decrease the sensitivity to this indole-alkylamine (Goldstein and Zsoster, 1978). This suggested that Mg$_o$ may directly modulate the 5-HT receptor of VSM. The data presented herein confirm and extend this observation. Contraction of the DMV by 5-HT and MSG, the antagonistic activity of 5-HT$_2$ receptor antagonists, and the K_D and maximal binding capacity for 5-[2-^{14}C]HT were directly dependent on [Mg$_o$] over the range 0–4.8 mM. This suggests that Mg$_o$ is directly involved in binding of 5-HT and antagonists to the 5-HT receptor of DMV. The inhibitory effect of decreases in [Mg$_o$] on 5-HT-induced contraction of DMV appears to be an expression of the decreased affinity of 5-HT for its receptor and a decrease in the total number of receptors available for contraction. This would suggest that Mg$_o$ may form a complex either within the 5-HT receptor, thereby maintaining the conformation of the 5-HT receptor complex, or between the receptor and 5-HT.

A decrease in the contractile responses of DMV to 5-HT occurs with [Mg$_o$] above 4.8 mM despite the increased binding of 5-[2-^{14}C]HT to

DMV. This anomalous action of Mg_0 may result from a nonspecific depressant effect of this ion on membrane excitability and subsequent calcium entry into, or mobilization within, DMV. The depressant effect of Mg_0 is also observed on the contractile responses to phenylephrine and on the responses of rat VSM to KCl, NA, and other agonists (Altura and Altura, 1981). Since reductions in $[Mg_0]$ do not affect the agonist–antagonist interaction of the α-adrenoceptors nor the contractile responses of DMV to phenylephrine, it is unlikely that Mg_0 is an integral moiety within the α-adrenoceptor complex. Thus, the suppression of the maximal contractions to phenylephrine, 5-HT, and MSG by elevated $[Mg_0]$ must reflect a nonspecific depressant action on the processes of excitation or contraction region of the receptor complex to which the indole moiety of the 5-HT molecule was bound, whereas the site of Mg_0 would be the region of the terminal amine group. The binding of divalent ions to these sites could decrease the affinity of the antagonists as well as the agonists.

According to the Kier–Korolkovas model of the 5-HT receptor, Ca_0 should bind to the portion of the 5-HT receptor to which the indole moiety was bound, since this should also be the anchoring site for antagonists. It is unlikely that Ca_0 would bind to the site in the region to which the terminal amino group attaches because this area would affect agonist-mediated contractions and Ca_0 is devoid of this action. A similar type of interaction has been postulated for the binding of β-adrenoceptor antagonists with the α adrenoceptor (Janis and Triggle, 1974; Olivares et al., 1967).

Extracellular magnesium ion should bind to the portion of the receptor to which the indole or terminal amino nitrogen is bound since the responses to both agonist (5-HT) and antagonists are altered by changes in $[Mg_0]$ and Mg_0 alters the binding of 5-$[2-^{14}C]HT$ to DMV. Since the three-point attachment appears to be obligatory for 5-HT binding to its receptors, a deficiency in Mg_0 at these sites could explain the capacity of magnesium to modulate the responses to $5-HT_2$ receptor agonists but not α-adrenoceptor agonists in DMV.

When the present study is viewed along with the previous studies of Altura and Altura (1981), Curro and Greenberg (1982a,b), Goldstein and Zsoster (1978), and Weiner et al. (1980), it becomes clear that the atypical $5-HT_2$ receptors of DMV are diverse and complex but do not differ from $5-HT_1$ receptors in their sensitivity to each of these interventions (Curro and Greenberg, 1982a).

In summary, then, four major factors determine the overall VSM response to 5-HT and its antagonists. These include calcium ion, magnesium ion, pH, and disulfide-reducing agents. The concentration of Mg_0 is of primary importance in determining the sensitivity of the DMV to 5-HT and its antagonists. This divalent ion can enhance the sensitivity and enhance or depress the contractile responses and pA_2 values of the antagonist, depending on its concentration in PSS and the sensitivity of the membrane to its stabilizing actions. The effects of Ca_o are more discreet, in that they alter the antagonist interaction with the 5-HT receptors rather than the agonist. Disulfide groups and ionizable, pH-labile peptide or perhaps disulfide linkages appear to play an important role in maintaining the integrity of the $5\text{-}HT_2$ receptor in DMV. The relationships between these factors and the functional integrity of the $5\text{-}HT_2$ receptor deserve careful consideration in the evaluation of responses of the microcirculation to 5-HT in both normal and pathophysiologic conditions. The absence of an effect of 5-HT antagonists may not indicate the absence of 5-HT receptors but rather the predominance of a specific type of 5-HT receptor in the microcirculation.

The following question must be raised. If little difference exists between the $5\text{-}HT_1$ and $5\text{-}HT_2$ receptors other than antagonist sensitivity, do these populations of receptors really differ? The contractile responses of VSM from different vascular beds within a multitude of species to 5-HT are inhibited by α-adrenergic receptor antagonists (Apperley et al., 1976, 1980; Clement et al., 1969; Curro and Greenberg, 1982a,b; Curro et al., 1978; Edvinsson et al., 1978; Humphrey, 1978; Innes and Kohli, 1970; Offermeier and Ariens, 1966a,b; van Neuten et al., 1981; Wilton and McCalden, 1977). Based on studies performed in canine DMV (Curro et al., 1978; Humphrey, 1978) and rabbit aortas and ear arteries (Apperley et al., 1976, 1980), the concept emerged that classical, MSG-inhibitable ($5\text{-}HT_1$) and atypical, MSG-resistant, α-adrenergic receptor-sensitive ($5\text{-}HT_2$) 5-HT receptors existed in VSM.

As an alternative to postulating distinct $5\text{-}HT_1$ and $5\text{-}HT_2$ receptors in VSM, the capacity of different antagonists to inhibit 5-HT responses in VSM could be explained on the basis of the Monod et al. (1965) and Karlin (1967) two-state model for agonist–antagonist binding to their specific receptors. According to this model an agonist and antagonist bind to two distinct conformations or states of the same receptor. These two states are interconvertible and in equilibrium to various degrees. It is possible that in some VSM the antagonist form of the receptor is converted to the agonist form. This would increase the binding of 5-[2-^{14}C]HT to the agonistic form of the receptor, thereby accounting for the increased 5-[2-^{14}C]HT binding. It would also account for the decreased blocking activity of cyproheptadine. Moreover, MSG is a partial agonist. According to the Monod–Karlin transition-state model MSG has affinity for both states of the receptor. A transition of the 5-HT receptor from the antagonist to the agonist state increases the contractile response to MSG and decreases its blocking potency. This transition model can also explain the blocking potency of α-adrenoceptor antagonists against 5-HT, if it is assumed that these antagonists possess affinity for the agonistic form of the receptor but not the antagonist form. Serotonin, under normal conditions, would have a greater affinity than 5-HT for the receptor. When many receptors are present, sufficient antagonist binds and overcomes the contractile responses to 5-HT. Further studies are required to delineate the mechanism of the change in 5-HT receptors in VSM.

The mechanism by which 5-HT elicits contraction of VSM appears to resemble that of NE. However, the responses to 5-HT appear to be more dependent on extracellular calcium ion and cell metabolism than are the responses to NE (Greenberg *et al.*, 1974; Altura and Altura, 1970; van Neuten *et al.*, 1980, 1981). 5-Hydroxytryptamine is a more potent contractor of venules than of arterioles and can cause venostasis (Altura and Hershey, 1967).

C. Angiotensin

Angiotensin II is a potent contractile substance in arteriolar and precapillary arteriolar VSM, as well as larger arteries, but is a poor agonist on most veins (Bohr and Uchida, 1967; Bohr, 1973; Bohr *et al.*, 1978; Peach, 1977; Messina *et al.*, 1975; Altura and Altura, 1977b). The notable exception to the venocontractile action of angiotensin II is the portal vein, in which angiotensin is a potent contractile agent. The order of sensitivity of most arterial smooth muscle to angiotensins is angiotensin II >>> angiotensin III >>> angiotensin I. Contractile responses to angiotensin I may be mediated by its conversion to angiotensin II by the endothelium or by the smooth muscle (Hofbauer, 1973; Itzkowitz and McGiff, 1974) or to an interaction of angiotensin I with angiotensin II receptors on the VSM. The maximal contractile responses of VSM to angiotensin II are usually significantly less than the contractile responses to other contractile substances (Vanhoutte, 1978; Bohr *et al.*, 1978) and may be related to the simultaneous stimulation of prostacyclin and/or PGE_2 from the endothelium and/or VSM (Aiken, 1973, 1974; for other references see Needleman and Isakson, 1980). Indomethacin and other inhibitors of prostanoid synthesis enhance the contractile responses to angiotensin II and prevent the characteristic "fade" response normally observed in VSM (Aiken, 1973; Needleman *et al.*, 1973a,b; McGiff *et al.*, 1975; Needleman and Isakson, 1980).

Angiotensin II exhibits two major characteristics in its contractile response of VSM fade: the diminution of the response despite the maintained concentration of angiotensin I at its receptor site and tachyphyllaxis, the diminution of the response to the repeated administration of the same concentration of angiotensin II (for references see Bohr *et al.,* 1978; Gross, 1976). Fade may be related to the simultaneous production of vasodilator prostanoids from the VSM which attenuates the pressor response to angiotensin II, which tachyphyllaxis appears to represent the maintained binding of angiotensin II to its receptor site, resulting in autoinhibition to subsequent challenges with angiotensin II. Khairallah *et al.* (1966) showed that washing the VSM with an acidic solution restored the responses of rabbit aorta to angiotensin II at a time when tachyphyllaxis was evident. This procedure resulted in a decline in the binding of angiotensin to the rabbit thoracic aorta. When the blood vessel was reincubated in normal PSS at pH 7.4, the responses to angiotensin II returned. This indicates that tachyphyllaxis is probably a physical phenomenon associated with excessive binding of angiotensin II at its receptor site.

In the microcirculation, angiotensin II seems to exhibit primarily fade (Messina and Kaley, 1982). The latter authors suggested that the *in vivo* system augments prostanoid production so that fade and tachyphyllaxis are readily evident and prostanoid dependent. Under *in vivo* conditions, in which prostanoid production is less than that *in vitro,* tachyphyllaxis and fade are both time and concentration phenomena and are prostanoid independent. Messina *et al.* (1976) evaluated tachyphyllaxis in the whole animal and showed that indomethacin did not interfere with tachyphyllaxis. Moreover, Messina *et al.* (1975) showed that angiotensin II contracted skeletal muscle microvascular smooth muscle only in damaged preparations but did not reduce arteriolar diameter in undamaged preparations. Their results seem to indicate that tachyphyllaxis and the degree of involvement of the prostanoid system in the vascular responses to angiotensin II may be dependent on the degree of vascular damage or unphysiologic nature of the preparation under study.

In addition to its capacity to affect the VSM of the microcirculation directly, angiotensin II may modify microvascular smooth muscle function, including that of the innervated venules, by enhancing the release of NE from adrenergic nerve terminals (Zimmerman *et al.,* 1973; Kadowitz *et al.,* 1975b) and by enhancing the postsynaptic, α-adrenergically mediated vasoconstrictor response to NE (Peach, 1977), as well as by inhibiting the uptake of NE into adrenergic nerves (Peach, 1977; Westfall, 1977). These secondary actions of angiotensin II occur in concentrations below that required to activate the angiotensin II receptors directly in the VSM, suggesting the possibility that these actions of angiotensin may be as important in modulating microcirculatory function as is its direct pressor action.

The receptors for angiotensin II are disulfide dependent, similar to those for 5-HT and neurohypophyseal peptides (see below) and some prostanoids (Greenberg et al., 1976; M. Johnson and Ramwell, 1973; M. Johnson et al., 1973, 1974a,b; E. Johnson et al., 1974), since dithiothreitol inhibits the responses to angiotensin II (Fleisch et al., 1973). The angiotensin II contraction of VSM is not only magnesium and sodium dependent, but also calcium dependent (Altura and Altura, 1971; Devynck and Meyer, 1976; Devynck et al., 1974). Increases in extracellular sodium enhance the pressor and contractile responses to angiotensin II, whereas decreases in extracellular sodium ion depress responses to this polypeptide (Wright et al., 1982). Moreover, alterations in sodium ion affect the specific binding of $2\text{-}^{14}C$- or ^{125}I-labeled angiotensin II to membrane fractions of VSM in a related manner. Thus, a disulfide-dependent, sodium-dependent moiety may be involved in the binding of angiotensin with its receptor. Freer (1977) suggested that calcium ion may be an integral component of the angiotensin II receptor in VSM because, in the absence of calcium ion, the contractile response to angiotensin II was maintained but was shifted to the right. Other studies would seem to suggest that the interaction of angiotensin II with its receptor results from a binding of calcium ion to both the histidyl residue of angiotensin II and perhaps a prolyl or related amino acid moiety on the VSM, which then results in angiotensin II displacing calcium ion from binding sites within the cell membrane (Freer, 1977). Angiotensin II has also been shown to stimulate the efflux of calcium from microsomal vesicles of VSM (Baudouin-Legros and Meyer, 1973; Baudouin-Legros et al., 1972), supporting the contention that angiotensin may release calcium ion from sequestered sites within the VSM. The contractile response to angiotensin then results from a biochemical mechanism similar to that of NE.

Wright et al. (1982) studied the regulation of angiotensin II receptors in rat mesenteric arteries. The binding of angiotensin II to membrane fractions of this preparation was stimulated by magnesium and calcium ion as well as sodium ion, whereas potassium ion inhibited the binding of angiotensin II to VSM. Guanosine triphosphate (GTP) and other nucleotides inhibited angiotensin II binding by a mechanism that appeared to be related to their capacity to chelate endogenous cations. This conclusion was reached because chelation of endogenous ions with EDTA inhibited the action of GTP. The monovalent and divalent ions affected receptor affinity, whereas GTP and its analogs affected the maximum binding capacity of the VSM for angiotensin II. Wright et al. (1982) concluded that cations and guanine nucleotides affected angiotensin II binding by controlling or modulating at least two distinct portions of the receptor complex. They also suggested that the interaction of these sites with cations and guanine nucleotides could be involved in the modulation of VSM responses to angiotensin II.

D. Neurohypophyseal Peptides

Krogh (1929) demonstrated that topical administration of extracts of posterior pituitary gland contracted the microvessels of the webbed feet of frogs and dog ears. The subsequent demonstration that hypophysectomy resulted in an increased microcirculatory blood flow led Krogh (1929) to postulate that the hormones from the posterior pituitary exerted a tonic vasoconstrictor influence on the peripheral vasculature and microcirculation.

1. Heterogeneity of Responses to Neurohypophyseal Peptides

Vascular smooth muscles exhibit a heterogeneity in their responses to oxytocin and arginine vasopressin, the neurohypophyseal peptides. Although it was generally believed that all VSM preparations were relatively insensitive to vasopressin (Douglas, 1975; Saameli, 1968; Sawyer, 1961; Mellander and Johansson, 1968), the experiments of Altura and Altura (1977b) demonstrated that rat terminal arterioles were sensitive to 1 fmol of vasopressin, three orders of magnitude greater than its sensitivity to angiotensin II (Altura, 1973; Altura and Altura, 1977b). Similar results were found in rat thoracic aortas (Altura and Altura, 1977b). In general, although different VSM from different sources within a single mammalian species exhibits a wide divergence of sensitivities to vasopressin, the smaller the VSM the more sensitive it is to vasopressin (for references see Altura, 1978a,b, 1981). It also appears that the muscle venules are the most sensitive of the microcirculatory blood vessels to vasopressin (Altura and Hershey, 1967; Altura, 1973, 1975a) and respond to circulating concentrations (0.1–1 fmol) of this peptide hormone (Lauson, 1974; Forsling, 1976).

Some of the potential mechanisms of the heterogeneity of response of VSM to vasopressin may result from the differential effects of sex hormones on the receptors for vasopressin within the different VSM preparations or on the VSM from discrete vascular beds. Estrogens may increase the concentration of internal sodium ion and subsequently internal calcium ion. This results is an increased or labilized intracellular calcium pool from which vasopressin may release intracellular calcium ion to elicit contraction, thereby potentiating the effects of vasopressin (Altura and Altura, 1971, 1976). Alternatively, the number and/or structure of the receptors for vasopressin and oxytocin (see Section III,C,4) may be highly individual for different VSM (Altura and Altura, 1971, 1976; Vanhoutte, 1978, 1980). Although it had been thought that neurohypophyseal peptides might act on receptors that mediated both relaxation and contraction, the data now suggest that the relaxant action on these polypeptides resulted from the preservative in the commercially available peptides and that these peptides act only on receptors that mediate contraction (Altura, 1978a,b, 1981).

2. Mechanism of Action of Neurohypophyseal Peptides

For both vasopressin and oxytocin, two fairly universal and somewhat unique characteristics appear to modulate the peptide–receptor complex interactions. These are (a) a requirement for magnesium ion (Somlyo et al., 1967; Altura and Altura, 1970) and (b) a requirement for an intact sulfhydryl group on the receptor (Martin and Schild, 1965; Altura and Altura, 1970). In the absence of magnesium ion the contractile responses of VSM to oxytocin and vasopressin are inhibited and/or abolished. Similarly, disulfide bond reduction inhibits the contractile response to these polypeptide vasoconstrictor agonists. Thus, it seems likely that magnesium ion and a disulfide group are integral moieties of the neurohypophyseal peptide–receptor complex.

The contractile responses of vasopressin and oxytocin are inhibited by ethanol, glucose deprivation, hypoxia, alterations in the external concentration of divalent cations, and male sex hormones but are enhanced by female sex hormones. Extracellular sodium concentrations and potassium ion concentrations do not appear to play a major role in the vasoconstrictor or vasopressor action of these hormones (Altura and Altura, 1977a,b; Altura, 1977, 1978a,b, 1981). Although the factors affecting the action of the neurohypophyseal peptides have been elucidated, little progress has been made in defining the mechanism of action of these substances at the cellular or molecular level in VSM. Both oxytocin and vasopressin, as well as ACh, contract uterine smooth muscle in vitro. Carsten (1974) showed that oxytocin may impair calcium sequestration by microsomal fractions of uterus, thereby affecting an increase in free, intracellular calcium ion. Similar actions may occur with vasopressin. The cellular action of these peptides differ from that of other contractile agents, such as ACh, in that they do not cause an increase in membrane permeability to potassium ion (Hodgson and Daniels, 1972). Thus, the neurohypophyseal peptides may contract VSM by combining with magnesium- and disulfide-dependent receptors to cause a decrease in intracellular or microsomal sequestration of calcium ion. This would lead to an increase in free calcium ion, which would then interact with calmodulin, activate the myosin light-chain kinase, and promote actomyosin ATPase activity and the sliding-filament mechanism involved in VSM contraction (see Section II,J). Further studies are necessary to resolve the mechanism of contraction of VSM by neurohypophyseal peptides.

3. Interaction of Neurohypophyseal Peptides with Vasopressor Substances

Vasopressin and oxytocin enhance the pressor responses of catecholamines in dogs, cats, and rats (Bartelstone and Nasmyth, 1965; Berde, 1965; Nakano, 1974; Nash et al., 1961) as well as the microcirculatory responses to epinephrine and NE (Altura et al., 1972; Altura, 1977; Altura and Hershey, 1967) in concentrations that do not exert a pressor or constrictor response themselves. Altura and Altura (1979b) suggested that the primary site of these interactions may be at the level of the microvasculature. This finding may be related either to the capacity of these peptide hormones to increase the level of ionized calcium to threshold levels within the VSM cell or to an inhibitory effect on the processes involved in the termination of action of these amines (uptake$_1$ or uptake$_2$). The mechanism remains to be defined. Nevertheless, the findings that elevated levels of vasopressin may play a role in the pathogenesis and/or maintenance of some forms of experimental hypertension (Berecek et al., 1980, 1982; McCaa et al., 1978), that venous smooth muscle reactivity and contractility are enhanced in hypertension (Greenberg et al., 1978, 1981; Greenberg and Bohr, 1975; Bevan et al., 1975; Simon et al., 1975), and that venous smooth muscle undergoes a decrease in diameter in the microcirculation (Bohlen and Gore, 1978) and hypertrophy (Greenberg et al., 1978; Greenberg and Wilborn, 1982; Greenberg, 1981d) in hypertension suggest that neurohypophyseal peptide–catecholamine interactions at the level of the microcirculation may play a role in the hemodynamic alterations in the pathogenesis of hypertension.

4. Neurohypophyseal Peptides and the Fetal–Maternal Microcirculation

That the umbilical arteries and veins, as well as some neonatal VSM, are sensitive to the actions of oxytocin and vasotocin is not an unexpected finding (Altura et al., 1972; Dyer and Gough, 1971; Dyer et al., 1972; Turlapaty and Altura, 1978). The actions of oxytocin and vasotocin are inhibited by low oxygen tensions and by the absence or reduction of estrogens (Altura, 1972b; Altura et al., 1972). The latter investigators have suggested that oxytocin may promote closure of the umbilical cord vessel at term by contracting these vessels in the presence of high oxygen tensions and the action of other hormones, such as the prostanoids. Determination of the exact role of oxytocin and vasotocin in regulating microcirculatory function in the fetal circulation must await the synthesis of specific antagonists of these substances. Moreover, these inhibitors, once developed, should be studied in the microcirculation of pregnant animals at term with established, vital microcirculatory techniques.

E. Kinins

Bradykinin, lysylbradykinin, and methionyllysylbradykinin are derived from kininogen in plasma and exist as both the prohormone and the active moiety. The synthesis and degradation are described in Section II,E. Kinins can also be released from leukocytes (leukokinins) by lysosomal enzyme activity and are believed to play a role in the microvascular response to tissue injury and anaphylaxis (for reference see Greenbaum, 1976; Movat and Habal, 1976). The kinins can initiate vasodilation and increased capillary permeability to fluids and other vasoactive agents, in addition to stimulating pain receptors (for references see Erdos, 1970; Rocha e Silva, 1970, 1974; Pisano and Austen, 1976). They are released in large quantity in response to anaphylaxis, circulatory shock, and tissue injury, and their synthesis and/or release are impaired by the action of nonspecific proteolysis inhibitors, such as aprotinin (for references see Amunsden, 1976).

Bradykinin (and other kinins) are among the most potent dilators of the microcirculation arteriolar smooth muscle, whereas they contract venular and umbilical arterial and venous smooth muscle *in vivo* in concentrations known to be present under physiologic conditions (Melmon et al., 1968; Altura and Altura, 1977a,b; Altura, 1978a,b, 1981). Moreover, bradykinin, in doses that do not affect the level of VSM tone, inhibits the vasoconstrictor responses of the microcirculation to NE, angiotensin II, and epinephrine, but not vasopressin (Altura, 1978a,b, 1981). Thus, kinins may alter microcirculatory function by a direct and indirect effect on the VSM. In addition, more recent studies suggest that bradykinin may inhibit the release of NE from adrenergic nerves, thereby modulating neurogenically mediated vasoconstriction (for references see Vanhoutte, 1978, 1980).

Bradykinin may contract venous smooth muscle and relax arterial smooth muscle by two potential mechanisms. Kinins have been shown to stimulate the release of vasodilator prostanoids from arterial smooth muscle and constrictor prostanoids from venous smooth muscle (Blumberg et al., 1977; Needleman et al., 1973a,b; Palmer et al., 1973; McGiff et al., 1972, 1975, 1976; Aiken, 1973). It has been suggested that kinins may directly activate phospholipase to promote the release of the prostanoids

(McGiff *et al.*, 1976; Needleman *et al.*, 1976, 1978). The prostanoids released from the endothelium or VSM then mediate the vasoconstrictor or vasodilator response to the kinins (for references see Needleman and Isakson, 1980). Evidence in support of this theory is that some inhibitors of prostanoid biosynthesis, such as indomethacin, reverse bradykinin-induced arterial relaxation and inhibit the venoconstriction produced by the kinins (McGiff *et al.*, 1972, 1975, 1976; Messina *et al.*, 1975, 1976; Needleman *et al.*, 1975). Wong *et al.* (1977) and Terragno *et al.* (1975, 1977, 1978) provided direct evidence for a differential effect of kinins on mesenteric artery and vein prostanoid synthesis. Greenberg and Kadowitz (1982) and Goldberg *et al.* (1975a,b, 1976) failed to inhibit bradykinin-induced venoconstriction in canine mesenteric arteries and veins with some inhibitors of prostanoid synthesis, yet found that indomethacin converted bradykinin-induced relaxation to contraction of the mesenteric arteries. Indomethacin-induced inhibition of bradykinin-mediated relaxation was associated with a reduction in prostanoid synthesis by the mesenteric vessels in response to bradykinin. To determine whether the effects of indomethacin were direct or indirect effects of the inhibitor (Northover, 1972, 1973, 1975), Greenberg and Kadowitz (1982) contracted the arteries with NE and obtained the relaxation in response to bradykinin before and after indomethacin, ETYA, or ETYA administered before indomethacin. The data are summarized in Figs. 20 and 21. Indomethacin inhibited bradykinin-induced relaxation in control mesenteric arteries and in blood vessels in which prostanoid synthesis had been already inhibited with ETYA (Table VII). Thus, the data suggest that bradykinin releases prostanoids, but it may not participate in the vasodilator response to the kinins in all species. Needleman *et al.* (1976) proposed another role for prostanoids released by kinins in the microcirculation of the heart. The kinins may mediate the pain and ischemic changes following anoxia and/or ischemia. The prostanoids may mediate the metabolic events subserving the interaction of kinins with their receptors on smooth muscle.

A second mechanism invoked to explain the actions of kinins on VSM presupposes that the endothelium is also obligatory for kinin-mediated relaxation of VSM (Furchgott *et al.*, 1981). This has been described in detail for Ach (see Section II, E). Although Altura and Chand (1981) failed to inhibit bradykinin-induced relaxation with inhibitors of lipoxygenase synthesis, they also found an endothelial obligation for kinin-mediated relaxation. Figure 15 summarizes the action of kinins and other substances on arterial smooth muscle in the presence and absence of the endothelium. It is quite clear, at least for larger arteries, that, in the absence of the endothelium, mesenteric arteries (0.5 mm OD) will not relax in response to kinins, substance P, or, to a limited extent, adenosine and ATP. The sig-

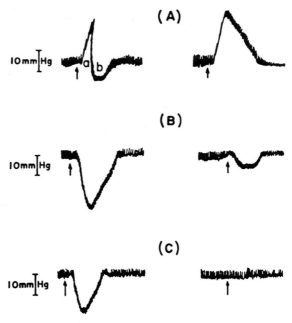

Fig. 20. Typical pressure responses to (A) angiotensin II, (B) bradykinin, and (C) arachidonic acid (controls left) and the effect of indomethacin (right) on these responses. (From Blumberg *et al.*, 1977, with permission.)

Dose	a	b	Indomethacin
		ΔP	
	Control		
Angiotensin II			
50	4 ± 2	−8 ± 1	9 ± 2*
100	17 ± 3	−11 ± 1	33 ± 7*
200	21 ± 4	−15 ± 4	37 ± 11*
		Control	
Bradykinin			
100		−26 ± 3	−8 ± 1*
200		−36 ± 6	−15 ± 4*
400		−37 ± 7	−16 ± 3*
Arachidonic acid			
100		−13 ± 2	0
250		−27 ± 3	−3 ± 3*
500		−42 ± 4	−3 ± 3*

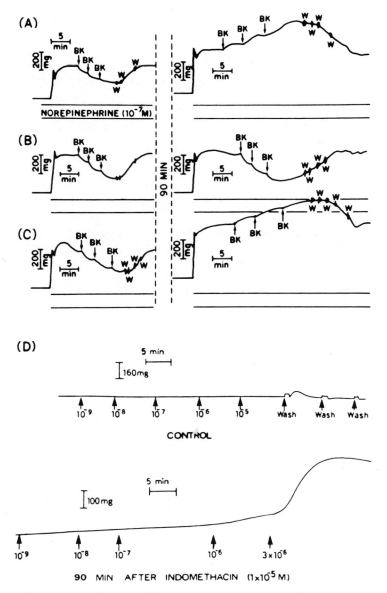

Fig. 21. Effect of indomethacin and eicosatetraynoic acid, alone and in combination, on responses of mesenteric arteries to bradykinin. BK, Bradykinin; W, wash. (From Greenberg and Kadowitz, 1982, with permission.)

TABLE VII

Effect of Indomethacin, Eicosatetraynoic Acid, and Tranylcypromine on Bradykinin- and Norepinephrine-Stimulated Prostaglandin and 6-Keto-PGF$_{1\alpha}$ Synthesis in Canine Arteries and Veins[a,b,c]

Agonist (concentration)	Preparation	INDO[c]	ETYA[c]	TCM[c]	% Inhibition at 10^{-5} M inhibitor			% Inhibition[d] at 10^{-5} M INDO together with 10^{-5} M ETYA
					INDO (PGE$_2$ + PGF$_{2\alpha}$)	ETYA	TCM (6-Keto-PGF$_{1\alpha}$)	
Bradykinin (10^{-5} M)	Splenic A	2.7 ± 0.6	2.1 ± 0.7	3.3 ± 0.2	99 ± 5	99 ± 3	100 ± 0	99 ± 6
	Mesenteric A	3.6 ± 0.4	3.3 ± 0.5	4.7 ± 0.3	98 ± 2	102 ± 4	100 ± 0	99 ± 7
	Splenic V	2.1 ± 0.5	2.6 ± 0.4	2.6 ± 0.5	98 ± 4	98 ± 4	100 ± 0	99 ± 5
	Mesenteric V	3.4 ± 0.2	2.9 ± 0.5	2.8 ± 0.7	99 ± 5	95 ± 4	100 ± 0	99 ± 4
	Portal V	4.1 ± 0.5	5.2 ± 0.6	2.1 ± 0.9	97 ± 3	99 ± 5	100 ± 0	98 ± 3
Norepinephrine (10^{-5} M)	Splenic A	2.9 ± 0.7	3.6 ± 0.6	2.9 ± 0.4	95 ± 4	101 ± 5	100 ± 0	98 ± 3
	Mesenteric A	3.1 ± 0.5	2.4 ± 0.2	3.7 ± 0.9	98 ± 6	99 ± 3	100 ± 0	99 ± 6
	Splenic V	2.4 ± 0.6	1.9 ± 0.3	2.2 ± 0.4	97 ± 5	98 ± 6	100 ± 0	97 ± 2
	Mesenteric V	4.5 ± 0.9	3.8 ± 0.2	2.6 ± 0.7	98 ± 3	94 ± 5	100 ± 0	99 ± 4
	Portal V	4.8 ± 0.6	5.2 ± 0.4	2.9 ± 0.5	97 ± 5	97 ± 3	100 ± 0	99 ± 3

[a] From Greenberg and Kadowitz (1982) with permission.

[b] Abbreviations: A, artery; ETYA, eicosatetraynoic acid; INDO, indomethacin; PG, prostaglandin; TCM, tranylcypromine; V, vein. Each mean represents the average values obtained from four to seven blood vessels.

[c] IC$_{50}$ = concentration of INDO and ETYA necessary to reduce agonist-induced stimulation of PGE$_2$ and PGF$_{2\alpha}$ and concentration of TCM necessary to inhibit by 50% the agonist-induced stimulation of 6-keto-PGF$_{1\alpha}$.

[d] Percent inhibition at 10^{-5} M prostaglandin synthesis with both INDO and ETYA present in incubate.

nificance of this finding to microcirculatory function remains to be examined.

F. Histamine

Histamine is a potent mediator of both vasodilation and peripheral edema in experimental animals and man. Although some controversy exists concerning whether histamine can dilate venules as well as arterioles and precapillary sphincters, the concept is generally accepted that the microvascular actions of histamine are mediated both by the classical histamine$_1$ (H$_1$) and histamine$_2$ (H$_2$) receptors (Chand and Eyre, 1975; Altura and Halevy, 1978; Owen, 1977; Simionescu et al., 1982). The histamine acting on the microcirculation may be histamine from mast cells, histamine stored in the vascular wall, or histamine released from histaminergic nerves (Beck and Brody, 1961). Alternatively, it has been suggested that adrenergic nerves may stabilize a non-mast-cell pool of histamine. Inhibition of sympathetic nerve activity would then result in a destabilization of this histamine pool, release of histamine, and subsequently histamine-mediated vasodilation and edema formation (Ryan and Brody, 1970; Boerth et al., 1970; Heitz and Brody, 1975) within the microcirculation.

Two distinct receptors mediate the action of histamine on the microcirculatory VSM: H$_1$ receptors blocked by classical antihistamine blocking agents and histamine receptors blocked by cimetidine and metiamide (for references see Black et al., 1972; Taylor and Richelson, 1982; Altura, 1978a,b, 1981; Vanhoutte, 1978). Altura and Halevy (1978) reported that equivalent topical doses of histamine increased vascular diameter in each of the components of the microcirculation. The order of magnitude of the dilation was arterioles > precapillary sphincters >> venules. The action of histamine is mediated by both H$_1$ and H$_2$ receptors since both pyribenzamine and metiamide inhibit the microcirculatory response to histamine (Chand and Eyre, 1975; Altura and Halevy, 1978; Owen, 1977). Antihistamines also contract microvascular VSM, both due to a direct effect on the smooth muscle and by virtue of their capacity to inhibit a dilator component of endogenous, circulating histamine (for references see Altura and Altura, 1974a,b; Altura, 1978, 1981; Vanhoutte, 1978). Thus, histamine released from mast cels, nonneuronal sources, or dietary sources may modify microcirculatory VSM function. In addition, because of the greater arterial versus venous effects, and by virtue of its capacity to increase membrane permeability, histamine can produce peripheral and/or microcirculatory edema and vascular damage.

The mechanism by which histamine relaxes VSM in vivo is speculative at present. In vitro, many blood vessels contract in response to histamine (see Vanhoutte, 1978), as do small veins *in vivo* (Shepherd and Vanhoutte, 1975). Microvascular responses to histamine are inhibited by steroids (Kalsner, 1970; Altura, 1966a,b), but this may be related to potentiation of the venoconstrictor action rather than due to a prostanoid-dependent mechanism. It has been suggested that the vasodilator effects of histamine may be mediated indirectly via inhibition of NE release from adrenergic nerves, an event mediated by H_2 receptors (McGrath and Shepherd, 1976). Histamine-mediated relaxation may also be a physical process secondary to the vascular permeability actions of this amine. Vanhoutte (1978) has speculated that histamine may cause endothelial contraction, resulting in fenestration of the endothelial lining and fluid loss from the extracellular space. This would change the osmolarity of the extracellular space, resulting in a hyperosmolar condition that has been shown to promote vasodilation and inhibition of adrenergic neurotransmission (Mellander and Lundvall, 1971; Haddy and Scott, 1968, 1975; McGrath and Shepherd, 1976).

In an attempt to elucidate the site and mechanism of histamine interaction with venular tissue, Simionescu *et al.* (1982) coupled histamine, methylhistamine, and a selective H_1 receptor agonist (4-pyridylethylamine) to ferritin. They measured the distribution of the radioactive forms of the complexes, as well as the electromicrographic localization of these substances in bovine pulmonary and human umbilical venous endothelial cells. They found that approximately 22% of the endothelial receptors for histamine were of the H_1 type, whereas 78% were of the H_2 type. Moreover, the H_2 binding sites were localized to the areas of the contractile proteins of the endothelial cells. It was speculated that contractions of these endothelial cells may allow gaps to form between the cells, increasing permeability. Moreover, since these sites were also associated with the areas of the coated pits and the Pastan (1982) receptosomes, sites of drug transport into the endothelial cell, the localization of histamine receptors at these sites could also play a role in increasing permeability by stimulating the opening of these "pore equivalents."

The biochemical mechanism of histamine action is unclear at present. Endothelial-obligatory relaxing factor does not appear to be important in the relaxation of VSM to histamine (Furchgott *et al.*, 1981). Histamine can stimulate the formation of both cyclic AMP and cyclic GMP. Desensitization to histamine is associated with a loss of the responses to histamine and a decrease in the maximum amount of cyclic GMP that can be formed. However, the affinity of histamine for its receptor is unaltered at the time of desensitization. This suggests that histamine-induced relaxation may be associated with an increase in cyclic GMP and that the number of receptors is important in determining the magnitude of the response. Moreover, it appears that H_1 receptor stimulation may be linked to the formation of cyclic GMP, whereas H_2 receptor stimulation may be linked to the formation of cyclic AMP (for references see Taylor and Richelson, 1982). Thus, histamine-mediated relaxation may be dependent on cyclic nucleotide-stimulated protein kinase-dependent dephosphorylation of myosin and phosphorylation of myosin light-chain kinase (see Section II,J).

G. Prostanoids, Thromboxanes, and Leukotrienes and Lipid Peroxides

The prostanoids and the other arachidonate-mediated metabolites represent such a vast family of compounds that entire monographs have been devoted to their action on the microcirculation. Therefore, this section briefly covers new information relating to the action of these substances on the microcirculation and the mechanism of prostanoid action. For a more detailed account the reader is referred to reviews on this subject (Karim, 1976; Messina et al., 1976; Samuelsson and Paoletti, 1982; Salmon, 1982; Heymann, 1980; Greenberg, 1982a,b).

The fatty acid precursors of prostanoids and leukotrienes are also the sources of prostacyclin and thromboxanes. However, the microvascular responses to endogenous prostanoid substances or exogenous fatty acids may not result only from the action of these substances on the microvasculature. The major sites of thromboxane A_2 synthesis are the platelets, whereas the circulating leukocytes metabolize arachidonic acids to hydroperoxides and leukotrienes. Prostacyclin is made primarily by the endothelial cells and VSM, whereas the smooth muscle synthesizes primarily prostanoids and prostacyclin. Thromboxane and prostacyclin have opposing actions on both the VSM and the platelet, whereas the leukotrienes appear to contract VSM and stimulate aggregation (Table VI, p. 74; Fig. 13). Moncada and Vane (1979a,b) suggested that the thromboxane–prostacyclin system acted as an important homeostatic mechanism in the regulation of platelet adherence to the vascular endothelium, platelet aggregation, and thrombi formation (Table VI, Fig. 13).

Prostaglandins of the E series decrease vascular diameter in the microcirculation with a greater effect on arterioles and precapillary arterioles than on venules. Moreover, prostanoids of the E series antagonize the vasoconstrictor action of angiotensin II, NE, and other agonists and enhance the dilator responses to bradykinin (Messina et al., 1976). Thromboxane A_2 and analogs of prostaglandin endoperoxides believed to stimulate thromboxane receptors (U44619) contract arterioles, precapillary

TABLE VIII

Glycogen Phosphorylase Activity, Oxygen Consumption, and Aerobic Glycolysis in Porcine Coronary Arteries[a,b]

Compound added	Change from basal (%)		
	J_{O_2}	J_{lac}	Phosphorylase activity[b]
KCl, 80 mM	68 ± 7	67 ± 8	55.8 ± 14.0
Ouabain, 10^{-5} M	21 ± 3.5	−47 ± 5	40.7 ± 18.6

[a] From Hellstrand and Paul (1982) with permission.
[b] Total activity in the presence of adenosine monophosphate was 0.14 ± 0.02 μmol/g per minute ($n = 20$).

arterioles, and venules (Higgs, 1982). Messina and Kaley (1982) incubated PHG$_2$ with platelet microsomes to generate thromboxane and found *in vivo* coronary dilation and *in vitro* contraction of VSM. Dusting *et al.* (1978) injected PGH$_2$ with microsomes into the mesenteric circulation of dogs and found only weak constriction. Injection of cold acetone extracts of thromboxane A$_2$ also resulted in weak responses of the mesenteric circulation. Thus, it is possible that an endogenous circulating inhibitor of thromboxnae action may be present *in vivo* or that *in vitro* concentrations of thromboxane cannot be achieved *in vivo*. Prostacyclin dilates arterioles and precapillary arterioles but does not affect venular tone (Higgs *et al.*, 1978a,b, 1979; Higgs, 1982). Indomethacin enhanced the sensitivity of the vasculature to prostacyclin, possibly by inhibiting endogenous production of prostacyclin. According to Higgs *et al.* (1978, 1979) prostacyclin is the most potent microcirculatory vasodilator agent, whereas Messina and Kaley (1982) suggest that PGE$_2$ is more potent than prostacyclin. Prostaglandin G$_2$ contracts microvascular VSM followed by a secondary dilation due to endogenous prostacyclin formation (Lewis *et al.*, 1977; Higgs, 1982; Higgs *et al.*, 1978a,b, 1979). The action of PGH$_2$ is similar to that of PGG$_2$. Thus, prostanoid production by VSM or endothelium may modulate microcirculatory VSM function by altering VSM tone or the subsequent effects of other modulators of the level of VSM constriction or dilation.

Prostanoids may also act to modulate leukocyte adherence *in vivo*. Weksler *et al.* (1977) showed that prostacyclin synthesized by endothelial cells modulated leukocyte function. Higgs *et al.* (1978) subsequently showed that the number of flow-moving leukocytes was reduced in hamster cheek pouch microvenules. Boxer *et al.* (1980) demonstrated that prostacyclin reduced the adherence of leukocytes to VSM *in vitro*. Using the hamster cheek pouch preparation, Higgs (1982) showed that prostacyclin reduced leukocyte margination by 90% in doses that reduced arterial pressure by 30 mm Hg. Equieffective concentrations of PGE on arterial pressure did not affect leukocyte adherence or margination in the hamster cheek pouch microvessels. Higgs (1982) suggested that prostacyclin inhibited leukocyte adherence to the VSM by increasing cyclic AMP. Moreover, he suggested that local production of prostacyclin by inflammed blood vessels enhances local vasodilation and plays a role in the early stages of inflammation to suppress leukocyte adherence and infiltration into the vascular wall.

The effect of prostanoids on thrombus formation in the microcirculation is dependent on the prostanoid under study. Prostacyclin and PGE_1 inhibit thrombus formation, whereas thromboxane and leukotrienes promote thrombus formation. In vitro PGG_2 stimulates platelet aggregation, whereas in vivo it is an inhibitor. This would indicate that, in vivo, prostacyclin is predominantly formed over that of thromboxane. Figure 13 summarizes the mechanism by which prostacyclin may oppose the action of thromboxane and inhibit thrombus formation (Boxer et al., 1980; Emmons et al., 1967; Gorman et al., 1977; Gorman, 1982; Hamberg et al., 1974; Higgs et al., 1978, 1979; Kloeze, 1967; Moncada et al., 1976a,b; Needleman et al., 1976; Tateson et al., 1977; Westwick, 1977).

The mechanism by which prostanoids may affect VSM tone is described below. However, it appears that the prostanoids may exert their action via discreet receptors located in or on the VSM cell membrane. Tachyphyllaxis to PGA is not associated with tachyphyllaxis to PGE or $PGF_{2\alpha}$, nor is tachphyllaxis to PGD_2 associated with tachyphyllaxis to other prostanoids. Thus, it appears that the receptors for individual prostanoids may differ from each other (for references see Fleisch, 1977; Greenberg et al., 1976). Wakeling and Wyngarden (1974) demonstrated the existence of a specific PGE-binding protein in myometrium. M. Johnson et al. (1973a,b, 1974a,b) subsequently showed that ultraviolet light inhibits prostanoid-dependent contraction of uterine smooth muscle, as do ouabain (Kadar and Sunahara, 1969; Greenberg et al., 1974) and inhibitors of disulfide of sulfhydryl groups (E. M. Johnson et al., 1974). Subsequent studies showed that reductions in extracellular magnesium ion concentration from normal (2.4 mM) to 0.6 or 0 mM inhibited prostanoid-induced contraction and relaxation of VSM (Altura and Altura, 1976; Greenberg and Bohr, 1975; Greenberg, 1981d, 1982a,b). These findings suggest that disulfide groups and magnesium ion are essential components of the prostanoid receptor and that the ouabain-inhibitable sodium transport ATPase of VSM may be an integral component of the contractile and relaxant mechanism activated by prostanoids.

Current data suggest that constrictor prostanoids may act by two distinct mechanisms. Conventional prostanoids may contract VSM by acting as a calcium ionophore and increase VSM permeability to calcium ion or inhibit (K,Na)-ATPase with a resultant increase in sodium and calcium ion (Greenberg et al., 1974a,b,c; Carsten, 1973, 1974; Carsten and Miller, 1977, 1978). The effects of thromboxanes and endoperoxide analogs, as well as leukotrienes, may be to inhibit intracellular calcium sequestration or promote release of intracellular calcium ion as well as inhibit magnesium uptake into VSM (van Breeman et al., 1979, 1980; McNamara et al., 1980; Greenberg, 1981d). The vasodilator responses to prostaglandins and prostacyclin may be related to an inhibition of calcium influx into the VSM cell and a stimulation of magnesium influx (Carsten and Miller, 1977, 1978; Greenberg et al., 1974; Greenberg, 1981d, 1982a,b). In addition, prostanoids that relax VSM stimulate adenylate cyclase and increase cyclic AMP, thereby potentially affecting the contractile and relaxation process as described above.

H. Acetylcholine

Acetylcholine has been implicated as a mediator and/or regulator of blood flow since the studies of Krogh (1929), which suggested that ACh increases microcirculatory blood flow. Cholinergic nerves innervate some vascular beds such as skeletal muscle (Mellander and Johansson, 1968), cerebral circulation (D'Alacy and Rose, 1977), kidney (Harkness and Brody, 1967), and coronary circulation (D'Alecy and Feigel, 1972). Moreover, ACh acts as a vasodilator to increase blood flow and decrease resistance in many vascular beds (Altura, 1966a,b, 1971a; Mellander and Johansson, 1968; Shepherd and Vanhoutte, 1975; Westfall, 1977). Finally, ACh can modulate the responses to other vasodilator and vasoconstrictor substances as well as nerve stimulation without directly affecting the VSM (Altura, 1978a,b, 1981; Vanhoutte, 1978, 1980). Although a large concentration of ACh is required to affect microcirculatory tone and blood flow in vivo, some evidence exists for a role of endogenous ACh in the modulation of microcirculatory VSM function.

Atropine is a selective, cholinergic, muscarinic receptor antagonist. Altura (1966a,b, 1971a) showed that atropine produced concentration-related contractions of precapillary sphincters and arterioles in concentrations that inhibited topically applied ACh-mediated dilation. However, these concentrations of atropine did not affect the vasodilator responses to bradykinin, histamine, or isoproterenol. This effect was not due to an artifact resulting from the topical administration of atropine, because intravenous administration of atropine, in concentrations sufficient to block topically administered ACh, also produced a decrease in the lumen size of metarterioles, arterioles, precapillary sphincters, and venules (Altura and Hershey, 1967). Since atropine does not contract VSM directly, the contractile responses to atropine may reflect inhibition of endogenous ACh-mediated vasodilation or, as suggested by Altura (1966a,b), the action of some other, unidentified choline–ester moiety.

The remaining evidence for ACh acting as a modulator of VSM tone in the microcirculation is inferred from its actions on larger arteries and the actions of subvasodilator concentrations of ACh on the microcirculation. Acetylcholine inhibits the postsynaptic responses to stimulation of adrenergic nerves by inhibiting the release of the neurotransmitter NE (Vanhoutte, 1974; Vanhoutte et al., 1973). Thus, ACh may modulate the level of VSM tone by altering the concentration of NE released from adrenergic nerves. In addition, subvasodilator concentrations of ACh attenuate the vasoconstrictor responses to NE, angiotension II, 5-HT, and a wide variety of other substances in venules, noninnervated precapillary sphincters, and other microvessels (Altura, 1978a,b, 1981). Thus, ACh may modulate the level of tone of both innervated and noninnervated VSM in the microcirculation.

1. Receptors for Acetylcholine

Previous work with large rabbit, rat, cat, and dog arteries (DeMey and Vanhoutte, 1978, 1981; Furchgott and Zawadski, 1980a,b,c; Furchgott et al., 1981; Altura and Chand, 1981) suggested that ACh acted on a muscarinic receptor on the endothelium to stimulate the release of an endothelial-derived relaxing factor, which in turn acted on the arterial smooth muscle to promote relaxation (see below). Greenberg et al. (1982a,b) confirmed the existence of endothelial-mediated relaxation of VSM in vitro and demonstrated the existence of distinct cholinergic, muscarinic receptors mediating the endothelial and smooth muscle actions of ACh. Moreover, data obtained with the cholinergic, muscarinic receptor antagonist cetiedil (Boissier et al., 1980; Cho et al., 1979) demonstrated that four distinct cholinergic receptors exist for ACh: two distinct cholinergic, muscarinic receptors on the venous and arterial endothelium and two on the venous and arterial smooth muscle. Cetiedil is avidly bound by VSM (Boissier et al., 1980). Differences in binding between artery and vein may require different concentrations of cetiedil to block cholinergic receptors. Alternatively, cetiedil may have the capacity to differentiate subclasses of cholinergic receptors not amenable to analyses with atropine. Further speculation is beyond the scope of this discussion. However, the data obtained from the atropine and the cetiedil studies clearly demonstrate that the muscarinic, cholinergic receptors of the endothelial-competent artery and vein cannot be the same receptor subtypes.

Estrada and Krause (1982) also reported that membrane fractions from bovine pia-arachnoid cerebral microvessels could be characterized by two specific binding sites. They speculated that the two binding sites were related to the cholinergic receptors present on the arterial smooth muscle and cerebral capillary endothelium. The data presented herein show that endothelial-dependent responses and responses independent of an intact endothelium can be characterized by two distinct kinetic constants. Moreover, the values obtained by Estrada and Krause (1982) for ACh interacting with the two receptors (2.67×10^{-7} and $1.65 \times 10^{-5}\ M$) are relatively the same as the ED_{50} concentrations for ACh-mediated relaxation and contraction of canine arteries in endothelial-intact and endothelial-deficient preparations, respectively. Thus, the existence of distinct cholinergic, muscarinic receptors mediating endothelial-dependent relaxation and smooth muscle contraction may be the rule, rather than the exception, in VSM. Further studies are needed to validate this concept.

2. Mechanism of Action of Acetylcholine

In contrast to the *in vivo* vasodilator action of ACh, the *in vitro* action of ACh generally results in a contraction of arterial and smooth muscle. Jeliffe *et al.* (1962), however, reported that rings of aortic smooth muscle relaxed in response to ACh. Furchgott and Zawadski (1979, 1980a,b,c) and DeMey and Vanhoutte (1978, 1981) demonstrated that ACh-mediated relaxation of arterial smooth muscle and some venous smooth muscles (Altura and Chand, 1981; Tanaka *et al.*, 1982a,b) was dependent on the presence of an intact endothelium. Furchgott *et al.* (1981) proposed that ACh-mediated relaxation of arterial smooth muscle is dependent on the release of hydroperoxide metabolites from the endothelium. These substances act on the smooth muscle to stimulate cyclic GMP, which in some manner promotes the relaxation of smooth muscle. This speculation was based on the findings that (*a*) lipoxygenase and cyclooxygenase inhibitors such as ETYA and nordihydroguaiaretic acid (NDGA) and hydroquinone antagonized by ACh-mediated relaxation of endothelial-competent arterial smooth muscle (Furchgott and Zawadski, 1980a,b,c); (*b*) analogs of cyclic GMP relaxed arterial smooth muscle (Schultz *et al.*, 1979); (*c*) ETYA and other lipoxygenase inhibitors inhibited the accumulation of cyclic GMP in smooth muscle (Spies *et al.*, 1980; Goldberg *et al.*, 1978); and (*d*) hydroperoxides and other peroxides derived from phospholipid stimulated the accumulation of cyclic GMP (Hidaka and Asano, 1977). This conclusion has been challenged by Diamond (1982) on the grounds that the changes in cyclic GMP with most vasodilator substances are insufficient to accommodate or promote relaxation and the temporal changes in cyclic GMP and relaxation do not appear to be temporally related to each other.

The studies of Greenberg *et al.* (1982a,b) with normal and rubbed canine mesenteric arteries and veins confirmed the observations of Furchgott and Zawadski (1978, 1980a,b,c,d) and Furchgott *et al.* (1981) that NDGA and ETYA as well as the other lipoxygenase inhibitors inhibit ACh-mediated relaxation. However, the following findings fail to support the speculation that ACh-mediated endothelial-dependent relaxation is initiated through the formation of endothelial-derived hydroperoxides that act on the smooth muscle to promote relaxation:

1.   Each of the lipoxygenase inhibitors inhibited both ACh-mediated relaxation of normal mesenteric arteries and contraction of normal and rubbed mesenteric veins.

2.   No significant differences existed in the concentrations of antagonists required to inhibit the concentration and relaxation processes.

3.   Arachidonic acid inhibited ACh-mediated relaxation and contraction.

4.   Each of the inhibitors inhibited NE-induced contraction in concentrations required to inhibit ACh-mediated relaxation of normal mesenteric arteries and contractions of normal mesenteric veins and rubbed mesenteric arteries and veins.

5.   Some lipoxygenase inhibitors inhibited ACh-mediated relaxation, whereas others were devoid of this activity.

6.   The concentrations of inhibitors required to block ACh-mediated contraction or relaxation were 10–300 times greater than the concentrations required to inhibit lipoxygenase (Samuelsson and Paoletti, 1982; Tappel *et al.*, 1953; Bray *et al.*, 1980; Volpi *et al.*, 1980).

7.   Ouabain, potassium-free saline solution, and high-potassium saline solution, which inhibit the (sodium–potassium)-activated, magnesium-dependent ATPase (electrogenic sodium pump), selectively inhibit ACh-mediated relaxation of endothelial-competent arteries (Greenberg *et al.*, 1982a; Webb *et al.*, 1981; DeMey and Vanhoutte, 1978; Jones, 1980; Haddy, 1978).

8.   Concentrations of metabolic inhibitors and hypoxia that do not affect the contractile responses to ACh or other vasoconstrictor agonists abolish ACh-mediated relaxation (DeMey and Vanhoutte, 1978; Furchgott *et al.*, 1981; Greenberg *et al.*, 1982b). The data represented support the conclusion that the effects of some of these inhibitors on ACh-mediated relaxation (and contraction) result from a nonspecific depressant effect of these substances on the processes that mediate both contraction and relaxation.

Some nonsteroidal antiinflammatory agents inhibit superprecipitation of actomyosin from VSM in concentrations that inhibit ACh-mediated contraction and relaxation (Gorog and Kovacs, 1972). This conclusion is also supported by the experiments of Tanaka *et al.* (1982a,b) which demonstrated that 10^{-4} *M* ETYA and NDGA suppress the relaxant effects of cetiedil on both normal and rubbed mesenteric arteries and veins. The relaxant effects of cetiedil are independent of (EDF) or cyclic GMP but depend on a direct stimulation of the electrogenic sodium pump on the smooth muscle of these VSM preparations (Tanaka *et al.*, 1982a,b). In addition, ETYA does not inhibit bradykinin-induced relaxation of canine mesenteric arteries (Greenberg and Kadowitz, 1982) or pulmonary vessels (Altura and Chand, 1981), responses dependent on the presence of an intact endothelium (Furchgott *et al.*, 1981). Furthermore, P. J. Kadowitz (personal communication) failed to block ACh-mediated pulmonary vascular relaxation in the perfused cat lung with 26 mg/kg ETYA. Thus, it is unlikely that ACh-mediated relaxation is dependent on the formation of ETYA- and NDGA-inhibitable hydroperoxides or prostanoids within the endothelium of the mesenteric arteries.

Cyanide and azide are fairly selective inhibitors of oxidative metabolism within VSM at low concentrations (Greenberg *et al.*, 1974a,b,c). The inhibitors decreased the concentration of ATP within the mesenteric arteries and veins and selectively inhibited or completely suppressed ACh-mediated relaxation but not ACh-mediated contraction of mesenteric arteries and veins, respectively. The data support the conclusion that energy derived from oxidative metabolism is obligatory for ACh-mediated relaxation of mesententeric arteries but anaerobic mechanisms or energy derived from the Embden–Myerhoff glycolytic pathway are sufficient to maintain ACh-mediated contraction of mesenteric veins. In support of this conclusion are the experiments of DeMey and Vanhoutte (1978, 1980a) and Furchgott *et al.* (1981), which show that anoxia suppresses ACh-mediated relaxation of canine and rabbit large arteries.

Guanosine triphosphate is essential for the formation of cyclic GMP (Goldberg *et al.*, 1978). A primary source of GTP is derived from the breakdown of glucose via the glycolytic pathway and the tricarboxylic acid cycle (Devlin, 1982). It is tempting to speculate that cyanide and azide inhibit ACh-mediated relaxation of normal mesenteric arteries by decreasing the concentration of GTP and thereby of cyclic GMP. This intriguing hypothesis generated the experiments with pyruvate and phosphoenolpyruvate (PEP), which should have increased the concentration of GTP and therefore of cyclic GMP. However, in the presence of PEP and pyruvate the responses to ACh were not enhanced, but depressed. Moreover, Murad *et al.* (1979) demonstrated that azide, in the presence of catalase, stimulates cyclic GMP accumulation. Cyanide inhibits cyclic GMP accumulation. However, both compounds inhibit ACh-mediated vasodilation. In addition, cyclic GMP derivatives and cyclic GMP itself relax VSM contracted by high-potassium ion solution. Physiologic salt solution with a high concentration of potassium ion inhibits ACh-mediated relaxation of mesenteric arteries. Therefore, it is unlikely that an inhibitory effect of hypoxia, azide, and cyanide on cyclic GMP formation can explain the inhibition of endothelial-dependent ACh-mediated relaxation of mesenteric arteries.

The findings summarized above clearly demonstrate that ACh-mediated relaxation of canine arteries and contraction of canine veins are two distinct processes mediated by different receptors and by different mechanisms. As summarized in Fig. 15, ACh-mediated relaxation is initiated by ACh interacting with distinct muscarinic receptors located on the endothelial cells. This interaction of ACh with these receptors stimulates the release of an unknown mediator, which appears to act directly on VSM to stimulate relaxation by an ouabain- and high-potassium-inhibitable mechanism. This mechanism appears to be related to the electrogenic sodium pump (Hendrickx and Casteels, 1974). Contraction appears to be related to a direct effect of ACh on the smooth muscle cells of mesenteric veins as well as by an indirect effect mediated through mesenteric vein EDF. These two actions appear to promote an increase in membrane permeability to extracellular calcium ion, as well as a mobilization of intracellular bound calcium. The nature of the EDF mediating VSM relaxation and contraction remains to be elucidated.

I. Adenosine and Nucleotides

Adenosine, ATP, AMP, and ADP relax arterioles, precapillary sphincters, and venules *in vivo*. The magnitude of relaxation depends on the level of VSM tone and follows the order arterioles > precapillary sphincters > venules. Adenosine may arise from the circulation or from tissues surrounding the vasculature during hypoxia, ischemia, or work (for references see Berne *et al.*, 1974; Berne and Rubio, 1974; Rubio and Berne, 1975; Rubio *et al.*, 1975).

The synthesis and degradation of adenosine are described above. Briefly, adenosine is taken up by endothelial cells. This action is inhibited by dipyridamole, a coronary and peripheral vasodilator. The enzyme involved in the degradation of adenine nucleotides, 5'-nucleotidase, is abundant along the luminal surface of endothelial cells primarily in association with caveolae and/or pinocytotic vesicles (Smith and Ryan, 1970, 1971; Ryan and Smith, 1971a,b). Adenosine diphosphate is degraded to

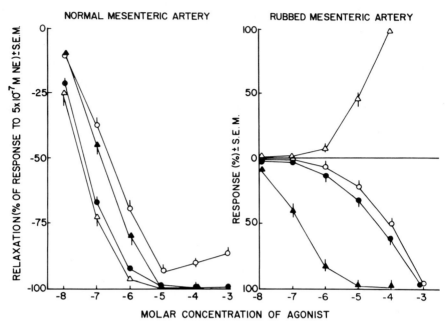

Fig. 22. Effect of endothelial rubbing on vascular relaxation of mesenteric arteries to ACh (△), adenosine (●), ATP (○), and isoproterenol (▲).

AMP, which in turn is metabolized to adenosine and inosine. The adenosine is taken up into the endothelial cell and resynthesized to ADP and ATP. Large arteries relax in response to adenosine and other nucleotides, as do the perfused vascular beds. Frohlich (1962) suggested that the relaxation in response to ATP and other nucleotides was dependent on their capacity to chelate calcium ion. The responses of large arteries to adenosine and other nucleotides appear to be independent of the endothelium, whereas small mesenteric arteries relax in response to adenosine and ATP, and destruction of the endothelium inhibits, but does not abolish, the relaxation (Fig. 22).

Adenine nucleotides produce biphasic effects on many VSM preparations. This is dependent on both the nucleotide under study and the level of VSM tone. Adenosine diphosphate and ATP contract isolated and intact arteries and veins, whereas high concentrations of adenosine enhance the excitatory activity of spontaneously active VSM (Furchgott, 1966; Somlyo and Somlyo, 1968, 1970; Shepherd and Vanhoutte, 1975; Walter and Bassenge, 1968; Sjoberg and Wahlstrom, 1975). The mechanism of the contraction can be explained by an increased permeability to calcium ion (Sjoberg and Wahlstrom, 1975), an increased ATP concentration, and perhaps an ionophoric action of the nucleotide transporting calcium ion across the cell. The vasodilator and relaxant actions in response to adenosine are greater than those to AMP > ATP > ADP (Walter and Bassenge, 1968; Somlyo and Somlyo, 1968, 1970; Norton *et al.*, 1972; Toda, 1974; Schnaar and Sparks, 1972; Verhaege *et al.*, 1977; Vanhoutte, 1978). The mechanism of the vasodilation produced by these nucleotides seems to be related to an increase in cellular calcium binding, which may result from a direct effect of the adenosine or an indirect effect caused by endothelial-derived relaxing factor, or it may be related to a prostanoid that may be released by adenosine. The vasodilating action of adenosine does not appear to result from its conversion to cyclic AMP. The magnitude and duration of action of adenosine depend on the degree of endothelial competency, the integrity of the transport and metabolizing systems, and the degree of uptake by the VSM (Berne and Rubio, 1974; Rubio and Berne, 1975). Adenosine and other nucleotides may modulate the level of VSM tone both directly and indirectly by altering neurotransmitter release (see Section II,B; for references see Vanhoutte, 1978, 1980).

Adenosine and adenine nucleotides have been implicated in the reactive hyperemia of working skeletal muscle, as well as the cerebral and coronary circulation following occlusion or ischemia (for references see Berne and Rubio, 1974; Rubio and Berne, 1975). Adenosine and other nucleotides are released from ischemic tissue and possibly from purinergic nerves. It has been suggested that adenosine and ATP may either alone, or as comodulators, mediate the cerebral and coronary vascular responses to hypoxia (Berne *et al.*, 1974, Rubio *et al.*, 1975) as well as pulmonary hypoxic vasoconstriction (Mentzer *et al.*, 1975). The question as to which of the mediators are involved is beyond the scope of this discussion and remains to be resolved (for references see Vanhoutte, 1978, 1980). However, if hypoxia damages the vascular endothelium and prevents the uptake and degradation of adenosine, then the amounts of adenosine and other nucleotides released by ischemic insults may modulate microcirculatory function.

J. Anesthetics and Alcohols

The effect of anesthetics and alcohols on the microcirculation has been covered extensively, and the interested reader is referred to Altura 1976, 1978a,b, 1981, 1982), and Longnecker and Harris (1980). Briefly, arterioles, precapillary sphincters, and venules relax in response to ethanol. The sensitivity to the vasodilator action of ethanol is equivalent in arterioles and venules, but the arterioles respond with a greater maximal in-

TABLE IX

Influence of Topical Anesthetic Agents on Arteriolar and Venular Diameters in Rat Mesentery[a]

	Microvessel	
Anesthetic	Arterioles	Muscular venules
Pentobarbital (10^{-4}–10^{-5} M)	Vasodilation	Vasodilation
Amobarbital (10^{-4}–10^{-5} M)	Vasodilation	Vasodilation
Ethanol (0.1–1%)	Vasodilation	Vasodilation
Procaine (100–1000 μg)	Vasodilation	0^b
Lidocaine (100–500 μg)	Vasodilation	0^b

[a] All animals were anesthetized with ketamine hydrochloride. Taken from data presented in Altura (1967), B. T. Altura and Altura (1978), and Altura *et al.* (1976, 1979).
[b] Signifies no effect.

crease in diameter. This is to be expected since the arterioles constrict more than the venules (Altura and Hershey, 1967; Altura, 1971a,b; Altura and Altura, 1974a; Altura *et al.,* 1979; Miller and Weigman, 1977; Longnecker and Harris, 1980; Fig. 23, Table IX). General and local anesthetics as well as barbiturate depressants affect microcirculatory function by depressing the vascular responses to vasoactive agents and by relaxing the VSM. Barbiturates and ethanol affect both arteries and veins but, according to Altura, lidocaine and procaine do not affect muscular venules (Altura, 1981). However, Tanaka *et al.* (1982a,b) showed that lidocaine inhibited adrenergic neurotransmission and relaxed small mesenteric veins *in vitro.* For the inhibitory effect on adrenergic neurotransmission 10^{-5} M of lidocaine was required, whereas 10^{-4} M lidocaine was required to inhibit or relax VSM contracted with NE or prostanoids. However, at higher concentrations lidocaine contracted the veins and, to a lesser extent, the arteries. Thus, the high concentrations (500 μg topically) of lidocaine used in topical application studies may mask the venodilator effects of lower concentrations. Alternatively, tone may have to be induced in the veins to unmask the relaxant response to local anesthetics.

The mechanism by which local and general anesthetics relax smooth muscle and inhibit microvascular responses to vasoactive agents remains obscure. Anesthetics may inhibit sodium channels to delay or block sodium conductance, and thereby calcium conductance, in VSM. Alternatively, anesthetics may interact with magnesium ion to enhance magnesium binding to the VSM cell, thereby decreasing calcium influx and suppressing reactivity. Finally, anesthetics may interfere with calcium release from sarcoplasmic reticulum and mitochondria or may substitute for

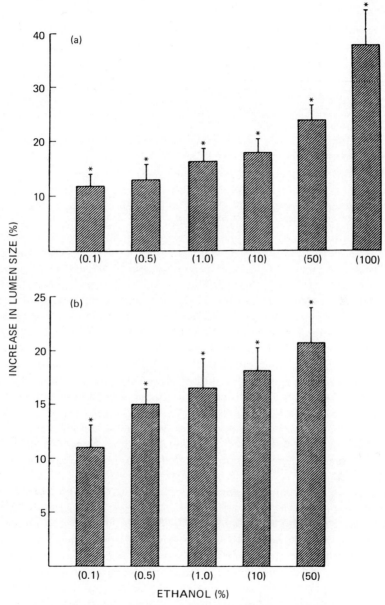

Fig. 23. Effect of ethanol on arteriolar (a) and venular (b) diameter. ▨, Ethanol; *, significantly different from control ($P < 0.02$). (From Altura, 1978, 1981, with permission.)

calcium ion on the VSM membrane, thereby preventing contraction and/or excitation. Further studies are necessary to evaluate the mechanism of anesthetic suppression of microvascular function (for references see Altura, 1981; Longnecker and Harris, 1980).

K. Antihypertensive Vasodilator Compounds

Thiazide diuretics lower blood pressure by a mechanism unrelated to the saliuretic or natriuretic action of thiazide. These diuretics depress both arteriolar and venular reactivity and tone after chronic administration, but acutely do not dilate VSM. Several mechanisms have been invoked to explain the antihypertensive actions of the thiazide diuretics. Thiazide diuretics may decrease the reactivity of the VSM by both inhibiting the release of neurotransmitter and desensitizing the postsynaptic receptors for NE, angiotensin II, and other vasoactive agents to their respective agonists. Evidence for this is derived from studies which show that thiazides inhibit the release of NE from adrenergic nerves and depress VSM responses to NE. Moreover, thiazides suppress the mobilization of calcium ion in VSM obtained from both animals and man. An inability of agonists to release calcium ion from within the cell or an exaggerated accumulation of calcium within the cell, after increased calcium entry from external pools of calcium ion, could diminish the magnitude of the subsequent contraction to vasoactive agents, despite the presence of an adequate stimulus and excitation contraction–coupling mechanism. Finally, the studies of Webster and Dollery (1981) and Watkins et al. (1980) suggest that thiazides may stimulate the formation of prostacyclin by the VSM or endothelium which modulates the level of vascular tone produced by the thiazides. The mechanism of action of these compounds remains to be resolved.

Both hydralazine and minoxidil are directly acting vasodilators that preferentially affect arteriolar versus venular tone. The mechanism of action of both compounds is unclear. Both drugs are considered together here since minoxidil appears to be a relative of hydralazine. Hydralazine and minoxidil reduce arterial pressure to equivalent levels (for references see Greenberg, 1980). However, hydralazine depresses vascular reactivity and responses to vasoactive agents, whereas minoxidil is devoid of this action. Thus, it is unlikely that suppression of VSM responsiveness in vitro accounts for the arterial smooth muscle effects of these compounds. Greenberg et al. (1980) and Pang and Sutter (1981) administered hydralazine and minoxidil chronically to spontaneously hypertensive rats (SHR) and found that despite equivalent reductions in pressure, minoxidil did not inhibit VSM tone or responses to vasoactive agents. Pang and Sutter (1981) showed that the action of hydralazine was independent of the calcium ion concentration. Thus, these effects of minoxidil and hydralazine on arterial pressure clearly seem unrelated to their incidental effects on vascular reactivity. Haeusler and Gerold (1978) measured an increase in PGE-like material after acute administration of these agents to dogs. Greenwalt *et al.* (1980) and Greenberg *et al.* (1982c) showed that hydralazine inhibited thromboxane A_2 generation in both the platelet and VSM, respectively. However, minoxidil was devoid of this action (Greenberg *et al.*, 1982a,b). Thus, although these drugs may inhibit prostanoid constrictor mechanisms, the relation to their antihypertensive action remains to be elucidated. It must be pointed out that minoxidil does not affect VSM tone unless it passes through the mesenteric–hepatic circulation (Ducharme, personal communication). It is possible that minoxidil forms a labile, hydroperoxide intermediate that affects the synthesis of leukotrienes or other lipid peroxides. Further studies are required to test this hypothesis.

Captopril is an angiotensin-converting enzyme inhibitor that inhibits the conversion of angiotensin I to angiotensin II and prevents the breakdown of bradykinin (Ondetti *et al.*, 1977). This drug decreases arteriolar and venular tone and lowers total peripheral resistance in patients with low, normal, or high renin hypertension (Bengis *et al.*, 1978; Brunner *et al.*, 1980; Gavras *et al.*, 1978; Swartz *et al.*, 1979, 1980; Williams and Hollenberg, 1977). However, the antihypertensive effect is due to factors other than its capacity simply to decrease angiotensin II or stimulate bradykinin accumulation. Bradykinin itself stimulates prostaglandin synthesis (McGiff *et al.*, 1972; Blumberg *et al.*, 1977). Captopril also stimulates prostaglandin and/or prostacyclin formation in VSM and the central nervous system (Dusting *et al.*, 1980; Swartz *et al.*, 1980), which may modulate the decrease in vascular resistance in hypertensive animals and man. Moreover, captopril can directly depress VSM function independent of its prostanoid-stimulating action. Each of these mechanisms may contribute to the antihypertensive and vasodilating effects of captopril.

Nitroprusside is believed to lower arteriolar and venular smooth muscle tone by effecting an increase in cyclic GMP in the VSM. This effect is independent of calcium ion and occurs in broken-cell preparations. Methylene blue inhibits nitroprusside-induced relaxation and the accumulation of cyclic GMP (Kukovetz *et al.*, 1981; Gruetter *et al.*, 1979). Moreover, drugs that inhibit phosphodiesterase potentiate the relaxant effects of nitroprusside (Kukovetz *et al.*, 1979a,b). The reported effects of nitroprusside and other compounds were not related to an increase in cellular calcium ion because (*a*) these compounds increased calcium efflux from VSM without increasing calcium influx (Zsoster *et al.*, 1977); (*b*) in the absence of extracellular calcium ion, nitrates and nitroprusside decreased calcium efflux from rabbit renal arteries and inhibited KCl-induced contraction, indicating that calcium sequestration was enhanced (Hester *et al.*, 1979); and (*c*) nitrites and nitroprusside do not inhibit directly calcium sequestration by sarcoplasmic reticulum from rabbit aorta (Thorens and Haeusler, 1979). Thus, although the evidence is at best circuitous and circumstantial, it is possible that nitroprusside stimulates cyclic GMP in VSM and that cyclic GMP regulates VSM relaxation by stimulating calcium sequestration by sarcoplasmic reticulum or enhancing calcium extrusion from the VSM cell (Fig. 17).

Diazoxide is a potent antihypertensive agent that relaxes arterial and venous smooth muscle when given by intravenous bolus injection. Because of its high capacity for binding to plasma proteins and the lack of control of the actions of the drug, once administered, its value in the treatment of hypertension is declining as newer drugs, such as minoxidil and the calcium-channel-blocking agents, are developed. The mechanism of this nondiuretic thiazide congener. This compound, like thiazides, depresses VSM reactivity and contractility (Wohl *et al.*, 1967, 1968a,b; McNeil *et al.*, 1969; Rhodes and Sutter, 1971; Janis and Triggle, 1973). Wohl *et al.* (1967) postulated that diazoxide may compete with calcium ion at a membrane site regulating the entry of this divalent ion. This was substantiated by Janis and Triggle (1973), but these investigators found that the competition was noncompetitive rather than competitive. In view of these findings and those of Rhodes and Sutter (1971), who also did not find competitive antagonism of potassium-depolarized portal vein with diazoxide, the postulate arose that diazoxide acted on a membrane-potential-dependent component of the excitation–contraction coupling mechanism. Although diazoxide increases cyclic AMP in VSM, it does not relax uterus by stimulating an increase in cyclic AMP (Polacek *et al.*, 1970; Tabachnik and Gulbekian, 1968). This finding and that of Wohl *et al.* (1968a) and Janis and Triggle (1973) that diazoxide is more effective in VSM from hypertensive than in VSM from normotensive animals suggested that diazoxide acts at a site of membrane derangement in VSM. In view of current knowledge this site may be the voltage-dependent calcium channel of VSM.

The newest class of antihypertensive agents affecting VSM tone consists of the calcium-channel-blocking agents (for references see Weiss, 1981a). These drugs are believed to lower arteriolar and venular vascular resistance, with greater effects on the arterioles than venules, by inhibiting both voltage-dependent and voltage-independent calcium channels in VSM (see Section II,H).

L. Peripheral Vasodilators

The nitrates (amyl nitrate, nitroglycerin, and organic nitrite compounds) are believed to act in a manner analogous to that of nitroprusside. The nitrite compounds affect arterial smooth muscle tone in lower concentrations than that required to affect arteriolar and/or venular smooth muscle tone (Schnaar and Sparks, 1972). The relaxation in response to nitroglycerin and other nitrates is believed to be mediated by an increase in cyclic GMP (for references and mechanism see Section III,K). The nitrites produce tachyphyllaxis with continued administration. Needleman and Johnson (1973) and Needleman *et al.* (1973a,b) showed that tolerance to nitrites could be prevented by dithiothreitol, a sulfide-protecting agent, and enhanced by furosemide, which alkylates sulfhydryl groups. They suggested that relaxation and tolerance depend on the interaction of nitrates and nitrites with sulfhydryl groups on the cell membrane. Fertel (1982) showed that tolerance to nitrites was associated with a capacity to stimulate cyclic GMP formation in VSM. Thus, it is possible that nitrites and nitrates stimulate guanylate cyclase through a sulhydryl-dependent receptor and that tolerance results from desensitization of the receptor and an inability to stimulate guanylate cyclase.

Dipyridamole is an arteriolar vasodilator with little effect on venous smooth muscle. This compound inhibits phosphorylation of adenosine by a direct mechanism and by inhibiting its uptake into endothelium and smooth muscle. It also interferes with phosphodiesterase, thus increasing the accumulation of cyclic AMP, and potentiates the action of prostacyclin on VSM, as well as stimulates prostacyclin production by VSM (McElroy and Philip, 1975; Masotii *et al.,* 1979; Philip and Lemeuix, 1969; Moncada and Korbut, 1978). The mechanism of its action remains to be defined.

Cetiedil is an effective new therapeutic modality for alleviating the pain and constriction associated with vasospastic disorders such as Raynauds' phenomenon (Haring *et al.,* 1980; Simaan and Aviado, 1976; Barbe *et al.,* 1980) and sickle cell disease (Asakura *et al.,* 1980; Berkowitz and Orringer, 1981; Glenn *et al.,* 1982). Cetiedil, in concentrations between 50 and 200 μmol/liter, has been found to reverse the sickling of the erythrocyte membrane obtained from patients with sickle cell disease (Asakura *et al.,* 1980), to inhibit the binding of calcium ion to calmodulin obtained from erythrocytes (E. P. Orringer, unpublished), to inhibit methacholine-induced bronchoconstriction in adult man suffering from asthma (Cho *et al.,* 1979), and to act as a nonspecific smooth muscle depressant and vasodilator (Boissier *et al.,* 1980; Simaan and Aviado, 1976). Despite the efficacy of cetiedil in alleviating the vasospasm and pain associated with the aforementioned vasospastic disorders, little is known about the effects of cetiedil on adrenergic neuroeffector mechanisms in vascular smooth muscle.

The actions of cetiedil in producing both relaxation and inhibition of NE- and KCl-mediated contractions differ from that of the calcium-channel-blocking agent verapamil (Tanaka et al., 1982a,b; Weiss, 1981a,b). Verapamil-induced relaxation of mesenteric arteries and veins is antagonized by increased concentrations of extracellular calcium but not by increasing concentrations of extracellular KCl (Weiss, 1981a,b). Verapamil inhibits the responses to KCl in lower concentration than is required to inhibit the contractile responses to NE (Weiss, 1981a,b; Greenberg et al., 1973a,b; Tanaka et al., 1982a,b). In contrast, cetiedil-induced relaxation of mesenteric arteries and veins is not affected by the concentration of extracellular calcium ion, is inhibited by contracting the muscle with 40 mM KCl, and is reduced by ouabain. Moreover, no significant differences exist in the concentration of cetiedil required to inhibit the contractile responses to NE and KCl (Tanaka et al., 1982a,b; Boissier et al., 1980). Finally, verapamil-induced inhibition of transmural nerve stimulation to VSM is inhibited by elevations in the concentration of extracellular calcium ion, whereas the inhibitory effect of cetiedil on adrenergic neuroeffector transmission to mesenteric arteries and veins is independent of the extracellular calcium ion concentration (Tanaka et al., 1982a,b). These findings support the conclusion that cetiedil is not a calcium-channel-blocking agent similar to verapamil.

It is also unlikely that cetiedil produces relaxation of mesenteric arteries and veins by stimulating the production of a vasodilator material from the vascular endothelium, in a manner similar to that of ACh and adenosine (Furchgott and Zawadski, 1980a,b,c; Furchgott et al., 1981; Greenberg et al., 1982b). This conclusion is based on the findings that (a) endothelial stripping does not affect the responses of the mesenteric arteries and veins to cetiedil but inhibits the relaxant responses to ACh; (b) concentrations of ETYA and NDGA that act as specific (relatively) inhibitors of lipoxygenase in other cells (Bray et al., 1980; Tappel et al., 1953; Volpi et al., 1980) do not inhibit cetiedil-induced relaxation of mesenteric arteries or veins; and (c) in concentrations that do not relax MA and MV, cetiedil inhibits the relaxant and contractile responses of the mesenteric arteries and veins to ACh (Greenberg et al., 1982b; Cho et al., 1979; Simaan and Aviado, 1976). It can be argued that cetiedil may act directly on the VSM, in a manner similar to that of the mediator released by ACh, to stimulate the production of cyclic GMP within the VSM cell (Furchgott et *al.*, 1981) and thereby promote relaxation of the mesenteric arteries and veins. Evidence in support of this argument is that, in high concentrations, ETYA and NDGA (unpublished) inhibit cetiedil-induced relaxation and the accumulation of cyclic GMP (Spies *et al.*, 1980). Moreover, cetiedil inhibits cyclic nucleotide phosphodiesterase in rat thoracic aortas (Boissier *et al.*, 1980). However, the concentrations of ETYA and NDGA that inhibit the responses to cetiedil also depress the responses of the mesenteric arteries and veins to NE, KCl, verapamil, and ACh, suggesting a nonspecific effect of these inhibitors on the integrity of the muscle. The capacity of cetiedil to inhibit phosphodiesterase occurs with concentrations of cetiedil in excess of 1 mM, much greater than that required to produce relaxation (Boissier *et al.*, 1980). Therefore, it is unlikely that cetiedil-induced increases in cyclic GMP can explain the mechanism of cetiedil-induced relaxation of mesenteric arteries and veins.

It is also unlikely that cetiedil relaxes VSM by suppressing the mobilization of calcium ion within the cell. A previous study demonstrated that small canine mesenteric veins were more dependent on the mobilization of intracellular calcium ion to sustain NE-induced tone than were the mesenteric arteries (Greenberg *et al.*, 1973a,b). KCl-induced contraction of mesenteric arteries and veins is dependent on an extracellular source of calcium ion and not on calcium mobilization within the cell (Bohr *et al.*, 1978; Bohr, 1973). If cetiedil acted to suppress calcium mobilization within the cell, then it would be highly unlikely that KCl-induced contracture would be suppressed by cetiedil. Moreover, a differential sensitivity of the mesenteric arteries and veins to cetiedil would exist, and no such evidence has been found.

Both high concentrations of KCl and concentrations of ouabain sufficient to inhibit the (sodium–potassium)-dependent, magnesium-activated ADPase activity of canine VSM (Jones, 1980) produce equivalent ($P > 0.05$) inhibition of cetiedil-induced relaxation of canine mesenteric VSM. Both of these interventions inhibit the sodium–potassium pumping mechanism. This would indirectly suggest that cetiedil may act to promote relaxation of mesenteric arteries and veins by stimulating a (sodium–potassium)-dependent electrogenic sodium transport mechanism and promoting potassium entry into the cell. Moreover, cetiedil did not relax canine mesenteric arteries and veins in PSS deficient in KCl. Potassium-deficient solutions inhibit the electrogenic sodium pump mechanism in VSM and thereby inhibit relaxation dependent on this mechanism (Webb *et al.*, 1981; Haddy, 1978; Jones, 1980). The greater inhibitory of KCl-deficient solution on cetiedil-induced relaxation of mesenteric arteries and veins may occur because cetiedil can overcome the block of the pump mechanism caused by high KCl and ouabain concentrations. However, in potassium-free PSS, there is an absolute deficiency in KCl and thereby an irreversible inhibition of the pump. Further studies are necessary to verify or refute this speculation.

It is also possible that cetiedil may relax canine mesenteric arteries and veins by inhibiting calcium binding to their calcium–calmodulin system. Our studies do not rule out this possibility. A positive correlation exists between the capacity of smooth muscle relaxants such as prenylamine and chlorpromazine to inhibit calcium binding to calmodulin and to promote relaxation of skinned smooth muscle (Cassidy *et al.*, 1980) as well as between the capacity of these drugs to bind to calmodulin, inhibit phosphorylation of myosin light-chain kinase, and promote relaxation of intact VSM *in vitro* (Hidaka *et al.*, 1979). Cetiedil (in concentrations greater than $5 \times 10^{-5} M$) inhibits the binding of calcium to calmodulin (E. P. Orringer, unpublished) and KCl-mediated calcium accumulation in erythrocytes (Berkowitz and Orringer, 1981). Further studies measuring the calcium-binding capacity of the VSM calmodulin obtained from cetiedil-treated animals are necessary to refute or verify the possibility that calmodulin is involved in the VSM relaxant action of cetiedil.

IV. Directions for Future Research

The mechanism of physiologic and pharmacologic control of microvascular VSM function has been ascertained by inference from the events that occur in larger vessels. Whether this is valid remains to be elucidated. Studies are required which will assess the capacity of microvessels to synthesize vasoactive compounds, relax in response to known stimulants of discreet metabolic pathways, and respond to specific calcium-channel-blocking agents. Moreover, microperfusion studies are required in which the effect of vasoactive agents on ion fluxes, metabolism, and prostanoid synthesis and release *in vivo* can be defined. In addition, studies in which physiologic humoral agents and pharmacologic moieties are administered *in vivo,* rather than topically, should be performed to ascertain the site of action of drugs under conditions of actual hemodynamic efficacy. Finally, studies of microvascular biochemistry are needed to elucidate the role of endothelium and smooth muscle mechanisms in microvascular function. With the current incipient stages of microvessel research, it is hoped that some of the questions raised in this review will find answers and provide new directions for the treatment of aberrant vascular function in pathologic disease states.

Acknowledgments

The authors' research was supported in part by grants HL 22216 and RCDAHL7K04-00428 from the National Heart, Lung, and Blood Institute. S. Greenberg was a recipient of Research Career Development Award 7-K04 HL00428 from the Hypertension Branch of the National Institutes of Health.

References

Adelstein, R. S. (1978). *Trends Biochem. Sci.* (*Pers. Ed.*) **3**, 27–30.
Adelstein, R. S., and Eisenberg, E. (1980). *Annu. Rev. Biochem.* **49**, 921–956.
Adelstein, R. S., and Klee, C. B. (1980). *In* "Calcium and Cell Function" (W. Y. Cheung, ed.), Vol. 1, pp. 167–182. Academic Press, New York.
Aiken, J. W. (1973). *J. Pharmacol. Exp. Ther.* **184**, 678–687.
Aiken, J. W. (1974). *Pol. J. Pharmacol. Pharm.* **26**, 217–227.
Alexander, R. S. (1968). *Microvasc. Res.* **3**, 3–17.
Alquist, R. P. (1948). *Am. J. Physiol.* **153**, 586–599.
Altura, B. M. (1966a). *Am. J. Physiol.* **211**, 1393–1397.
Altura, B. M. (1966b). *Am. J. Physiol.* **212**, 1447–1454.
Altura, B. M. (1971a). *Microvasc. Res.* **3**, 361–384.
Altura, B. M. (1971b). *Proc. Soc. Exp. Biol. Med.* **138**, 273–276.
Altura, B. M. (1972a). *Microvasc. Res.* **4**, 319
Altura, B. M. (1972b). *Eur. J. Pharmacol.* **19**, 171–179.
Altura, B. M. (1973). *Eur. J. Pharmacol.* **24**, 49–60.
Altura, B. M. (1975a). *J. Pharmacol. Exp. Ther.* **193**, 403–412.
Altura, B. M. (1975b). *Circ. Res.* **36–37** (Suppl. I), 233–240.
Altura, B. M. (1975c). *Am. J. Physiol.* **228**, 1615–1620.
Altura, B. M. (1976). *Artery* (*Fulton, Mich.*) **2**, 18–25.
Altura, B. M. (1977). *Fed. Proc. Fed. Am. Soc. Exp. Biol.* **36**, 1840–1847.
Altura, B. M. (1978a). *Microvasc. Res.* **16**, 91–117.
Altura, B. M. (1978b). *In* "Microcirculation" (G. Kaley and B. M. Altura, eds.), Vol. 2, pp. 431–502. Univ. Park Press, Baltimore, Maryland.
Altura, B. M. (1979). *In* "Current Concepts in Kinin Research" (G. L. Haberland, and U. Hamberg, eds.), pp. 47–55. Pergamon, Oxford.
Altura, B. M. (1981). *In* "Microcirculation, Current Physiologic, Medical and Surgical Concepts" (R. M. Effros, H. Schmid-Shonbein, and J. Ditzel, eds.), pp. 52–105. Academic Press, New York.
Altura, B. M., and Altura, B. T. (1970). *Am. J. Physiol.* **219**, 1698–1705.
Altura, B. M., and Altura, B. T. (1971). *Am. J. Physiol.* **220**, 938–944.
Altura, B. M., and Altura, B. T. (1974a). *Anesthesiology* **41**, 197–214.
Altura, B. M., and Altura, B. T. (1974b). *Microvasc. Res.* **7**, 145–155.
Altura, B. M., and Altura, B. T. (1976). *Fed. Proc. Fed. Am. Soc. Exp. Biol.* **35**, 2360–2366.
Altura, B. M., and Altura, B. T. (1977a). *Fed. Proc. Fed. Am. Soc. Exp. Biol.* **36**, 1853–1860.
Altura, B. M., and Altura, B. T. (1977b). *In* "Excitation–Contraction Coupling in Smooth Muscle" (R. Casteels, T. Godfraind, and J. C. Ruegg, eds.), pp. 137–144. Elsevier, Amsterdam.

Altura, B. M., and Altura, B. T. (1981). *Fed. Proc. Fed. Am. Soc. Exp. Biol.* **39**, 234–241.
Altura, B. M., and Chand, N. (1981). *Br. J. Pharmacol.* **68**, 245–247.
Altura, B. M., and Halevy, S. (1978). *Proc. Natl. Acad. Sci. USA* **75**, 2941–2944.
Altura, B. M., and Hershey, S. G. (1967). *Angiology* **18**, 428–439.
Altura, B. M., Malaviya, D., Reich, C. F., and Orkin, L. R. (1972). *Am. J. Physiol.* **222**, 345–355.
Altura, B. M., Altura, B. T., and Waldemar, Y. (1976). *Artery (Fulton, Mich.)* **2**, 326–336.
Altura, B. M., Ogunkoya, A., and Gebrewold, A., and Altura, B. T. (1979). *J. Cardiovasc. Pharmacol.* **1**, 97–113.
Amer, M. S. (1973). *Science (Washington, D.C.)* **179**, 807–809.
Amer, M. S. (1977). *In* "Cyclic 3'5'-Nucleotides: Mechanism of Action" (H. Kramer and J. Schultz, eds.), pp. 381–396. Wiley, New York.
Amer, M. S., Doba, M., and Reis, D. J. (1974). *Proc. Natl. Acad. Sci. USA,* **72**, 2135–2139.
Amunsden, E. (1976). *In* "Chemistry and Biology of the Kallekrein-Kinin System in Health and Disease" (J. J. Pisano, and K. F. Austen, eds.), pp. 517–524. US Govt. Printing Office, Washington, D.C.
Anderson, D. K. (1976). *Fed. Proc. Fed. Am. Soc. Exp. Biol.* **35**, 1294–1297.
Andersson, R., Lundholm, L., Mohme-Lundholm, E., and Nilsson, K. (1972). *Adv. Cyclic Nucleotide Res.* **1**, 213–230.
Angles-d'Auriac, G., Badouin, M., and Meyer, P. (1972). *Circ. Res.* **31**, (Suppl. II), 151–157.
Apperley, E., Humphrey, P. P. A., and Levey, G. P. (1976). *Br. J. Pharmacol.* **58**, 211–221.
Apperley, E., Humphrey, P. P. A., and Levey, G. P. (1977). *Br. J. Pharmacol.* **61**, 465P
Apperley, E., Humphrey, P. P. A., and Levey, G. P. (1980). *Br. J. Pharmacol.* **58**, 211–221.
Armstrong, J. M. (1982). *In* "Cardiovascular Pharmacology of the Prostaglandins" (A. G. Herman, P. M. Vanhoutte, H. Denolin, and A. Goosens, eds.), pp. 51–64. Raven, New York.
Asakura, T., Ohnishi, S. T., Adachi, K., Oxuc, M., Hashimoto, K., Singer, M., Russell, M. O., and Schwartz, E. (1980). *Proc. Natl. Acad. Sci. USA* **77**, 2955–2959.
Ashton, F. T., Somlyo, A. V., and Somlyo, A. P. (1975). *J. Mol. Biol.* **98**, 17–29.
Axelsson, J., Johansson, B., Jonsson, O., and Wahstrom, B. (1967). *Bibl. Anat.* **8**, 16–20.
Bar, H. P. (1974). *Adv. Cyclic Nucleotide Res.* **54**, 195–238.
Barbe, R., Amiel, M., Pouzeratte, B., Veyre, B., Villard, J., and Grivet, G. (1980). *Clin. Trials J.* **17**, 1–25.
Bartelstone, H. J., and Nasmyth, P. A. (1965). *Am. J. Physiol.* **208**, 754–762.
Baudouin-Legros, M., and Meyer, P. (1973). *Br. J. Pharmacol.* **47**, 377–385.
Baudouin-Legros, M., and Meyer, P., Fermandijan, S., and Morgat, J. (1972). *Nature (London)* **235**, 336–338.
Beck, L., and Brody, M. J. (1961). *Angiology* **12**, 202–221.
Bell, R. L., and Majerius, P. W. (1980). *J. Biol. Chem.* **255**, 1790–1792.
Bell, R. L., and Baenziger, N. L., and Majerius, P. W. (1980). *Prostaglandins* **20**, 269–274.
Belleau, B. (1967). *Ann. N.Y. Acad. Sci.* **139**, 580–605.
Bengis, R. G., Coleman, T. G., Young, D. B., and McCaa, R. E. (1978). *Circ. Res.* **43**, (Suppl. I), 45–53.
Berde, B. (1965). *Oxytocin Res. Proc. Symp.* pp. 11–35.
Berecek, K. H., Stocker, M., and Gross, F. (1980). *Circ. Res.* **46**, 619–624.
Berecek, K. H., Stocker, M., and Gross, G. (1982). *Hypertension (Dallas)* **4**,
Berkowitz, L. R., and Orringer, E. P. (1981). *J. Clin. Invest.* **68**, 1215–1220.

Berkowitz, B. A., Lee, C. H., and Spector, S. (1975). *Clin. Exp. Pharmacol. Physiol.* **1**, 397–400.

Berne, R. M., and Rubio, R. (1974). *Adv. Cardiol.* **12**, 303–317.

Berne, R. M., Rubio, R., and Curnish, R. R. (1974). *Circ. Res.* **35**, 262–271.

Berridge, M. J. (1975). *Adv. Cyclic Nucleotide Res.* **6**, 1–98.

Bertelsen, S., and Pettinger, W. A. (1977). *Life Sci.* **21**, 595–606.

Bevan, J. A. (1982). *In* "Prostaglandins Organ and Tissue Specific Actions" (S. Greenberg, P. J. Kadowitz, and T. F. Burks, eds.), pp. 1–11. Dekker, New York.

Bevan, J. A., and Su, C. (1973). *Annu. Rev. Pharmacol.* **13**, 269–285.

Bevan, J. A., Gartska, W., Su, C., and Su, M. O. (1973). *Eur. J. Pharmacol.* **22**, 47–53.

Bevan, J. A., Bevan, R. D., Chang, P. C., Pegram, B. L., Purdy, R. E., and Su, C. (1975). *Circ. Res.* **37**, 183–198.

Bito, L. Z., and Barody, R. A. (1975). *Prostaglandins* **10**, 633–638.

Black, J. L., French, R. J., and Mylecharane, E. J. (1981). *Br. J. Pharmacol.* **74**, 619–626.

Black, J. W., Duncan, W. A. M., Durant, C. J., Ganellin, C. R., and Parsons, E. M. (1972). *Nature (London)* **236**, 385–390.

Blackwell, G. J., Flower, R. J., Nijkamp, F. P., and Vane, J. R. (1978). *Br. J. Pharmacol.* **62**, 79–89.

Blackwell, G. J., Carnucio, R., DiRosa, M., Flower, R. J., Parente, L., and Perisco, P. (1980). *Nature (London)* **287**, 147–149.

Bloom, D. S., Cole, A. W. G., and Palmer, T. N. (1979). *Br. J. Pharmacol.* **65**, 587–592.

Blumberg, A. L., Denny, S. F., Marshall, G. R., and Needleman, P. (1977). *Am. J. Physiol.* **232**, H305–H310.

Boerth, R. C., Ryan, M. J., and Brody, M. J. (1970). *J. Pharmacol. Exp. Ther.* **172**, 52–61.

Bohlen, P., and Gore, M. B. (1978). *Am. J. Physiol.* **235**, 886–892.

Bohr, D. F. (1973). *Circ. Res.* **32**, 665–672.

Bohr, D. F., and Uchida, E. (1967). *Circ. Res.* **21**, (Suppl. II), 135–143.

Bohr, D. F., Greenberg, S., and Bonacorrsi, A. (1978). *In* "Microcirculation" (G. Kaley and B. Altura, eds.), Vol. 2, pp. 311–348. Univ. Park Press, Baltimore, Maryland.

Boissier, J. R., Aurousseau, M., Guidicelli, J. F., and Duval, D. (1980). *Arzneim. Forsch.* **28**, 2222–2228.

Bonaccorsi, A., Hermsmeyer, K., Aprigliano, O., Smith, C. B., and Bohr, D. F. (1977). *Blood Vessels* **14**, 261–276.

Boxer, L. A., Allen, J. M., Schmidt, M., Yoder, M., and Baehner, R. L. (1980). *J. Lab. Clin. Med.* **95**, 672–678.

Bray, M. A., Ford-Hutchinson, A. W., Shipley, M. E., and Smith, M. J. H. (1980). *Br. J. Pharmacol.* **71**, 507–512.

Brown, M. S., and Goldstein, J. L. (1979). *Proc. Natl. Acad. Sci. USA* **76**, 3330–3337.

Brunner, H. R., Gavras, H., Waeber, B., Turini, G. A., and Wauters, J. P. (1980). *Arch. Int. Pharmacodyn. Ther.* **247**, (Suppl. 2), 188–212.

Burnstock, G. (1976). *Neuroscience* **1**, 239–248.

Carsten, M. E. (1973). *Gynecol. Invest.* **4**, 95–105.

Carsten, M. E. (1974). *Prostaglandins* **5**, 33–40.

Carsten, M. E., and Miller, J. D. (1977). *J. Biol. Chem.* **252**, 2576–2582.

Carsten, M. E., and Miller, J. D. (1978). *Arch. Biochem. Biophys.* **185**, 282–295.

Cassidy, P., Hoar, P. E., and Kerrick, W. G. L. (1980). *Pfleugers Arch.* **387**, 115–120.

Chand, N., and Eyre, P. (1975). *Agents Actions* **5**, 277–295.

Chernukh, A. M., and Timkina, M. I. (1976). *In* "Physiology of Smooth Muscle" (E. Bulbring, and M. F. Shuba, eds.), pp. 403–410. Raven, New York.

Chin, A. K., and Evonuk, E. (1971). *J. Appl. Physiol.* **30**, 205–207.

Cho, Y. W., Han, H. C., Oh, S. Y., and Kuemmerle, H. P. (1979). *Int. J. Tissue React.* **1,** 155–158.

Clement, D., Vanhoutte, P. M., and Leusen, I. (1969). *Arch. Int. Physiol. Biochim.* **77,** 73–87.

Conti, M. A., and Adelstein, R. S. (1980). *Fed. Proc. Fed. Am. Soc. Exp. Biol.* **39,** 1569–1573.

Crain, K. R., and Appleman, M. M. (1978). *Adv. Cyclic Nucleotide Res.* **9,** 221–230.

Curro, F. A., and Greenberg, S. (1982a). *J. Pharmacol. Exp. Ther.*

Curro, F. A., and Greenberg, S. (1982b). *Methods Findings Clin. Exp. Pharmacol. Physiol.* (in press).

Curro, F. A., Greenberg, S., Verbeuren, T., and Vanhoutte, P. M. (1978). *J. Pharmacol. Exp. Ther.* **207,** 936–949.

Dabrowska, R., Aromatorio, D., Sherry, J. M. F., and Hartshorne, D. J. (1978). *Biochemistry* **17,** 253–258.

D'Alecy, L. G., and Feigel, E. (1972). *Circ. Res.* **30,** 214–224.

D'Alecy, L. G., and Rose, C. J. (1977). *Circ. Res.* **41,** 324–331.

DeMey, J. G., and Vanhoutte, P. M. (1978). *Arch. Int. Pharmacodyn. Ther.* **234,** 339 (Abs.)

DeMey, J. G., and Vanhoutte, P. M. (1980a). *Blood Vessels* **17,** 27–40.

DeMey, J. G., and Vanhoutte, P. M. (1980b). *Circ. Res.* **46,** 826–835.

DeMey, J. G., and Vanhoutte, P. M. (1980c). *Eur. J. Pharmacol.* **67,** 159–164.

DeMey, J. G., and Vanhoutte, P. M. (1980d). *Pharmacologist* **22,** 282. (Abs.).

DeMey, J. G., and Vanhoutte, P. M. (1981). *Br. J. Pharmacol.* **72,** 501P. (Abs.).

DeMey, J. G., Burnstock, G., and Vanhoutte, P. M. (1979). *Eur. J. Pharmacol.* **55,** 401–405.

Devlin, T. M. (ed.) (1982). "Textbook of Biochemistry with Clinical Correlations" Wiley, New York.

Devynck, M. A., and Meyer, P. (1976). *Am. J. Med.* **61,** 758–767.

Devynck, M. A., Pernollet, M. G., Meyer, P., Fermandijan, S., Fromageot, P., and Bumpus, M. (1974). *Nature* (*London*) **249,** 67–69.

Diamond, J. (1978). *Adv. Cyclic Nucleotide Res.* **9,** 327–340.

Diamond, J. (1982). *Fed. Proc. Fed. Am. Soc. Exp. Biol.* **41,**

Douglas, W. W. (1975). *In* "The Pharmacological Basis of Therapeutics" (L. S. Goodman and A. Gilman, eds.), pp. 630–652. MacMillan, New York.

Dunham, E. W., Haddox, M. K., and Goldberg, N. D. (1974). *Proc. Natl. Acad. Sci. USA* **71,** 815–819.

Dusting, J. G., Moncada, S., and Vane, J. R. (1978). *Eur. J. Pharmacol.* **49,** 65–72.

Dusting, J. G., Mullins, E. M., and Doyle, A. E. (1980). *Adv. Prostaglandin Thromboxane Res.* **7,** 815–819.

Dyer, D. C., and Gough, E. D. (1971). *Am. J. Obstet. Gynecol.* **111,** 820–825.

Dyer, D. C., Ueland, K., and Eng, M. (1972). *Arch. Int. Pharmacodyn. Ther.* **200,** 213–221.

Ebashi, S., Mikawa, T., Hirata, M., and Nonomura, Y. (1978). *Ann. N.Y. Acad. Sci.* **307,** 451–461.

Edvinsson, L., Hardebo, J. E., and Owman, C. (1978). *Circ. Res.* **42,** 143–151.

Eling, T. E., and Anderson, M. W. (1976). *Agents Actions* **6,** 543–547.

Emmons, P. R., Hampton, J. R., Harrison, M. J. C., Honour, A. J., and Mitchell, R. J. A. (1967). *Br. Med. J.* **2,** 468–472.

Erdos, E. G. (1970). *Handb. Exp. Pharmacol.* **25,**

Estrada, C., and Krause, D. N. (1982). *J. Pharmacol. Exp. Ther.* **221,** 85–90.

Evensen, S. A. (1979). *Haemostasis* **8**, 203–210.

Fertel, R. (1982). *J. Pharmacol. Exp. Ther.*

Fleisch, J. R. (1977). *In* "Factors Influencing Vascular Reactivity" (O. Carrier, and S. Shibata, eds.), pp. 78–95. Igaku-Shoin, Tokyo.

Fleisch, J. H., and Hooker, C. S. (1976). *Circ. Res.* **38**, 243–249.

Fleisch, J. H., Krzan, M. C., and Titus, E. (1973). *Circ. Res.* **33**, 284–290.

Forsling, M. L. (1976). "Anti-Diuretic Hormone." Edan, Montreal.

Freer, R. J. (1977). *Am. J. Physiol.* **232**, 231–239.

Freidman, M. (1973). "Chemistry and Biochemistry of the Sulfhydryl Group in Amino Acids, Peptides and Proteins." Pergamon, New York.

Freyburger, W. A., Graham, B. E., Rapport, M. M., Seay, P. H., Govier, W. N., Swoap, O. F., and Vanderbrook, M. J. (1952). *J. Pharmacol. Exp. Ther.* **101**, 80–86.

Frohlich, E. D. (1962). *Am. J. Physiol.* **203**, 162–166.

Funaki, S. (1961). *Nature (London)* **191**, 1102–1103.

Funaki, S., and Bohr, D. F. (1964). *Nature (London)* **203**, 192–194.

Furchgott, R. F. (1955). *Pharmacol. Rev.* **7**, 183–265.

Furchgott, R. F. (1966). *Bull. N.Y. Acad. Med.* **42**, 996–1006.

Furchgott, R. F., and Zawadski, J. V. (1979). *Pharmacologist* **21**, 271 (Abs.).

Furchgott, R. F., and Zawadski, J. V. (1980a). *Fed. Proc. Fed. Am. Soc. Exp. Biol.* **39**, 581 (Abs.).

Furchgott, R. F., and Zawadski, J. V. (1980b). *Nature (London)* **288**, 373–376.

Furchgott, R. F., and Zawadski, J. V. (1980c). *Pharmacologist* **22**, 271 (Abs.).

Furchgott, R. F., Zawadski, J. V., and Cherry, P. D. (1981). *In* "Vasodilation" (P. M. Vanhoutte, and I. Leusen, eds.), pp. 49–66. Raven, New York.

Furness, J. B., and Marshall, J. M. (1974). *J. Physiol. (London)* **239**, 75–88.

Gabella, G. (1981). *In* "Smooth Muscle: An Assessment of Current Knowledge" (E. Bulbring, A. F. Brading, A. W. Jones, and T. Tomita, eds.), pp. 1–46. Univ. of Texas Press, Austin.

Gavras, H., Brunner, H. R., Turini, G. A., Kershaw, G. R., Tifft, C. P., Cuttlelod, S., Gavras, I., Vukovich, R. A., and McKinstry, D. N. (1978). *N. Engl. J. Med.* **298**, 991–995.

Gellai, M., Norton, J. M., and Detar, R. (1973). *Circ. Res.* **32**, 279–289.

Gerritsen, M. (1982). *Fed. Proc. Fed. Am. Soc. Exp. Biol.* **41**, 879 (Abs.).

Glenn, T. M., Sakane, Y., and Cho, Y. W. (1982). *J. Clin. Pharmacol.*

Gluck, E. V., and Paul, R. J. (1977). *Pfleugers Arch.* **370**, 9–18.

Goldberg, M. R., Joiner, P. D., Greenberg, S., Hyman, A. L., and Kadowitz, P. J. (1975a). *Prostaglandins* **9**, 385–390.

Goldberg, M. R., Kadowitz, P. J., and Greenberg, S. (1975b). *Pharmacologist* **17**, 221 (Abs.).

Goldberg, M. R., Chapnick, B. M., Joiner, P. D., Hyman, A. L., and Kadowitz, P. J. (1976). *J. Pharmacol. Exp. Ther.* **198**, 357–365.

Goldberg, N. D., Haddox, M. K., Hartle, D. K., and Hadden, J. W. (1973). *In* "Pharmacology and the Future of Man: Proceedings of the 5th International Conference on Pharmacology" (R. A. Maxwell, and G. H. Acheson, eds.), pp. 149–169. Karger, Basle.

Goldberg, N. D., Graff, G., Haddox, M. K., Stephenson, J. H., Glass, D. B., and Moser, M. E. (1978). *Adv. Cyclic Nucleotide Res.* **9**, 101–130.

Goldstein, S., and Zsoster, T. T. (1978). *Br. J. Pharmacol.* **62**, 507–514.

Golenhofen, K., and Lammel, E. (1972). *Pflugers Arch.* **331**, 233–243.

Golenhofen, K., Hermstein, N., and Lammel, E. (1973). *Microvasc. Res.* **5**, 73–80.

Gorman, R. R. (1982). *In* "Prostaglandins: Cardiovascular and Cardiopulmonary Actions" (S. Greenberg, and T. M. Glenn, eds.). Academic Press, New York.

Gorman, R. R., Bunting, S., and Miller, O. V. (1977). *Prostaglandins* **13**, 377–388.

Gorog, P., and Kovacs, I. B. (1972). *Biochem. Pharmacol.* **21**, 1713–1723.

Greenbaum, L. M. (1976). *In* "Chemistry and Biology of the Kallekrein-Kinin System in Health and Disease" (J. J. Pisano, and K. F. Austen, eds.), pp. 455–462. U.S. Govt. Printing Office, Washington, D.C.

Greenberg, S. (1980). *J. Pharmacol. Exp. Ther.* **215**, 279–286.

Greenberg, S. (1981a). *Am. J. Physiol.* **242**, H525–H538.

Greenberg, S. (1981b). *Circ. Res.* **48**, 895–906.

Greenberg, S. (1981c). *J. Pharmacol. Exp. Ther.* **219**, 326–337.

Greenberg, S. (1981d). *J. Pharmacol. Exp. Ther.* **219**, 279–292.

Greenberg, S. (1982a). *In* "Prostaglandins: Tissue and Organ Specific Actions" (S. Greenberg, P. J. Kadowitz, and T. F. Burks, eds.). Dekker, New York.

Greenberg, S. (1982b). *In* "Prostaglandins: Cardiovascular and Cardiopulmonary Actions" (S. Greenberg, and T. M. Glenn, eds.). Academic Press, New York.

Greenberg, S., and Bohr, D. F. (1975). *Circ. Res. Suppl.* **36**, 213–218.

Greenberg, S., and Curro, F. A. (1982a). *Hypertension (Dallas)* (in press).

Greenberg, S., and Curro, F. A. (1982b). *Circ. Res.* (in press).

Greenberg, S., and Kadowitz, P. J. (1982). *Methods Find. Exp. Clin. Pharmacol.* **4**, 7–24.

Greenberg, S., and Wilborn, W. M. (1982). *Arch. Int. Pharmacodyn. Ther.* (in press).

Greenberg, S., Wilson, W. R., and Long, J. P. (1973a). *Arch. Int. Pharmacodyn. Ther.* **206**, 213–228.

Greenberg, S., Diecke, F. P. J., and Long, J. P. (1973b). *J. Pharmacol. Exp. Ther.* **185**, 493–503.

Greenberg, S., Heitz, D. C., Brody, M. J., Diecke, F. P. J., Wilson, W. R., and Long, J. P. (1974a). *J. Pharmacol. Exp. Ther.* **191**, 458–467.

Greenberg, S., Heitz, D., and Long, J. P. (1974b). *Can. J. Physiol. Pharmacol.* **52**, 649–650.

Greenberg, S., Englebrecht, J., Howard, L., and Long, J. P. (1974c). *Prostaglandins* **5**, 49–61.

Greenberg, S., Kadowitz, P. J., Diecke, F. P. J., and Long, J. P. (1974d). *Proc. Soc. Exp. Biol. Med.* **143**, 1008–1013.

Greenberg, S., Kadowitz, P. J., Long, J. P., and Wilson, W. R. (1976). *Circ. Res.* **39**, 66–76.

Greenberg, S., Palmer, E. C., Palmer, S. J., and Wilborn, W. (1978). *Clin. Sci. Molec. Med.* **51**, 31–36.

Greenberg, S., Glenn, T. M., Eddy, L. J., and Rebert, R. R. (1980). *Adv. Shock Res.* **3**, 238–263.

Greenberg, S., Glenn, T. M., and McGowan, C. (1981a). *Am. J. Physiol.* H528–H535.

Greenberg, S., Gaines, K., and Sweatt, D. (1981b). *Am. J. Physiol.* H343–H352.

Greenberg, S., Kadowitz, P. J., Hyman, A. L., and Curro, F. A. (1981a). *Am. J. Physiol.* **9**, 274–285.

Greenberg, S., McGowan, C., and Gaida, M. M. (1982a). *Clin. Exp. Hypertens.* (in press).

Greenberg, S., McGowan, C., and Gaida, M. M. (1982b). *Can. J. Physiol. Pharmacol.* (in press).

Greenberg, S., Tanaka, T. P., and Peevey, K. (1982c). *Proc. Soc. Exp. Biol. Med.* (in press).

Greenberg, S., Tanaka, T. P., Peevey, K., and Blackburn, W. (1982b). *Circ. Res.* (in press).

Greenberg, S., Gaines, K., and Glenn, T. M. (1982e). *Proc. Symp. Hydroxamic Acids Biol.* (in press).

Greenwalt, J. E., Wong, L. K., Alexander, M., and Bianchine, J. R. (1980). *Adv. Prostaglandin Thromboxane Res.* **6**, 293–296.

Gross, F. (1976). *Handb. Exp. Pharmacol.* **35**, 378–456.

Gruetter, C. A., Barry, B. K., McNamara, D. B., Gruetter, D. Y., Kadowitz, P. J., and Ignarro, L. J. (1979). *J. Cyclic Nucleotide Res.* **5**, 211–224.

Guignard, J. P., and Friedman, S. (1970). *Circ. Res.* **27**, 505–512.

Gyermek, L. (1966). *Handb. Exp. Pharmacol.* **19**, 471–528.

Haddy, F. J. (1978). *In* "Mechanisms of Vasodilation" (P. M. Vanhoutte, and I. Leusen, eds.), pp. 200–205. Karger, Basel.

Haddy, F. J., and Scott, J. B. (1968). *Physiol. Rev.* **48**, 688–707.

Haddy, F. J., and Scott, J. B. (1975). *Fed. Proc. Fed. Am. Soc. Exp. Biol.* **34**, 2006–2011.

Haddy, F. J., Gordon, P., and Emmanuel, D. (1959). *Circ. Res.* **7**, 123–130.

Haeusler, G. (1972). *J. Pharmacol. Exp. Ther.* **180**, 672–682.

Haeusler, G. (1973). *Experientia* **29**, 762–763.

Haeusler, G., and Gerold, M. (1978). *Proc. Int. Congr. Pharmacol. 7th*, p. 806. (Abs).

Haeusler, G., and Thorens, S. (1980a). *J. Physiol. (London)* **303**, 203–224.

Haeusler, G., and Thorens, S. (1980b). *J. Physiol. (London)* **303**, 225–241.

Hagen, I. H., and White, R. L. (1978). *Stroke* **4**, 68–71.

Hamberg, M., Svensson, J., Wakabayashi, T., and Samuelsson, B. (1974). *Proc. Natl. Acad. Sci. USA* **71**, 345–349.

Haring, J., Mesangeau, D., Huet, Y., and Aurousseau, M. (1980). *Int. J. Clin. Pharmacol. Ther. Toxicol.* **18**, 467–481.

Harkness, H., and Brody, M. J. (1967). *Am. J. Physiol.* **213**, 424–428.

Hedquist, P. (1977). *Annu. Rev. Pharmacol. Toxicol.* **17**, 259–279.

Heistad, D. D., and Marcus, M. L. (1978). *Circ. Res.* **42**, 295–302.

Heitz, D. C., and Brody, M. J. (1975). *Am. J. Physiol.* **228**, 1351–1357.

Hellstrand, P., and Paul, R. J. (1980). *Physiologist* **23**, 95 (Abs.).

Hellstrand, P., and Paul, R. J. (1982). *In* "Vascular Smooth Muscle: Metabolic, Ionic and Contractile Mechanisms" (M. F. Crass, and C. D. Barnes, eds.), pp. 1–35. Academic Press, New York.

Henderson, R. M. (1975). *In* "Methods in Pharmacology" (E. E. Daniel, and D. M. Paton, eds.), Vol. 3, pp. 47–77. Plenum, New York.

Hendrickx, H., and Casteels, R. (1974). *Pfluegers Arch.* **346**, 299–306.

Hester, R. K., Weiss, G. B., and Fry, W. Y. (1979). *J. Pharmacol. Exp. Ther.* **208**, 155–160.

Heymann, M. A. (1980). "Prostaglandins in the Perinatal Period." Grune & Stratton, New York.

Hidaka, H., and Asano, T. (1977). *Proc. Natl. Acad. Sci. USA* **74**, 3657–3661.

Hidaka, H., Yamaki, T., Tatsuka, T., and Asano, M. (1979). *Mol. Pharmacol.* **15**, 49–59.

Higgs, G. A. (1982). *In* "Cardiovascular Pharmacology of the Prostaglandins" (A. G. Herman, P. M. Vanhoutte, H. Denolin, and A. Goosens, eds.), pp. 315–325. Raven, New York.

Higgs, E. A., Higgs, G. A., Moncada, S., and Vane, J. R. (1978a). *Br. J. Pharmacol.* **63**, 535–539.

Higgs, G. A., Moncada, S., and Vane, J. R. (1978b). *J. Physiol. (London)* **280**, 30–31P.

Higgs, G. A., Moncada, S., and Vane, J. R. (1978c). *J. Physiol.* (*London*) **280**, 55–56P.
Higgs, G. A., Cardinale, D. C., Moncada, S., and Vane, J. R. (1979). *Microvasc. Res.* **18**, 245–254.
Hinke, J. A. M. (1965). *In* "Muscle" (W. M. Paul, E. E. Daniel, C. M. McKay, and G. Monckton, eds.), pp. 269–285. Pergamon, Oxford.
Hirst, G. D. S. (1977). *J. Physiol* (*London*) **273**, 263–275.
Hodgson, B. J., and Daniels, E. E. (1972). *Can. J. Physiol. Pharmacol.* **50**, 725–730.
Hofbauer, J. H. (1973). *Clin. Sci. Mol. Med.* **39**, 263–278.
Horrobin, D. F., Mtajabi, J. P., and Manku, M. S. (1976). *Med. Hypotheses* **2**, 219–226.
Hoult, J. R. S., and Moore, P. K. (1982). *In* "Cardiovascular Pharmacology of the Prostaglandins" (A. G. Herman, P. M. Vanhoutte, H. Denolin, and A. Goosens, eds.), pp. 35–49. Raven, New York.
Hudgins, P. M., and Weiss, G. B. (1968). *J. Pharmacol. Exp. Ther.* **159**, 91–97.
Hughes, J., Gillis, C. N., and Bloom, F. E. (1969). *J. Pharmacol. Exp. Ther.* **169**, 237–248.
Humphrey, P. P. A. (1978). *Br. J. Pharmacol.* **63**, 671–675.
Huxley, J., and Hanson, J. (1954). *Nature* (*London*) **154**.
Innes, I. R. (1962). *Br. J. Pharmacol. Chemother.* **19**, 427–441.
Innes, I. R., and Kohli, J. D. (1970). *Arch. Int. Pharmacodyn. Ther.* **188**, 287–297.
Itzkowitz, H. D., and McGiff, J. C. (1974). *Circ. Res.* **34–35** (Suppl.), 65–73.
Janis, R. A., and Triggle, D. J. (1973). *Can. J. Physiol. Pharmacol.* **51**, 621–626.
Janis, R. A., and Triggle, D. J. (1974). *Pharmacol. Res. Commun.* **6**, 55–60.
Jarrot, B., McQueen, A., Graf, L., and Louis, W. J. (1975). *Clin. Exp. Pharmacol. Physiol.* **3** (Suppl. 2), 65–73.
Jeliffe, R. W. (1962). *J. Pharmacol. Exp. Ther.* **135**, 349–353.
Johansson, B., Jonsson, O., Axelsson, J., and Wahlstrom, B. (1967). *Circ. Res.* **21**, 619–633.
Johnson, E. M., Jr., Marshall, G. R., and Needleman, P. (1974). *Br. J. Pharmacol.* **51**, 541–547.
Johnson, M., and Ramwell, P. W. (1973). *Prostaglandins* **3**, 703–723.
Johnson, M., Jessup, R., and Ramwell, P. (1973a). *Prostaglandins* **4**, 593–605.
Johnson, M., Jessup, R., and Ramwell, P. (1974a). *Prostaglandins* **5**, 125–136.
Johnson, M., Jessup, R., Jessup, S., and Ramwell, P. (1974b). *Prostaglandins* **6**, 433–449.
Joiner, P. D., Kadowitz, P. J., Hughes, J. P., and Hyman, A. L. (1975). *Proc. Soc. Exp. Biol. Med.* **150**, 414–421.
Jones, A. W. (1973). *Circ. Res.* **33**, 563–572.
Jones, A. W. (1980). *Handb. Physiol. Sect. 2 Cardiovasc. Sys.* **2**, 253–299.
Junod, A. F. (1972a). *J. Pharmacol. Exp. Ther.* **183**, 182–187.
Junod, A. F. (1972b). *J. Pharmacol. Exp. Ther.* **183**, 341–344.
Kadar, D., and Sunahara, F. A. (1969). *Can. J. Physiol. Pharmacol.* **47**, 871–879.
Kadowitz, P. J., and Hyman, A. L. (1973). *Circ. Res.* **32**, 221–227.
Kadowitz, P. J., Sweet, C. S., and Brody, M. J. (1973). *Adv. Biosci.* **9**, 243–252.
Kadowitz, P. J., Joiner, P. D., and Hyman, A. L. (1975a). *J. Pharmacol. Exp. Ther.* **191**, 432–505.
Kadowitz, P. J., Joiner, P. D., and Hyman, A. L. (1975b). *Annu. Rev. Pharmacol.* **15**, 285–306.
Kadowitz, P. J., Knight, D. S., Hibbs, R. G., Elbson, J. P., Joiner, P. D., Brody, M. J., and Hyman, A. L. (1976). *Circ. Res.* **39**, 191–198.
Kadowitz, P. J., Greenberg S., Knight, D. S., Gruetter, C. A., Greenberg, S., and Hyman, A. L. (1981). *In* "Microcirculation: Current Physiologic, Medical and Surgical Con-

cepts'' (R. M. Effros, H. Schmid-Shonbein, and J. Ditzel, eds.), pp. 107–124. Academic Press, New York.

Kadowitz, P. J., Greenberg, S., and Hyman, A. L. (1982a). In "Prostanoids, Cardiopulmonary and Cardiovascular Actions" (S. Greenberg, and T. M. Glenn, eds.). Academic Press, New York.

Kadowitz, P. J., Knight, J. P., Greenberg, S., and Hyman, A. L. (1982b). In "Prostaglandins: Organ and Tissue Specific Actions" (S. Greenberg, P. J. Kadowitz, and T. F. Burks, eds.). Dekker, New York.

Kaley, G., and Altura, B. M. (1978). "Microcirculation" Vol. 2 Univ. Park Press, Baltimore, Maryland.

Kalsner, S. (1970). Can. J. Physiol. Pharmacol. 48, 443–449.

Karim, S. M. M. (1976). "Prostaglandins: Physiological, Pharmacological and Pathological Aspects." Lancester MTP Press, Lancester, England.

Karlin, A. (1967). J. Theor. Biol. 16, 306–320.

Katsuki, S., Arnold, W., Mittal, C., and Murad, F. (1977). J. Cyclic Nucleotide Res. 3, 23–35.

Keatinge, W. R. (1964). J. Physiol. (London) 174, 184–205.

Keatinge, W. R. (1968a). J. Physiol. (London) 194, 169–182.

Keatinge, W. R. (1968b). J. Physiol. (London) 194, 183–200.

Keatinge, W. R. (1976). J. Physiol. (London) 258, 73P–74P.

Keatinge, W. R. (1977). In "Excitation Contraction Coupling in Smooth Muscle" (R. Casteels, T. Godfraind, and J. C. Ruegg, eds.), pp. 47–52. Elsevier–North Holland Biomedical Press, Amsterdam.

Keatinge, W. R. (1978). J. Physiol. (London) 279, 275–289.

Keatinge, W. R. (1979). Br. Med. Bull. 35, 249–254.

Khairallah, P. A., Page, I. H., Bumpus, F. M., and Turker, R. K. (1966). Circ. Res. 14, 247–254.

Kier, L. B. (1968). J. Pharm. Sci. 57, 1188–1191.

Kimura, H., Mittal, C., and Murad, F. (1975). J. Biol. Chem. 250, 8016–8022.

Kloeze, J. (1967). In "Prostaglandins" (S. Bergstrom, and B. Samuelsson, eds.), Vol. 2, pp. 241–252. Armquist & Wiksell, Stockholm.

Korolkovas, A. (1970). "Essentials of Molecular Pharmacology: Background for Drug Design." Wiley, New York.

Krogh, A. (1929). "The Anatomy and Physiology of Capillaries." Yale Univ. Press, New Haven, Connecticut.

Kukovetz, W. R., Holtzmann, S., Wurm, A., and Poch, G. (1979a). J. Cyclic Nucleotide Res. 5, 469–476.

Kukovetz, W. R., Holtzmann, S., Wurm, A., and Poch, G. (1979b). Naunyn Schmiedebergs Arch. Pharmacol. 310, 129–138.

Kukovetz, W. R., Poch, G., and Holtzmann, S. (1981). In "Vasodilation" (P. M. Vanhoutte, and I. Leusen, eds.), pp. 339–351. Raven, New York.

Kumamoto, M. (1977). In "Factors Influencing Vascular Reactivity" (O. Carrier and S. Shibata, eds.), pp. 106–131. Igaku-Shoin, Tokyo.

Kuriyama, H., and Suzuki, H. (1978). Br. J. Pharmacol. 64, 493–501.

Langer, S. Z., Shepperson, N. B., and Massingham, R. (1981). Hypertension (Dallas) 3 (Suppl.), 112–118.

Lauson, H. D. (1974). Handb. Physiol. Sect. 7 Endocrinol. 4, 287–393.

Lee, T. J. F., Hume, W. R., Su, C., and Bevan, J. A. (1978). Circ. Res. 42, 535–542.

Levitt, B., and Westfall, D. P. (1982). Blood Vessels 19, 30–40.

Lewis, G. P., Westwicke, J., and Williams, T. J. (1977). Br. J. Pharmacol. 59, 442P (Abs.).

Limas, C. J., and Cohn, J. N. (1974). *Circ. Res.* **35,** 601–607.

Longnecker, D., and Harris, P. D. (1980). *In* "Microcirculation" (G. Kaley, and B. M. Altura, eds.), Vol. 3, pp. 384–405. Univ. Park Press, Baltimore, Maryland.

Majno, G. (1965). *Handb. Physiol. Sect. 2 Cardiovasc. Sys.* **3,** 2293–2375.

Marcus, A. J., Broekman, M. J., Weksler, B. B. Jaffe, E. A., Safier, L. B., Ullman, H. L., and Tack-Goldman, K. (1982). *In* "Cardiovascular Pharmacology of the Prostaglandins" (A. G. Herman, P. M. Vanhoutte, H. Denolin, and A. Goosens, eds.), pp. 125–136. Raven, New York.

Martin, P. J., and Schild, H. O. (1965). *Br. J. Pharmacol.* **25,** 418–431.

Masotti, G., Poggessi, L., Galanti, G., and Neri Serneri, G. G. (1979). *Thromb. Haemostasis* **42,** 197 (Abs.).

McCaa, R. E., Hall, J. E., and McCaa, C. S. (1978). *Circ. Res.* **43** (Suppl. 1), 32–39.

McElroy, F. A., and Philip, R. B. (1975). *Life Sci.* **17,** 1479–1493.

McGiff, J. C., Terragno, N. A., Malik, K. A., and Lonigro, A. J. (1972). *Circ. Res.* **31,** 36–43.

McGiff, J. C., Itskowitz, H. D., and Terragno, N. A. (1975). *Clin. Sci. Mol. Med.* **49,** 125–128.

McGiff, J. C., Itskowitz, H. D., Terragno, A., and Wong, P. K. Y. (1976). *Fed. Proc. Fed. Am. Soc. Exp. Biol.* **35,** 175–180.

McGrath, M. M. (1977). *Circ. Res.* **41,** 428–435.

McGrath, M. M. (1978). *Fed. Proc. Fed. Am. Soc. Exp. Biol.* **37,** 187–193.

McGrath, M. M., and Shepherd, J. T. (1976). *Circ. Res.* **39,** 566–573.

McNamara, D. B., Roulet, M. J., Gruetter, C. A., Hyman, A. L., and Kadowitz, P. J. (1980). *Prostaglandins* **20,** 311–320.

McNeil, J. H., Barnes, R. V., Davis, R. S., and Hook, J. B. (1969). *Can. J. Physiol. Pharmacol.* **47,** 663–669.

Mekata, F. (1971). *J. Gen. Physiol.* **57,** 738–751.

Mekata, F., and Niu, H. (1972). *J. Gen. Physiol.* **59,** 92–102.

Mellander, S., and Johansson, B. (1968). *Pharmacol. Rev.* **20,** 117–196.

Mellander, S., and Lundvall, J. (1971). *Circ. Res.* **28–29** (Suppl. I), 39–45.

Melmon, K. L., Kline, M. J., Hughes, T., and Nies, A. S. (1968). *J. Clin. Invest* **47,** 1295–1302.

Mentzer, R. M., Jr., Rubio, R., and Berne, R. M. (1975). *Am. J. Physiol.* **229,** 1625–1631.

Messina, E. J., and Kaley, G. (1982). *In* "Prostaglandins: Cardiovascular and Cardiopulmonary Actions" (S. Greenberg, and T. M. Glenn, eds.). Academic Press, New York.

Messina, E. J., Weiner, R., and Kaley, G. (1975). *Circ. Res.* **37,** 430–437.

Messina, E. J., Weiner, R., and Kaley, G. (1976). *Fed. Proc. Fed. Am. Soc. Exp. Biol.* **35,** 2367–2375.

Miller, F. N., and Harris, P. D. (1975). *Microvasc. Res.* **10,** 340–351.

Miller, F. N., and Weigman, D. L. (1977). *Eur. J. Pharmacol.* **44,** 331–337.

Moncada, S., and Korbut, R. (1978). *Lancet* **1,** 1286–1289.

Moncada, S., and Vane, J. R. (1979a). *In* "Prostacyclin" (J. R. Vane, and S. Bergstrom, eds.), pp. 5–16. Raven, New York.

Moncada, S., and Vane, J. R. (1979b). *Pharmacol. Rev.* **30,** 293–331.

Moncada, S., Gryglewski, R. J., Bunting, S., and Vane, J. R. (1976a). *Prostaglandins* **12,** 715–737.

Moncada, S., Gryglewski, R. J., Bunting, S., and Vane, J. R. (1976b). *Nature (London)* **263,** 663–665.

Monod, J., Wyman, J., and Changeux, J. P. (1965). *J. Mol. Biol.* **12,** 88–118.

Moretti, R. L., and Abraham, S. (1978a). *Circ. Res.* **42**, 317–323.
Moretti, R. L., and Abraham, S. (1978b). *Prostaglandins* **15**, 603–622.
Moretti, R. L., and Lin, C. Y. (1980). *Prostaglandins* **19**, 99–108.
Moretti, R. L., Abraham, S., and Ecker, R. R. (1976). *Circ. Res.* **39**, 231–238.
Movat, H. Z., and Habal, F. M. (1976). *In* "Chemistry and Biology of the Kallekrein-Kinin System in Health and Disease" (J. J. Pisano and F. K. Austen, eds.), pp. 463–469. US Govt. Printing Office, Washington, D.C.
Moylan, R. D., and Westfall, T. C. (1979). *Blood Vessels* **16**, 302–310.
Murad, F., Arnold, W. P., Mittal, C. K., and Braughler, J. M. (1979). *Adv. Cyclic Nucleotide Res.* **2**, 175–204.
Nakajima, A., and Horn, L. (1967). *Am. J. Physiol.* **213**, 25–30.
Nakano, J. (1974). *Handb. Physiol. Sect. 7 Endocrinol.* **4**, 395–442.
Namm, D. H. (1971). *J. Pharmacol. Exp. Ther.* **178**, 299–310.
Nash, C. B., Boyaji, L. D., and Manley, E. S. (1961). *Arch. Int. Pharmacodyn. Ther.* **133**, 433–443.
Needleman, P. (1976). *Fed. Proc. Fed. Am. Soc. Exp. Biol.* **35**, 2376–2383.
Needleman, P., and Isakson, P. C. (1980). *Handb. Physiol. Sect. 2 Cardiovasc. Sys.* **2**, 613–634.
Needleman, P., and Johnson, E. M. (1973). *J. Pharmacol. Exp. Ther.* **184**, 709–715.
Needleman, P., Jakschik, B., and Johnson, E. M., Jr. (1973a). *J. Pharmacol. Exp. Ther.* **187**, 324–331.
Needleman, P., Kauffman, A. H., Douglas, J. R., Jr., Johnson, E. M., Jr., and Marshall, G. R. (1973b). *Am. J. Physiol.* **224**, 1415–1419.
Needleman, P., Douglas, J. R., Jakschik, B., Stoechlein, P. B., and Johnson, E. M. (1974). *J. Pharmacol. Exp. Ther.* **188**, 453–465.
Needleman, P., Keys, S. L., Denny, S. E., Isaksson, P. C., and Marshall, G. R. (1975). *Proc. Natl. Acad. Sci. USA* **72**, 2060–2063.
Needleman, P., Moncada, S., Bunting, S., Vane, J. R., Hamberg, M., and Samuelsson, B. (1976). *Nature (London)* **261**, 558–560.
Needleman, P., Bronson, S. D., Wyche, A., Sivakoff, M., and Nichalou, K. C. (1978). *J. Clin. Invest.* **61**, 839–846.
Nishiki, K., Erecinska, M., and Wilson, D. F. (1978). *Am. J. Physiol.* **234**, C73–C81.
Nishino, K., Irikura, T., and Takayanagi, I. (1970). *Nature (London)* **228**, 564–565.
Northover, B. J. (1972). *Br. J. Pharmacol.* **45**, 651–659.
Northover, B. J. (1973). *Br. J. Pharmacol.* **48**, 496–504.
Northover, B. J. (1975). *Br. J. Pharmacol.* **53**, 113–120.
Norton, J. M., Gellai, M., and Detar, R. (1972). *Pfleugers Arch.* **335**, 279–286.
Offermeier, J., and Ariens, E. J. (1966a). *Arch. Int. Pharmacodyn. Ther.* **164**, 192–215.
Offermeier, J., and Ariens, E. J. (1966b). *Arch. Int. Pharmacodyn. Ther.* **164**, 216–245.
Olivares, G. J., Smith, N. T., and Aranow, L. (1967). *Br. J. Pharmacol. Chemother.* **30**, 240–250.
Ondetti, M. A., Rubin, B., and Cushman, D. W. (1977). *Science (Washington, D.C.)* **196**, 441–444.
Orton, T. C., Anderson, M. W., Pickett, R. D., Eling, T., and Fouts, J. R. (1975). *J. Pharmacol. Exp. Ther.* **186**, 482–497.
Owen, D. A. A. (1977). *Gen. Pharmacol.* **8**, 141–156.
Page, I. H. (1968). "Serotonin." Yearbook Publ. Chicago, Illinois.
Palmer, M. A., Piper, P. J., and Vane, J. R. (1973). *Br. J. Pharmacol.* **49**, 226–242.
Pang, C. C. Y., and Sutter, M. C. (1981). *Blood Vessels* **17**, 293–301.
Paul, R. J. (1980). *Handb. Physiol. Sect. 2 Cardiovasc. Sys.* **2**, 174–239.

Peach, M. J. (1977). *Physiol. Rev.* **57,** 313–370.

Pearson, J. D. (1982). *In* "Cardiovascular Pharmacology of the Prostaglandins" (A. G. Herman, P. M. Vanhoutte, H. Denolin, and A. Goosens, eds.), pp. 23–34. Raven, New York.

Pearson, J. D., Carleton, J. S., Hutchins, A., and Gordon, J. L. (1978). *Biochem. J.* **170,** 265–271.

Perry, S. V., and Grand, R. J. A. (1979). *Br. Med. Bull.* **35,** 219–226.

Peterson, J. W., and Paul, R. J. (1974). *Biochim. Biphys. Acta* **357,** 167–176.

Philip, R. B., and Lemieux, J. P. V. (1969). *Nature (London)* **221,** 1162

Pisano, J. J., and Austen, F. K. (eds.) (1976). "Chemistry and Biology of the Kallekrein-Kinin System in Health and Disease." US Govt. Printing Office, Washington, D.C.

Polacek, I. J., Bolan, J., and Daniel, E. E. (1970). *Can. J. Physiol. Pharmacol.* **49,** 999–1004.

Popescu, L. M. (1974). *Stud. Biophys.* **44,** S141–S153.

Rhodes, H. J., and Sutter, M. C. (1971). *Can. J. Physiol. Pharmacol.* **49,** 276–287.

Rhodin, J. A. G. (1968). *J. Ultrastruct. Res.* **25,** 452–500.

Rhodin, J. A. G. (1974). *In* "Histology, a Text and Atlas" (J. A. G. Rhodin, ed.). Oxford Univ. Press, London.

Rhodin, J. A. G. (1980). *Handb. Physiol. Sect. 2 Cardiovasc. Sys.* **2,** 1–31.

Rhodin, J. A. G. (1981). *In* "Microcirculation: Current Physiologic, Medical and Surgical Concepts" (R. M. Effros, H. Schmid-Shonbein, and J. Ditzel, eds.), pp. 11–17. Academic Press, New York.

Rocha e Silva, M. (1970). "Kinin Hormones." Springfield, Illinois.

Rocha e Silva, M. (1974). *Life Sci.* **15,** 7–22.

Rubio, R., and Berne, R. M. (1975). *Prog. Cardiovasc. Dis.* **18,** 105–122.

Rubio, R., Berne, R. M., Bockman, E. L., and Curnish, R. R. (1975). *Am. J. Physiol.* **228,** 1896–1901.

Ryan, M. J., and Brody, M. J. (1970). *J. Pharmacol. Exp. Ther.* **174,** 123–132.

Ryan, J. W., and Ryan, U. S. (1977a). *Am. J. Med.* **63,** 595–603.

Ryan, J. W., and Ryan, U. S. (1977b). *Fed. Proc. Fed. Am. Soc. Exp. Biol.* **36,** 2683–2691.

Ryan, J. W., and Ryan, U. S. (1980). *In* "Enzymatic Release of Vasoactive Peptides" (F. Gross, and H. F. Vogel, eds.), pp. 259–274. Raven, New York.

Ryan, J. W., and Ryan, U. S. (1981). *In* "Microcirculation: Current Physiologic, Medical and Surgical Concepts" (R. M. Effros, H. Schmid-Shonbein, and J. Ditzel, eds.), pp. 147–169. Academic Press, New York.

Ryan, J. W., and Smith, U. (1971a). *Biochim. Biophys. Acta* **249,** 177–180.

Ryan, J. W., and Smith, U. (1971b). *Trans. Assoc. Am. Physicians* **84,** 297–306.

Saameli, K. (1968). *Handb. Exp. Pharmacol.* **23,** 545–612.

Salmon, J. A. (1982). *In* "Cardiovascular Pharmacology of the Prostaglandins" (A. G. Herman, P. M. Vanhoutte, H. Denolin, and A. Goosens, eds.), pp. 7–22. Raven, New York.

Salmon, J. A., Smith, D. R., Flower, R. J., Moncada, S., and Vane, J. R. (1978). *Biochim. Biophys. Acta* **523,** 250–262.

Samuelsson, E., and Paoletti, R. (1982). *Adv. Prostaglandin Thromboxane Leukotriene Res.* **9,** 1–343.

Sawyer, W. H. (1961). *Pharmacol. Rev.* **13,** 225–277.

Schnaar, R. L., and Sparks, H. V. (1972). *Am. J. Physiol.* **223,** 223–228.

Schultz, K. D., Bohme, E., Kreye, V. W., and Schultz, G. (1979). *Naunyn Schmiedebergs Arch. Pharmacol.* **301,** 1–9.

Shepherd, J. T., and Vanhoutte, P. M. (1975). "Veins and Their Control." Sauders, Philadelphia, Pennsylvania.

Shepro, D., Batbouta, J. C., Carson, M. P., Robblee, L., and Belamarich, F. A. (1975). *Circ. Res.* **36,** 799–806.

Sigurdsson, S. B., Uvelius, B., and Johansson, B. (1975). *Acta Physiol. Scand.* **95,** 263–269.

Simaan, J. A., and Aviado, D. M. (1976). *J. Pharmacol. Exp. Ther.* **198,** 176–186.

Simionescu, N., Heltianu, C., Antohe, F., and Simionescu, M. (1982). *N.Y. Acad. Sci.*

Simon, G. M., Pamnami, G., Dunkel, J. F., and Overbeck, H. W. (1975). *Circ. Res.* **36,** 791–798.

Sjoberg, B., and Wahlstrom, B. A. (1975). *Acta Physiol. Scand.* **94,** 46–53.

Small, J. V., and Sobieszek, A. (1977). *Eur. J. Biochem.* **76,** 521–530.

Small, J. V., and Sobieszek, A. (1980). *Int. Rev. Cytol.* **64,** 241–306.

Smith, A. D., and Winkler, H. (1972). *Handb. Exp. Pharmacol.* **33,** 538–617.

Smith, U., and Ryan, J. W. (1970). *Adv. Exp. Med. Biol.* **8,** 249–262.

Smith, U., and Ryan, J. W. (1971). *Chest* **59,** 13.

Snipes, R. L., Thoenen, H., and Tranzer, J. P. (1968). *Experientia* **20,** 1026–1027.

Somlyo, A. P., and Somlyo, A. V. (1968). *Pharmacol. Rev.* **20,** 197–272.

Somlyo, A. V., and Somlyo, A. P. (1970). *Pharmacol. Rev.* **22,** 249–253.

Somlyo, A. P., Somlyo, A. V., and Woo, C. Y. (1967). *J. Physiol. (London)* **192,** 657–668.

Speden, R. N. (1964). *Nature (London)* **202,** 193–194.

Spies, C., Schultz, K. D., and Schultz, G. (1980). *Naunyn Schmiedebergs Arch. Pharmacol.* **311,** 71–77.

Stalcup, S. A. (1982). *Ann. N.Y. Acad. Sci.*

Stalcup, S. A., Lipset, J. S., Legant, P. M., Leuenberger, P. J., and Mellins, R. B. (1979a). *J. Appl. Physiol.* **46,** 227–234.

Stalcup, S. A., Lipset, J. S., Woam, J. M., Leuenberger, P. J., and Mellins, R. B. (1979b). *J. Clin. Invest.* **63,** 966–976.

Strum, J. M., and Junod, A. F. (1972). *J. Cell Biol.* **54,** 456–467.

Stull, J. T., and Sanford, C. F. (1981). *In* "New Perspectives on Calcium Antagonists" (G. B. Weiss, ed.), pp. 35–46. Amer. Physiol. Soc., Bethesda, Maryland.

Su, C. (1975). *J. Pharmacol. Exp. Ther.* **195,** 159–166.

Su, C. (1977). *J. Pharmacol. Exp. Ther.* **204,** 351–361.

Su, C., and Bevan, J. A. (1976). *Pharmacol. Ther. Part B.* **2,** 275–288.

Su, C., Bevan, R. D., Duckles, S. D., and Bevan, J. A. (1978). *Microvasc. Res.* **15,** 37–44.

Swartz, S. L., Williams, G. H., Hollenberg, N. K., Moore, T. J., and Dluhy, R. G. (1979). *Hypertension (Dallas)* **1,** 106–111.

Swartz, S. L., Williams, G. H., Hollenberg, N. K., Levin, L., Dluhy, R. G., and Moore, T. J. (1980). *J. Clin. Invest.* **65,** 1257–1264.

Tabachnik, U. I. A., and Gulbekian, A. (1968). *Ann. N.Y. Acad. Sci.* **150,** 204–218.

Tanaka, P., Greenberg, S., Glenn, T. M., Peevy, K. J., and Cho, Y. W. (1982a). *Eur. J. Pharmacol.* (in press).

Tanaka, P., Greenberg, S., Glenn, T. M., and Cho, Y. W. (1982b). *J. Pharmacol. Exp. Ther.*

Tani, E., Yamagama, S., and Ito, Y. (1977). *Cell Tissue Res.* **179,** 131–142.

Tappel, A. L., Lundberg, W. O., and Boyer, P. D. (1953). *Arch. Biochem. Biophys.* **33,** 293–303.

Tateson, J. E., Moncada, S., and Vane, J. R. (1977). *Prostaglandins* **13,** 389–399.

Taylor, J. E., and Richelson, E. (1982). *In* "Receptors and Recognition" (H. I. Yamamura, and S. J. Enna, eds.), pp. 71–100. Chapman & Hall, Cambridge.

Terragno, D. A., Crowshaw, K., Terragno, N. A., and McGiff, J. C. (1975). *Circ. Res.* **36–37** (Suppl. I), 76–80.

Terragno, N. A., Terragno, D. A., and McGiff, J. C. (1977). *Circ. Res.* **40,** 590–598.

Terragno, N. A., Terragno, D. A., Early, J. A., Roberts, M. A., and McGiff, J. C. (1978). *Clin. Sci. Mol. Med.* **55**, s199–s202.
Thoa, N. A., Eccleston, D., and Axelrod, J. (1969). *J. Pharmacol. Exp. Ther.* **169**, 68–73.
Thorens, S., and Haeusler, G. (1979). *Eur. J. Pharmacol.* **54**, 79–91.
Toda, N. (1974). *J. Pharmacol. Exp. Ther.* **191**, 139–146.
Todd, A. S. (1959). *J. Pathol. Bacteriol.* **78**, 281–283.
Todd, A. S. (1964). *J. Clin. Pathol.* **17**, 324–327.
Triggle, D. J. (1976). *In* "Chemical Pharmacology of the Synapse" (D. J. Triggle, and C. R. Triggle, eds.), pp. 431–594. Academic Press, New York.
Triggle, D. J. (1981). *Chest* **84**, 278–283.
Turlapaty, P., and Altura, B. M. (1978). *Eur. J. Pharmacol.* **52**, 421–423.
van Breeman, C., Aaronson, P., and Loutzenhiser, R. (1979). *Pharmacol. Rev.* **30**, 167–208.
Vanhoutte, P. M. (1974). *Circ. Res.* **34**, 317–326.
Vanhoutte, P. M. (1978). *In* "Microcirculation" (G. Kaley, and B. M. Altura, eds.), Vol. 3, pp. 181–309. Univ. Park Press, Baltimore, Maryland.
Vanhoutte, P. M. (1980). *Handb. Physiol. Sect. 2 Cardiovasc. Sys.* **2**, 443–474.
Vanhoutte, P. M. (1981a). *In* "New Perspectives on Calcium Antagonists" (G. B. Weiss, ed.), pp. 109–121. Amer. Physiol. Soc., Bethesda, Maryland.
Vanhoutte, P. M. (1981b). *In* "Vasodilation" (P. M. Vanhoutte, and I. Leusen, eds.), pp. 67–72. Raven, New York.
Vanhoutte, P. M. (1982). *J. Cardiovasc. Pharmacol.* **4** (Suppl. 1), S91–S96.
Vanhoutte, P. M., and Leusen, I. (eds.) (1981). "Vasodilation" Raven, New York.
Vanhoutte, P. M., Lorenz, R. R., and Tyce, G. M. (1973). *J. Pharmacol. Exp. Ther.* **185**, 386–394.
Van Nueten, J. M., Van Beek, J., and Janssen, P. A. J. (1978). *Arch. Int. Pharmacodyn. Ther.* **232**, 42–52.
Van Nueten, J. M., Van Beek, J., and Vanhoutte, P. M. (1980). *J. Pharmacol. Exp. Ther.* **213**, 179–187.
Van Nueten, J. M., Janssen, P. A. J., Van Beek, J., Xhonneux, R., Verbeuren, T. J., and Vanhoutte, P. M. (1981). *J. Pharmacol. Exp. Ther.* **218**, 217–230.
Verhaege, R. H., Vanhoutte, P. M., and Shepherd, J. T. (1977). *Circ. Res.* **40**, 208–215.
Volpi, M., Naccache, P. H., and Sha'afi, R. I. (1980). *Biochem. Biophys. Res. Commun.* **92**, 1231–1237.
Von Loh, D., and Bohr, D. F. (1973). *Proc. Soc. Exp. Biol. Med.* **144**, 513–516.
Wakade, A. R., Kanwar, R. S., and Gulati, O. D. (1970). *J. Pharmacol. Exp. Ther.* **175**, 189–196.
Wakeling, A. E., and Wyngarden, L. J. (1974). *Prostaglandins* **5**, 291–301.
Walter, P., and Bassenge, E. (1968). *Pfleugers Arch.* **299**, 52–65.
Watkins, J., Abbot, E. C., Hensby, C. N., Webster, J., and Dollery, C. T. (1980). *Br. Med. J.* **281**, 702–705.
Webb, R. C., Lockette, W. E., Vanhoutte, P. M., and Bohr, D. F. (1981). *In* "Vasodilation" (P. M. Vanhoutte, and I. Leusen, eds.), pp. 319–330. Raven, New York.
Webster, J., and Dollery, C. T. (1981). *Br. J. Clin. Pharmacol.* **4**, 201–203.
Weibel, E. R. (1974). *Microvasc. Res.* **8**, 218–235.
Weiner, R., Turlapaty, P., and Altura, B. M. (1980). *Eur. J. Pharmacol.* **63**, 241–249.
Weiss, G. B. (1977). *Adv. Gen. Cell. Pharmacol.* **2**, 71–154.
Weiss, G. B. (1978). *In* "Calcium in Drug Action" (G. B. Weiss, ed.), pp. 57–74. Plenum, New York.
Weiss, G. B. (1981a). *In* "Vasodilation" (P. M. Vanhoutte, and I. Leusen, eds.), pp. 307–310. Raven, New York.

Weiss, G. B. (1981b). *In* "New Perspectives on Calcium Antagonists" (G. B. Weiss, ed.), pp. 83–94. Amer. Physiol. Soc., Bethesda, Maryland.

Weiss, G. B., and Rosecrans, J. A. (1971a). *Eur. J. Pharmacol.* **13,** 197–207.

Weiss, G. B., and Rosecrans, J. A. (1971b). *Eur. J. Pharmacol.* **14,** 130–139.

Weksler, B. B., Knapp, J. M., and Jaffe, E. A. (1977). *Blood* **50** (Suppl. 1), 287S (Abs.).

Westfall, T. C. (1977). *Physiol. Rev.* **57,** 659–728.

Weston, A. H. (1972). *Br. J. Pharmacol.* **45,** 95–103.

Westwick, J. (1977). *Br. J. Pharmacol.* **61,** 138P–139P (Abs.).

White, R. (1982). *In* "Prostanoids: Cariopulmonary and Cardiovascular Actions" (S. Greenberg, and T. M. Glenn, eds.). Academic Press, New York.

Wikberg, J. E. S. (1979). *Acta Physiol. Scand.* (Suppl. 468), 1–89.

Williams, G. H., and Hollenberg, N. K. (1977). *N. Engl. J. Med.* **297,** 184–188.

Williamson, J. R., Vogler, N. J., and Kilo, C. (1969). *Diabetes* **18,** 567–568.

Wilton, P. B., and McCalden, T. A. (1977). *Eur. J. Pharmacol.* **46,** 213–219.

Wohl, A. J., Haeusler, L. M., and Roth, F. E. (1967). *J. Pharmacol. Exp. Ther.* **158,** 531–539.

Wohl, A. J., Hausler, L. M., and Roth, F. E. (1968a). *J. Pharmacol. Exp. Ther.* **162,** 109–114.

Wohl, A. J., Hausler, L. M., and Roth, F. E. (1968b). *Life Sci.* **7,** 381–387.

Wong, P. K. Y., Terragno, D. A., Terragno, N. A., and McGiff, J. C. (1977). *Prostaglandins* **13,** 1113–1125.

Wright, G. B., Alexander, R. W., Ekstein, L. S., and Gimbrone, M. A., Jr. (1982). *Circ. Res.* **50,** 462–469.

Zimmerman, B. G. (1973). *J. Pharmacol. Exp. Ther.* **168,** 303–309.

Zimmerman, B. G., Ryan, M. J., Gomer, S., and Kraft, E. (1973). *J. Pharmacol. Exp. Ther.* **187,** 315–323.

Zimmerman, B. G., Ryan, M. J., Gomer, S., and Kraft, E. (1974). *Life Sci.* **11,** 1104–1112.

Zins, G. R. (1975). *Am. J. Med.* **58,** 14–24.

Zsoster, T. T., Heneim, N. F., and Wolchinsky, C. (1977). *Eur. J. Pharmacol.* **45,** 7–12.

3 Fluid Exchange in the Microcirculation

Nicholas A. Mortillaro
Aubrey E. Taylor

I. Introduction

Under normal circumstances interstitial fluid volume is kept fairly constant via a regulated plasma–interstitial fluid balance. Whereas plasma volume is regulated through mechanisms involving water intake and renal secretion of salt and water, the regulation of interstitial fluid volume is by and large a local one that is directly coupled to transcapillary fluid exchange.

In 1896, Starling proposed that the rate and direction of fluid movement across capillaries was a function of the capillary hydrostatic pressure and the plasma colloid osmotic pressure, the former acting as the driving force responsible for filtration and the latter for absorption. When the forces are in balance, net fluid exchange is zero. Although Starling recognized that a small amount of fluid is continuously filtered across the capillary barrier to form lymph, he assumed that this was so small that the filtering and absorbing forces were at, or near, a balanced state.

THE PHYSIOLOGY AND PHARMACOLOGY
OF THE MICROCIRCULATION, VOLUME 1

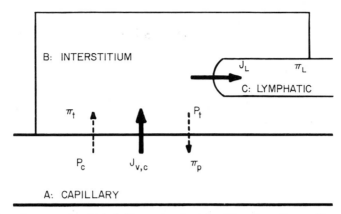

Fig. 1. Type I system, in which fluid entering the interstitium from the capillary (net filtration) can exit only via the lymphatic. The lymphatic acts as a primary "overflow" compartment. J_{vc} is the transcapillary volume flow, P_c and P_t are the capillary hydrostatic and interstitial fluid pressure, π_p, π_t, and π_L the plasma, interstitial, and lymph colloid osmotic pressures, respectively, and J_L is the lymph flow. The type I system is represented by skin or skeletal muscle. – – –, Pressure gradient; —, direction of volume flow.

Starling's basic concept of forces associated with transcapillary fluid exchange was later extended to include the interstitial fluid pressure and the colloid osmotic pressure of the interstitial fluid (Iverson and Johansen, 1929; Landis, 1927, 1928, 1934; Pappenheimer and Soto-Rivera, 1948; Kedem and Katchalsky, 1958; Landis and Pappenheimer, 1963). More recently, the concept of a negative interstitial fluid pressure and the physiochemical construct of the interstitial matrix as well as a greater understanding of the physical properties of the capillary membrane have added considerably to our knowledge and understanding of the interplay of those forces and associated parameters in the overall regulation of transcapillary fluid exchange (Guyton, 1963; Guyton *et al.*, 1966; Taylor, 1981; Aukland and Nicolaysen, 1981).

Presented in this chapter is an overview describing the mechanisms involved in the regulation of transcapillary fluid exchange.

II. Starling Forces Defined

A. Starling Hypothesis

The present concept of the relationship among the several forces at the microcirculatory level has evolved into what is commonly referred to as the Starling hypothesis. Figure 1 represents an idealized capillary–tissue

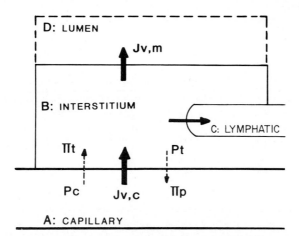

Fig. 2. Type II system, in which a second "overflow" compartment exists, here shown as the lumen of the intestine. J_{vm} is the volume flow from the interstitial compartment into the luminal compartment. In addition to the intestine, the type II system is represented by the lung (containing alveoli as the second overflow compartment).

–lymphatic system in which fluid entering into the interstitial compartment from the vascular compartment may exit only via the lymphatics, assuming a net filtering capillary. Such a type I system is representative of skin or skeletal muscle. The transcapillary volume flow may be represented by the relationship (Kedem and Katchalsky, 1958)

$$J_{vc} = K_{fc}[(P_c - P_t) - \sigma_d(\pi_p - \pi_t)], \tag{1}$$

where J_{vc} is the transcapillary volume flow, K_{fc} the capillary filtration coefficient, P_c the capillary hydrostatic pressure, P_t the interstitial fluid pressure, σ_d the colloid osmotic reflection coefficient, and π_p and π_t are the colloid osmotic pressure of plasma and interstitial fluid, respectively.

Figure 2 represents a type II system in which a second "overflow" compartment, in addition to the lymphatic compartment, is present. Such an overflow compartment is representative of the lumen of the intestine or the alveoli of the lung. With the addition of a volume term, Eq. (1) becomes (shown here for the intestine)

$$J_{vc} = K_{fc}[(P_c - P_t) - \sigma_d(\pi_p - \pi_t)] + J_{vm}, \tag{2}$$

where J_{vm} is the volume flow from the interstitial compartment across the mucosal surface and into the intestinal lumen.

Both types I and II system equations represent steady-state equations, requiring that K_{fc} and σ_d be constant and that the forces P_c, P_t, π_p, and π_t be steady-state values for a given condition or set of conditions.

B. Capillary Hydrostatic Pressure

Under normal circumstances, the single most important force influencing the moment-to-moment exchange of transcapillary fluid in any given capillary bed is P_c (measured in mm Hg). As an intravascular hydrostatic pressure, P_c's existence results from the generation of an arterial systemic pressure coupled to the state of the precapillary and postcapillary resistances. Because microvascular resistance is readily influenced by myogenic, metabolic, humoral, or drug factors, factors that are themselves continuously changing, P_c in a single capillary would be expected to also be continuously changing.

Attempts at estimating P_c in single capillaries have been made, employing direct-micropuncture techniques (Wiederhielm, 1968; Zweifach and Intaglietta, 1968). Direct measurements obtained from single capillaries (Wiederhielm, 1968) have shown that fluctuations in P_c result from the rhythmic contraction and relaxation (vasomotion) of precapillary sphincters; filtration occurs during the relaxation phase (high P_c) and absorption occurs during the constrictor phase (low P_c).

P_c measurements in whole organs has been employed using the stop-flow isogravimetric or isovolumetric method (Pappenheimer and Soto-Rivera, 1948; Johnson and Hanson, 1966; Gaar et al., 1967; Diana and Laughlin, 1974; Mortillaro and Taylor, 1976; Chen et al., 1976). In comparison to the direct measurement of P_c in single capillaries, the whole-organ approach yields a composite value for P_c, that is, a functional average for the part of the microvascular bed participating in fluid exchange (Aukland and Nicolaysen, 1981). Functional averages obtained from whole-organ studies have been lower than the P_cs reported from single capillaries. It should be noted that the capillary as defined by the physiologist encompasses that functional zone of the microvasculature that participates in solute and solvent exchange and, as such, includes the venules. It is the belief of many investigators that, because the surface area of a venule exceeds that of the capillary it drains, the major exchange site is weighted toward the terminal capillaries and venules, if not within the venules themselves (Intaglietta and Zweifach, 1971).

C. Interstitial Fluid Pressure

Several methods have been employed in an attempt to measure P_t (in mm Hg): needle insertion into tissue spaces (McMaster, 1946; Wiederhielm, 1967; Brace et al., 1975; Nicoll and Hogan, 1978), cotton wicks inserted into tissue spaces (Scholander et al., 1968; Snashall et al., 1971;

TABLE I

Summary of Interstitial Fluid Pressure P_t

Organ	Method	P_t (mm Hg)	Reference
Subcutaneous	Needle	2	McMaster (1946)
Subcutaneous	Needle	−3	Brace et al. (1975)
Renal	Capsule	6.1	Ott et al. (1975)
Gastric	Capsule	0.53	Altamirano et al. (1975)
Subcutaneous	Capsule	−6.4	Guyton (1963)
Ileum	Calculated	1.8	Mortillaro and Taylor (1976)
Ileum	Capsule	3.6	Mortillaro and Taylor (1982)
Subcutaneous	Wick	−1.0	Fadnes et al. (1977)
Hindlimb	Capsule	−4.7	Chen et al. (1976)
Subcutaneous	Wick	−2.0	Scholander et al. (1968)
Subcutaneous	Capsule	−4.4	Stromberg and Wiederhielm (1970)

Fadnes *et al.*, 1977; Hargens *et al.*, 1978), and chronically implanted capsules (Guyton, 1963; Stromberg and Wiederhielm, 1970; Prather *et al.*, 1971; Ott *et al.*, 1975; Chen *et al.*, 1976; Brace and Guyton, 1977; Mortillaro and Taylor, 1982). A most striking observation is the lack of consistency among all the values reported for P_t employing these methods of measurement (see Table I).

Tissue compliance plays a role in the development and effectiveness of P_t. The pressure–volume curve for both subcutaneous and ileal tissues are biphasic, that is, a zone of low compliance followed by a zone of higher compliance (Guyton, 1963; Chen *et al.*, 1976; Mortillaro and Taylor, 1976). For the ileum the initial compliance has been measured as 0.4 ml (mm Hg)$^{-1}$, increasing some 10-fold to 4 ml (mm Hg)$^{-1}$ at the higher end, the point of inflection occurring at a P_t of 3.6 mm Hg (Mortillaro and Taylor, 1976), whereas the point of inflection reported for subcutaneous tissue occurred at a P_t of 0 mm Hg (Guyton, 1963; Chen *et al.*, 1976).

D. Plasma and Interstitial Fluid Colloid Osmotic Pressures

Obtaining blood samples and, hence, plasma samples presents very few problems for investigators. Plasma colloid osmotic pressure (mm Hg) can be readily obtained by direct measurement on a Prather-type osmometer (Prather *et al.*, 1968). Alternatively, values for plasma protein concentration can be measured by refractometry and converted to pressure values,

TABLE II
Typical Values for Interstitial Colloid Osmotic Pressure π_t

Organ	Method	π_t (mm Hg)	Reference
Subcutaneous	Capsule	6.0	Szabo et al. (1980)
Subcutaneous	Capsule	6.1	Liebermann et al. (1972)
Subcutaneous	Capsule	4.4	Taylor et al. (1973)
Subcutaneous	Wick	6.4	Szabo et al. (1980)
Skeletal muscle	Wick	8.0	Reed (1981)
Renal	Micropipette	5.5	Wolgast et al. (1973)
Subcutaneous	Micropipette	6.4	Rutili and Arfors (1975)

utilizing the empirically developed cubic equation given by Landis and Pappenheimer (1963). Navar and Navar (1977) have demonstrated that great care must be taken in converting plasma protein concentration to pressure values, insofar as the relative concentration of the several protein fractions in plasma as well as the temperature at which the refractometer readings are made can greatly influence the final values obtained.

Theoretically, obtaining the colloid osmotic pressure (mm Hg) of interstitial fluid may be arrived at by applying the same technique as that for plasma. However, because of the highly limited free fluid in the interstitial spaces, obtaining samples of such fluid from normal (versus edematous) tissues has proven to be a most formidable problem. Nevertheless, attempts have been made and protein concentrations reported (Table II). The methods used have included micropipette sampling of interstitial fluid (Creese et al., 1962; Rutili and Arfors, 1977), wicks (Aukland and Fadnes, 1973; Fadnes and Aukland, 1977), implanted capsules (Taylor et al., 1973; Haljamae et al., 1974), and implanted colloid osmometers (Stromberg and Wiederhielm, 1976; Reed, 1979).

Because of the great difficulty in obtaining interstitial fluid for protein-concentration analysis and pressure determination, many investigators use lymph fluid as an indicator of the values for interstitial fluid from which lymph originated. However, a long-standing controversy exists in equating lymph-fluid protein concentration to that of interstitial fluid.

E. Capillary Filtration Coefficient

In the Starling equation there are two coefficients that play an essential role in the extent to which an imbalance in forces is effective in fluid exchange. These two "weighting" functions are represented by the capillary filtration coefficient (K_{fc}) and the colloid osmotic reflection coefficient (σ_d).

K_{fc} is equal to the product of the hydraulic conductivity of the capillary membrane and the capillary surface area of the organ under consideration. Thus K_{fc} may be taken as an index of the capillary surface area available for fluid exchange as well a reflection of the composite exchange properties of the capillary membrane. K_{fc}, as an indicator of capillary exchange capacity, has been used extensively in studies of capillary fluid exchange in various organs (Landis and Gibbons, 1933; Pappenheimer and Soto-Rivera, 1948; Folkow *et al.*, 1963; Johnson and Hanson, 1966; Mortillaro and Taylor, 1976; Chen *et al.*, 1976; Granger *et al.*, 1979; Kvietys *et al.*, 1980).

The filtration coefficient may be estimated from

$$K_{fc} = J_{vc}/\Delta P, \tag{3}$$

where J_{vc} is the instantaneous transcapillary volume flow and ΔP the instantaneous imbalance in forces acting across the capillary, that is, $\Delta P = (P_c - P_t) - \sigma_d(\pi_p - \pi_t)$. Hence, for a given net pressure gradient ΔP, the greater the capillary filtration coefficient, the greater the rate of fluid exchange.

Several methods have been used to determine K_{fc}, among which is the recording of tissue volume or weight increase following an increase in capillary hydrostatic pressure. The resulting volume curve typically is in two phases. The first or rapid phase reflects a passive distention of the capacitance vessels, increase in regional blood volume, whereas the succeeding slower second phase results from fluid being filtered from the capillaries into the interstitial spaces. The initial slope of the slower phase divided by the estimated change in P_c yields a value for K_{fc}. However, this method suffers from the disadvantage that it is difficult to precisely delineate when the blood shift ends and the filtration phase begins (see Granger *et al.*, 1979). Table III presents a summary of K_{fc} values from a variety of organs. It should be noted that K_{fc}, as an indicator of capillary exchange capacity, is subject to wide variations and, in some organs, changes as much as fourfold (Mortillaro and Taylor, 1976).

F. Colloid Osmotic Reflection Coefficient

The reflection coefficient, the second of the two coefficients found in the Starling equation, is a unitless term that establishes the effectiveness of the colloid osmotic pressure gradient ($\pi_p - \pi_t$) existing across the capillary membrane. It may take on a value ranging from 0 to 1. A value of

TABLE III
Capillary Filtration Coefficient K_{fc}

Organ	K_{fc}[ml min^{-1} (mm Hg)$^{-1}$ 100 g^{-1}]	Reference
Hindpaws	0.028	Chen et al. (1976)
Hindpaws	0.030	Arturson and Mellander (1964)
Skeletal muscle	0.01	Eliasson et al. (1973)
Skeletal muscle	0.008	Diana (1970)
Hindlimbs	0.025	Pappenheimer and Soto-Rivera (1948)
Lung	0.21	Drake et al. (1978)
Colon	0.20	Kvietys et al. (1980)
Colon	0.33	Richardson et al. (1980)
Ileum	0.17	Folkow et al. (1963)
Ileum	0.08	Mortillaro and Taylor (1976)
Ileum	0.10	Wallentin (1966)
Ileum	0.06	Granger et al. (1979)
Ileum	0.11	Johnson and Hanson (1966)
Pancreas	0.1	Eliasson et al. (1973)
Liver	0.060	Greenway and Lautt (1970)
Liver	0.080	Laine et al. (1979)
Spleen	5.0	Davies et al. (1979)
Spleen	1.0	Witherington et al. (1979)
Stomach	0.06	Jannson et al. (1970)

$\sigma_d = 1$ indicates a membrane system impermeable to plasma proteins, whereas $\sigma_d = 0$ indicates one that is freely permeable. Hence, a capillary system having $\sigma_d = 1$ would demonstrate a colloid osmotic pressure gradient that is fully effective, whereas the system having $\sigma_d = 0$ would theoretically have a nonexistent osmotic pressure gradient.

In the past, because of the absence of any reliable data regarding σ_d, most investigators have assumed $\sigma_d = 1$. More recently, a mathematical approach, coupled to the appropriate experimental method, has been used to estimate σ_d in several organ systems (Patlak et al., 1963; Taylor et al., 1977; Granger and Taylor, 1980; Rutili et al., 1979; Parker et al., 1980; Mortillaro et al., 1981; Richardson et al., 1980). A detailed discussion of the method used in estimating σ_d using lymph protein fluxes will be found in Chapter 4.

G. Lymph Flow

Lymphatics, where they exist, play an important role in the overall regulation of fluid exchange, by removing excess fluid from the interstitial spaces as well as removing proteins that have escaped into the tissue spaces. However, the capability of the lymphatic system to oppose tissue volume expansion following increases in capillary filtration is variable and limited.

Lymph flow (J_L) has been measured in several organ systems (Johnson and Richardson, 1974; Chen *et al.*, 1976; Mortillaro and Taylor, 1976; Taylor and Drake, 1977; Laine *et al.*, 1979), and estimates of the steady-state Starling forces have been made. In an organ system that contains lymphatic drainage and that is in an isogravimetric or isovolumetric state (type I system), Eq. (1) may be rewritten using the following assumptions: $J_{vc} = J_L$, and $\pi_t = \pi_L$ (π_L is the colloid osmotic pressure of lymph draining the area under study). Therefore

$$J_L = K_{fc}[(P_c - P_t) - \sigma_d(\pi_p - \pi_L)]. \tag{4}$$

From an experimental standpoint, the relationship encompassed in Eq. (4) lends itself very easily in estimating the Starling force imbalance. In most organs, most if not all of the parameters of Eq. (4) can be measured directly and at different filtration rates and levels of steady-state (Mortillaro and Taylor, 1976; Chen *et al.*, 1976). In a type II system, the same relationship may be used with the addition of the second overflow compartment. As such, the rate of flow into the second overflow compartment may be estimated by measuring all remaining parameters of Eq. (4), that is, for the intestine

$$J_{vm} = K_{fc}[(P_c - P_t) - \sigma_d(\pi_p - \pi_L)] - J_L. \tag{5}$$

III. Interactive Relationship among the Starling Forces

A. Elevation in Capillary Hydrostatic Pressure

When P_c is elevated in a step-wise manner, fluid is initially filtered at a relatively high rate, but after some time the rate is reduced, and a new steady state (isovolumetric) is achieved, in which $J_{vc} = J_L$. The achievement of a new steady state in the face of a continued elevation in P_c suggests that a readjustment of the Starling forces has occurred in a direction and of a magnitude so as to oppose the filtration force. For the ileum these adjustments have been shown to be an increase in P_t and lymph flow and a decrease in K_{fc} and π_L, all related to the transfer of fluid from the vascular compartment to the surrounding interstitial spaces (Mortillaro and Taylor, 1976) and all in a manner so as to offset the changes in P_c. The eleva-

TABLE IV

Edema Safety Factor

Organ	Change in P_c (mm Hg)	Contribution to the safety factor (%)			Reference
		P_t	$(\pi_p - \pi_L)$	J_L	
Hindpaw	29	62	14	24	Chen et al. (1976)
Hindlimb	7	71	29	0	Brace and Guyton (1977)
Colon	12	44	52	4	Richardson et al. (1980)
Ileum	20	30	50	20	Mortillaro and Taylor (1976)
Ileum	9	0	80	20	Johnson and Richardson (1974)
Liver	24	58	0	42	Laine et al. (1979)
Lung	18	39	33	28	Drake and Taylor (1977)
Lung	18	0	50	50	Erdmann et al. (1975)

tion in P_c in this series of experiments was induced by elevating the venous outflow pressure of the ileal segment, of which 70% of the increase in venous outflow pressure was transmitted to the capillaries and was reflected as an increase in P_c. The volume expansion occasioned by the increase in the filtration force (P_c) resulted in an increased P_t; concomitantly, lymph flow increased as a result of an increase in lymphatic filling, no doubt resulting from the increased pressure gradient from interstitium to the terminal lymphatics. In addition, the volume expansion resulted in the dilution of the interstitial proteins (decrease in π_L). The increased P_c caused a myogenic closure of precapillary sphincters, thereby reducing the surface area of capillaries available for exchange; that is, K_{fc} was reduced. A similar pattern has been reported for the canine hindpaw (Chen et al., 1976).

B. Edema Safety Factor

When the forces can no longer accommodate the change in filtration force, an excessive amount of fluid accumulates in the interstitial spaces, resulting in the condition known as edema. However, most tissues have the ability to accommodate and thereby offset changes in filtration forces. This ability has been described as the *margin of safety* (Krogh et al., 1932), or the *edema safety factor* (Guyton and Coleman, 1968; Taylor et al., 1973). The edema safety factor, derived from several studies, is given in Table IV for several organs.

IV. Drug Effects

It is most probably true that a whole host of drugs are available that can affect changes in the Starling force balance of most capillary beds. Although studies are lacking in which the specific aim was to develop data on the effects of drugs specifically on the Starling force balance, nevertheless, studies are available that give some indication of these effects.

In the ileum, administration of histamine has resulted in a significant reduction in the reflection coefficient, from a control of 0.92 to 0.57 (Mortillaro *et al.*, 1981). Histamine also caused a significant vasodilation, resulting most probably in an increase in K_{fc}. Thus, for a given change in P_c and because the capillary surface area available for exchange was expanded and the effectiveness of the osmotic gradient was considerably reduced, the ability of such a histamine-treated organ in opposing the filtration force was severely compromised. In a similar ileal preparation, glucagon decreased σ_d, but not to the same extent as histamine (Granger *et al.*, 1980); bradykinin decreased δ_d (Granger *et al.*, 1979) while increasing K_{fc}, P_c, and P_t (Barrowman *et al.*, 1981); and isoprenaline had no effect on σ_d but did increase K_{fc} (Granger *et al.*, 1979). On the other hand, in the colon both norepinephrine and vasopressin reduced K_{fc}, and isoproterenol increased it (Richardson *et al.*, 1980).

It would thus seem apparent that the drugs affecting capillary exchange would fall into two very broad categories: (1) vasoconstrictors or vasodilators, the vasoactive drugs, and/or (2) those drugs that have a direct effect on capillary permeability. It is not too unreasonable to expect that a vasodilator drug would increase capillary surface area available for exchange (increase K_{fc}) and increase the functional average filtration force P_c, whereas a vasoconstrictor would most probably have the opposite effect.

VI. Future Endeavors

The efforts placed by investigators into the study of capillary exchange in the 1970s and 1980s have been highly noteworthy. However, much of it has been piecemeal in its approach. Insofar as reliable methods are now available, future emphasis should be in the direction of studying the interactions of the Starling forces under specifically prescribed set of conditions. This holds true, most emphatically, for the effects of specific drugs on capillary exchange.

References

Altamirano, M., Requena, M., and Perez, T. C. (1975). *Am. J. Physiol.* **229,** 1414–1429.
Arturson, G., and Mellander, S. (1964). *Acta Physiol. Scand.* **62,** 457–463.
Aukland, K., and Fadnes, H. O. (1973). *Acta Physiol. Scand.* **88,** 350–358.
Aukland, K., and Nicolaysen, G. (1981). *Physiol. Rev.* **61,** 556–643.
Barrowman, J. A., Perry, M. A., Kvietys, P. R., Ulrich, M., and Granger, D. N. (1981). *Can. J. Physiol. Pharmacol.* **59,** 786–789.
Brace, R. A., and Guyton, A. C. (1977). *Am. J. Physiol.* **233,** H136–H140.
Brace, R. A., Guyton, A. C., and Taylor, A. E. (1975). *Am. J. Physiol.* **229,** 603–607.
Chen, H. I., Granger, H. G., and Taylor, A. E. (1976). *Circ. Res.* **39,** 245–254.
Creese, R., D'Silva, J. L., and Shaw, D. M. (1962). *J. Physiol.* (*London*) **162,** 44–53.
Davies, B. N., Richardson, P. D. I., and Witherington, P. G. (1979). *J. Physiol.* (*London*) **295,** 37–38.
Diana, J. N. (1970). *Am. J. Physiol.* **219,** 1574–1584.
Diana, J. N., and Laughlin, M. H. (1974). *Circ. Res.* **35,** 77–101.
Drake, R. E., and Taylor, A. E. (1977). *Prog. Lymphol.* [*Sel. Lect. Int. Congr.*], *4th, 5th, 1973, 1975,* pp. 13–17.
Drake, R. E., Gaar, K. A., and Taylor, A. E. (1978). *Am. J. Physiol.* **234,** H226–H274.
Eliasson, E., Folkow, B., and Hilton, S. M. (1973). *Acta Physiol. Scand.* **87,** 11–12.
Erdmann, A. J., Vaughn, T., Brigham, W., and Staub, N. C. (1975). *Circ. Res.* **37,** 271–284.
Fadnes, H. O., and Aukland, K. (1977). *Microvasc. Res.* **14,** 11–25.
Fadnes, H. O., Reed, R. K., and Aukland, K. (1977). *Microvasc. Res.* **14,** 27–36.
Folkow, B., Lundgren, O., and Wallentin, I. (1963). *Acta Physiol. Scand.* **57,** 270–283.
Gaar, K. A., Taylor, A. E., Owens, L. J., and Guyton, A. C. (1967). *Am. J. Physiol.* **213,** 79–82.
Granger, D. N., and Taylor, A. E. (1980). *Am. J. Physiol.* **238,** H457–H464.
Granger, D. N., Richardson, P. D. I., and Taylor A. E. (1979). *Pfluegers Arch.* **381,** 25–33.
Granger, D. N., Kvietys, P. R., Wilborn, W. H., Mortillaro, N. A., and Taylor, A. E. (1980). *Am. J. Physiol.* **239,** G30–G38.
Greenway, C. V., and Lautt, W. W. (1970). *Circ. Res.* **26,** 697–703.
Guyton, A. C. (1963). *Circ. Res.* **12,** 399–414.
Guyton, A. C., and Coleman, T. G. (1968). *Ann. N.Y. Acad. Sci.* **150,** 537–547.
Guyton, A. C., Scheel, K., and Murphree, D. (1966). *Circ. Res.* **19,** 412–419.
Haljamae, H., Linde, A., and Amundson, B. (1974). *Am. J. Physiol.* **227,** 1199–1205.
Hargens, A. R., Scholander, P. F., and Orris, W. L. (1978). *Microvasc. Res.* **15,** 239–244.
Intaglietta, M., and Zweifach, B. W. (1971). *Circ. Res.* **28,** 593–600.
Iverson, P., and Johansen, E. H. (1929). *Klin. Wochenschr.* **8,** 1311–1319.
Jannson, G., Lundgren, O., and Martinson, J. (1970). *Gastroenterology* **58,** 424–429.
Johnson, P. C., and Hanson, K. M. (1966). *Circ. Res.* **19,** 766–773.
Johnson, P. C., and Richardson, D. R. (1974). *Microvasc. Res.* **7,** 296–306.
Kedem, O., and Katchalsky, A. (1958). *Biochim. Biophys. Acta* **27,** 229–246.
Krogh, A., Landis, E. M., and Turner, A. H. (1932). *J. Clin. Invest.* **11,** 63–95.
Kvietys, P. R., Miller, T., and Granger, D. N. (1980). *Am. J. Physiol.* **238,** G478–G484.
Laine, G. A., Hall, J. T., Laine, S. H., and Granger, H. J. (1979). *Circ. Res.* **45,** 317–323.
Landis, E. M. (1927). *Am. J. Physiol.* **82,** 217–238.
Landis, E. M. (1928). *Am. J. Physiol.* **83,** 523–542.
Landis, E. M. (1934). *Physiol. Rev.* **14,** 404–481.

Landis, E. M., and Gibbon, J. H. (1933). *J. Clin. Invest.* **12**, 105–138.
Landis, E. M., and Pappenheimer, J. R. (1963). *Handb. Physiol. Sect. 2 Cardiovasc. Sys.* **2**, 961–1034.
Liebermann, I.M., Gonzalez, F., Brazzuna, H., Garcia, H., and Labuonora, D. (1972). *J. Appl. Physiol.* **33**, 751–756.
McMaster, P. D. (1946). *J. Exp. Med.* **84**, 473–494.
Mortillaro, N. A., and Taylor, A. E. (1976). *Circ. Res.* **39**, 348–358.
Mortillaro, N. A., and Taylor, A. E. (1982). *Microvasc. Res.* **23**, 268.
Mortillaro, N. A., Granger, D. N., Kvietys, P. R., Rutili, G., and Taylor, A. E. (1981). *Am. J. Physiol.* **240**, G381–G386.
Navar, P. D., and Navar, L. G. (1977). *Am. J. Physiol.* **233**, H295–H298.
Nicoll, P. A., and Hogan, R. D. (1978). *Microvasc. Res.* **15**, 257–259.
Ott, C. E., Cuche, J., and Knox, F. G. (1975). *J. Appl. Physiol.* **38**, 937–941.
Pappenheimer, J. R., and Soto-Rivera, A. (1948). *Am. J. Physiol.* **152**, 471–491.
Parker, J. C., Roselli, R. J., and Brigham, K. L. (1980). *Fed. Proc. Fed. Am. Soc. Exp. Biol.* **39**, 279.
Patlak, C. S., Goldstein, D. A., and Hoffman, J. F. (1963). *J. Theor. Biol.* **5**, 426–442.
Prather, J. W., Gaar, K. A., and Guyton, A. C. (1968). *J. Appl. Physiol.* **24**, 602–605.
Prather, J. W., Bowes, B. N., Warrell, D. A., and Zweifach, B. W. (1971). *J. Appl. Physiol.* **31**, 942–945.
Reed, R. K. (1981). *Acta Physiol. Scand.* **112**, 1–5.
Richardson, P. D. I., Granger, D. N., and Kvietys, P. R. (1980). *Gastroenterology* **78**, 1537–1544.
Rutili, G., and Arfors, K. E. (1975). *Bibl. Anat.* **13**, 70–71.
Rutili, G., and Arfors, K. E. (1977). *Acta Physiol. Scand.* **99**, 1–8.
Rutili, G., Granger, D. N., Mortillaro, N. A., Parker, J. C., and Taylor, A. E. (1982). *Microvasc. Res.* **23**, 347–360.
Scholander, P. F., Hargens, A. R., and Miller, S. L. (1968). *Science (Washington, D.C.)* **161**, 321–328.
Snashall, P. D., Lucas, J., Guz, A., and Floyer, M. A. (1971). *Clin. Sci.* **41**, 35–53.
Starling, E. H. (1896). *J. Physiol. (London)* **19**, 312–326.
Stromberg, D. D., and Wiederhielm, C. A. (1970). *Am. J. Physiol.* **219**, 928–932.
Stromberg, D. D., and Wiederhielm, C. A. (1976). *Am. J. Physiol.* **231**, 888–891.
Szabo, G., Posch, E., and Magyar, Z. (1980). *Acta Physiol. Acad. Sci. Hung.* **56**, 367–378.
Taylor, A. E. (1981). *Circ. Res.* **49**, 557–575.
Taylor, A. E., and Drake, R. E. (1977). *In* "Lung Biology in Health and Disease" (N. C. Staub, ed.), Vol. 9, pp. 129–182. Dekker, New York.
Taylor, A. E., Gibson, W. H., Granger, H. J., and Guyton, A. C. (1973). *Lymphology* **6**, 192–208.
Taylor, A. E., Granger, D. N., and Brace, R. A. (1977). *Microvasc. Res.* **13**, 297–313.
Wallentin, I. (1966). *Acta Physiol. Scand.* **68**, 304–315.
Wiederhielm, C. A. (1967). *In* "Physical Basis of Circulatory Transport: Regulation and Exchange" (E. B. Reeve, and A. C. Guyton, eds.), pp. 313–326. Saunders, Philadelphia, Pennsylvania.
Wiederhielm, C. A. (1968). *J. Gen. Physiol.* **52**, 29–63.
Witherington, P. G., Richardson, P. D. I., and Davies, B. N. (1979). *Microvasc. Res.* **17**, S17.
Wolgast, M. E., Persson, J., Schnermann, H., Ulfendahl, H., and Wunderlich, P. (1973). *Pfluegers Arch.* **340**, 123–131.

Zweifach, B. W., and Intaglietta, M. (1968). *Microvasc. Res.* **1,** 83–101.

4 Permeability Characteristics of the Mircocirculation

D. Neil Granger
Michael A. Perry

I. Introduction

The basic function of the microcirculation is to allow rapid exchange of nutrients, gases, waste products, and water between the blood and tissue cells. This exchange of fluid and solutes across the microcirculation is generally considered to occur at the capillaries. During the past 30 years considerable effort has been made to define the mechanisms and pathways involved in the exchange of solutes across capillaries. From this effort a wealth of information has been generated regarding the characteristics of the permeability of capillaries to small and large molecules in a variety of tissues. The details of the permeability properties of capillaries in specific tissues are presented in subsequent chapters in this monograph. In this chapter we present a brief description of the techniques most commonly employed for studying vascular permeability. The various applications of vascular permeability data to pore theory are also described. This is followed by a brief review of the ultrastructural character-

THE PHYSIOLOGY AND PHARMACOLOGY
OF THE MICROCIRCULATION, VOLUME 1

istics of the various capillary types and an attempt to relate the structurally defined pathways for solute exchange to physiologic estimates of vascular permeability.

II. Methods for Studying Vascular Permeability

A. Indicator-Dilution Technique

The principle of indicator dilution has been used to measure the permeability characteristics of capillaries in many organs. The application of this technique became possible with the advent of radioisotopes, because this allowed the blood concentrations of different solutes to be measured with ease and accuracy. The tracer molecules are introduced into the circulation either as a single injection or as a constant infusion, and their concentration curves in venous blood are recorded as a function of time. The information obtained from indicator-dilution curves has been analyzed to produce estimates of the permeability–surface-area product (PS), the extravascular volume of distribution, and the rate of cellular metabolism of a wide variety of molecules. The use of this technique has led to a greater understanding of the processes involved in transcapillary exchange of small molecules.

1. Theory

The indicator-dilution technique involves the injection of a mixture of tracers into the arterial supply of an organ and the collection of venous samples. The injected mixture contains both a vascular tracer and one or more tracers that cross the capillary wall. The vascular tracer does not leave the vasculature during passage through an organ, whereas the other solutes leave the circulation and are distributed in both the intravascular volume and part of the extravascular volume (Fig. 1a). Figure 1b depicts an outflow curve following the injection of a single bolus containing both a vascular and a diffusible marker. Note that the vascular marker attains a higher relative concentration more rapidly than the diffusible marker. This is because the diffusible marker leaves the circulation and distributes itself in a larger volume that incorporates part of the interstitium. The decline in the concentration of the vascular marker is more rapid than that of the diffusible marker due to back diffusion of the diffusible tracer from the interstitium into the circulation.

Comparison of the relative concentration (relative to its concentration in the injected solution) of the diffusible tracer (C_{diff}) with that of the vas-

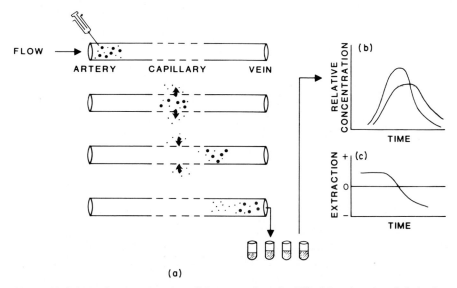

Fig. 1. (a) Schematic representation of the extraction of a diffusible solute (small dot) relative to a vascular tracer (large dot) as the bolus of injected material passes through the vasculature; (b) relative concentrations of the two tracers in venous samples; (c) pattern of extraction of the smaller tracer.

cular tracer (C_{ref}) gives the proportion of the diffusible solute that has left the circulation. This proportional loss is termed "extraction" (Fig. 1c) and is calculated as

$$E = (C_{ref} - C_{diff})/C_{ref}. \tag{1}$$

The total flux of the diffusible solute (J_s) across the capillary bed is

$$J_s = \dot{Q}_p (C_{ref} - C_{diff}), \tag{2}$$

where $\dot{Q}_p$ is plasma flow rate through the organ. Given certain conditions, which will be discussed later, J_s represents a unidirectional flux of the diffusible tracer from blood to interstitium and is influenced by the permeability (P) of the solute across the capillary wall and the available capillary surface area for exchange (S). The solute flux may also be described as

$$J_s = PS \, \triangle \bar{C}, \tag{3}$$

where $\triangle \bar{C}$ is the average concentration difference across the capillary wall and is equal to $(C_{ref} - C_{diff})/\ln(C_{ref}/C_{diff})$ (see Crone and Christensen, 1979). Combining Eqs. (2) and (3) yield

$$PS = \dot{Q}_p \ln(C_{ref}/C_{diff}). \tag{4}$$

Because $C_{diff}/C_{ref} = 1 - E$,

$$\ln(C_{ref}/C_{diff}) = -\ln(1 - E). \tag{5}$$

Substitution of Eq. (5) into Eq. (4) gives the equation originally described by Renkin (1959):

$$PS = \dot{Q}_p \ln(1 - E). \tag{6}$$

The addition of two diffusible solutes to the injectate allows a comparison of the simultaneous estimates of PS for each solute. Under these conditions capillary surface area and plasma flow rate are common for both solutes and $P_1/P_2 = \ln(1 - E_1)/\ln(1 - E_2)$. If both solutes diffuse freely from the circulation without restriction at the capillary wall into a large extravascular volume, then P_1/P_2 will be equal to the ratio of their respective free diffusion coefficients (D_1/D_2). However, if the larger of the two solutes $(P_2$ in this example) is restricted to some degree by the capillary wall, then P_1/P_2 will be greater than D_1/D_2. The way in which this degree of restricted diffusion, $(P_1/P_2)/(D_1/D_2)$, can be used to calculate an "equivalent" or "effective" pore radius for the capillary wall is discussed in Section III.

Certain criteria must be met before the indicator-dilution technique can provide meaningful permeability data:

1.   The diffusible tracer must not be metabolized during a single pass through the circulation.

2.   The diffusibility of the solute should not be so high or the flow rate so low that the test tracer equilibrates with the interstitium during a single passage through the organ. These conditions will produce PS values that increase with flow. The magnitude of PS is then governed by flow rate and not by the permeability characteristics of the endothelial membrane; that is, the substance is *flow-limited*.

3.   Highly diffusible solutes may also undergo lateral diffusion known as the *Taylor effect* (Taylor, 1953). This results from the diffusible tracer moving from the fast transit pathway in the center of the vessel into slower pathways near the vessel wall. The substance then reenters the fast pathway once the bolus of injected tracers has passed (Fig. 2). This results in apparent extraction values that are first positive, then negative, and again positive (Fig. 3). This effect is most likely to occur with highly diffusible tracers such as sodium and under conditions in which the flow rate is sufficiently slow to allow time for the tracer to diffuse toward the wall of the vessel. The Taylor effect may occur in both the vascular system and the extracorporeal circuits required for sample collection.

4.   The vascular bed should be homogeneous with respect to both the permeability characteristics and the time required for the tracers to move

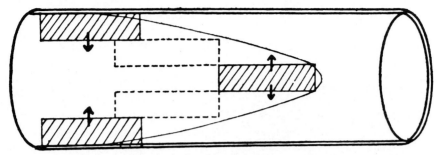

Fig. 2. Diagrammatic representation of interlaminar diffusion. The parabolic line represents the velocity profile within the vessel. Following a bolus injection of two tracer molecules, the smaller molecule will diffuse from the center of the vessel to a slower-flowing layer on the periphery of the vessel, producing an apparent positive extraction. Once the bolus has passed along the vessel, the smaller solute will diffuse from the periphery and reenter the fast axial stream, producing an apparent negative extraction. The last of the bolus will have lost most of the smaller tracer to the fast pathway in the center of the vessel and will therefore display a positive extraction. (From Lassen and Crone, 1970.)

through the various vascular pathways. Inhomogeneity, of either flow or permeability, generally causes PS to be underestimated.

   5.   Extraction should not be influenced by back diffusion of the tracer from the interstitium into the blood.

   Conditions 4 and 5 represent the most formidable theoretical problems associated with using the indicator-dilution technique for assessing capillary permeability. When this technique is used, both reference and diffusible tracers require complete mixing with blood perfusing the organ to ensure uniform exposure of the test solute to the vascular wall. The sampling catheter must be located close to the venous outflow of the organ and should be as short as possible. This allows the indicator curve to be measured with minimal distortion and avoids mixing of early and later samples of different concentrations. In addition, the flow rate through the sampling catheter must be sufficiently high to allow an adequate number of samples to be collected. This ensures that the shape of the indicator curves are well defined.

2. Developments in the Application of the Indicator-Dilution Technique

   In early studies Chinard and Enns (1954) investigated the permeability of pulmonary capillaries by making a rapid injection of a vascular and two diffusible tracers into the jugular vein of the dog and collecting samples from the carotid artery. They found only a small difference in the relative concentration of the vascular tracer, either labeled red blood cells or

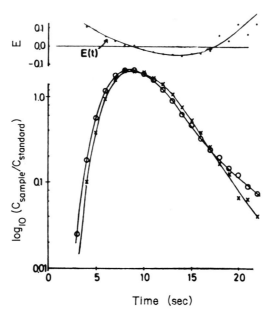

Fig. 3. Indicator-dilution curves for T-1824 albumin (○) and $^{24}Na^+$ (×) in human brain (lower panel) and extraction (E) of $^{24}Na^+$, illustrating the Taylor effect. (From Lassen and Crone, 1970.)

T-1824 albumin, and diffusible tracers such as $^{22}Na^+$, inulin, and thiocyanate. The authors concluded that either the lung capillaries were impermeable to these small diffusible tracers, or only a small extravascular volume of distribution existed in the lung tissue. However, these findings could also be due to the use of injection and sampling sites distant from the lung.

Crone (1963a) estimated extraction values for sucrose and inulin in the dog hindlimb and calculated PS values for these solutes using Eq. (6). The extraction values obtained in successive venous samples were initially constant but decreased in later samples; therefore, initial extraction values that displayed a plateau were used to calculate PS. Since the sucrose-to-inulin permeability ratio was similar to the ratio of their free diffusion coefficients, Crone concluded that muscle capillaries offered no restriction to the diffusion of these small molecules.

Crone also found that in liver and kidney the extraction of sucrose and inulin decreased with time. This decreasing extraction was thought to be a result of back diffusion of the tracers from the interstitium. In order to use Eqs. (1)–(6), the concentration of diffusible tracer in the interstitium must be zero; that is, there must be no back diffusion. To avoid the effect of back diffusion, Crone extrapolated the extraction values to the time at which the tracers first appeared in venous samples, which was thought to represent the extraction when the interstitial concentration of the tracer was zero.

Because in the lung there was little or no extraction of either sucrose or inulin, Crone concluded that the technique could not be applied to organs with a high perfusion rate. However, in these experiments injection of tracers and collection of samples were made at sites distant from the lung. This factor as well as the high flow rates caused the low extraction values. Subsequent studies in the dog (Yipintsoi, 1976) and the rabbit (Perry and Garlick, 1978), using pulmonary venous collection sites, indicated that the extractions of sodium, raffinose, and inulin in the lung decreased with time. This suggests that the markers escaped the circulation and displayed rapid back diffusion.

The magnitude of back diffusion from the interstitium is greater with highly diffusible tracers because the extravascular volume available for diffusion is rapidly saturated. Although extrapolated extraction values offer a simple solution, there are uncertainties as to the time at which tracers first appear in the venous samples. Martin de Julian and Yudilevich (1964) proposed a method of graphic analysis that could be used when E was not constant, but declined with time, and when the tracer was confined to a single extravascular compartment:

$$E = k \int_0^t \frac{(C_{ref} - C_{diff})\, dt}{C_{ref}} - \frac{C_{diff}}{C_{ref}} + 1, \qquad (7)$$

where C_{ref} is concentration at time t of the vascular tracer, C_{diff} is concentration at time t of the diffusible tracer, and k is the fractional turnover rate of the interstitial space. The values of k and E are obtained from a graph of $\int_0^t (C_{ref} - C_{diff})dt/C_{ref}$ versus C_{diff}/C_{ref}. Using this approach, Yudilevich and Alvarez (1967) found that ^{22}Na was more restricted than ^{3}H$_2$O in the coronary circulation and proposed that water could cross the endothelial cells, whereas ^{22}Na was restricted to passage through the intercellular clefts. Later, Alvarez and Yudilevich (1969) found that highly diffusible tracers such as ^{22}Na were flow-limited; that is, as flow increased, the PS value increased. However, with diffusible tracers ranging in size from glucose to inulin, constant PS values were obtained at modest flow rates. Their estimates of capillary permeability for sucrose and inulin in heart muscle were similar to values obtained by Crone (1963b) in skeletal muscle. Since the permeability values for the diffusible tracers were a constant proportion of their respective free diffusion coefficients, it was concluded that none of these molecules were restricted by the capillary wall. The absence of restriction to diffusion of inulin at the capillary wall requires a minimum effective small-pore radius of 80–100 Å in cardiac muscle. This is larger than the dimensions commonly accepted as representing the small-pore radius of skeletal muscle capillaries (40–45 Å).

Extraction may be influenced by several factors other than capillary permeability. Early extraction values may be influenced by both heterogeneity of flow (Trap-Jensen and Lassen, 1971) and interlaminar diffusion (Lassen and Crone, 1970). With heterogeneous flow patterns, the initial extraction values represent samples that have passed rapidly through the vasculature, and E, which is inversely related to flow, will be low. Later samples represent slower flow pathways in which E will be higher. An extraction pattern that shows an increase in the early samples indicates flow heterogeneity. If samples with different extractions are mixed, true capillary permeability will be underestimated. Interlaminar diffusion will also result in erroneous extraction values, although it is likely to occur only with smaller, more diffusible solutes. In order to minimize the effects of flow heterogeneity and the Taylor effect, extraction values have been used that are based on the differences between the areas beneath the reference and the diffusible tracer curves. These values are obtained by integrating the area difference over a given time. The upper limits that have been chosen for integration are (a) the peak of the reference tracer curve (t_{peak}), (b) the time at which extraction values start to decline ($t_{plateau}$), (c) the time at which the reference tracer curve has decreased to 40% of its peak value ($t_{40\%}$), or (d) the time at which the reference and diffusible tracer curves cross (t_{cross}). These limits are illustrated on the abscissa in Fig. 4. Experiments in exercising human forearm using ^{51}Cr-EDTA as the diffusible tracer (Lassen and Trap-Jensen, 1970) reveal no difference in the values obtained for E using any of the four upper limits for integration.

Trap-Jensen and Lassen (1971) calculated capillary diffusion capacities (CDC) for inulin and ^{51}Cr-EDTA in exercising human forearm. The values of E were obtained by the previously described method of area difference analysis. The ratio of the CDCs for the diffusible tracers was 6.39 compared with the ratio of their free diffusion coefficients of 3.2. Such a restriction in diffusion supported the existence of pores of radius 40 Å, which had previously been proposed by Landis and Pappenheimer (1963). This finding was at variance with that of Crone (1963b), possibly due to the heterogeneity of flow in the resting hindlimb of the dog. Evidence of restricted diffusion of sucrose as compared with inulin was also found by Garlick (1970) in the isolated gastrocnemius muscle of the cat.

The mean extraction values obtained by area difference analysis are applicable to studies in skeletal muscle because there is likely to be heterogeneity of flow, interlaminar diffusion because of the low flow rate (in the

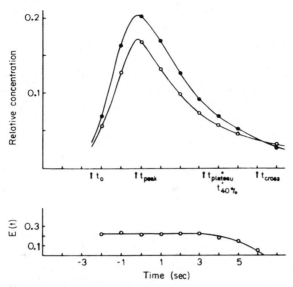

Fig. 4. Indicator-dilution curves for T-1824 albumin (●) and ^{51}Cr-EDTA (○) in exercising human forearm. The different points in time to which the area difference between the tracer curves are integrated are shown on the abscissa. The lower panel shows the instantaneous extraction of ^{51}Cr-EDTA in each sample. (From Lassen and Trap-Jensen, 1970.)

resting state), and delayed back diffusion for all but the most highly diffusible tracers. In tissues such as the lung, where the extraction pattern decreases with time (Nicolaysen, 1971; Perry and Garlick, 1978; Yipintsoi, 1976), it is not appropriate to use mean extraction values. In the lung the initial extraction value will give a more accurate estimate of PS because it is more likely to represent extraction when the interstitial concentration of the tracer is zero.

The previously discussed methods for analyzing indicator-dilution data represent attempts to minimize the errors introduced by heterogeneity of flow, the Taylor effect, and back diffusion of tracer. However, they do not quantify the influence of the individual factors on extraction. Numerous mathematical models have been developed to refine further the permeability estimates obtained using indicator-dilution techniques (Bassingthwaighte, 1974; Goresky et al., 1970; Harris et al., 1976; Johnson and Wilson, 1966; Levitt, 1970; Perl, 1970, 1971, 1973; Perl and Chinard, 1968). The limitations of a model approach for analyzing indicator-dilution data are related to the inherent assumptions, the completeness of the model, and the degree of complexity involved in describing the phenomena. However, they provide a means of describing the complex events that may be occurring during transcapillary exchange of solutes. For example, Harris and associates (1976) used a model approach to increase the sensitivity for detecting PS changes during various pathologic conditions.

Other models provide useful guidelines to the conditions at which reliable permeability values may be obtained from experimental data. For example, Bassingthwaighte (1974) found that the most accurate estimates of capillary permeability were obtained when $PS/\dot{Q}_p$ ratios were between 0.2 and 1.0 or when peak extraction values were between 0.1 and 0.6. For large hydrophilic solutes, extraction values should be greater than 0.05. Levitt (1970) found that permeability values obtained using early extraction methods underestimate the actual permeability if the extravascular volume of the tracer is less than three times capillary volume.

Guller *et al.* (1975) obtained PS values for sodium in the heart using several different calculation methods. They compared the observed data with values obtained by fitting the dilution curves with predictions obtained from a Krogh capillary-tissue cylinder model. This approach produced a modification of the Renkin equation in which the extraction was multiplied by 1.15 to correct for back diffusion of sodium in cardiac muscle:

$$PS = -\dot{Q}_p \ln(1 - 1.15E). \qquad (8)$$

The appropriate mathematics are available to describe the events occuring during transcapillary exchange of solutes, and many investigators have used the indicator-dilution technique to study the permeability characteristics of different vascular beds. The PS values may be calculated when extraction of the solute is contant for several successive samples. However, when extraction is not constant, a model approach is required to interpret the data.

3. General Findings in Different Tissues

Indicator-dilution techniques have been used to estimate vascular permeability in a variety of organs throughout the body, particularly the lung, heart, and skeletal muscle. Values for PS and permeability coefficients have been obtained for a spectrum of molecules ranging in size from water to albumin. In reviewing this extensive literature, it is apparent that permeability estimates from different laboratories are not calculated in the same fashion; for example, extraction values have been calculated by different methods, and different values for capillary surface area have been used even for the same organ. In order to facilitate comparison of the published data presented in Tables I–V, the data were recalculated using standard values for capillary surface area and, when available, we chose to use extraction values that could be computed from the published data. The value of S and the method of computing E are given in the tables for each set of data. Published values for PS calculated using blood flow instead of plasma flow were corrected by assuming a blood hematocrit of 0.35.

An overview of the results obtained with the indicator-dilution technique in different tissues is presented in this section. For a more comprehensive analysis of the data obtained in individual tissues the reader is referred to a review by Parker *et al.* (1983).

a. Lung. The lung is probably the most difficult organ in which to assess vascular permeability with the indicator-dilution technique. It is a tissue with an extremely high blood flow and a low extraction for all but the most diffusible of tracer molecules. Rapid back diffusion of the tracer molecule occurs because many of the capillaries in the lung septum are surrounded by only a thin band of interstitium. When larger tracer molecules are used in order to avoid the problems associated with early back diffusion, the extraction values soon become too small to measure. A rapid decline in extraction of solutes ranging in size from $^{22}Na^+$ (Nicolaysen, 1971; Yipintsoi, 1976) to inulin (Perry and Garlick, 1978) has been observed. The absence of a plateau in the extraction versus time relationship has led to extraction being calculated by a variety of methods including extraction at appearance time, extraction by integration of the area difference between reference and diffusible tracer curves, and extraction values derived following modeling of the data. The PS values and permeability coefficients (P) calculated for the lung are given in Table I. In general, the permeability coefficients for the larger solute molecules are greater than values reported in skeletal muscle. This suggests that the lung is a slightly more permeable vascular bed than muscle. Smaller solutes up to the size of mannitol generally demonstrate lower permeabilities in lung than in muscle. However, this may reflect the fact that the indicator-dilution technique underestimates the true permeability for small solutes because of the problems described above.

The indicator-dilution technique has been used to assess pathologic changes in lung vascular permeability (Harris *et al.*, 1976). Although the underlying mechanisms are not understood, it appears that urea is a suitable tracer for this purpose, possibly because of the partial lipid solubility of urea, giving this tracer greater access to pockets of fluid in edematous lungs, which lipid insoluble solutes cannot reach during a single transit. The same technique has also been used to evaluate [^{14}C]urea PS in human subjects (Brigham *et al.*, 1979b).

TABLE I
Permeability Characteristics of Lung Capillaries for Small Solutes[a]

Species (age/treatment)	PS H₂O	P H₂O	PS Na⁺	P Na⁺	PS urea	P urea	PS gluc	P gluc	PS sucr	P sucr	PS raff	P raff	PS inulin	P inulin	S	Extraction, E	Ref.[b]
Rat							270	1.5	396	2.2					3000 cm² g⁻¹	E integrated to peak	1
Rat									108	0.6					3000 cm² g⁻¹	E integrated to peak	2
Dog (control)	774	4.3							174	1.0					72 m²/lung[c]	E_max by numerical deconvolution	3
(isopro-terenol)	888	4.9							168	0.9					72 m²/lung		
(alloxan)	1176	6.5							240	1.3					72 m²/lung		
Dog (control)	450	2.5			66	0.4									72 m²/lung[d]	E integrated to peak	4
(increased pressure)	378	2.1			90	0.5											
Dog (control)	660	3.7			138	0.8									72 m²/lung[d]	E integrated to peak	4
(alloxan)	792	4.4			192	1.1											
Dog (control)			18–84	0.1–0.5											3000 cm² g⁻¹	E peak of tracer curve	5
Dog (control)			72	0.4											3000 cm² g⁻¹	E peak of tracer curve	6
Dog (control)	4500	25	198	1.1											3000 cm² g⁻¹	E model	7, 8
Sheep (control)					270	1.5									3000 cm² g⁻¹	E integrated to peak	9
(histamine)					402	2.2									3000 cm² g⁻¹		

168

Sheep									
(control)	138	0.8	60	0.3			$3000\ \mathrm{cm^2\,g^{-1}}$[e]	E integrated to peak	10
(histamine)	168	0.9	54	0.3					
Newborn lambs									
(control)	312	1.7	138	0.8			$3000\ \mathrm{cm^2\,g^{-1}}$	E integrated to peak	11
Sheep									
(control)	150	0.8	54	0.3			$3000\ \mathrm{cm^2\,g^{-1}}$[e]	E integrated to peak	12
Rabbit									
(adult)			234	1.3	84	0.5	$3000\ \mathrm{cm^2\,g^{-1}}$[f]	E at appearance	13
(adult)			192	1.1	102	0.6	$3000\ \mathrm{cm^2\,g^{-1}}$	E at appearance	
(6 weeks)			318	1.8	144	0.8	$3000\ \mathrm{cm^2\,g^{-1}}$	E at appearance	
(3 weeks)			282	1.6	150	0.8	$3000\ \mathrm{cm^2\,g^{-1}}$	E at appearance	
(neonate)			342	1.9	180	1.0	$3000\ \mathrm{cm^2\,g^{-1}}$	E at appearance	
(fetal)			198	4.1	66	1.4	$800\ \mathrm{cm^2\,g^{-1}}$[f]	E at appearance	
Man									
(control)	408	4.9	108	1.3			$70\ \mathrm{m^2/lung}$[g]	$E_{\max}$ by numerical deconvolution	14
(isoproterenol)	516	6.1	102	1.2			$70\ \mathrm{m^2/lung}$		
Man									
(cardiac failure)	24–270	0.3–3.5					$70\ \mathrm{m^2/lung}$[g]	E integrated to peak	15

[a] Abbreviations: PS, permeability surface-area product (ml min⁻¹ 100 g⁻¹); P, permeability coefficient (cm sec⁻¹ × 10⁻⁶); gluc, glucose (mannitol); sucr, sucrose; raff, raffinose; S, capillary surface area (cm² g⁻¹).

[b] References: 1, Basset et al. (1976); 2, Basset et al. (1975); 3, Neufeld et al. (1976); 4, Harris et al. (1975); 5, Yipintsoi (1976); 6, Tancredi and Yipintsoi (1980); 7, Chinard et al. (1977); 8, Perl et al. (1976); 9, Harris et al. (1978); 10, Brigham et al. (1977a); 11, Brigham et al. (1978); 12, Brigham et al. (1977b); 13, Perry and Garlick (1978); 14, Neufeld et al. (1975); 15, Brigham et al. (1979b).

[c] Assumed dog lung weight was 240 g (Yipintsoi, 1976) and $S = 3000\ \mathrm{cm^2\,g^{-1}}$.

[d] Weight of dog lung assumed to be 240 g (Yipintsoi, 1976).

[e] Lung weight calculated from Brigham et al. (1978).

[f] Capillary surface-area values for adult and fetal rabbits taken from Perry (1980).

[g] Assumed lung weight in man was 500 g (Staub, 1974) and $S = 70\ \mathrm{m^2}$ (Weibel, 1973).

TABLE II
Permeability Characteristics of Skeletal Muscle Capillaries for Small Solutes[a]

Species (treatment)	Muscle	PS K+	P K+	PS Na+	P Na+	PS gluc	P gluc	PS sucr	P sucr	PS raff	P raff	PS inulin	P inulin	Type of experiment	Extraction, E	Ref.[b]
Rat (rest)	Hind-quarters							5.7[c]	1.36[c]					Bolus	$E_{50\%}$	1
Cat (rest)	Gastroc-nemius	2.7	0.6											Constant infusion	[d]	2
(exercise)	Gastroc-nemius	4.9	1.2													
Cat (rest)	Gastroc-nemius							5.5[c]	1.3[c]					Bolus	$E_{40\%}$	3
Cat (isolated, perfused)	Gastroc-nemius					4.0	0.9							Bolus	E_{plateau}	4
Cat (isolated, perfused)	Gastroc-nemius					20.0	4.8	18.6	4.4			4.5	1.1	Bolus	E_0	5
						17.6	4.2	9.2	2.2			0.7	0.17	Bolus	E_{peak}	
						13.7	3.3	9.6	2.3			1.2	0.29	Washout	E_{washout}	
Cat (rest)								6.2[c]	1.5[c]	3.3[e]	0.8[e]			Bolus	E_{total}	6

170

Species (condition)	Tissue	PS / P values by solute	E values	E type	Method	Ref
Cat (rest)			0.89	$E_{\text{total curve}}$	Bolus	7
Dog (rest)	Gracilis	4.5 / 1.1	0.21	E_0^d	Constant infusion	8
Dog (rest)	Hindlimb	2.0 / 0.48	0.71 / 0.17	E_0^d	Bolus	9
Man (exercise)	Forearm	17.6 / 4.2; 4.5^c / 1.07^c		E_{plateau}	Bolus	10
Man (exercise)	Forearm	16.5 / 3.9; 5.9 / 1.4; 4.0^c / 0.95^c; 2.36 / 0.56; 3.7 / 0.88	0.37 / 0.09	E_{plateau}^f	Bolus	11
Man (exercise)	Forearm	7.2 / 1.71		E_{plateau}^f	Bolus	10
(diabetes)		20.7 / 4.9	1.04 / 0.25			

[a] Abbreviations: PS, permeability surface-area product (ml min⁻¹ 100 g⁻¹); P, permeability coefficient (cm sec⁻¹ × 10⁻⁵); gluc, glucose; sucr, sucrose; raff, raffinose. Capillary surface area S was assumed to be 70 cm² g⁻¹ in all calculations.

[b] References: 1, Rippe et al. (1978); 2, Hilton et al. (1974); 3, Sejrsen (1979); 4, Crone (1973); 5, Garlick (1970); 6, Paaske (1977); 7, Paaske and Sejrsen (1977); 8, Yudilevich et al. (1968); 9, Crone (1963a); 10, Lassen and Trap-Jensen (1970); 11, Lassen and Trap-Jensen (1969).

[c] Values for Cr-EDTA, a molecule similar in dimensions to sucrose.

[d] Values calculated using plasma flow and assuming blood hematocrit of 0.35.

[e] Values for cyanocobalamin, MW 1353.

[f] Calculated from published capillary diffusion coefficients by dividing by 0.89 for charged solutes and 0.94 for uncharged solutes.

b. Skeletal Muscle. In skeletal muscle the extraction pattern for diffusible tracers generally displays a plateau, indicating an absence of significant back diffusion in early samples. This simplifies the interpretation of indicator-dilution data in this tissue. Early studies in which the indicator-dilution technique was used to assess the permeability of the vasculature in resting skeletal muscle revealed no restriction to the diffusion of solutes as large as inulin (Crone, 1963a; Yudilevich *et al.*, 1968). However, more recent evidence suggests that at blood flow rates observed in resting muscle (below 10–15 ml min^{-1} 100 g^{-1}) there is flow limitation of small tracer molecules (Rippe *et al.*, 1978; Trap-Jensen and Lassen, 1970). When blood flow to the muscle is high, for example, during exercise, there is evidence for restricted diffusion of inulin, a finding consistent with an effective small-"pore" radius of 40–45 Å in skeletal muscle capillaries. Pathologic changes in skeletal muscle vascular permeability have also been investigated with this technique (Trap-Jensen and Lassen, 1970). The results suggest that diabetes mellitus produces an increase in the effective radius of the small-pore population in muscle capillaries. Some investigators have also used the indicator-dilution technique to investigate the presence of an active transport mechanism within the muscle vasculature (Crone, 1973).

Data obtained with the indicator-dilution technique in skeletal muscle beds of different species are shown in Table II.

c. Cardiac Muscle. The PS values obtained in cardiac muscle are greater than those obtained in skeletal muscle for two reasons: (*a*) cardiac muscle has a greater capillary surface area for exchange (500 cm^2 g^{-1}) (Bassingthwaighte, 1974) and (*b*) the permeability coefficients for small molecules appear to be greater in heart muscle. Results obtained with the indicator-dilution technique in cardiac muscle are shown in Table III.

In the heart early extraction values often increase until a plateau is reached. This pattern of extraction is most likely due to heterogeneity of flow; that is, the earliest samples represent fast transit pathways in which extraction is low, whereas later samples approximate the mean transit time with slightly higher extraction values. However, extensive analysis of indicator-dilution curves obtained in the heart support the use of plateau extraction values for calculating PS in this tissue (Guller *et al.*, 1975).

Flow limitation for all but the largest solutes occurs in the heart at plasma flow rates below 40 ml min^{-1} 100 g^{-1} (Duran and Yudilevich, 1978). For small solutes such as sodium flow limitation may persist even at very high plasma flow rates (Mann, 1981). With large molecules, PS increases with increasing flow, even at flow rates above 100 ml min^{-1} 100 g^{-1}. This pattern of increasing PS with increasing flow under conditions in which flow limitation is not a factor has been interpreted as a progressive recruitment of capillary surface area for exchange (Guller *et al.*, 1975).

There is little evidence of restricted diffusion of small solutes in cardiac muscle capillaries. Mann (1981) found only modest restriction to insulin (MW 5807, r = 15 Å). The results of this and other studies (Bassingthwaighte *et al.*, 1975; Laughlin and Diana, 1975) suggest that the effective radius of the small pores in cardiac capillaries is greater than in skeletal muscle capillaries. Comparison of the permeability coefficients reported in Table II (skeletal muscle) with those in Table III (cardiac muscle) supports this contention.

Future indicator-dilution studies incorporating large solutes as the tracers may provide more definite information on the restrictive properties of cardiac capillaries.

d. Digestive Tract. The ultrastructural appearance of the fenestrated capillaries found in the mucosal and submucosal regions of the stomach and intestine suggests that these vascular beds may be very permeable to small solutes. Perry and Granger (1981) reported PS values for raffinose and inulin in the small intestine that are 20 times larger than values observed in hyperemic skeletal muscle. Calculated permeability coefficients indicate that the intestinal capillaries are 5–7 times more permeable to raffinose and inulin than skeletal muscle capillaries. In the stomach the reported PS values are 3 times larger than those obtained in the intestine (Perry *et al.*, 1981). There was no evidence of restricted diffusion of inulin in either intestine or stomach vascular beds. However, β-lactoglobulin A (r = 28 Å) was restricted; the degree of restriction was consistent with effective small-pore radii of 53–59 Å. In one study (Perry *et al.*, 1981) the equivalent small-pore radius of gastric capillaries was calculated both from indicator-dilution data and by lymphatic protein flux analysis. The two techniques predicted similar effective small-pore dimensions.

In the digestive organs studied the diffusible tracers display a plateau in extraction values up to or beyond the peak of the vascular indicator curve (Fig. 5). However, these vascular beds represent a mixture of continuous capillaries in muscular layer and fenestrated capillaries in the mucosa and submucosa. Because the combined mucosa–submucosa receives 80–85% of the total blood flow to these organs (Delaney and Grim, 1964; Lundgren, 1967), it is likely that the reported values represent predominantly the permeability characteristics of the fenestrated type of capillary. By selective dilation of the muscular layer of the small intestine Perry and Granger (1981) presented limited evidence that the permeability charac-

TABLE III

Permeability Characteristics of Cardiac Muscle Capillaries for Small Solutes[a]

Species (treatment)	PS H_2O	P H_2O	PS K^+	P K^+	PS Na^+	P Na^+	PS urea	P urea	PS gluc	P gluc	PS sucr	P sucr	PS inulin	P inulin	Extraction, E	Ref.[b]
Dog	1800	60									66–99	2.2–3.3			E_{model}	1
Dog															E_{model}	2
Dog					75	2.5					52	1.7			E_{model} (PS max)	3
Dog			110	3.7					45	1.5	40	1.3			E_{max}	4
Dog					100	3.3			50	1.7	36	1.2			$E_{max} \times 1.136$	5
Dog (isol dilated)					83	2.8									$E \times 1.14$	6
Dog (isol)			106	3.5	54	1.8									$E_{max} \times 1.136$	7
Dog (isol)	231	7.7			74	2.5									$E_{\lim t \to 0}$	8
Dog							60	2.0	20	0.7	16	0.5	5.2	0.17	$E_{\lim t \to 0}$	9
Dog (dilated)					67	2.2			37	1.2					$E_{plateau}$	10

Dog (dilated)	117	3.9							$E_{plateau}$	11
Dog			64	2.1	26	0.9			E_{peak}	11
Dog (control)	68	2.3			24	0.8	7.0	0.23	$E_{plateau}^c$ or E_{peak}	12
(exercise)	75	2.5			26	0.9	9.4	0.31		
(tricusp insuff)	128	4.3			48	1.6	34.0	1.13		
Rabbit	218	7.3			59	2.0			$E_{plateau}$	13
Rabbit (isol plasma perfused)	315	10.5			106^d	3.5^d	6.3^e	0.21^e	$E_{plateau}$	14
					63^f	2.1^f				

[a] Abbreviations: PS, permeability surface-area product (ml min^{-1} 100 g^{-1}); P, permeability coefficient (cm sec^{-1} × 10^{-5}); gluc, glucose; sucr, sucrose; isol, isolated heart preparation; dilated, vasodilated preparation; tricusp insuff, tricuspid insufficiency. Capillary surface area was assumed to be 500 cm^2 g^{-1} in all calculations.

[b] References: 1, Rose and Goresky (1976); 2, Rose et al. (1977); 3, Ziegler and Goresky (1971); 4, Yipintsoi et al. (1970); 5, Bassingthwaighte et al. (1975); 6, Guller et al. (1975); 7, Tancredi et al. (1975); 8, Yudilevich and Alvarez (1967); 9, Alvarez and Yudilevich (1969); 10, Duran et al. (1973); 11, Duran and Yudilevich (1978); 12, Laughlin and Diana (1975); 13, Bassingthwaighte et al. (1979); 14, Mann (1981).

[c] Assumed hematocrit of 0.35 to convert blood flow to plasma flow.

[d] Values for Cr-EDTA, a molecule similar in dimensions to sucrose.

[e] Values for insulin (MW = 5860), a molecule similar in dimensions to inulin.

[f] Values for cyanocobalamin (MW = 1353).

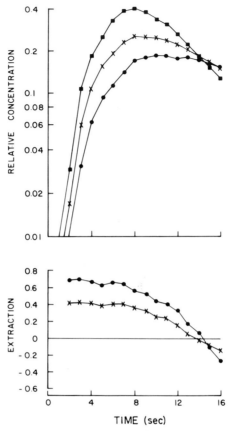

Fig. 5. Relative concentrations of vascular tracer (^{125}I-γ-globulin, ■) and two diffusible tracers ([^{3}H]raffinose, ●, and [^{14}C]inulin, ×) in venous blood samples collected from the cat
small intestine. Extraction of diffusible tracers shown in the lower panel displays a pronounced plateau up to the peak of the reference tracer curve. (From Perry and Granger,
1981.)

teristics of capillaries in smooth muscle are similar to those reported by
others for skeletal muscle capillaries.

Another fenestrated vascular bed that has been studied with the indicator-dilution technique is the salivary gland (Mann *et al.,* 1979a,b). The PS
values for this tissue (which possesses only fenestrated capillaries) are 10
times larger than values reported for the small intestine (Table IV). These
higher PS values may be due in part to a greater vascular permeability
because the calculated effective pore radius is approximately 120 Å in the
salivary gland (Mann *et al.,* 1979a) compared with approximately 60 Å in
the small intestine.

TABLE IV

Permeability Characteristics of Capillaries in the Digestive Tract for Small Solutes[a,b]

Species (tissue/treatment)	PS gluc	P gluc	PS sucr	P sucr	PS raff	P raff	PS inulin	P inulin	PS lactogl	P lactogl	Extraction, E	Ref.[c]
Cat (salivary gland)			>800[d]		411[e]		176 180[f]				$E_{\lim t \to 0}$	1
Cat (salivary gland) (duct obstruction)			526[d] 420[d]		322[e] 202[e]		152[f] 72[f]				$E_{\lim t \to 0}$	2
Cat (small intestine)					42	5.6[g]	23	3.1[g]	3.5	0.47[g]	E_{plateau}	3
Rabbit (small intestine)					55	7.3[g]	26	3.5[g]			E_{plateau}	4
Dog (stomach)	23.2[h]										E_0	5
Dog (stomach)					140		70		8		E_{plateau}	6

[a] All values were obtained following bolus injections of the tracers.

[b] Abbreviations: PS, permeability surface-area product (ml min⁻¹ 100 g⁻¹); P, permeability coefficient (cm sec⁻¹ × 10⁻⁵); gluc, glucose; sucr, sucrose; raff, raffinose; lactogl, lactoglobulin. Capillary surface area S (cm² g⁻¹) not known for all organs in the digestive tract.

[c] References: 1, Mann et al. (1979a); 2, Mann et al. (1979b); 3, Perry and Granger (1981); M. A. Perry (unpublished observations); 5, Yudilevich et al. (1968); 6, Perry et al. (1981).

[d] Values for Cr-EDTA, a molecule similar in size to sucrose.

[e] Values for cyanocobalamin (MW 1353).

[f] Values for insulin (MW 5807).

[g] Capillary surface area for cat jejunum assumed to be 125 cm² g⁻¹ (Casley-Smith et al., 1975).

[h] Calculated from blood flow assuming hematocrit of 0.35.

e. Liver. The capillaries of the liver, spleen, and bone marrow represent the most permeable vascular beds in the body. The only barrier to the exchange of solutes between plasma and cells is the interstitium. In the liver the exchange of all solutes studied, including albumin, is flow-limited (Goresky, 1963, 1965). This is due not only to the permeable nature of the vascular bed but also to the long transit time of solutes through the liver vasculature. Because there is thought to be complete equilibration of tracers during a single transit through the liver, the indicator-dilution technique has been used in this organ to measure the volumes of distribution of various solutes as well as the degree of exclusion of these solutes from the liver interstitium, both under normal conditions and during cirrhosis (Huet *et al.*, 1980). The technique has also been used to measure the rate of cellular uptake of blood-borne substances (Goresky *et al.*, 1973; Goresky and Nadeau, 1974).

f. Brain. Application of indicator-dilution methodology to analysis of the permeability characteristics of cerebral capillaries (Table V) has shown that the blood–brain barrier is remarkably impermeable even to small, lipid-insoluble solutes (Crone, 1963a; Yudilevich and DeRose, 1971). The technique has also revealed the presence of a specific transport mechanism for D-glucose in the cerebral circulation (Crone, 1965; Murray and Plioplys, 1972). However, this mechanism may be located in the choroid plexus rather than the endothelial cell (Wright and Prather, 1970).

B. Osmotic Transient Technique

The first description of the effects of hypertonic solutions on the rate of fluid exchange across the microcirculation was provided by Starling in 1896. In his epochal study on capillary filtration, Starling noted that the hemodilution resulting from intravascular injection of a hypertonic solution was some function of solute size. He noted a relatively greater hemodilution with Na_2SO_4 than with NaCl solutions of equivalent osmolarity. Although Starling did not concisely ascribe the differential responsiveness of the microvasculature to a graded selectivity of the capillary wall to solutes on the basis of size, his study represented the first description of the osmotic transient technique (Starling, 1896).

A more sophisticated application of the osmotic transient method was described by Pappenheimer *et al.* (1951). They estimated the net solute flows from the blood into the tissues from the product of blood flow and the arteriovenous concentration. The mean concentration gradient across the capillary wall was estimated from the osmotic pressure resulting from it. The test solute was added to the perfusion system and, when it reached

TABLE V

Permeability Characteristics of Capillaries in the Brain for Small Solutes[a,b]

Species	PS H$_2$O	P H$_2$O	PS ethanol	P ethanol	PS antipyrene	P antipyrene	PS urea	P urea	PS fructose	P fruc	PS raff	PS inulin	Extraction, E	Ref.[c]
Rat	150	10.4											E_{peak}	1
Dog											0	0		2
Dog			144^d	10^d	39^{d,e}	2.7^{d,e}	4.2^{d,f}	0.29^{d,f}	1.5^{d,f}	0.1^{d,f}	0	0	$E_{upslope}$	3
Monkey	114	7.9											E by extrapolation	4
Monkey	110^e	6.9											E by extrapolation	5

[a] All values were obtained following bolus injection of tracers.

[b] Abbreviations: PS, permeability surface-area product (ml min^{-1} 100 g^{-1}); P, permeability coefficient (cm sec^{-1} × 10^{-5}); fruc, fructose; raff, raffinose. Capillary surface area was assumed to be 240 cm²/cm³ in all calculations (Crone, 1963a).

[c] References: 1, Bolwig and Lassen (1975); 2, Crone (1963a); 3, Crone (1965); 4, Eichling et al. (1974); 5, Raichle et al. (1974).

[d] Assumed blood flow of 54 ml min^{-1} 100 g^{-1}.

[e] Assumed water content of blood as 0.81 ml/ml blood (Bolwig and Lassen, 1975).

[f] Assumed hematocrit of 0.35 to convert blood flow to plasma flow.

the capillary bed, the osmotic pressure gradient across the capillary wall caused fluid to shift from the tissues into the blood. The fluid movement was detected as a fall in the weight of the tissue (hindlimb), and it was opposed by raising the hydrostatic pressure in the capillaries. Using this approach Pappenheimer *et al.* (1951) were able to follow the changing transcapillary osmotic pressure.

The osmotic pressure gradient ($\Delta\pi$) achieved during the osmotic transient was converted to the mean concentration gradient using van't Hoff's law, that is,

$$\Delta C = \Delta\pi/RT, \tag{9}$$

where R represents the universal gas constant and T is the absolute temperature.

Having estimated the net flux of solute (J_s) and ΔC, Pappenheimer *et al.* (1951) calculated the product of permeability and capillary surface area as

$$D_s A_s/\Delta X = J_s/\Delta C, \tag{10}$$

where D_s is the solute free diffusion coefficient, A_s is the total area available for the solute, and ΔX is the thickness of the membrane (length of pores).

Using this approach, Pappenheimer and co-workers obtained values for capillary permeability for a wide range of lipid-insoluble molecules. These results led to the theory of restricted diffusion through pores and the proposal that the capillary wall is penetrated by pores with an equivalent cylindrical radius of 30–35 Å or by rectangular slits 37 Å in width. The major criticism of Pappenheimer's osmotic transient approach was the assumption that the concentration gradient could be calculated from the osmotic gradient without reference to the reflection coefficient (Michel, 1972). Landis and Pappenheimer (1963) calculated the influence of the reflection coefficient on these results and obtained a modified set of values for permeability, which altered the original conclusions only slightly.

Vargas and Johnson (1964) described a rather different osmotic transient technique that allowed for direct estimation of the reflection coefficient in accordance with the principles laid down by Kedem and Katchalsky in 1958. In their original study, they employed an isolated rabbit heart preparation that was perfused at a high flow rate and was weighed continuously. Osmotic transients for test solutes were expressed as flow across the capillary wall per unit concentration difference ($J_v/\Delta C$) and plotted as a function of time. The values for $J_v/\Delta C$ was extrapolated to zero time to obtain the initial concentration of the test solute (Kedem and Katchalsky, 1958). It was assumed that, when this initial concentration gradient was established, the mean concentration of test solute in the capillaries was equal to the inflow concentration on the grounds that flow rate was very high and the extravascular concentration of solute was zero. The hydraulic conductance of the capillary bed (LpS) was determined from a separate osmotic transient when test perfusate contained albumin (for which it was assumed that σ equals 1). The mathematical relationship between the reflection coefficient (σ) and osmotic fluid movement across the capillary wall is

$$-J_v = -LpS\sigma RT \ \Delta C \tag{11}$$

or

$$\sigma = J_v/(LpSRT \ \Delta C). \tag{12}$$

The values obtained for σ in Vargas and Johnson's study are presented in Table VI along with values reported subsequently by other investigators for different tissues. It is noteworthy that the equivalent pore radius predicted by Vargas and Johnson in heart is nearly identical (35 Å) to that predicted by Pappenheimer and associates for skeletal muscle, in spite of the fact that the latter ignored σ in their analysis.

The osmotic transient approach described by Vargas and Johnson has been subsequently used by several investigators to study capillary permeability. Whereas some investigators have employed the osmotic transient approach in an identical fashion to that described by Vargas and Johnson (1964), others have modified the technique to include an actual measurement of LpS using volumetric/gravimetric methods (Taylor and Gaar, 1970). This modification negates the use of albumin transients to obtain LpS and the assumption that the σ for albumin equals 1.0. Studies employing other techniques indicate that σ for albumin is significantly less than 1 in most capillary beds.

There are several serious criticisms and limitations of the osmotic transient technique. These include (a) overestimation of the $\Delta\pi$ acting across the capillary wall at zero time, (b) overestimation of LpS using volumetric/gravimetric approaches, (c) osmotic removal of water from cells, (d) capillary heteroporosity, (c) local vascular resistance and blood volume changes in response to an increase in plasma osmolality, (f) heterogeneity of capillary types within a tissue, and (g) osmotically induced changes in capillary permeability. The most common criticism of the technique concerns the assumption that the mean concentration gradient across the capillary walls at zero time is equal to the inflowing concentration of test solutes. It is frequently suggested that the concentration gradient across the capillary wall at "zero time" may be substantially less than the capillary concentration. For rapidly penetrating solutes (e.g., urea), it is likely that the gradient across the arterial end of the capillary wall would be con-

TABLE VI
Reflection Coefficients Obtained Using the Osmotic Transient Technique in Various Tissues

Tissue, solute	Solute radius (Å)	Reflection coefficient	Predicted equivalent pore size (Å)	Reference
Skeletal muscle			39	Diana *et al.* (1972)
Urea	2.3	0.055		
Glucose	3.7	0.092		
Sucrose	4.8	0.106		
Raffinose	5.7	0.139		
Inulin	9–12	0.542		
Dextran 10	22	1.000		
Brain			7–9	Fenstermacher and
Urea	2.7	0.44		Johnson (1966)
Glucose	4.4	0.89		
Sucrose	5.3	0.98		
Raffinose	6.1	1.00		
Heart			35	Vargas and Johnson
Urea	1.7–2.6	0.11		(1964)
Sucrose	5.2	0.30		
Raffinose	6.0	0.38		
Inulin	11–15	0.69		
Lung			40–58	Taylor and Gaar (1970)
Urea	2.7	0.018		
Glucose	4.3	0.026		
Sucrose	5.2	0.044		
Intestine			200–350	Granger *et al.* (1979a)
Urea	2.7	0.0006		
Glucose	4.3	0.0017		
Mannitol	4.3	0.0014		
Maltose	5.2	0.0014		
Mesentery[a]			—	Curry *et al.* (1976)
Sodium chloride	2.3	0.068		
Urea	2.6	0.071		
Sucrose	4.8	0.115		
Vitamin B_{12}	8.0	0.100		

[a] Values obtained from individual capillaries.

siderably below its initial value by the time the unextracted solutes have reached the venous end of the capillary. This problem is compounded in tissues (e.g., lung, intestine) where the interstitial compartment surrounding the capillaries is small. The errors introduced by the uncertainty of the mean concentration gradient across the capillary wall would generally lead to an underestimation of σ and consequently an overestimation of equivalent pore size.

An equally serious criticism of the osmotic transient approach is that a larger proportion of the fluid entering the vasculature during an osmotic transient is extracted from cells. Thus, it may be incorrect to assume that water and small solutes cross the capillary walls by the same pathway during an osmotic transient. The error introduced by fluid withdrawal from cells during an osmotic transient is likely to lead to an overestimation of σ and an underestimation of pore sizes. The cell pathway for fluid movement during an osmotic transient is generally used to explain the frequent observation that there is no correlation between σ and solute size for such solutes as sodium chloride, urea, glucose, and sucrose (Michel, 1978).

Another criticism of the osmotic transient approach is that the increased plasma osmolality imposed during a transient increases vascular permeability. An increase in plasma osmolality by as little as 20 mOsm (using glucose) has been shown to increase the leakage of proteins across intestinal capillaries (Granger et al., 1979a). Hypertonic sucrose solutions have been shown to increase the permeability of capillaries to both urea and albumin (Rasio et al., 1981). If such changes in vascular permeability occur during an osmotic transient experiment, the estimates of σ would be underestimates. This serious limitation may well invalidate the technique.

For a more detailed description and evaluation of the factors that influence the osmotic transient method, the reader is referred to a series of articles by Johnson and co-workers (Bloom and Johnson, 1981; Johnson and Bloom, 1981; Johnson et al., 1981).

C. Lymphatic Protein Flux Analyses

Since the time of Starling (1915) it was known that the concentration of protein in lymph varied from tissue to tissue. Although Starling realized that the tissue-to-tissue variability of lymph protein content most likely represented regional differences in capillary permeability, the technique of using lymph solute concentrations as an estimate of capillary permeability was not introduced until the mid-1900s by Grotte (1956) and Mayerson et al. (1960). Since that time lymph solute analyses have become the most popular technique for studying capillary permeability to macromolecules.

Grotte introduced the method of using the relationship between lymph-to-plasma solute concentration ratio (L/P) and molecular radius for sev-

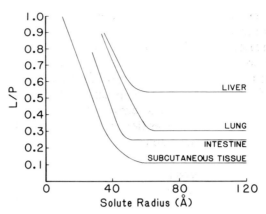

Fig. 6. Relationship between lymph-to-plasma solute concentration ratio (L/P) and solute radius for subcutaneous tissue (Rutili and Arfors, 1977), small intestine (Granger and Taylor, 1980), lung (Parker *et al.*, 1981a), and liver (Granger *et al.*, 1979b).

eral solutes to study vascular permeability. This approach has been frequently used to compare the permeability of one capillary bed with that of another. Figure 6 illustrates the relationship between L/P and solute radius for several organs. On the basis of the assumption that steady-state L/P values provide an estimate of capillary permeability to a molecule, the data presented in Fig. 6 would indicate that the liver sinusoids are the most permeable microvessels, followed by pulmonary and intestinal capillaries, with subcutaneous capillaries being the least permeable. These conclusions are generally consistent with results obtained using more sophisticated analyses (Taylor and Granger, 1982). Although this approach appears to provide a reasonably good assessment of regional differences in vascular permeability, there are problems with the analysis that may limit its usefulness as a measure of vascular permeability.

Although it is generally assumed that differences in L/P for a given solute between capillary beds represent corresponding differences in vascular permeability, they may also result from variations in capillary surface area and/or capillary filtration rate. For example, tissues with identical capillary permeability and capillary filtration rates yet differing capillary surface areas will have different L/Ps; the tissue with the highest capillary surface area will exhibit the highest L/P. Comparable variations in L/P for a given solute can result from tissues with identical capillary surface areas and permeabilities yet differing capillary filtration rates. Since the steady-state L/P is influenced by factors other than capillary permeability, the interpretation of L/P data at normal filtration rates (Fig. 6) may not be as straightforward as previously suggested. For example, it is conceivable

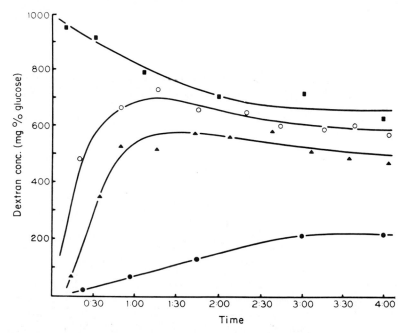

Fig. 7. Plot of dextran (MW 35,000) concentration in plasma (■), hepatic lymph (○), intestinal lymph (▲), and cervical lymph (●) in dog from studies by Mayerson. (From Mayerson *et al.*, 1960.)

that pulmonary capillaries are as impermeable to macromolecules as intestinal capillaries. However, due to an extremely large capillary surface area relative to capillary filtration rate in the lung, its L/P values would exceed that of intestine.

Another method used to assess regional differences in vascular permeability involves the determination of equilibration time of macromolecules in the lymph. This approach was introduced and subsequently refined by Mayerson *et al.* (1960). Figure 7 illustrates the results obtained in Mayerson's original study. The data clearly indicate differences in equilibration time of a dextran (molecular radius 41 Å) in lymph-draining liver, intestine, and skeletal muscle. On the basis of these findings, Mayerson and co-workers suggested that capillary permeability followed the order liver > intestine > skeletal muscle. This approach is very similar to the L/P versus molecular radius method, in that it generally provides only qualitative information regarding regional differences in vascular permeability. Furthermore, the difference in lymph equilibration times between tissues could result from differences in capillary filtration rate, capillary surface area, and interstitial volumes rather than variations in vascular permeability. Newer applications of the lymph equilibrium technique allow for the estimation of capillary membrane parameters such as the reflection coefficient or PS (Parker *et al.*, 1981a). Estimates of σ derived from lymph equilibration data require some assumptions (or independent estimations) of the volume of distribution of the solute in the interstitium and the PS.

The first method for analyzing lymphatic protein data in terms of the PS was developed by Renkin (1964). This method of estimating PS was based on the assumption that the movement of macromolecules across capillaries occurs entirely by diffusion, that is,

$$J_s = J_L C_L = PS(C_p - C_L),$$

or

$$PS = \frac{J_L C_L}{C_p - C_L}, \qquad (13)$$

where J_s represents lymphatic solute flux, J_L is lymph flow, C_L is the lymph protein concentration, and C_p is the plasma protein concentration. The analysis therefore requires steady-state determinations of J_L, C_L, and C_p. Renkin (Carter *et al.*, 1974; Renkin, 1979a) and others (Brigham *et al.*, 1974, 1979a; Brigham and Owen, 1975) have used this method of PS determination to assess regional differences in vascular permeability. However, in recent years the technique has been extensively criticized because of the inherent assumption that there is no convective movement of macromolecules across the capillary wall (Taylor and Granger, 1982). By ignoring convective exchange, this technique leads to an overestimation of PS.

It is generally considered that both diffusive and convective processes are involved in the movement of macromolecules across capillary walls. Therefore, methods have been developed for the determination of both the reflection coefficient and PS using lymphatic protein flux data (Taylor *et al.*, 1977; Renkin *et al.*, 1977a; Brace *et al.*, 1977, 1978). These methods are based on the formulations of Kedem and Katchalsky (1958, 1961), which describe solvent (J_v) and solute (J_s) flows across porous barriers:

$$J_s = J_v(1 - \sigma)\bar{C}_s + PS\,\Delta C, \qquad (14)$$

where $\bar{C}_s$ is an expression of the concentration profile of a solute within the porous structure of the membrane, and ΔC is the solute concentration gradient.

One method used to estimate σ and PS involves the acquisition of lymph flux data (C_L and C_p) at two capillary filtration rates. Since Eq. (14) is linear, a single value for σ and PS can be obtained which describes the two flux states by solving two equations for two unknowns. These values can be graphically derived from the intersection of two linear equations relating $1 - C_L/\bar{C}_s$ and $(J_v \times C_L)/(C_p - C_L)$. An assumption inherent in this approach is that membrane parameters (σ and PS) are unchanged by the imposed experimental conditions required to alter capillary filtration rate (e.g., venous congestion, plasma volume expansion). Estimates of σ and PS for a wide range of capillary filtration rates [using Eq. (14)] suggest that both σ and PS increase as capillary filtration is enhanced (Taylor and Granger, 1982). Although the rise in PS with capillary filtration rate could result from a "stretched pore" effect due to venous pressure elevation, the concomitant rise in σ makes this explanation an unlikely one. However, solute movement across a heteroporous membrane with nonuniform pressure gradients could result in a rise in both PS and σ without altering membrane porosity.

Other methods have been developed from estimating σ and PS using Eq. (14) and several lymph flux states (Renkin et al., 1977a; Perl, 1975). These approaches also take advantage of the linear nature of Eq. (14), and they assume that σ and PS are filtration rate independent. The latter assumption has led to extensive criticism of these approaches.

As a group, the methods developed for estimating σ and PS from Eq. (14) yield relatively little information regarding regional differences in capillary permeability. This is due primarily to the influence of capillary filtration rate on the estimated values for σ and PS. Furthermore, there is growing evidence that the Kedem–Katchalsky equation [Eq. (14)] cannot accurately describe solute exchange across capillaries because it was derived for a membrane–solute–solvent system at near equilibrium (Taylor and Granger, 1982).

A technique has been developed for determining the osmotic reflection coefficient (σ_d) using the relationship between L/Ps and lymph flow (Granger and Taylor, 1980). As illustrated in Fig. 8, when lymph flow is increased from its normal value (by elevating venous pressure), L/P decreases (filtration rate dependent) until sufficiently high lymph flows are obtained at which L/P is no longer influenced by further increases in lymph flow (filtration rate independent). When L/P becomes filtration rate independent, it can be assumed that convective exchange accounts for all solute movement across the capillaries and the L/P represents the true separative capacity of the capillary membrane. Therefore, when L/P is filtration rate independent, σ_d is equal to $1 - L/P$.

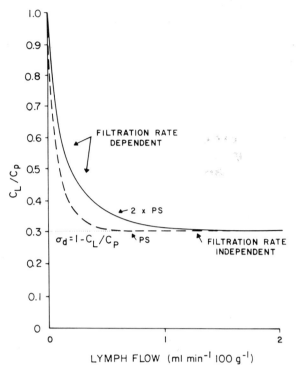

Fig. 8. Theoretical relationship between C_L/C_P and lymph flow at two capillary surface areas predicted by Eq. (15). Theoretically, the osmotic reflection coefficient (σ_d) can be estimated using $\sigma_d = 1 - C_L/C_P$ when C_L/C_P is filtration rate independent. $\sigma_d = 0.70$; PS = 0.05. (From Granger and Taylor, 1980.)

There is both theoretical (Bresler and Groome, 1981; Granger and Taylor, 1980) and experimental evidence to support the contention that σ_d can be estimated using $1 - L/P$ at high capillary filtration rates. The theoretical curve in Fig. 8 was derived from the equation (Granger and Taylor, 1980)

$$L/P = (1 - \sigma)/(1 - \sigma e^{-x}), \qquad (15)$$

where $x = (1 - \sigma)J_L/PS$ and J_L is lymph flow. Comparable curves have been obtained experimentally from a variety of tissues (Granger and Taylor, 1980; Parker *et al.*, 1981a,b; Perry and Granger, 1981; Richardson *et al.*, 1980; Rutili *et al.*, 1982). Figure 9 depicts total protein L/P data obtained from the small intestine of cat and rat. Assuming $\sigma_d = 1 - L/P$ when L/P is filtration rate independent, a value of 0.92 is predicted for intestinal capillaries from Fig. 9. Table VII summarizes the values of σ_d

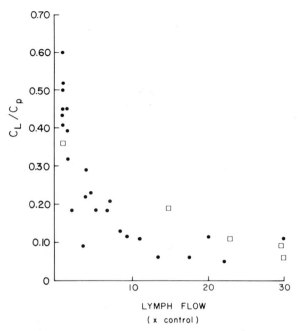

Fig. 9. Steady-state relationship between C_L/C_P for total proteins and lymph flow in the small intestine of cat (●) and rat (□). (Data from Granger and Taylor, 1980, and Lee, 1981.)

obtained using this approach in several tissues. This technique has proved useful for the development of pore models because σ_d values have been obtained for a number of solutes of differing size (see Section III,C, for a description of analysis). In addition to its application to the delineation of regional differences in vascular permeability, this approach has been extensively used to study physiologic, pharmacologic, and pathologic changes in vascular permeability (Taylor and Granger, 1982).

The major assumptions implicit in all analyses employing lymph to study vascular permeability are that (a) lymph provides a true sample of interstitial fluid and (b) the capillary is the limiting membrane restricting the movement of macromolecules to lymph. It has long been assumed that the composition of lymph is identical to that of interstitial fluid under steady-state conditions (Rusznyak *et al.,* 1967; Yoffey and Courtice, 1970). Numerous investigators have provided indirect data to support or refute this assumption. Direct comparisons of interstitial fluid samples with lymph collected simultaneously from the same tissue generally support the contention that the concentrations of macromolecules in lymph and interstitial fluid are identical. Interstitial fluid samples collected by

TABLE VII
Reflection Coefficients Calculated Using L/P Data Obtained at High
Capillary Filtration Rates

Organ	Solute radius (Å)	Reflection coefficient	Reference
Small intestine	Total protein	0.92	Granger and Taylor (1980)
	37	0.90	
	38	0.92	
	39	0.94	
	42	0.96	
	96	0.98	
	120	0.99	
Stomach	Total protein	0.78	Perry et al. (1981)
	37	0.73	
	38	0.77	
	39	0.78	
	42	0.79	
	96	0.91	
	120	0.91	
Colon	Total protein	0.85	Richardson et al. (1980)
	37	0.75	
	40	0.82	
	44	0.87	
	48	0.88	
	100	0.95	
	120	0.98	
Lung	Total protein	0.62	Parker et al. (1981a)
	37	0.50	
	40	0.59	
	44	0.67	
	53	0.72	
	100	0.94	
	120	0.96	
Liver	Total protein	0.15	Granger et al. (1979b)
Subcutaneous tissue	Total protein	0.90	Rutili et al. (1982)
Pancreas	Total protein	0.85	P. R. Kvietys (unpubl. observ.)

micropipette appear to be closest in composition to prenodal lymph (Rutili and Arfors, 1977). Indirect sources of interstitial fluid (i.e., capsule and wick samples) frequently exhibit a higher protein content than lymph due to inflammation (Aukland and Fadnes, 1973; Haljamäe and Fredén, 1970; Libermann et al., 1972; Reed and Aukland, 1977; Szabo et al., 1976). However, when steps are taken to minimize the influence of inflammation, the difference in protein content between capsular fluid and lymph is small (Reed and Aukland, 1977; Renkin, 1979b; Taylor and Gibson, 1975; Taylor *et al.*, 1973).

The possibility that the composition of lymph may be modified after it has entered the collecting lymphatic has been addressed by several investigators (Renkin, 1979b). The bulk of the data indicates that the exchange of solutes and water between lymphatic vessels and interstitial spaces is probably very small. However, there is considerable evidence suggesting that the composition of lymph is modified within lymph nodes (Courtice, 1971; Quinn and Shannon, 1977; Renkin, 1979b). Thus, the concentration of macromolecules in postnodal lymph may not be representative of interstitial fluid. The available data therefore suggest that lymph can provide an estimate of interstitial fluid composition under steady-state conditions given that the source of lymph is a prenodal lymphatic. Lymph acquired under non-steady-state conditions and/or from a postnodal lymphatic is of questionable value when assumed to represent interstitial fluid.

An assumption inherent in most lymph protein flux studies is that the capillary is the limiting membrane restricting the movement of molecules from blood to lymph. Anatomically, the macromolecule must traverse several barriers, that is, capillary pores, basement membrane, interstitial gel, and lymphatic wall, before exiting the tissue via lymph. Although the lymphatic wall can be ruled out as a significant barrier to blood–lymph protein transport, the interstitial gel and basement membrane could play an important role in restricting the blood–lymph movement of macromolecules. Estimates of equivalent pore sizes in dense connective tissue suggest that the normally hydrated interstitium possesses an equivalent pore radius of 250 Å; that is, for albumin $\sigma_d \leq 0.30$. Increasing the matrix hydration results in a significant diminution of the restrictive properties of the interstitium, and σ_d should fall accordingly. These observations suggest that the interstitial matrix could account for some of the selectivity observed at normal filtration rates. Estimates of vascular permeability based on L/P data at high capillary filtration rates are least likely to be influenced by the interstitium.

III. Applications of Vascular Permeability Data to Pore Theory

A. Indicator-Dilution Technique

A permeability ratio (P_1/P_2) is obtained if two diffusible solutes are used during indicator-dilution experiments (see Section II,A). If both diffusible tracers leave the circulation freely without restriction at the capillary wall and the extravascular volume of distribution of the tracers is large (and neither tracer is flow-limited), then P_1/P_2 will be equal to the ratio of the free diffusion coefficients of the two molecules (D_1/D_2). Under these conditions pore theory predicts that the pore radius is infinitely large. However, if the larger tracer of the pair (P_2) is restricted to some degree by the capillary wall, then P_1/P_2 will be greater than D_1/D_2. The degree of restriction, $(P_1/P_2)/(D_1/D_2)$, can be used to calculate an "equivalent" or "effective" pore radius for the capillary wall as follows. The permeability of a porous membrane to a solute can be expressed as

$$P = D(A_s/S) \, \Delta x^{-1}, \tag{16}$$

where A_s is the pore or slit area available to the solute and Δx is the diffusion path length across the membrane (Landis and Pappenheimer, 1963). For two solutes

$$P_1/P_2 = D_1(A_{s,1}/D_2)A_{s,2}, \quad \text{or} \quad (P_1/P_2)/(D_1/D_2) = A_{s,1}/A_{s,2}. \tag{17}$$

Renkin (1954) derived an equation for the effects of steric hindrance and frictional resistance to the diffusion of a solute through a cylindrical pore in the absence of flow through the pore:

$$A_s/A_p = (1 - a/r)^2[1 - 2.104(a/r) + 2.09(a/r)^3 - 0.95(a/r)^5 \,...], \tag{18}$$

where A_p is total pore area, a is the radius of the solute molecule, and r is the pore radius. Combining Eqs. (17) and (18) for the case in which two diffusible solutes are injected simultaneously,

$$\frac{P_1/P_2}{D_1/D_2} = \frac{(1 - \alpha)^2(1 - 2.104\alpha + 2.09\alpha^3 - 0.95\alpha^5)}{(1 - \beta)^2(1 - 2.104\beta + 2.09\beta^3 - 0.95\beta^5)}, \tag{19}$$

where $\alpha = a_1/r$ and $\beta = a_2/r$ and a_1 and a_2 refer to the radii of solutes 1 and 2, respectively, and r refers to the radius of the equivalent or effective pore in the capillary wall. Although the relationship between calculated effective radii and their morphologic counterparts in the capillary wall has not been established, they represent a convenient way of comparing the permeability characteristics of capillaries in different vascular beds.

B. Osmotic Transient Technique

Reflection coefficients obtained using the osmotic transient approach can be used to estimate equivalent pore sizes. The relationship between solute radius (a), capillary pore radius (r), and the reflection coefficient (σ) has

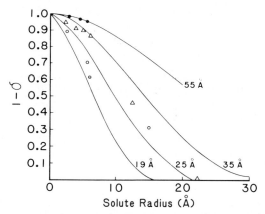

Fig. 10. Plot of 1 minus the reflection coefficient $(1 - \sigma)$ against solute radius for skeletal muscle ($\triangle$), lung ($\bullet$), and heart ($\bigcirc$). The reflection coefficients were obtained using the osmotic transient technique (see Table VI), and the curves representing different pore sizes were generated using Eq. (20).

been defined by several hydrodynamic formulations (Renkin and Curry, 1978). One such formulation was described by Drake and Davis (1978):

$$\sigma = \tfrac{16}{3}(a/r)^2 - \tfrac{20}{3}(a/r)^3 + \tfrac{7}{3}(a/r)^4. \tag{20}$$

Assuming a fixed radius for the pore and water molecules, $1 - \sigma$ becomes a function of solute radius. To estimate equivalent pore sizes from σ values obtained with the osmotic transient, the experimental values for $1 - \sigma$ are plotted among curves generated from the hydrodynamic formulation. Figure 10 illustrates such an analysis using Eq. (20) and data reported for skeletal muscle, lung, and heart (from Table VI). The analysis suggests that the σ data for lung, skeletal muscle, and heart are consistent with equivalent pores of 55, 25–35, and 19–25 Å, respectively.

The approach used to estimate equivalent pores from osmotic transient data has the advantage of computational simplicity. However, the predictive value of the analysis is limited to either a single pore size or a range of sizes. The analysis does not allow for correction of the effects of fluid withdrawal from cells or the influence of "large pores."

C. Lymphatic Protein Flux Analyses

Two approaches have been extensively employed for predicting capillary pore sizes from lymph flux data. One approach involves the use of L/P data for molecules of different sizes at normal lymph flows. From the relationship between L/P and molecular radius the small-pore radius is determined from the portion of the curve exhibiting a steep fall in L/P (in Fig. 6, for example, small pores of approximately 45, 52, 76, and 78 Å would be predicted for subcutaneous tissue, intestine, lung, and liver, respectively). The dimension of the large pore is then generally assumed to represent a value larger than the size of the biggest molecule displaying a constant residual permeability (in Fig. 6, for example, the large pores in all tissues must significantly exceed 120 Å). Having predicted the size of the small and large pores, one can then estimate the relative number of large to small pores using:

$$N_1/N_2 = r_l^2/[r_s^2(L/P)_l^{-1}], \tag{21}$$

where r_l is the radius of the large pores, r_s is the radius of the small pores, and $(L/P)_l^{-1}$ is the extrapolated L/P for the molecules displaying a constant residual permeability.

Estimating capillary pore sizes using the relationship between L/P and molecular radius at normal lymph flow has several limitations. A major limitation is imposed by the use of L/P data obtained under conditions in which diffusive exchange is an important determinant of transcapillary solute exchange. Another shortcoming is the fact that the dimensions of the large pores cannot be determined using this approach. The accuracy of the prediction of small-pore sizes appears reasonable when compared to values obtained for the same tissue using more sophisticated approaches.

Renkin et al. (1977b) introduced a method by which pore dimensions can be derived using a simple graphic solution when the σ_d values of several macromolecules of different sizes are measured using lymph. This method is based on equations that relate the membrane reflection coefficient to the sum of the hydraulic conductances occurring through each set of pores. The analysis is applied to lymph data by plotting $1 - \sigma_d$ as a function of solute radius. The resulting plot can be described by fitting the data with two sets of equivalent pores. This is done by first fitting a theoretical large-pore line to the points representing the larger solutes. Then, by a curve-peeling process, the resulting values of $1 - \sigma_d$ for smaller molecules are fitted with another theoretical pore curve. In addition to giving two populations of pores, the analysis also predicts the percentage of total conductance occurring through each set of pores. This is easily estimated from the ordinate intercept.

An example of this type of pore analysis is shown in Fig. 11. This figure represents $1 - \sigma_d$ values for different-sized protein fractions (range 37–120 Å) obtained from stomach lymph and plotted as a function of molecu-

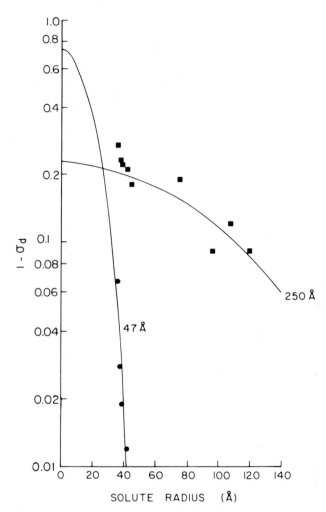

Fig. 11. Pore stripping analysis for lymphatic protein data from cat stomach. (From Perry *et al.*, 1981.)

lar size (Perry *et al.*, 1981). In this example, the pore radii that best fit the data were 47 and 250 Å. The relative hydraulic conductances through the small- (F_s) and large-pore (F_l) populations were 0.75 and 0.23, respectively. The ratios of large- to small-pore areas (A_l/A_s) and pore numbers (N_l/N_s) can be determined by assuming Pouisielle flow through the pores and using the equations

$$A_l/A_s = (r_s^2/r_l^2)(F_l/F_s) \qquad (22)$$

and

$$N_1/N_s = (A_1/A_s)(r_s^2/r_1^2). \tag{23}$$

The latter approach has proved to be very useful for predicting equivalent pore sizes in capillaries using lymph data. Nonetheless, the accuracy of the technique is predicated to a large extent on the reliability of σ_d estimates and the number of solutes studied. A frequent problem with the application of this technique is the use of inappropriate values for σ_d. This usually represents the use of L/P data that are not filtration rate independent. For example, in lung lymph studies (Parker *et al.*, 1981a) molecules the size of albumin do not reach filtration rate independence, and the application of these data to the pore analysis leads to an overestimation of the size of the small pores. The technique also suffers from its failure to identify more than two pore populations. This problem can be eliminated by the use of a larger number and wider size range of solutes.

IV. Ultrastructural Basis for Capillary Permeability

The pore theory of capillary permeability predicts that the capillary wall possesses at least two populations of "pores" or pathways for exchange. With the advent of the electron microscope many investigators have attempted to define the ultrastructural equivalents of the small and large pores. Morphologic analyses and ultrastructural tracer studies have produced a detailed description of the nature, organization, and functional role of the structures that contribute to the permeability characteristics of the capillary wall (Bennett *et al.*, 1959; Karnovsky, 1968; Palade *et al.*, 1979; Simionescu *et al.*, 1976). There are significant variations in the ultrastructural appearance of the capillaries in different tissues, which presumably accounts for the observed differences in capillary permeability among the organs throughout the body. Figure 12 illustrates the basic structural features of continuous, fenestrated, and discontinuous type of capillaries. For each capillary type, specific pathways (or barriers) are designated which may play a role in governing transcapillary exchange of fluid and solutes. Physiologically defined transport pathways and their relative frequencies are presented in Table VIII for several different organs. Following a morphologic description of the different exchange pathways in a given capillary type, we will attempt to correlate the structural feature of the capillary wall (Fig. 12) that best describes the physiologically defined pathways (Table VIII). It should be remembered, however, that the physiologic estimates of the dimensions of the exchange pathways are

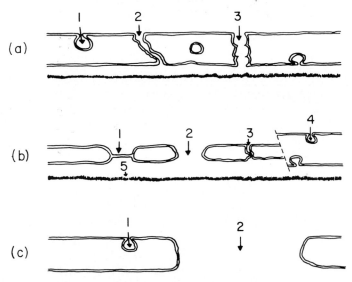

Fig. 12. Diagrammatic representation of possible transport pathways for macromolecules across continuous (a), fenestrated (b), and discontinuous (c) capillaries. For the continuous capillary, pathways 1–3 denote pinocytotic vesicles, intercellular junction, and a transendothelial channel, respectively. For the fenestrated capillary, pathways 1–5 denote diaphragmed fenestrae, open fenestrae, intercellular junctions, pinocytotic vesicles, and basement membrane, respectively. For the discontinuous capillary, pathways 1 and 2 represent pinocytotic vesicles and intercellular gaps, respectively. (From Taylor and Granger, 1982.)

based on the assumption that such pathways are uniform cylindrical pores, whereas the ultrastructural pathways appear to be irregular structures with numerous different widths. It is unlikely, therefore, that the physiologically defined pores will have an exact ultrastructural counterpart. The pore dimensions calculated from physiologic data most likely represent the most restrictive portion of the ultrastructural pathway.

A. *Continuous Capillaries*

Continuous capillaries are the most widely distributed in mammalian tissues. They are found in skeletal, heart, and smooth muscles, lung, skin, subcutaneous tissue, and serous and mucous membranes (Bennett *et al.*, 1959; Karnovsky, 1968). The following transport pathways may play an important role in macromolecule exchange in these capillaries:

1.   Pinocytotic vesicles. A relatively large volume of the endothelial cell is occupied by vesicles with an internal radius of approximately

TABLE VIII

Predicted Pore Sizes and Distribution in Several Capillary Beds[a]

Organ	Species	Small-pore radius (Å)	Large-pore radius (Å)	Fraction of hydraulic conductance			Ratio of large- to small-pore	
				Through small pores	Through large pores	Other	Areas	Numbers
Paw	Dog	47	195	0.82	0.13	0.05	1:114	1:2060
Lung	Dog	80	200	0.80	0.16	0.04	1:31	1:195
Skeletal muscle	Rat	67	220	0.65	0.018	0.33[b]	1:361	1:3610
Blood–cerebrospinal fluid barrier	Man	70	180	0.86	0.10	0.04	1:52	1:345
Small intestine	Cat	46	200	0.90	0.05	0.05	1:340	1:6400
Stomach	Cat	47	250	0.75	0.23	0.02	1:92	1:2600
Colon	Dog	53	180	0.71	0.17	0.12	1:48	1:550
Liver	Cat	90	330	0.20	0.80	—	1:3.4	1:46

[a] Values derived from published data using the method of graphic analysis of Renkin et al. (1977b). The sources of the data are for the paw (Taylor et al., 1982), lung (Parker et al., 1981a), skeletal muscle (Youlten, 1969), blood–cerebrospinal fluid barrier (Felgenhauer, 1974), small intestine (Granger and Taylor, 1980), stomach (Perry et al., 1981), colon (Richardson et al., 1980), and liver (Granger et al., 1979b).

[b] Value probably represents dilution caused by superfusion of muscle.

250 Å. The vesicles are considered to move freely (by thermal kinetic energy) from one side to another and fuse with the plasma membrane, carrying either plasma or interstitial fluid. Ultrastructural tracer studies indicate that the vesicles participate in the transport of particles as large as 300 Å diameter. The population density of vesicles within the endothelium increases from arterial to venous ends of the capillary. The overall density of vesicles also varies from one continuous type of capillary bed to another, that is, vesicle population in muscle > lung > brain (Palade and Bruns, 1968; Palade, 1960, 1961; Palade et al., 1979; Reese and Karnovsky, 1969; Simionescu et al., 1974, 1978; Weibel, 1970).

2. Intercellular junctions. Open intercellular junctions (maculae occludentes) have been described in muscle capillaries (endothelial junctions in brain are closed). Ultrastructural tracer studies suggest that open intercellular junctions measure 20–60 Å in width. Intercellular junctions of arteriolar and capillary endothelium appear morphologically closed and functionally impermeable to solutes of 20 Å diameter. However, 25–30% of the junctions appear open in the endothelium of postcapillary venules (Palade et al., 1979; Reese and Karnovsky, 1969; Schneeberger, 1976; Simionescu et al., 1973, 1975; Williams and Wissig, 1975).

3. Transendothelial channels. Patent transendothelial channels are formed by one or more vesicles open simultaneously on both sides of the endothelium. The maximal internal diameter of these transient channels approaches that of a single vesicle (i.e., 500 Å), yet they have strictures at their necks and points of fusion between vesicles, which reduce the internal diameter to 100–400 Å. Occasionally, the channel opening is provided with the equivalent of a stomatal diaphragm. (The diaphragms have a porosity with an exclusion limit between 50 and 110 Å molecular diameter.) The relative frequency of transendothelial channels increases from arterial to venous ends of the capillary (Bruns and Palade, 1968; Palade and Bruns, 1968; Palade et al., 1979; Simionescu et al., 1976).

The physiologic estimates of transport pathways for macromolecules in continuous capillaries are generally consistent with small- and large-pore populations (Table VIII). Small-pore estimates range between 67 and 80 Å radius, whereas channels of radius 200–280 Å are predicted for the large pores. Equivalent pore estimates based on osmotic transients using macromolecules in heart, adipose tissue, lung, and mesentery generally fall within the range 55–70 Å radius. Morphologic correlates to the physiologically defined transport pathways are not readily apparent. The intercellular junctions, as described above, behave as if they have an effective radius of less than 20 Å and are unlikely candidates for the small-pore equivalency. It is conceivable that there is a population of intercellular channels with dimensions comparable to the physiologic estimates of the large pores, yet the rarity of such pathways makes it unlikely that they could be systematically found and identified. The pinocytotic vesicles and transendothelial channels, however, may well be the structural equivalents to both large- and small-pore systems, respectively. The large-pore estimates (200–280 Å) for continuous capillaries are in reasonable agreement with the inner radius of an average vesicle ($\sim$250 Å). Evidence for and against vesicular transport as a major pathway has been presented for continuous capillary beds (Crone, 1980; Renkin *et al.*, 1977b; Rippe *et al.*, 1979). Another structural feature that may represent both the small- and the large-pore pathways is the transendothelial channel. Transendothelial channels free of size-limiting structures (diaphragms and strictures) would possess an internal radius of approximately 200–250 Å and thus could be plausible candidates for the large-pore system involved in convective transport. The size-limiting structures of the transendothelial channels (particularly the stomatal diaphragms) may allow a proportion of these structures to function as the small-pore system. The minimal internal radius of the channels produced by strictures (50–100 Å) and the limiting porosity of the stomatal diaphragms (up to 55 Å radius) are in reasonable agreement with the physiologic estimates of small-pore size (67–80 Å). Although the transendothelial channel provides one of the few reasonable correlates between morphologic and physiologic data, the significance of this transient pathway cannot be defined until more definitive data regarding their duration and frequency of occurrence are acquired.

B. Fenestrated Capillaries

Fenestrated capillaries are generally found in the intestinal mucosa, endocrine and exocrine glands, and the glomerular and peritubular capillaries of the kidney (Bennett *et al.*, 1959; Karnovsky, 1968). Due to the unique structure of fenestrated capillaries in the kidney, the following description of morphologic transport pathways will be limited primarily to observations on gastrointestinal capillaries. The reader is referred to several treatises for a detailed description of morphologic transport pathways across glomerular capillaries (Farquhar, 1975; Karnovsky, 1979; Rennke and Venkatachalam, 1977; Venkatachalam and Rennke, 1978). The following features of the fenestrated capillary wall may be transport pathways for macromolecules:

1. Diaphragmed fenestrae. Fenestrae are circular openings of 200–300 Å radius within the attentuated body of endothelial cells. Over 60% of the fenestrae are provided with an aperture or diaphragm similar in appearance to the stomatal diaphragm of the transendothelial channels. Al-

though the porosity of the diaphragm is unknown, these structures are considered to account for the observation that tracer molecules of 100 Å diameter or larger exit only through a relatively small fraction of the fenestral population. In this regard, it is interesting that large dextran particles appear to unravel when passing through the fenestral diaphragm (Bennett *et al.*, 1959; Casley-Smith *et al.*, 1975; Clementi and Palade, 1969; Karnovsky, 1968; Palade *et al.*, 1979; Simionescu *et al.*, 1972, 1976).

2. Open fenestrae. Fenestrae not subtended by a diaphragm appear to offer minimal restriction to transcapillary movement of macromolecules. Tracer molecules ranging in radius between 25 and 150 Å readily permeate open fenestrae. The frequency of fenestrae (both open and diaphragmed) increases from arterial to venous ends of the capillary (Clementi and Palade, 1969; Palade *et al.*, 1979; Simionescu *et al.*, 1972, 1976).

3. Intercellular junctions. Tracer molecules as small as 25 Å radius do not permeate the intercellular junctions of intestinal capillaries (Clementi and Palade, 1969; Simionescu *et al.*, 1972).

4. Pinocytotic vesicles. Vesicles are found in relatively large numbers in fenestrated endothelium. Tracers ranging in radius between 25 and 150 Å gain access to the vesicles. Ultrastructural tracer studies indicate that transport of macromolecules by vesicles is, at best, three to eight times slower than through the fenestrae (Clementi and Palade, 1969; Palade *et al.*, 1979; Simionescu *et al.*, 1972, 1976).

5. Basement membrane. The basement membrane surrounding fenestrated capillaries is formed by a layer of fine fibrillar material similar to that surrounding other capillaries. Although there are no structurally recognizable pathways across the basement membrane, there is evidence that this structure reduces the rate of transport of large tracer particles. After penetration through the fenestrae, tracer particles (62–150 Å radius) transiently accumulate in the subendothelial space against the basement membrane to form small clusters opposite permeable fenestrae. Particles ranging in radius between 25 and 55 Å are not temporarily retained by the basement membrane (Clementi and Palade, 1969; Simionescu *et al.*, 1972).

The physiologic estimates of transport pathways for the fenestrated capillaries of stomach, small intestine, and colon are presented in Table VIII. The data are consistent with small- and large-pore populations of 46–53 and 180–250 Å radius, respectively. The morphologic equivalent of the large pores must clearly reside, to a large extent, at the open fenestrae (200–400 Å radius). The internal radius of the cytoplasmic vesicles

($\sim$250 Å) is also in reasonable agreement with the physiologic large-pore estimates. Thus, this structure may play a role, albeit small, in the transport of macromolecules across the fenestrated capillary. It is also plausible that differential porosities within the fibrillar structure of the basement membrane account for a component of the large-pore equivalency. Although the correlation of morphologically and phyiologically defined pathways is reasonably clear for the large-pore system (Simionescu *et al.*, 1972, 1976), the morphologic equivalent to the small-pore system is not as readily apparent. The intercellular junctions are impermeant to solutes of 25 Å radius, making these structures unlikely candidates for the small-pore equivalency. Although the porosity of the fenestral diaphragms is unknown, it is generally considered that the porosity of this structure provides the morphologic correlate to the small-pore system. The concept that the presence or absence of size-limiting structures within the fenestral diaphragms differentiates subpopulations that correspond to small- and large-pore systems (Palade *et al.*, 1979; Simionescu *et al.*, 1976) seems tenable, yet the relative frequency of open and diaphragmed fenestrae appears to be much higher than the relative frequency of small and large pores predicted by the physiologic data (Table VIII).

C. Discontinuous Capillaries

The distribution of discontinuous capillaries is more limited than that of other capillary types; these capillaries are found almost exclusively in liver, spleen, and bone marrow (Bennett *et al.*, 1959; Karnovsky, 1968). They are characterized by an absence of a basement membrane. The following features of discontinuous capillaries may represent transport pathways for macromolecules:

1. Pinocytotic vesicles. These structures are present in significant numbers in the endothelium of discontinuous capillaries. However, they are considered to play a negligible role in macromolecule transport relative to the endothelial gap (Bennett *et al.*, 1959).
2. Endothelial gaps. The intercellular junctions in these capillaries range in diameter between 1000 and 10,000 Å (Bennett *et al.*, 1959; Kardon and Kessel, 1980; Poulsen, 1974).

Correlation of physiologic and morphologic transport pathways across sinusoidal endothelial is more difficult than for other capillary types. The presence of extremely large intercellular gaps, coupled with the absence of a basement membrane, leads one to conclude that the sinusoidal wall exercises no selective filtering effect on even the largest proteins. However, the physiologic data acquired when sieving is maximal between liver lymph and blood is consistent with a small- and large-pore population of 90 and 330 Å radius, respectively. The inconsistency between ultrastructural and physiologic data suggests that barriers lying past the sinusoidal wall, possibly the interstitial matrix, account for the physiologic pore predictions.

As a result of the early physiologic studies of Pappenheimer *et al.* (1951) and morphologic studies of Karnovsky (1968), it was long considered that the intercellular junctions were the morphologic counterpart to the small-pore system. However, in recent years the dimensions of the physiologic small pores have been revised upward, whereas newer ultrastructural tracer studies have led to a reduction in the predicted dimension of the capillary intercellular junction (Palade *et al.*, 1979). The effective radius of the intercellular junctions determined using electron-dense tracers is now considerably less than the effective radius of the small-pore system predicted from physiologic data. It is not possible, therefore, to correlate the intercellular junctions with the small-pore system in any capillary bed.

For continuous and fenestrated type of capillaries, size-limiting structures within transendothelial channels (diaphragms, strictures) and fenestrae (diaphragms) are invoked to explain the small-pore system predicted from physiologic data (Palade *et al.*, 1979). However, the porosity and frequency of such structures remain uncertain.

Pinocytotic vesicles and leaks (large intercellular gaps) were once the obvious candidates for the large-pore system. After many years of searching, the routine existence of leaks in continuous capillaries remains unconfirmed. Therefore, patent transendothelial channels may be a viable alternative. The contribution of vesicles to the large-pore system is controversial, yet it remains a likely candidate for the large-pore system in continuous capillaries. For fenestrated and discontinuous type of capillaries the morphologic equivalents of the large-pore system appear to be reasonably clear.

It is difficult to find a degree of reasonable agreement between structural and physiologic postulates for small- and large-pore systems. This results from the many inherent limitations of the structural and physiologic techniques employed. Methodolgic problems associated with tissue fixation, exogenous electron-dense markers, and interpretation of tracer concentration profiles may limit the accuracy of morphologic findings (Bundgaard, 1980). Equally limiting are the problems associated with physiologic studies. A heterogeneity of capillary types within a tissue (e.g., lung and intestine), restriction of macromolecules by barriers between capillary wall and lymphatic, a lymphatic concentrating capacity, and non-steady-state conditions may in turn limit functional–structural correlations. Many of the physiologic data (paw, lung, skeletal muscle, kidney) acquired thus far do not lend themselves to accurate pore estimates because reliable σ_d values are unavailable. Progress toward a more definitive correlation between structural and functional data must rely on the development of new approaches and the refinement of existing techniques in both fields.

References

Alvarez, O. A., and Yudilevich, D. (1969). *J. Physiol.* (*London*) **202**, 45–48.
Aukland, K., and Fadnes, H. O. (1973). *Acta Physiol. Scand.* **88**, 350–358.
Basset, G., Fulla, Y., Moreau, F., and Turiaf, J. (1975). *Bibl. Anat.* **13**, 17–20.
Basset, G., Moreau, F., Trenule, D., and Turiaf, J. (1976). *Ann. N.Y. Acad. Sci.* **278**, 308–320.
Bassingthwaighte, J. B. (1974). *Circ. Res.* **35**, 483–503.
Bassingthwaighte, J. B., Yipintsoi, T., and Grabowski, E. F. (1975). Bibl. Anat. **13**, 24–27.
Bassingthwaighte, J. B., Yipintsoi, T., and Knopp, T. J. (1979). *Microvasc. Res.* **17**, S85.
Bennett, H. S., Luft, J. H., and Hampton, J. C. (1959). *Am. J. Physiol.* **196**, 381–390.
Bloom, G., and Johnson, J. A. (1981). *Microvasc. Res.* **22**, 64–79.
Bolwig, T. G., and Lassen, N. A. (1975). *Acta Physiol. Scand.* **93**, 415–422.
Brace, R. A., Granger, D. N., and Taylor, A. E. (1977). *Microvasc. Res.* **14**, 215–226.
Brace, R. A., Granger, D. N., and Taylor, A. E. (1978). *Microvasc. Res.* **16**, 297–303.
Bresler, E. H., and Groome, L. J. (1981). Am. J. Physiol. **241**, F469–F476.
Brigham, K. L., and Owen, P. J. (1975). *Circ. Res.* **37**, 647–657.
Brigham, K. L., Woolverton, W. C., Blake, L. H., and Staub, N. C. (1974). *J. Clin. Invest.* **54**, 792–804.
Brigham, K. L., Harris, T. R., and Owen, P. J. (1977a). *J. Appl. Physiol. Respir. Environ. Exercise Physiol.* **43**, 99–101.
Brigham, K. L., Harris, T. R., Rowlett, R. D., and Owen, P. J. (1977b). *Microvasc. Res.* **13**, 97–105.
Brigham, K. L., Sundell, H., Harris, T. R., Catterton, Z., Kovar, I., and Stahlman, M. (1978). *Circ. Res.* **42**, 851–855.
Brigham, K. L., Bowers, R. E., and Haynes, J. (1979a). *Circ. Res.* **45**, 292–297.
Brigham, K. L., Snell, J. D., Harris, T. R., Marshall, S., Haynes, J., Bowers, R. E., and Perry, J. (1979b). *Circ. Res.* **44**, 523–530.
Bruns, R. R., and Palade, G. E. (1968). *J. Cell. Biol.* **37**, 277–299.
Bundgaard, M. (1980). *Annu. Rev. Physiol.* **42**, 325–326.
Carter, R. D., Joyner, W. L., and Renkin, E. M. (1974). *Microvasc. Res.* **7**, 31–48.
Casley-Smith, J. R., O'Donoghue, P. J., and Crocker, K. W. J. (1975). *Microvasc. Res.* **9**, 78–100.
Chinard, F. P., and Enns, T. (1954). *Am. J. Physiol.* **178**, 197–202.
Chinard, F. P., Ritter, A. B., and Chowdhury, P. (1977). *Proc. IUPS* **13**, 137.
Clementi, F., and Palade, G. (1969). *J. Cell Biol.* **41**, 33–58.
Courtice, F. C. (1971). *Lymphology* **4**, 9–17.
Crone, C. (1963a). *Acta Physiol. Scand.* **58**, 292–305.
Crone, C. (1963b). *Proc. Soc. Exp. Biol. Med.* **112**, 454–455.

Crone, C. (1965). *Acta Physiol. Scand.* **64,** 407–417.

Crone, C. (1973). *Acta Physiol. Scand.* **87,** 138–144.

Crone, C. (1980). *Microvasc. Res.* **20,** 133–149.

Crone, C., and Christensen, O. (1979). *Int. Rev. Physiol.* **18,** 149–213.

Curry, F. E., Mason, J. C., and Michel, C. C. (1976). *J. Physiol. (London)* **261,** 319–336.

Delaney, J. P., and Grim, E. (1964). *Am. J. Physiol.* **207,** 1195–1202.

Diana, J. N., Long, S. C., and Yao, H. (1972). *Microvasc. Res.* **4,** 413–437.

Drake, R. and Davis, E. (1978). *Microvasc. Res.* **15,** 259.

Duran, W. N., and Yudilevich, D. L. (1978). *Microvasc. Res.* **15,** 195–205.

Duran, W. N., Alvarez, O. A., and Yudilevich, D. L. (1973). *Microvasc. Res.* **6,** 347–359.

Eichling, J. O., Raichle, M. E., Grubb, R. L., and Terpogossian, M. M. (1974). *Circ. Res.* **35,** 358–364.

Farquhar, M. G. (1975). *Kidney Int.* **8,** 197–211.

Felgenhauer, K. (1974). *Klin. Wochenschr.* **52,** 1158–1164.

Fenstermacher, J., and Johnson, J. (1966). *Am. J. Physiol.* **211,** 341–346.

Garlick, D. G. (1970). *In* "Capillary Permeability" (C. Crone, and N. A. Lassen, eds)., pp. 228–238. Munksgaard, Copenhagen.

Goresky, C. A. (1963). *Am. J. Physiol.* **204,** 626–640.

Goresky, C. A. (1965). *Can. Med. Assoc. J.* **92,** 517–522.

Goresky, C. A., and Nadeau, B. E. (1974). *J. Clin. Invest.* **53,** 634–646.

Goresky, C. A., Ziegler, W. H., and Bach, G. C. (1970). *Circ. Res.* **27,** 739–764.

Goresky, C. A., Bach, G. G., and Nadeau, B. E. (1973). *J. Clin. Invest.* **52,** 991–1009.

Granger, D. N., and Taylor, A. E. (1980). *Am. J. Physiol.* **238,** H457–H464.

Granger, D. N., Granger, J. P., Brace, R. A., Parker, R. E., and Taylor, A. E. (1979a). *Circ. Res.* **44,** 335–344.

Granger, D. N., Miller, T., Allen, R., Parker, R. E., Parker, J. C., and Taylor, A. E. (1979b). *Gastroenterology* **77,** 103–109.

Grotte, G. (1956). *Acta Chir. Scand.* **211** (Suppl.), 1–84.

Guller, B., Yipintsoi, T., Orvis, A. L., and Bassingthwaighte, J. B. (1975). *Circ. Res.* **37,** 359–378.

Haljamäe, H., and Fredén, H. (1970). *Microvasc. Res.* **2,** 163–171.

Harris, T. R., Rowlett, R. D., and Brigham, K. L. (1976). *Microvasc. Res.* **12,** 177–196.

Harris, T. R., Brigham, K. L., and Rowlett, R. D. (1978). *J. Appl. Physiol. Respir. Environ. Exercise Physiol.* **44,** 245–253.

Hilton, S. M., Hudlicka, O., and Jackson, J. R. (1974). *J. Physiol. (London)* **239,** 98P–99P.

Huet, P. M., Goresky, C. A., and Lough, J. O. (1980). *Gastroenterology* **79,** 1073.

Johnson, J. A., and Bloom, G. (1981). *Microvasc. Res.* **22,** 80–92.

Johnson, J. A., and Wilson, T. A. (1966). *Am. J. Physiol.* **210,** 1299–1303.

Johnson, J. A., Bloom, G., Anderson, S., and McEvoy, K. (1981). *Microvasc. Res.* **22,** 93–109.

Kardon, R. H., and Kessel, R. G. (1980). *Gastroenterology* **79,** 72–81.

Karnovsky, M. J. (1968). *J. Gen. Physiol.* **52,** 641–696.

Karnovsky, M. J. (1979). *In* "Kidney Disease—Present Status" ( ), pp. 1–41. Williams & Wilkins, Baltimore, Maryland.

Kedem, O., and Katchalsky, A. (1958). *Biochem. Biophys. Acta* **27,** 229–246.

Kedem, O., and Katchalsky, A. (1961). *J. Gen. Physiol.* **45,** 143–179.

Landis, E. M., and Pappenheimer, J. R. (1963). *Handb. Physiol. Sect. 2 Cardiovasc. Sys.* **2,** 961–1034.

Lassen, N. A., and Crone, C. (1970). *In* "Capillary Permeability" (C. Crone, and N. A. Lassen, eds.), pp. 48–59. Munksgaard, Copenhagen.

Lassen, N. A., and Trap-Jensen, J. (1969). *Acta Physiol. Scand.* **76,** 9A–10A.
Lassen, N. A., and Trap-Jensen, J. (1970). *Eur. J. Clin. Invest.* **1,** 118–123.
Laughlin, M. H., and Diana, J. N. (1975). *Am. J. Physiol.* **229,** 838–846.
Lee, J. S. (1981). *In* "Tissue Fluid Pressure and Composition" (A. R. Hargen, ed.), pp. 165–172. Williams & Wilkins, Baltimore, Maryland.
Levitt, D. G. (1970). *Circ. Res.* **27,** 81–95.
Libermann, I. M., Gonzalez, F., Brazzuna, H., Garcia, H., and Labuonora, D. (1972). *J. Appl. Physiol.* **33,** 751–756.
Lundgren, O. (1967). *Acta Physiol. Scand.* **303** (Suppl.), 5–42.
Mann, G. E. (1981). *J. Physiol.* (*London*) **319,** 311–323.
Mann, G. E., Smaje, L. H., and Yudilevich, D. L. (1979a). *J. Physiol.* (*London*) **279,** 335–354.
Mann, G. E., Smaje, L. H., and Yudilevich, D. L. (1979b). *J. Physiol.* (*London*) **297,** 355–367.
Martin de Julian, P., and Yudilevich, D. (1964). *Am. J. Physiol.* **207,** 162–168.
Mayerson, H. S., Wolfram, C. G., Shirley, H. H., and Wasserman, K. (1960). *Am. J. Physiol.* **198,** 155–160.
Michel, C. C. (1972). *In* "Cardiovascular Fluid Dynamics" (D. H. Bergel, ed.), pp. 241–298. Academic Press, New York and London.
Michel, C. C. (1978). *Arch. Int. Physiol. Biochem.* **86,** 657–667.
Murray, J. E., and Plioplys, A. (1972). *J. Appl. Physiol.* **33,** 681–683.
Neufeld, G. F., Williams, J. J., Graves, D. J., Soma, L. R., and Marshall, B. E. (1975). *Microvasc. Res.* **10,** 192–207.
Nicolaysen, G. (1971). *Acta Physiol. Scand.* **82,** 393–405.
Paaske, W. B. (1977). *Acta Physiol. Scand.* **101,** 1–14.
Paaske, W. B., and Sejrsen, P. (1977). *Acta Physiol. Scand.* **100,** 437–445.
Palade, G. E. (1960). *Anat. Rec.* **136,** 254.
Palade, G. E. (1961). *Circulation* **24,** 368.
Palade, G. E., and Bruns, R. R. (1968). *J. Cell Biol.* **37,** 633–649.
Palade, G. E., Simionescu, M., and Simionescu, N. (1979). *Acta Physiol. Scand.* **463,** 11–32.
Pappenheimer, J. R., Renkin, E. M., and Borrero, L. M. (1951). *Am. J. Physiol.* **167,** 13–46.
Parker, J. C., Parker, R. E., Granger, D. N., and Taylor, A. E. (1981a). *Circ. Res.* **48,** 549–561.
Parker, R. E., Rosseli, R. J., Harris, T. R., and Brigham, K. L. (1981b). *Circ. Res.* **49,** 1164–1172.
Parker, J. C., Perry, M. A., and Taylor, A. E. (1983). *In* "Edema" (N. C. Staub, and A. E. Taylor, eds.). Raven, New York.
Perl, W. (1970). *In* "Capillary Permeability" (C. Crone, and N. A. Lassen, eds.), pp. 185–201. Munksgaard, Copenhagen.
Perl, W. (1971). *Microvasc. Res.* **3,** 233–251.
Perl, W. (1973). *Microvasc. Res.* **6,** 169–193.
Perl, W. (1975). *Microvasc. Res.* **10,** 83–94.
Perl, W., and Chinard, F. P. (1968). *Circ. Res.* **22,** 273–298.
Perl, W., Silverman, F., Delea, A. C., and Chinard, F. P. (1976). *Am. J. Physiol.* **230,** 1708–1721.
Perry, M. A. (1980). *Microvasc. Res.* **19,** 142–157.
Perry, M. A., and Garlick, D. G. (1978). *Clin. Exp. Pharmacol. Physiol.* **5,** 361–377.
Perry, M. A., and Granger, D. N. (1981). *Am. J. Physiol.* **4,** G24–G30.
Perry, M. A., Crook, W. J., and Granger, D. N. (1981). *Am. J. Physiol.* **4,** G478–G486.

Poulsen, H. L. (1974). *Scand. J. Clin. Lab. Invest.* **34**, 119–122.

Quinn, J. W., and Shannon, A. D. (1977). *J. Physiol. (London)* **264**, 307–321.

Raichle, M. E., Eichling, J. O., and Grubb, R. L. (1974). *Arch. Neurol. (Chicago)* **30**, 319–321.

Rasio, E. A., Bendayan, M., and Goresky, C. A. (1981). *Circ. Res.* **49**, 661–676.

Reed, R. K., and Aukland, K. (1977). *Microvasc. Res.* **14**, 37–43.

Reese, T. S., and Karnovsky, M. J. (1969). *J. Cell Biol.* **34**, 207–217.

Renkin, E. M. (1954). *J. Gen. Physiol.* **38**, 225–243.

Renkin, E. M. (1959). *Am. J. Physiol.* **197**, 1205–1210.

Renkin, E. M. (1964). *Physiologist* **7**, 13–28.

Renkin, E. M. (1979a). *Acta Physiol. Scand.* **463**, (Suppl.), 81–91.

Renkin, E. M. (1979b). *In* "Pulmonary Edema" (A. P. Fishman, and E. M. Renkin, eds.), pp. 145–159. Williams & Wilkins, Baltimore, Maryland.

Renkin, E. M., and Curry, F. E. (1978). *In* "Handbook of Epithelial Transport" (G. Giebisch, and D. C. Tosteson, eds.), Vol. IV, pp. 1–45. Springer, New York.

Renkin, E. M., Joyner, W. L., Sloop, C. H., and Watson, P. D. (1977a). *Microvasc. Res.* **14**, 191–204.

Renkin, E. M., Watson, P. D., Sloop, C. H., Joyner, W. L., and Curry, F. E. (1977b). *Microvasc. Res.* **14**, 205–214.

Rennke, H. G., and Venkatachalam, M. A. (1977). *Fed. Proc. Fed. Am. Soc. Exp. Biol.* **36**, 2619–2626.

Richardson, P. D. I., Granger, D. N., Mailman, D., and Kvietys, P. R. (1980). *Am. J. Physiol.* **239**, G300–G305.

Rippe, B., Kamiya, A., and Folkow, B. (1978). *Acta Physiol. Scand.* **104**, 318–336.

Rippe, B., Kamiya, A., and Folkow, B. (1979). *Acta Physiol. Scand.* **105**, 171–187.

Rose, C. P., and Goresky, C. A. (1976). *Circ. Res.* **39**, 541–554.

Rose, C. P., Goresky, C. A., and Bach, G. G. (1977). *Circ. Res.* **41**, 515–533.

Rusznyak, I., Foldi, M., and Szabo, G. (1967). Lymphatics and Lymph Circulation: Physiology and Pathology (2nd ed.), pp. 196–366. Pergamon, Oxford.

Rutili, G., and Arfors, K.-E. (1977). *Acta Physiol. Scand.* **99**, 1–8.

Rutili, G., Granger, D. N., Parker, J. C., Taylor, A. E., and Mortillaro, N. A. (1982). *Microvasc. Res.* **23**, 347–360.

Schneeberger, E. E. (1976). *Ciba Found. Symp.* **38**, 3–21.

Sejrsen, P. (1979). *Acta Physiol. Scand.* **105**, 73–92.

Simionescu, N., Simionescu, M., and Palade, G. E. (1972). *J. Cell Biol.* **53**, 365–392.

Simionescu, N., Simionescu, M., and Palade, G. E. (1973). *J. Cell Biol.* **57**, 424–452.

Simionescu, M., Simionescu, N., and Palade, G. E. (1974). *J. Cell Biol.* **60**, 128–137.

Simionescu, M., Simionescu, N., and Palade, G. E. (1975). *J. Cell Biol.* **67**, 863–885.

Simionescu, N., Simionescu, M., and Palade, G. E. (1976). *Thromb. Res.* **8**, 257–269.

Simionescu, N., Simionescu, M., and Palade, G. E. (1978). *Microvasc. Res.* **15**, 17–36.

Starling, E. H. (1896). *J. Physiol. (London)* **19**, 312–326.

Starling, E. H. (1915). "Principles of Human Physiology." Lea & Febiger, Philadelphia, Pennsylvania.

Staub, N. C. (1974). *Am. Rev. Respir. Dis.* **109**, 358–372.

Szabo, G., Magyar, Z., and Posch, E. (1976). *Lymphology* **9**, 145–149.

Tancredi, R. G., and Yipintsoi, T. (1980). *Circ. Res.* **46**, 669–680.

Tancredi, R. G., Yipintsoi, T., and Bassingthwaighte, J. B. (1975). *Am. J. Physiol.* **229**, 537–544.

Taylor, A. E., and Gaar, K. A., Jr. (1970). *Am. J. Physiol.* **218**, 1133–1140.

Taylor, A. E., and Gibson, H. (1975). *Lymphology*, **8**, 43–49.

Taylor, A. E., and Granger, D. N. (1982). *Handb. Physiol.* (in press).

Taylor, A. E., Gibson, W. H., Granger, H. J., and Guyton, A. C. (1973). *Lymphology* **6**, 192–208.

Taylor, A. E., Granger, D. N., and Brace, R. A. (1977). *Microvasc. Res.* **13**, 297–313.

Taylor, A. E., Perry, M. A., Shin, D. W., Granger, D. N., and Parker, J. C. (1982). *Microvasc. Res.* **23**, 276.

Taylor, G. (1953). *Proc. R. Soc. London Ser. A* **219**, 186–203.

Trap-Jensen, J., and Lassen, N. A. (1970). *In* "Capillary Permeability" (C. Crone, and N. A. Lassen, eds.), pp. 135–152. Munksgaard, Copenhagen.

Trap-Jensen, J., and Lassen, N. A. (1971). *Am. J. Physiol.* **220**, 371–376.

Vargas, F., and Johnson, J. A. (1964). *J. Gen. Physiol.* **47**, 667–677.

Venkatachalam, M. A., and Rennke, H. G. (1978). *Circ. Res.* **43**, 337–347.

Weibel, E. R. (1970). *Prog. Respir. Res.* **5**, 2–12.

Weibel, E. R. (1973). *Physiol. Rev.* **53**, 419–495.

Williams, M. C., and Wissig, S. L. (1975). *J. Cell Biol.* **66**, 531–555.

Wright, E. M., and Prather, J. W. (1970). *J. Memb. Biol.* **2**, 127–149.

Yipintsoi, T. (1976). *Circ. Res.* **39**, 523–531.

Yipintsoi, T., Tancredi, R., Richmond, D., and Bassingthwaighte, J. B. (1970). *In* "Capillary Permeability" (C. Crone, and N. A. Lassen, eds.), pp. 153–156. Munksgaard, Copenhagen.

Yoffey, J. M., and Courtice, F. C. (1970). "Lymphatics, Lymph and the Lymphomyeloid Complex." Academic Press, New York and London.

Youlten, L. J. F. (1969). *J. Physiol. (London)* **204**, 112P–113P.

Yudilevich, D. L., and Alvarez, O. A. (1967). *Am. J. Physiol.* **213**, 308–314.

Yudilevich, D. L., and DeRose, N. (1971). *Am. J. Physiol.* **220**, 841–846.

Yudilevich, D. L., Renkin, E. M., Alvarez, O. A., and Bravo, I. (1968). *Circ. Res.* **23**, 325–336.

Ziegler, W. H., and Goresky, C. A. (1971). *Circ. Res.* **29**, 181–207.

5 Microcirculatory Control Systems

Harris J. Granger
Jeffrey L. Borders
Gerald A. Meininger
Anthony H. Goodman
George E. Barnes

I. Introduction

The microvasculature is the site of control of tissue perfusion, blood–tissue exchanges, and tissue blood volume. As illustrated in Fig. 1 each of these functions can be associated with specific microvascular segments. Because intravascular pressure measurements demonstrate that a major fraction of total pressure dissipation occurs in precapillary microvessels, the arterioles are designated as resistance vessels. At any given moment local and extrinsic stimuli impinge on the wall of the arteriole and exert control over the caliber of the microvessel. In so doing these signals modulate the blood flow through the tissue. The capillaries are the major exchange vessels; across the surface of these microvessels flow all the nutrients required to sustain the cells of the body. In most tissues only a fraction of the capillaries are perfused under normal conditions. We shall use the term *precapillary sphincter* to describe those precapillary microvascular elements that exert control over the number of perfused capillar-

209

THE PHYSIOLOGY AND PHARMACOLOGY
OF THE MICROCIRCULATION, VOLUME 1

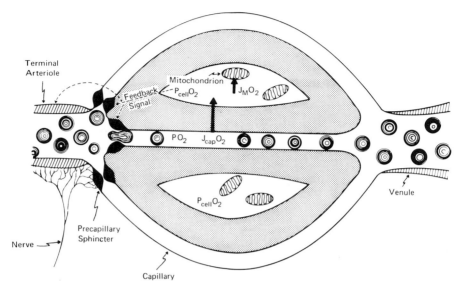

Fig. 1. Schematic representation of the functional segments of the microvasculature. (From Shepherd and Granger, 1973, by permission.)

ies. Finally, the venules are classified as capacitance vessels because most of the tissue blood volume is localized in these microvessels.

The purpose of this chapter is to provide an overview of the control mechanisms that modulate microcirculatory dynamics. We shall emphasize the role of local and remote controllers of arteriolar and precapillary sphincter tone. Although it often is difficult in biological systems to define the controlled variables, we emphasize the role of local microvascular control systems in the regulation of tissue oxygenation and transvascular water flux. The role of remote regulators of microvascular function is viewed mainly in the context of arterial pressure control.

II. Local Microcirculatory Control Systems

Many tissues of the body are endowed with the capacity to regulate their own microvasculature after removal of the organ from the organism and elimination of all nervous and hormonal influences (Johnson, 1964). These local or intrinsic microvascular control systems allow the microcirculation to respond to the specific needs of the tissue that it subserves. Local vascular reactions can be elicited by applying a number of stresses to the isolated tissue. The most commonly used perturbations are alterations in

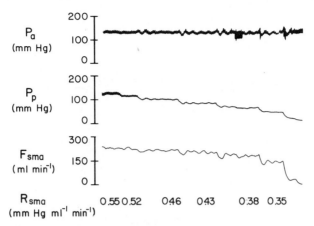

Fig. 2. Autoregulation of blood flow in small intestine. P_a, Systemic arterial pressure; P_p, intestinal perfusion pressure; F_{sma}, superior mesenteric blood flow; R_{sma}, vascular resistance. (From Norris *et al.*, 1979, by permission.)

arterial pressure, venous pressure, arterial oxygen concentration, and parenchymal activity. Changes in arterial perfusion pressure elicit local resistance responses that tend to stabilize flow in spite of altered input pressure (Fig. 2); this local control phenomenon is known as *autoregulation of blood flow*. Another intrinsic vascular reaction is evinced after release of an arterial occlusion; the term *reactive hyperemia* is used to describe the transient blood flow overshoot resulting from an intrinsic vasodilation elicited by total obstruction of the arterial inflow (Fig. 3). Venous pressure elevation also initiates automatic vascular reactions in isolated organs (Fig. 4). In some tissues perfusion with blood containing a lower than normal concentration of oxygen elicits an intrinsic vasodilation; the resultant flow increase is termed *hypoxemic hyperemia* (Fig. 5). Finally, the rate of blood flow is enhanced in most isolated organs when the functional activity of the tissue is increased; this local control phenomenon is known as *functional hyperemia* (Fig. 6).

A. Intrinsic Microvascular Control of Tissue Oxygenation

At present the metabolic and myogenic theories of local vasoregulation can be invoked to explain these local control responses (Johnson, 1964). We now consider the conceptual bases of these two theories. The metabolic hypothesis proposes that a feedback linkage exists between cell metabolism and the tone of the microvessels exerting control over blood per-

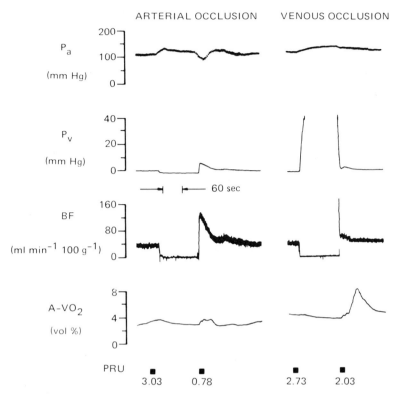

Fig. 3. Reactive hyperemia in small intestine following release of arterial or venous occlusion. P_a, Arterial pressure; P_v, venous pressure; BF, blood flow; A–VO$_2$, arteriovenous O$_2$ difference; PRU, intestinal vascular resistance (mm Hg/ml min 100 g). (From Mortillaro and Granger, 1977, by permission.)

fusion and its distribution. Before examining the homeostatic significance of metabolic control of the microcirculation, it is important to understand the dynamics of tissue oxygen transport and utilization. The rationale for doing so is based on the idea that oxygen or some metabolite associated with parenchymal oxidative processes in the essential linkage that couples the microcirculation to cell metabolism.

The translocation of oxygen from the main supply artery to its final destination in the mitochondria of the parenchymal cells involves three separate processes: (*a*) convection, (*b*) diffusion, and (*c*) chemical reaction. First, oxygen is carried from the major artery to the capillaries by convection in the stream of blood that courses through the microcirculation. Consequently, the rate of oxygen delivery ($J_A O_2$) to the capillary level is

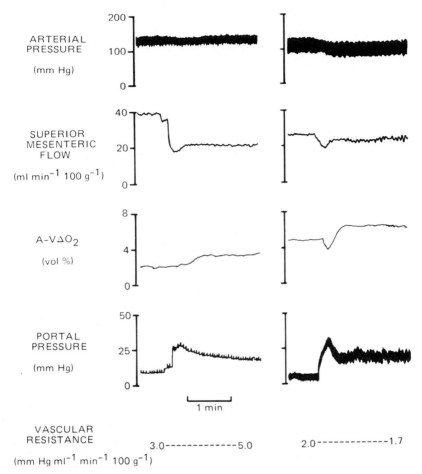

Fig. 4. Local vascular responses in small intestine subjected to sudden venous hypertension. (From Granger and Norris, 1980, by permission.)

dependent on the blood flow (F_A) and the concentration $[O_2]_A$ of the gas in arterial blood, or

$$J_A O_2 = F_A [O_2]_A . \tag{1}$$

Physiologic control of O_2 convection is achieved by modulation of blood flow via appropriate alterations in vascular resistance. The homeostatic importance of flow control in the regulation of O_2 transport can best be appreciated by solving the Fick equation for venous O_2 concentration $[O_2]_V$; the result is

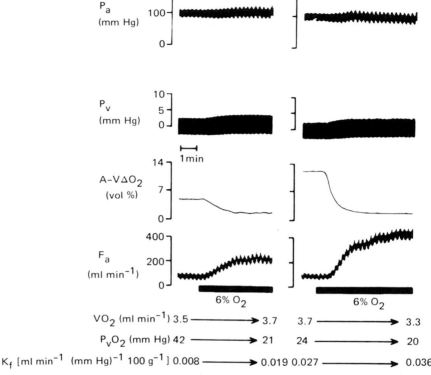

Fig. 5. Hypoxemic vasodilation in skeletal muscle following induction of 6% O_2 breathing in a reflexic dog. P_a, Arterial pressure; P_v, venous pressure; A–VΔO_2, arteriovenous O_2 difference; F_a, blood flow; $\dot{V}O_2$, muscle O_2 uptake; P_vO_2, venous PO_2; K_f, capillary filtration coefficient. (From Granger *et al.*, 1976, by permission.)

$$[O_2]_V = [O_2]_A - (J_DO_2/F_A), \qquad (2)$$

where J_DO_2 is the transcapillary O_2 flux. Assume for the moment that venous O_2 concentration reflects capillary oxygenation (i.e., capillary PO_2). Equation (2) states that for a constant $[O_2]_A$, the O_2 uptake/blood flow ratio is a primary determinent of capillary PO_2. In other words, by modulating convection in accordance with O_2 needs, the flow control system serves to stabilize the source PO_2, which drives O_2 out of the blood into the tissues.

The movement of O_2 from the capillaries into the cells is governed by laws of diffusion. The major determinents of diffusive O_2 flux (J_DO_2) are the capillary O_2 tension ($P_{cap}O_2$), the O_2 tension in the cell ($P_{cell}O_2$), and

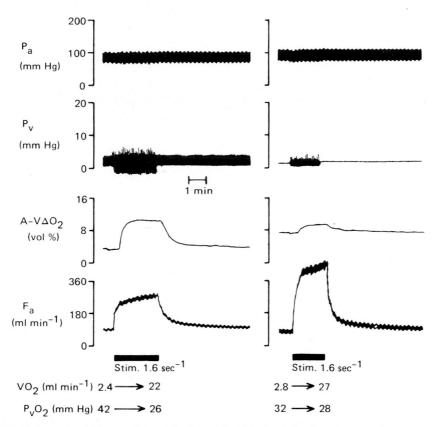

Fig. 6. Functional hyperemia in skeletal muscle following induction of contractions at rate of 1.6 per second. For definition of symbols see Fig. 5. (From Granger *et al.*, 1976, by permission.)

diffusion parameters including capillary surface area (A) and capillary-to-cell diffusion distance (ΔX), or

$$J_D O_2 = K_1 A (P_{cap}O_2 - P_{cell}O_2)/\Delta X, \qquad (3)$$

where K_1 is a constant and includes the solubility and diffusion coefficients. In muscle tissue the capillary distribution pattern with relationship to the parenchymal cells allows changes in both A and ΔX when the number of open capillaries (N) is altered (Granger and Shepherd, 1973). Thus, in muscle, A changes in proportion to capillarity (i.e., number of open capillaries) and ΔX is inversely proportional to the square root of N. As a consequence, the diffusive O_2 flux is proportional to $N^{3/2}$, and the rate of diffusion increases eightfold for a fourfold increment of functional capillary density. Therefore, for skeletal muscle Eq. (3) reduces to

$$J_{\mathrm{D}}O_2 = K_2 N^{3/2}(P_{\mathrm{cap}}O_2 - P_{\mathrm{cell}}O_2). \tag{4}$$

The vascular and parenchymal organization of other organs suggests that the arguments used to generate Eq. (4) from Eq. (3) are not appropriate. With this consideration in mind, diffusive O_2 flux in tissues may be better described by

$$J_{\mathrm{D}}O_2 = K_3 N^k(P_{\mathrm{cap}}O_2 - P_{\mathrm{cell}}O_2), \tag{5}$$

where $k \geq 1$ and is determined by tissue geometry.

After O_2 diffuses into the cell, the gas acts as an electron acceptor and removes reducing equivalents from the terminal oxidase of the respiratory chain. Thus, the final stage of O_2 transport involves the process of chemical reaction. The rate of mitochondrial O_2 utilization ($J_{\mathrm{M}}O_2$) is dependent on the concentration of electron acceptor (i.e., oxygen) and the concentration of reduced cytochrome $a \cdot a_3$, the electron donor (Jobsis, 1964). Hence,

$$J_{\mathrm{M}}O_2 = K[a \cdot a_3]_{\mathrm{R}} P_{\mathrm{cell}}O_2, \tag{6}$$

where K is a constant. Within the mitochondrion, cytochrome $a \cdot a_3$ exists in the interchangeable reduced and oxidized forms. At a resting metabolic rate, the fraction of $a \cdot a_3$ in the reduced form is small (e.g., 0.1 or less). In such a state, reductions in cell PO_2 elicit a temporary decrease in conversion of reduced cytochrome oxidase to oxidized cytochrome oxidase. Consequently, $[a \cdot a_3]_{\mathrm{R}}$ rises to compensate for the reduced cell PO_2, and mitochrondrial O_2 uptake remains unchanged. With further reductions in cell PO_2, elevated $[a \cdot a_3]_{\mathrm{R}}$ continues to stabilize $J_{\mathrm{M}}O_2$ until a cell oxygen tension is reached at which all of the cytochrome $a \cdot a_3$ is reduced (Fig. 7). Lowering of cell PO_2 below this critical level results in a reduction of oxygen utilization because further compensatory increases in $[a \cdot a_3]_{\mathrm{R}}$ are not possible. As a consequence of Eq. (6), the kinetics of mitochondrial O_2 utilization can be described by

$$J_{\mathrm{M}}O_2 = [P_{\mathrm{cell}}O_2/(K_{\mathrm{M}} + P_{\mathrm{cell}}O_2)]J_{\max}O_2, \tag{7}$$

where K_{M} is the cell PO_2 at which O_2 uptake is half the maximum rate (JO_2) possible in the given metabolic state. In most tissues, K_{M} is less than 0.1 mm Hg (Jobsis, 1972). Therefore, cell PO_2 in these tissues exceeds the K_{M} by one to two orders of magnitude, and $J_{\mathrm{M}}O_2$ is independent of cell PO_2 until the oxygen tension in the tissue falls below 1 mm Hg.

Although Eqs. (2), (3), and (7) provide a basis for examining the interactions of O_2 supply and demand, many physiologists are more comfortable with, and have a clearer understanding of, graphic analyses of functional

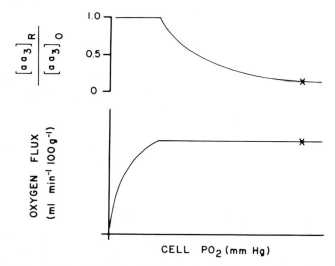

Fig. 7. Mitochondrial O_2 utilization and oxidation–reduction state of cytochrome oxidase as functions of cell PO_2 [Eq. (6)]. The $[a \cdot a_3]_R$ and $[a \cdot a_3]_0$ are the concentrations of reduced and total cytochrome oxidase, respectively. (From Granger and Nyhof, 1982, by permission.)

relationships. Therefore, we present a simple graphic representation of the basic concepts summarized above. The approach consists of separating the diffusion and chemical reaction stages of O_2 transport at the level of the cell and utilizing cell PO_2 as the primary variable common to both processes. Figure 8 illustrates the method. The reader will recognize that

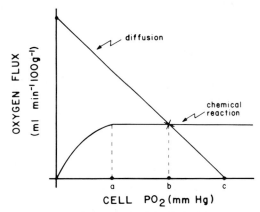

Fig. 8. Basic O_2 supply/uptake curves for graphic analysis of tissue oxygenation. Point a, critical cell PO_2; b, normal cell PO_2; c, capillary PO_2; $b - a$, cell PO_2 reserve; $c - b$, capillary-to-cell PO_2 difference. (From Granger and Nyhof, 1982, by permission.)

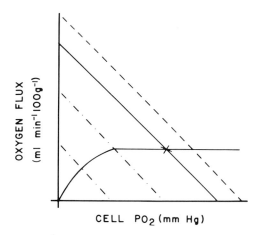

Fig. 9. Effect of changes in blood flow and arterial PO_2 on tissue O_2 supply/uptake balance. Key: ---, increase in flow or P_AO_2; —·—, decrease in flow or P_AO_2. (From Granger and Nyhof, 1982, by permission.)

the chemical reaction curve is a restatement of the basic relationship between mitochondrial O_2 uptake and cell PO_2. The diffusion curve simply states that, all other factors being constant, the rate of O_2 supply to the cell decreases in inverse linear fashion as the O_2 tension in the cell rises. In the steady state, supply and uptake are equal, as indicated by the intersection of the two curves. The *x*- and *y*-axis values of the intersection point represent the prevailing cell PO_2 (point *b*) and O_2 utilization rate, respectively. The intersection of the supply curve with the *x*-axis (point *c*) identifies the prevailing capillary PO_2; at this point, cell and capillary PO_2 are equal, and diffusive O_2 flux is zero. Thus, the magnitude of the sector between points *b* and *c* provides a measure of the capillary-to-cell PO_2 difference. Finally, the length of the segment between points *a* (i.e., the critical PO_2) and *b* reflects the cell PO_2 reserve against the development of tissue hypoxia.

Having established the basic relationships, let us consider the effects of different factors on the supply/uptake curves. As illustrated in Fig. 9, changes in blood flow and arterial PO_2 simply produce parallel shifts in the supply curve; increasing blood flow or arterial O_2 tension shifts the curve to the right, whereas a shift to the left occurs with reduced arterial PO_2 or blood flow. Consider the graded effects of a reduction in blood flow. For both hypoperfusion states shown in Fig. 9, the capillary and cell PO_2 are reduced, the former reflecting augmented extraction of O_2 from the bloodstream. At moderate levels of reduction in flow, the capillary-to-cell PO_2 difference remains normal and the cell PO_2 stabilizes above the

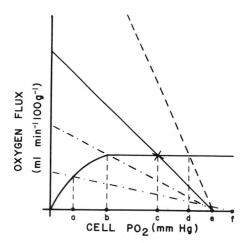

Fig. 10. Effect of changes in functional capillary density on tissue O_2 supply/uptake relationships. Key: ---, increase in capillarity; —·—, decrease in capillarity. (From Granger and Nyhof, 1982, by permission.)

critical value. Thus, O_2 uptake is maintained at the normal level due to a passive increase in O_2 extraction made possible by the preexisting cell PO_2 reserve. In other words, the cell PO_2 reserve provides a "margin of safety" against the development of tissue hypoxia. This safety factor is inherent in the cell and is available even in the absence of local vascular compensations. With more severe reductions in flow, the reserve is depleted, cell PO_2 falls below the critical level, and the capillary-to-cell PO_2 difference falls; consequently, O_2 uptake is compromised. Thus, in the second case the increase in O_2 extraction is not sufficient to compensate for the flow reduction, and cell hypoxia results. By contrast, the hyperperfusion curve clearly illustrates that O_2 uptake does not increase with augmented flow because the capillary-to-cell PO_2 difference remains constant in spite of dramatic increases in the prevailing tissue and capillary O_2 tensions. From these examples, the value of an intrinsic flow control system is evident. Stabilization of flow at an appropriate level helps to prevent the development of tissue hypoxia and also eliminates the need for providing excessive resting flow as a means of effecting such protection.

As indicated earlier in this section, functional capillary density is an important determinant of transmicrovascular O_2 flux. The impact on the supply curve of changes in the number of perfused capillaries is illustrated in Fig. 10. As indicated in the figure, changes in capillarity modify the slope of the supply relationship, as long as the intersection of the supply/uptake relations occurs in the plateau region of the uptake curve. In this region augmentation of capillary density increases the slope of the supply curve and the magnitude of the prevailing cell PO_2 (point d). By contrast, capillary PO_2 is unchanged (point e), and the capillary-to-cell PO_2 difference is reduced ($e - d$). However, due to changes in diffusion parameters, the PO_2 gradient remains constant in the face of a reduced PO_2 difference, and O_2 uptake is unaltered. Thus, with constant flow perfusion, O_2 extraction is unchanged in the face of increased capillarity density; under these circumstances, changes in extraction do not provide a measure of altered capillarity. With small reductions in capillary density, the capillary-to-cell PO_2 difference is increased ($e - b$) in the face of a constant capillary PO_2. Tissue PO_2 (point b) falls but not to the critical level; thus, in this situation also, O_2 extraction and consumption remain normal. With further reductions in capillary density, the critical level is reached and O_2 uptake is compromised (intersection extending from point a). Under these conditions, not only is the slope reduced, but the supply curve is shifted to the right. The reason for the parallel shift can be appreciated by examination of Eqs. (2) and (3), the underlying bases for the supply curve. Note that the capillary PO_2 is dependent on the venous O_2 concentration described in Eq. (2), which in turn includes O_2 uptake as an independent variable. Thus, whenever the supply and uptake curves intersect at an O_2 uptake different from control, the supply curve shifts to the left if O_2 uptake is increased or to the right if O_2 uptake is increased or to the right if O_2 uptake is decreased. Thus, in our example of a dramatic reduction in capillary density, capillary PO_2 is elevated above control (point f), O_2 extraction is reduced, and O_2 uptake falls in spite of a large capillary-to-cell PO_2 differences ($f - a$).

The impact of changes in O_2 demand is illustrated in Fig. 11. As expected, elevated O_2 demand results in an upward shift in the uptake curve. In addition, there is some evidence that the K_M is elevated; therefore, the critical PO_2 rises. As indicated above, the supply curve is shifted to the left when uptake increases above normal. The net effect is a decrease in tissue (point a) and capillary O_2 tensions (point c) with a greater reduction in the former than in the latter; consequently, the capillary-to-cell PO_2 difference ($c - a$) and gradient are increased and O_2 consumption is accelerated. With reductions in O_2 demand, the uptake curve is lowered and the supply curve is shifted to the right. Thus, the O_2 tensions in the cells (point e) and capillaries (point f) are elevated, with the former rising more than the latter. Hence, PO_2 difference is reduced ($f - e$), and O_2 consumption is diminished.

A reexamination of Figs. 8–11 reveals an additional major feature of tissue O_2 dynamics. Under normal conditions, cell PO_2 is higher than the critical level, and O_2 flux is reaction-limited. In other words augmentation

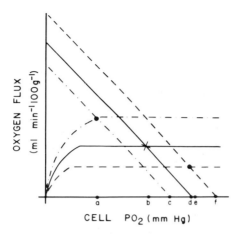

Fig. 11. Effect of altered O_2 demand on supply/uptake curves. Key: ---, decrease in O_2 demand; —·—, increase in O_2 demand. (From Granger and Nyhof, 1982, by permission.)

of tissue perfusion or exchange capacity does not alter O_2 uptake in the normal state. By contrast, tissue O_2 dynamics are transport-limited when O_2 uptake can be increased by elevating blood flow or opening more capillaries. Transport limitation is evident if the prevailing cell PO_2 is lower than the critical value. At such a low level of tissue oxygenation, improvement of the O_2 supply leads to accelerated mitochondrial uptake of O_2.

The foregoing analyses clearly demonstrate the powerful impact of blood flow and functional capillarity density as major determinants of tissue O_2 delivery. These considerations led to the formulation of a fundamental conceptual and mathematical framework for analysis of vascular control of tissue oxygenation (Granger and Shepherd, 1973). The basic tenets of the model are simple, as illustrated in Fig. 12. According to the metabolic theory of local vasoregulation, the tone of microvascular smooth muscle is modulated directly or indirectly by the prevailing level of tissue oxygenation. As a consequence of this metabolic linkage, tissue PO_2 is stabilized in the face of any stress tending to alter the balance between O_2 supply and demand. Active microvascular buffering of tissue oxygenation can be accomplished by local modulation of tissue blood flow and/or microvascular O_2 exchange capacity. In many tissues of the body, the major site of vascular resistance is in the small to medium-sized arterioles. Thus, local modulation of arteriolar tone at these loci allows intrinsic regulation of total blood flow through the microvascular network. In turn, the arteriolar flow control system serves to buffer tissue oxygenation by stabilizing capillary PO_2; this is achieved by matching blood flow to the oxygen demands of the tissue. Control of microvascular

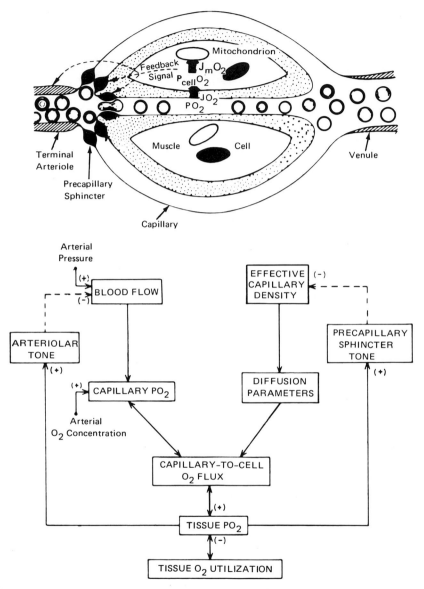

Fig. 12. Local metabolic feedback mechanisms responsible for stabilization of tissue oxygenation in the face of various stresses.

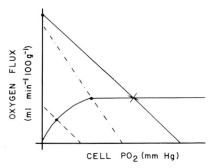

Fig. 13. Initial and final response of the O_2 delivery system to a sudden reduction in arterial pressure (P_a). After an initial reduction in O_2 flux, cell PO_2 rises above the critical level as a result of flow autoregulation (rightward shift of supply curve) and increased capillarity (increase in slope of supply curve). Key: —, control; ---, initial response to reduction in P_a; —·—, final response to reduction in P_a. (From Granger and Nyhof, 1982, by permission.)

O_2 exchange capacity resides in the terminal ramifications of the precapillary network (i.e., terminal arterioles and precapillary sphincters). These microvascular effectors modulate the number of capillaries perfused at a given moment. The exchange control system stabilizes tissue oxygenation by modifying surface area and effective capillary-to-cell diffusion distance. This component of the local vasoregulatory system provides buffering capability even in the face of reduced capillary PO_2. By working in unison the flow and exchange controllers provide a wide "margin of safety" against the development of tissue hypoxia during stress.

Let us consider the local control phenomena in terms of the metabolic theory of intrinsic vasoregulation. With a sudden decrease in perfusion pressure, O_2 transport to the capillary is reduced as blood flow falls. Consequently, the reduced tissue PO_2 induces relaxation of arterioles and precapillary sphincters; thus, vascular conductance and capillarity rise and tissue oxygenation returns toward normal. Figure 13 presents a graphic analysis of the autoregulatory response. Reactive hyperemia is a manifestation of the severest form of a hypotensive stress. That is, arterial perfusion pressure is reduced to venous pressure levels, flow falls to zero, and O_2 transport to the tissues is precluded. The resultant local vasodilation, due to a dramatic fall in tissue PO_2, is evinced as a flow overshoot upon restitution of the arterial perfusion pressure. As normal tissue oxygenation is reinstated, blood flow returns to normal. According to the metabolic theory, hypoxemic vasodilation is a natural consequence of compromising tissue oxygenation via reduction of arterial O_2 concentration. Finally, the hyperemia and augmented capillarity elicited by a sudden elevation in metabolic rate can be understood in terms of the reduction in

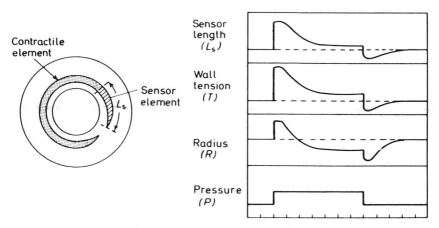

Fig. 14. Two-element model of myogenic mechanism of local microvascular control. $T = PR$, $L_s = f(T)$. The model is based on a series arrangement of the contractile element and a tension-sensing element in the arteriolar wall. (From Johnson, 1974b.)

tissue PO_2 resulting from a temporary imbalance between O_2 transport and uptake. Thus, as a result of these local vascular adjustments, cell PO_2 is maintained above the critical level in the face of changes in perfusion pressure, arterial O_2 concentration, and metabolic rate.

B. Intrinsic Microvascular Control of Transvascular Fluid Flux

The myogenic theory of local vasoregulation is based on an inherent property of vascular smooth muscle. Stretch of isolated smooth muscle fibers elicits an increase in the rate and intensity of intrinsic contractile activity (Bulbring, 1955). When extrapolated to blood vessels *in situ,* this myogenic property allows the microvasculature to respond actively to changes in transmural pressure in such a manner than active vascular tone is a direct function of the difference between intravascular and extravascular pressures (Johnson, 1981). From a mechanistic viewpoint, the myogenic response can be understood best in terms of a sensor element connected in series with the contractile elements of the vascular wall. Also, we assume that stretch of the sensor elicits a direct excitatory action on the contractile element. Figure 14 depicts the dynamics of the response to elevated intravascular pressure. With elevated transmural pressure, the vessel and sensor elements are stretched. In turn, distension of the sensor element stimulates the contractile element, and active tension rises. With the increase in active tension, the vessel constricts until total wall tension is returned toward the control level. According to the law of Laplace (i.e., tension = pressure × radius), a reduction in vessel radius below control is required to return wall tension to normal in the face of an elevated intravascular pressure (Johnson, 1974a).

From the viewpoint of microcirculatory homeostasis, the myogenic theory of local vasoregulation proposes that the intrinsic control system is designed to stabilize the rate of fluid movement across the capillary wall. At any moment transvascular fluid flux (J_v) is determined by the filtration coefficient (K_f), the protein reflection coefficient (σ), capillary hydrostatic pressure (P_c), interstitial hydrostatic pressure (P_i), and the oncotic pressures of plasma (π_c) and interstitial fluid (π_i), or

$$J_v = K_f[(P_c - P_i) - \sigma(\pi_c - \pi_i)]. \tag{8}$$

Consideration of Eq. (8) suggests that regulation of transcapillary water flux by the precapillary microvessels can be achieved by modulating K_f and P_c (Chen et al., 1976). Since K_f is a direct function of capillary surface area, the rate of fluid filtration at any given capillary pressure can be modified by the vascular elements that exert control over the number of perfused capillaries. Capillary hydrostatic pressure, on the other hand, is regulated by appropriate adjustments in precapillary resistance, as indicated by

$$P_c = [(R_v/R_a)P_a + P_v]/[1 + (R_v/R_a)], \tag{9}$$

where P_a is arterial pressure, P_v is venous pressure, R_v is postcapillary resistance, and R_a is precapillary resistance (Landis and Pappenheimer, 1963). Thus, a stress tending to increase P_c can be counterbalanced by an increase in R_a; in this manner, the transvascular filtration rate is stabilized. Equation (9) predicts that the change in R_a required to stabilize P_c increases dramatically as the prevailing P_c approaches venous pressure (Table I). For arterial and venous pressures of 100 and 0 mm Hg, respectively, a twofold rise in precapillary resistance must occur to maintain capillary pressure at 10 mm Hg following an increment in venous pressure of only 5 mm Hg. Because pressure in most peripheral capillaries is in the range 10–20 mm Hg (Guyton et al., 1975), large changes in precapillary resistance are required to buffer the effects of small elevations in venous pressure. By contrast, glomerular capillary pressure can be stabilized at 50 mm Hg with much smaller increases in precapillary resistance.

In terms of the myogenic theory, autoregulation of blood flow is an indirect manifestation of a local control system seeking to stabilize capillary pressure in the face of altered perfusion pressure. For a reduction in perfusion pressure, the rate of transcapillary fluid flux is initially diminished as capillary hydrostatic pressure falls. However, the reduction in disten-

TABLE I

Effect of Initial Capillary Pressure on Precapillary
Vasoconstriction Required to Prevent Capillary
Hypertension Following an Elevation in Venous
Pressure of 5 mm Hg[a]

Initial capillary pressure (mm Hg)	Change in precapillary resistance (x − control)
10	2.00
20	1.33
30	1.20
40	1.14
50	1.11

[a] Assumptions: (1) Capillary pressure is perfectly autoregulated at
initial value; (2) arterial and initial venous pressures are 100 and 0 mm
Hg, respectively.

sion force operating on the arterioles and precapillary sphincters elicits a
decrease in precapillary resistance and an increase in capillary density.
The partial recovery of capillary pressure and the rise in K_f tend to return
the rate of transcapillary filatration toward normal. In skeletal muscle and
heart the myogenic hypothesis can also be invoked to explain the hyperemia associated with increased contractile activity. As the rate or intensity
of muscle contraction is augmented, extravascular pressure rises due to
compression of the interstitium by the muscle fibers. With an elevation in
extravascular pressure, transmural pressure falls and a myogenic dilation
of the arterioles and precapillary sphincters occurs. Thus, the initial tendency of transvascular fluid flux to fall due to an increase in interstitial
pressure is negated by a rise in capillary pressure and filtration coefficient.

C. Interaction of Metabolic and Myogenic Control Systems

In tissues subserved by metabolic and myogenic control systems operating in parallel, the two feedback mechanisms may produce directionally
similar vascular reactions under certain stresses. Under other conditions
the myogenic and metabolic feedback signals may compete with each
other for ultimate control of microvascular tone. A reduction in arterial
perfusion elicits decreases in both cell PO_2 and transmural pressure. Consequently, the myogenic and metabolic signals can act in a synergistic
fashion to produce a substantial vasodilation and excellent stabilization of

blood flow (Morff and Granger, 1982). By contrast, an elevation in venous pressure induces a reduction in cell PO_2 and an increase in arteriolar transmural pressure. Thus, the metabolic feedback signal urges the arteriole to dilate, whereas the myogenic controller implores it to constrict. The final response of the blood vessel underlies the relative potency of the two parallel control systems. Indeed, venous pressure elevation has become the primary perturbation for characterizing the relative roles of myogenic and metabolic feedback mechanisms in the intrinsic regulation of microvascular perfusion. Tissues exhibiting vasoconstrictor responses to elevated venous pressure often are considered to possess a predominant myogenic control system (Johnson, 1964); vasodilation during acute venous hypertension usually is interpreted to reflect strong metabolic modulation of microvascular tone (Jones and Berne, 1964).

III. Remote Control of the Microcirculation

As discussed above some of the control signals impinging on the smooth muscle cells of microvessels originate outside of the region subserved by a particular microvascular bed. In general, these signals originate from brain and endocrine glands. These nervous and hormonal control systems act on pre- and postcapillary microvessels in an effort to stabilize a systemic variable, such as blood pressure, which is of primary importance for the survival of the whole organism. Thus, remote control systems tend to ignore the needs of the individual tissues subserved by individual microvascular beds. Instead, the low-priority microcirculations (i.e., muscle, skin, splanchnic organs) are commanded to respond in such a fashion that the integrity of the vital organs (i.e., brain and heart) is maintained in the face of life-threatening stresses.

A. Nervous Control of the Microvasculature

The junction of a sympathetic nerve terminal with vascular smooth muscle is shown in Fig. 15. In terminals located several hundred angstroms from the smooth muscle cell, norepinephrine is synthesized from tyrosine and stored in membrane-bound vesicles (von Euler, 1972). The rate-limiting reaction is catalyzed by tyrosine hydroxylase. Regulation of transmitter synthesis is achieved via feedback inhibition of tyrosine hydroxylase by norepinephrine (von Euler, 1972). Thus, a reduction of the norepinephrine pool in the terminal leads to a stimulation of transmitter synthesis and a return of norepinephrine levels to control levels. The release of norepi-

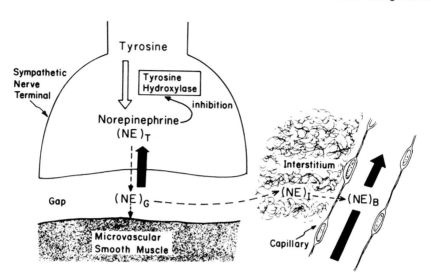

Fig. 15. Schematic representation of neurovascular junction. (From Granger and Shephard, 1979, by permission.)

nephrine into the neurovascular gap is initiated by the arrival of an action potential at the terminal. In some manner not yet understood, depolarization causes the norepinephrine vesicles to coalesce with the neuronal membrane, and the transmitter is extruded into the gap by the process of exocytosis (Drapeau and Blaustein, 1982). Upon entering the neurovascular gap, the transmitter may (*a*) bind to the smooth muscle receptor, (*b*) reenter the terminal via an active transport mechanism, (*c*) enter the vascular smooth muscle cell for inactivation, and (*d*) diffuse away from the gap into the blood capillaries (Folkow *et al.*, 1967). In general, the rate of norepinephrine release from the terminals is proportional to the stimulation frequency and the concentration of norepinephrine in the nerve ending. More than 50% of the transmitter released into the gap is reabsorbed at a rapid rate by active transport. Another 15–25% of the released catecholamine diffuses into the interstitium, then into the blood, and is finally carried out of the tissue via the venous circulation. The vasoconstrictor action of norepinephrine is brought about by the binding of a small fraction of the released norepinephrine molecules to receptors located on the surface of the vascular smooth muscle cells (Somlyo and Somlyo, 1968). Stimulation of the adrenergic receptor elicits an increase in calcium movement into the cytoplasm of the muscle cell (Somlyo and Somlyo, 1968); consequently, the interaction of myosin and actin is enhanced, and microvascular tone rises. Figure 16 illustrates the response of a mathe-

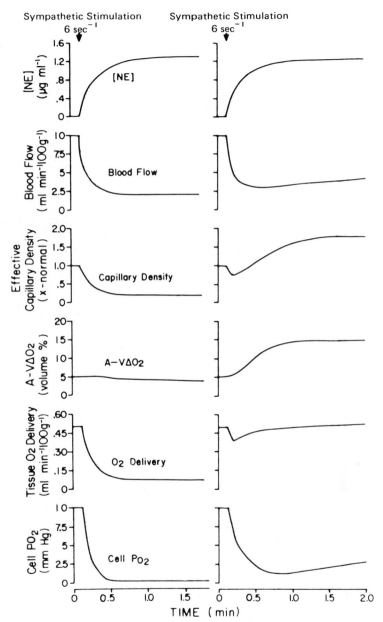

Fig. 16. Vascular and oxygenation responses to sympathetic stimulation at rate of 6 impulses per second. (From Granger and Shephard, 1979, by permission.)

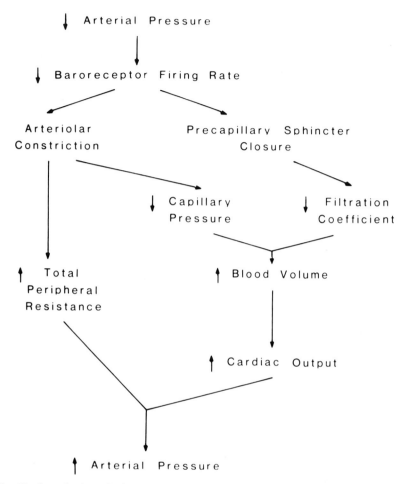

Fig. 17. Contribution of microcirculatory responses to operation of baroreceptor reflex.

matical model of neurovascular·interactions to stimulation of the sympathetic nerve in skeletal muscle at a rate of 6 impulses per second. Within 15 sec after the beginning of stimulation, the norepinephrine concentration in the gap rises to 1 μg ml^{-1}. This high level of catecholamine produces vasoconstriction great enough to lower blood flow and capillary density to less than one-fourth of normal values. In addition, increased tone of the venules and veins leads to a displacement of blood volume from the tissue (not shown in figure).

The role of neural control of microcirculatory function in whole-body homeostasis can best be appreciated by considering the microvascular reactions elicited via the baroreceptor, chemoreceptor, and volume re-

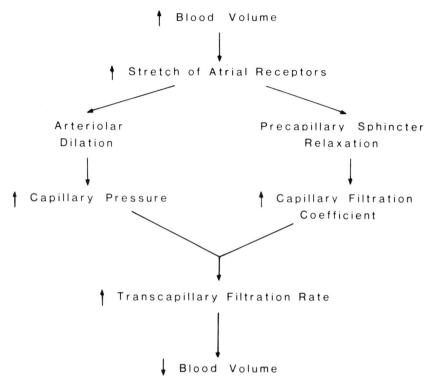

Fig. 18. Role of microcirculation in reflex control of blood volume via atrial stretch receptors.

flexes. As shown in Fig. 17, a reduction in systemic arterial pressure causes a decrease in baroreceptor firing rate, which in turn initiates a neurogenic constriction of peripheral arterioles and precapillary sphincters (Mellander and Johansson, 1968). Consequently, capillary pressure and filtration area fall, fluid is absorbed into the capillaries, blood volume rises, and cardiac output is accelerated. Arteriolar constriction also leads to an elevation of total peripheral resistance. The increases in cardiac output and total peripheral resistance allow the systemic arterial pressure to return toward control. The microvascular responses to stimulation of the volume reflex are summarized in Fig. 18. With an increase in blood volume, the atria are distended, the atrial stretch receptors are activated, and the sympathetic outflow to the peripheral microvasculature is diminished (Guyton *et al.*, 1975). As a result of arteriolar and precapillary sphincter dilation, capillary pressure and filtration surface area rise. In turn, fluid leaves the circulation and blood volume returns toward normal. Finally, microcirculatory responses to chemoreceptor stimulation are shown in

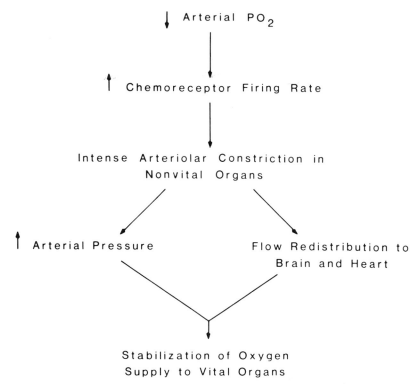

Fig. 19. Microcirculatory responses following initiation of chemoreceptor stimulation.

Fig. 19. As arterial PO_2 falls, chemoreceptor activation initiates an intense neurogenically mediated vasoconstriction in the nonvital organs such as skin, muscle, and splanchnic region (Folkow and Neil, 1971). As a consequence, cardiac output is redistributed to the heart and brain because the microvessels of the vital organs are relatively insensitive to adrenergic stimuli. In addition, the vasoconstriction in nonvital tissues elevate systemic arterial pressure and enhances the perfusion of brain and heart. Thus, the net effect of the chemoreceptor response pattern is to ensure adequate delivery of oxygen to the vital organs in systemic hypoxemia.

B. Endocrine Control of the Microvasculature

The major endocrine organs involved in cardiovascular homeostasis are the adrenal medulla, the posterior pituitary gland, and the kidney. The ac-

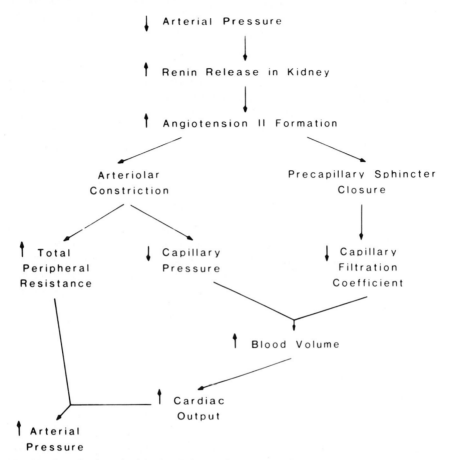

Fig. 20. Contribution of microcirculation to functioning of renin–angiotensin system as a regulator of systemic arterial pressure.

tions of the norepinephrine and epinephrine released by the adrenal gland resemble the patterns elicited by stimulation of sympathetic adrenergic nerves. The release of the pituitary hormone, vasopressin, is to some extent controlled by the volume receptors described above (Guyton *et al.,* 1975). With reductions in blood volume and the degree of atrial stretch, the volume receptor inhibition of vasopressin release is diminished and the vasoconstrictor pours into the bloodstream. As a result capillary pressure falls and fluid is reabsorbed from the interstitium into the bloodstream. Consequently, blood volume and atrial pressure return toward normal. Finally, the release of renin by the kidney elicits a series of microvascular reactions that help to stabilize systemic blood pressure (Folkow and Neil, 1971). The effects of the renin–antiotensin system on microcirculatory dynamics are summarized in Fig. 20. A reduction in systemic arterial pressure results in a decrease in renal perfusion and renin release from the kidney. Renin catalyzes the first step in a series of reactions that eventually lead to the formation of angiotensin II, a powerful vasoconstrictor. The enhancement of microvascular tone by angiotensin II is the result of several actions of the hormone at the neurovascular junction (Shepherd and Vanhoutte, 1979). At low plasma concentrations, angiotensin II increases the norepinephrine concentration in the neurovascular gap by stimulating release and inhibiting reuptake of norepinephrine by the nerve terminal. At higher concentrations, angiotensin II has a direct stimulatory effect on vascular smooth muscle. In addition, the hormone potentiates the interaction of norepinephrine with the vascular adrenergic receptor. Through these mechanisms arteriolor constriction is achieved and capillary pressure falls. With capillary fluid reabsorption, blood volume and cardiac output rise. The increases in cardiac output and total peripheral resistance contribute to the reestablishment of a normal systemic arterial pressure.

IV. Conclusions

In this brief chapter we have sketched the control mechanisms responsible for modulating microcirculatory function in accordance with the local needs of the tissue and the requirements for systemic homeostasis. We have examined regulators concerned with tissue oxygenation, transvascular fluid balance, and maintenance of a stable systemic arterial pressure. Under numerous circumstances conflicts arise over the local needs of individual tissues versus the necessity of ensuring the survival of the organism. The outcome of this competition between local and remote controllers of microcirculatory behavior varies from organ to organ, as is discussed in later chapters. At this point it is sufficient to say that the interactions between local and remote regulation of the microvasculature allow a large variety of response patterns to a specific stress; the response at a given moment is dependent on the prevailing conditions at the local and systemic levels. In the final analysis it is this mutability of control behavior that guarantees the survival of the organism and its components over a wide range of stresses.

Acknowledgments

The authors' original investigations were supported by grants HL-25387, HL-21498, and HL-24315 from the National Heart, Lung, and Blood Institute and by a grant-in-aid (79-767) from the American Heart Association. H. J. Granger and J. L. Borders are recipients of Research Career Development (K04-HL00409) and National Research Service (F32-HL06576) Awards, respectively. The authors were indebted to Mildred Markse and Elizabeth Green for secretarial assistance.

References

Bulbring, E. (1955). *J. Physiol* (*London*) **128,** 200–221.
Chen, H. I., Granger, H. J., and Taylor, A. E. (1976). *Circ. Res.* **39,** 245–254.
Drapeau, P., and Blaustein, M. P. (1982). *In* "Trends in Autonomic Pharmacology" (S. Kalsner, ed.), Vol. 2, pp. 117–130. Urban & Schwarzenberg, Baltimore.
Folkow, B., and Neil, E. (1971). "Circulation." Oxford Univ. Press, London.
Folkow, B., Haggendal, H., and Lisander, B. (1967). *Acta Physiol. Scand.* (Suppl. 307), 1–38.
Granger, H. J., and Norris, C. P. (1980). *Am. J. Physiol.* **238,** H836–H843.
Granger, H. J., and Nyhof, R. A. (1982). *Am. J. Physiol.* **243,** G91–G96.
Granger, H. J., and Shepherd, A. P. (1973). *Microvasc. Res.* **5,** 49–72.
Granger, H. J., and Shepherd, A. P. (1979). Adv. Biomed. Eng. **7,** 1–63.
Granger, H. J., Goodman, A. H., and Granger, D. N. (1976). *Circ. Res.* **38,** 379–385.
Guyton, A. C., Taylor, A. E., and Granger, H. J. (1975). "Circulatory Physiology: Dynamics and Control of the Body Fluids," Vol. 2. Saunders, Philadelphia, Pennsylvania.
Jobsis, F. F. (1964). *Sect. 3 Respir.* **1,** 63–124.
Jobsis, F. F. (1972). *Fed. Proc. Fed. Am. Soc. Exp. Biol.* **31,** 1404–1413.
Johnson, P. C. (1964). *Circ. Res.* **15,** (Suppl. I), 12–19.
Johnson, P. C. (1974). *In* "Cardiovascular Physiology" (A. C. Guyton, and C. E. Jones, eds.), pp. 163–195. Univ. Park Press, Baltimore, Maryland.
Johnson, P. C. (1981). *In* "Advances in Physiological Sciences. Cardiovascular Physiology, Microcirculation and Capillary Exchange" (A. G. B. Kouach, J. Hamar, and L. Szabo, eds.), Vol. 7, pp. 17–34. Pergamon, New York.
Jones, R. D., and Berne, R. M. (1964). *Circ. Res.* **15,** (Suppl. I), 130–138.
Landis, E. M., and Pappenheimer, J. R. (1963). *Handb. Physiol. Sect. 2 Cardiovasc. Sys.* **2,** 961–1034.
Mellander, S., and Johansson, B. (1968). *Pharmacol. Rev.* **20,** 117–196.
Morff, R. J., and Granger, H. J. (1982). *Circ. Res.*
Mortillaro, N. A., and Granger, H. J. (1977). *Circ. Res.* **41,** 859–865.
Norris, C. P., Barnes, G. E., Smith, E. E., and Granger, H. J. (1979). *Am. J. Physiol.* **237,** H174–H177.
Shepherd, J. T., and Granger, H. J. (1973). *Gastroenterology* **65,** 77–91.
Shepherd, J. T., and Vanhoutte, P. M. (1979). "The Human Cardiovascular System: Facts and Concepts." Raven, New York.

Somlyo, A. P., and Somlyo, A. V. (1968). *Pharmacol. Rev.* **20,** 197–272.
von Euler, U. S. (1972). *Pharmacol. Rev.* **24,** 365–379.

6 Microcirculation of the Brain

Richard J. Traystman

I. Introduction

The literature concerning the cerebral circulation, its regulation in health and disease, is enormous and involves a remarkable number of books, articles, and reviews. Many experimental techniques to measure cerebral blood flow have been employed, and many species of animals have been used. In fact these two aspects, techniques and species of animals used, may in part be the source of some of the confusion relating to cerebral circulatory control, even though the use of these same techniques and species has increased our knowledge and understanding of the cerebral circulation. The purpose of this chapter is to review briefly several areas relating to the cerebral circulation and its control and to express our cur-

THE PHYSIOLOGY AND PHARMACOLOGY
OF THE MICROCIRCULATION, VOLUME 1

rent understanding of these areas. Specifically, we consider cerebral vascular anatomy, methods of studying the cerebral circulation, and regulation of cerebral blood flow in the adult, neonate, and fetus.

II. Anatomic Considerations

A. Arterial System

The brain of essentially all mammalian species is supplied with blood from several major sources, that is, internal and external carotid, vertebral, and spinal anterior arteries. However, the relative importance of these channels in any species is unclear (Schmidt, 1950). Although the internal carotid leads directly to the brain, in some species this vessel is unimportant, and it may be the external carotid that carries the major proportion of blood reaching the brain. In general, in human beings the anterior three-fifths of the cerebrum, except for parts of the occipital and temporal lobes, is supplied by the carotid arteries. The posterior two-fifths of the cerebrum, the cerebellum, and the brainstem are supplied by the vertebrobasilar system. The carotid and vertebral arteries unite at the base of the brain to form the circle of Willis. In addition, there are a number of possible arterial anastomotic vessels on each side of the head between the intracranial and extracranial circulations. These include (a) a connection between the vertebral and occipital arteries, (b) a communication between the ascending pharyngeal and internal carotid arteries, (c) the middle meningeal artery branching off from the internal maxillary artery and connecting with the internal carotid artery, (d) the anastomotic artery between the internal maxillary and internal carotid arteries, (e) pathways between the external and internal ophthalmic arteries, (f) anastomosis between the external and internal ethmoidal arteries, (g) collaterals between the vertebral and the omocervical arteries, and (h) connections between the spinal anterior and vertebral arteries (Jewell, 1952; Kaplan and Ford, 1966; Green and Denison, 1956).

In certain species the external carotid system branches into a complicated network of arteries, the rete mirable, prior to its entrance to the circle of Willis. This rete system has been proposed to be involved in a heat-exchange countercurrent mechanism, which acts to lower the temperature of the blood entering the brain (Baker and Chapman, 1977; Nagel et al., 1968). The hexagonal structural arrangement of the circle of Willis connects the two carotid arteries with each other and with the basilar artery. Several main arteries leave the circle and course toward the brain (anterior, middle, and posterior cerebral arteries) and to extracranial structures. Under certain circumstances the circle may carry blood from one side of the brain to the other; however, under normal circumstances there is little or no mixing between the right and left sides (Wellens *et al.*, 1975). As these major arteries leave the circle of Willis they reduce their diameter to become arterioles and pial vessels. Pial arteries then plunge at a 90° angle into the brain parenchyma. There is much evidence that there is a close relationship between pial vessels and the leptomeninges. These vessels, as they enter the parenchyma, are invested with a leptomeningeal sheath and are surrounded by a cerebrospinal-fluid-containing space (Purves, 1972). It should be mentioned here that most studies of cerebral vessels using methods of staining and light microscopy have not shown any differences between brain vessels and vessels in other organs.

B. Venous System

Blood is drained from the brain via two primary sets of veins: the external group and the deep or internal group. These drain into the dural sinuses and then the internal jugular veins. The external venous system is divided into the superior, middle, inferior, and occipital cerebral veins, which drain the outer portion of the cerebral hemispheres. The superior cerebral vein drains the cortex and underlying white matter above the corpus callosum. Several veins on each side merge to form three large trunks, which enter the superior sagittal sinus or straight sinus. The most prominent superior cerebral vein is the great anastomotic vein of Trolard connecting the superior sagittal sinus with the Sylvian vein. The internal cerebral or deep veins include a variety of small transcerebral veins draining the bulk of white matter from the anterior and middle group of the brain. This system eventually drains through the great vein of Galen and the straight sinus. Veins from all parts of the brain drain into many sinuses situated between two layers of dura, that is, superior sagittal sinus, inferior sagittal sinus, occipital sinus, superior petrosal sinus, cavernous sinus, and transverse sinus. Very extensive intervenous collateral anastomoses exist between the two main venous draining systems and with the extracranial venous draining system.

C. Capillary System

The brain contains a rich network of capillaries; however, the density of capillaries within the central nervous system is less than that in the heart, kidney, and muscle (Sjostrand, 1935). Gray matter contains about two and one-half times as many capillaries as does white matter; that is, cerebral cortex has about 1000 capillaries/mm^3 and white matter about 300 capillaries/mm^3 (Craigie, 1920; Dunning and Wolff, 1937). Dunning and Wolff (1937) proposed that capillary density is correlated with the number of synapses in a particular brain region. The high density of capillaries in the cervical sympathetic ganglion, which contains synapses, compared to that in the trigeminal ganglion, which lacks them, demonstrates this point. Oxygen consumption may be the link between capillary density and synaptic frequency. Support for this hypothesis comes from the work of Sokoloff (1977), which demonstrated that the glucose utilization of gray matter is greater than that of white matter by a factor similar to the ratio of capillary densities for the two tissues. Exposure of experimental animals (rats and rabbits) to hypoxia for a long period leads to an increase in capillary density (Diemer, 1968). Thus, oxygen lack must be either a direct or indirect stimulus to capillary growth; however, the precise mechanism responsible for this increased vascularity remains unknown. Cerebral capillary density also varies with age. Diemer (1968) demonstrated that capillary density at birth is about 30% of that in the adult and is even lower in the premature infant.

D. Blood–Brain Barrier and Capillary Permeability

The concept of a blood–brain barrier arose from the work of a number of investigators who demonstrated that certain dyes and pharmacologically active compounds did not enter the brain but could enter most other organs. The barrier had to be a vascular one because the same substances would readily enter the brain when injected directly into the cerebrospinal fluid. It was subsequently shown that the dyes that could not penetrate the brain from the vascular side were bound to plasma proteins, so that the barrier was actually to dye–protein complexes. A complete description of the morphologic localization of the barrier to circulating protein was given by Reese and Karnovsky (1967) and Brightman and Reese (1969), who used horseradish peroxidase, a protein that could be localized by electron microscopy.

The blood–brain barrier separates two of the major compartments of the central nervous system, the brain and cerebrospinal fluid, from the third compartment, the blood. The sites of the barrier are the interfaces between the blood and these two compartments: the choroid plexus, the blood vessels of the brain and subarachnoid space, and the arachnoid membrane. All barrier sites are characterized by cells connected by tight junctions, which restrict intercellular diffusion. These cells are represented by endothelia of blood vessels, epithelia of the choroid plexus, and cells of the arachnoid layer. When the cells are connected via tight junctions, they act as if they were one single layer of cells, and solute exchange occurs transcellularly. These cells thus determine the solubility and transport functions of the entire layer of cells. Lipid-soluble substances penetrate easily and equilibrate between brain and blood quickly. It has also been shown that there is only minimal transport by pinocytotic vessels at the barrier site (Reese and Karnovsky, 1967), and this in addition to the tight junctions limits protein transport into the extracellular fluid (Bradbury, 1979; Rapoport, 1976).

Whereas the passage of the more permeable substances (sugars and amino acids) into the brain is determined by both the cerebral blood flow and the permeability characteristics, the permeability of ions and large molecules depends largely on the characteristics of the blood–brain barrier membrane rather than the blood flow. Nonelectrolytes of small molecular weight penetrate faster than their lipid solubilities and diffusion coefficients would predict. Thus, the presence of water channels across the barrier is likely (Bradbury, 1979). This blood–brain barrier may not be equally permeable in all areas of the brain. For example, the area postrema, choroid plexus, hypophysis, pineal, and areas in the hypothalamus have no blood–brain barrier at all. Peters *et al.* (1976) showed that in these areas the cerebral capillaries have fenestrations, and there are a large number of pinocytotic vesicles in the endothelial cells. Besides these areas, within the brain there are moderate differences in apparent barrier permeability of different regions. The entry of most solutes into gray matter is about three to four times faster than into white matter. This may be correlated with a similar difference in the length of capillaries per unit volume of gray compared to white matter.

Breakdown of the blood–brain barrier can be caused by mechanisms that either alter the tension in the walls of small vessels or damage the vessel wall in other ways, that is, chemically or by radiation. Several investigators have shown that inhalation of a high concentration of CO_2 (20%) increases the penetration of labeled proteins into the brain (Clemedson *et al.*, 1958; Goldberg *et al.*, 1961). The effect of CO_2 on blood–brain barrer permeability is reversible and, if the associated rise in blood pressure is abolished as CO_2 is administered, blood–brain barrier function is unaltered. Repeated seizure activity also gives rise to extreme cerebral vasodilation, and again the barrier may be opened (Bauer and Leonhardt, 1956). As with CO_2 administration the breakdown is enhanced by elevated blood pressure. Hypertension itself also disrupts the barrier. Johansson *et al.* (1970) demonstrated that when blood pressure was elevated by more than 90 mm Hg extravasation of dye occurred. This effect is due to a breakdown of the small vessels of the brain. In a classic paper

Rapoport *et al.* (1972) characterized the properties of osmotic opening of the barrier. The degree of opening was determined by the amount of extravasation of dye (Evan's blue) as hyperosmolar solutions of different concentrations were applied to the surface of the cerebral cortex. The major conclusions of their study were that the barrier opening was reversible and that the degree of opening increased with increases in osmolality. These authors suggested that the hyperosmolar solutions shrink the endothelial cells and open the tight junctions. However, Bradbury (1979) and Westergaard (1977) suggested that hyperosmolar solutions increase vesicular transport in endothelial cells.

The structural integrity of cerebral endothelium is immediately dependent on metabolism, and endothelia resist hypoxia and ischemia much longer than do other cells of the brain (Broman, 1949; Goodale *et al.*, 1970). Broman (1949) showed that barrier impermeability to dye is retained for up to 12 h after an animal is killed. However, histochemical and biochemical studies have shown that cerebral cortical neurons do not survive O_2 deprivation for more than 3 to 8 min (Blackwood *et al.*, 1963). Following occlusion of the blood supply to a region of the brain the cerebral endothelial cells swell or flatten, but the endothelium continuity is undisturbed (Hossmann and Olsson, 1970). Vascular disruption develops after several hours and is preceded by irreversible metabolic and cytologic changes in cells of the surrounding parenchyma (Siesjo and Ljundggren, 1973). Thus, hypoxia and ischemia are not potent causes of barrier breakdown.

A large number of other miscellaneous insults may increase barrier permeability. These include physical, chemical, infective, allergic, and neoplastic processes, and they generally result in barrier opening by sensitizing or damaging directly the cerebral vessels.

III. Methods of Studying the Cerebral Circulation

There have been many reviews concerning the methods of measuring responses of the cerebral circulation (Edvinsson and MacKenzie, 1977; Purves, 1972). However, because much controversy over cerebral responsiveness may be accounted for by the use of different methodologies, a brief discussion and account of the advantages and disadvantages of some of the frequently used techniques will be given.

The ideal anatomic condition for a hemodynamic study of a vascular bed is fulfilled when an organ has a single arterial input or venous output. Because neither of these conditions can be attained in the brain, the study of the cerebral vascular bed becomes quite complicated. The technical problems involved in measuring cerebral blood flow were pointed out as early as 1890 by Roy and Sherrington. Subsequent reviews by Wolff (1936), Schmidt (1950), and Lassen (1959) discussed the various methods that were applied to the study of cerebral circulation. The methods used for studying the cerebral circulation are diverse in both principle and reliability. However, they may be grouped into four general categories: (*a*) direct observation of changes in vascular diameter, (*b*) application of the Fick principle using diffusible indicators, (*c*) application of the indicator-concentration technique using nondiffusible indicators, and (*d*) direct arterial or venous blood flow measurement using electromagnetic flow probes.

A. *Pial Artery Diameter*

Measurement of pial artery diameter is a classic method of evaluating variations in the responsiveness of cerebral blood vessels. This method provides a direct measure of cerebral vessel responsiveness and has been shown to be accurate and reproducible, especially since the introduction of the television microscopy image-splitting technique (Baez, 1966). This technique has been especially useful in examining the responsiveness of pial vessels to locally administered agents, for example, ions, autonomic agonists, and blocking agents (Wei *et al.*, 1980a,b; Kontos *et al.*, 1977a; Kuschinsky *et al.*, 1972; Fog, 1939a,b). The effects of pharmacologic agents on pial vessels can be studied directly, because the agents are applied locally and systemic effects are minimal. The effects of nerve stimulation and alterations in perfusion pressure have also been studied effectively with this technique. In addition, this technique allows for the separation of responses from different-sized pial vessels. Although the technique has proved to be very useful for many years, its disadvantage is that it measures pial artery diameter, not blood flow. Thus, it provides only indirect information about cerebral blood flow since there is no suitable method for converting changes in arteriole diameter into changes in blood flow.

More recently, this pial diameter technique has been used simultaneously with a pulsed doppler technique (Marcus *et al.*, 1981). By placing a piezoelectric crystal under the vessel in which diameter is measured, one can calculate the flow in the vessel because flow is equal to the velocity times the diameter. In this way flow can be monitored almost continuously in a pial artery.

B. Diffusible Indicator Techniques

The most well known of the diffusible indicator methods is the Kety–Schmidt nitrous oxide technique (Kety and Schmidt, 1948a,b). This technique utilizes an inert gas, such as nitrous oxide, which is taken up by the brain in a known relationship to the blood concentration of the gas. The gas is inhaled until approximate equilibrium is attained between the arterial blood and the brain content of the gas. During the time of gas uptake, the cerebral venous blood has a lower concentration of the gas than docs the simultaneously measured arterial blood. By taking sufficient simultaneous samples of arterial and cerebral venous blood during the period of gas uptake by the brain, one obtains data that allow plotting of curves of arterial and venous blood concentration of the gas with time. The concentration of nitrous oxide in the brain at equilibrium divided by the area between the two curves gives the cerebral blood flow (milliliters per minute per 100 g). The brain concentration of nitrous oxide is calculated from the cerebral venous concentration of the gas at equilibrium corrected for the partition coefficient for the relative solubility of the gas in brain tissue versus blood.

The advantage of this technique is that it can be used in human beings; however, a number of criticisms must be dealt with. Several assumptions are made in the use of the technique that may introduce significant errors in results. First, the assumption that the partition coefficient of nitrous oxide, which is the ratio of the solubility of the gas in the brain to its solubility in whole blood, is a constant value is merely an approximation because neither brain tissues nor whole blood are homogeneous. The coefficient varies with hematocrit and also with different brain tissues. Second, the assumption that the venous sample from the superior bulb of the internal jugular vein in human beings is free of extracerebral blood is also an approximation. Extracranial contamination has been found to be as high as 7%; however, Lassen (1959) supported the validity of this technique by finding that only 5% of 67 samples were grossly contaminated. Finally, the assumption that cerebral blood flow remains constant during the measurement is also somewhat questionable.

One modification of the Kety–Schmidt technique involves the use of a diffusible radioactive indicator. The indicator is infused intravenously. Count rates are made simultaneously and continuously from blood withdrawn continuously from an artery and the jugular vein; simultaneously, count rates are recorded with a collimated external counter focused on the brain. Repeated flows are calculated for periods as short as 1 min by dividing the 1-min increase in brain count rate by the 1-min integrated area (concentration × time) between the arterial and venous blood concentrations of the isotope for the same time interval (Scheinberg, 1965).

Cerebral blood flow has also been studied by modifications of the sodium clearance technique. In this case a radioactive substance such as ^{85}Kr or ^{133}Xe, which is taken up by the brain, is inhaled or injected either intravascularly or directly into the brain. The exponential rate of rise of the count during uptake or the exponential rate of decline of count rate after cessation of uptake, that is, the rate of desaturation, is recorded by collimated external counters arranged to focus on the brain. Flow is expressed as a function of the slope of the rise or fall when plotted or computed exponentially (Hoedt-Rasmussen et al., 1966; Ingvar and Lassen, 1962). The use of ^{85}Kr or ^{133}Xe (radioactive inert gases) obviates the need for arterial and venous cannulation, because the clearance of the isotope from the brain could be measured via external detectors. However, one of the difficulties with this technique is that, since the external detectors must be placed over the head of the animal, gross extracranial contamination may be involved.

C. Nondiffusible Indicator Techniques

Cerebral blood flow has also been estimated by the use of radioactive indicators or dyes that remain in the blood. The substances are injected into one or both internal carotid arteries. The jugular venous concentration versus time curve of the substance is obtained by withdrawing cerebral venous blood separately from each jugular bulb at a constant rate through separate continuous analyzing cuvettes (Nylin, 1958). By the use of this indicator-concentration method, one can also determine differences in transit times of the indicator through the two sides of the brain by injecting alternately into each internal carotid artery (Scheinberg, 1965). Quantitative flow measurement by this method, however, is complicated due to both uncertainty as to the degree of mixing of the blood from the injected artery with blood from the opposite internal carotid and the two vertebral arteries, and uncertainty regarding the degree and variability of admixture of venous blood from areas that received the indicator with blood from cerebral and extracerebral areas that did not receive the indicator (Schmidt, 1950).

The circulation time for nondiffusible indicators (^{131}I[iodo]albumin, [^{131}I]iodohippuran) has been used as an index of cerebral flow (Fedoruk and Feindel, 1960; Oldendorf, 1962). The indicator is injected intravenously, and an activity curve is obtained from γ counting with a scintillation counter placed externally over the head region. The curve is then differentiated, and the circulation time measured. The information gained from the method, however, must be treated with caution. It is a measurement of velocity and cannot yield quantitative data about cerebral blood flow unless cerebral blood volume is known. Harper *et al.* (1968) demonstrated that this method is dependent on a constant cerebral blood volume. Therefore, unless cerebral blood volume is independently measured the technique may be inadequate and could lead to erroneous interpretations.

The calculation of cerebral blood flow from the radiolabeled microsphere technique is based on the bolus fractionation principle developed by Sapirstein (1962). Sapirstein's method consists of injecting a known quantity of isotope intravenously and measuring the concentration (activity per gram) in a variety of organs post mortem. If the cardiac output is also known, the distribution of isotope can be expressed as blood flow, that is, as a fraction of cardiac output. In using the labeled microsphere technique to measure total and regional cerebral blood flow several major assumptions must be made: (*a*) that the microspheres are well mixed when injected into the left heart and then distributed according to the blood flow, (*b*) that essentially all the microspheres are trapped in the microcirculation, (*c*) that the blood flow is not significantly altered during the time period in which the spheres are trapped, and (*d*) that the cardiac output, or reference flow, can be accurately measured. The validity of using radiolabeled microspheres to assess the distribution of cardiac output to various organs including the brain has been well established and described in detail (Buckberg *et al.*, 1971; Marcus *et al.*, 1976; Rudolph and Heymann, 1972). The major advantages of the microsphere technique are that it allows for the measurement of cerebral blood flow in discrete regional areas of the brain as well as flow in other organs, it avoids the extracranial contamination problem that plagues so many of the other techniques, and it does not involve great surgical trauma to the animal. The disadvantages are that only a limited number of labeled spheres are available and can be separated by differential spectroscopy, and only steady-state measurements (no transients) can be made.

D. Direct Arterial or Venous Blood Flow Measurement

The cephalic circulation can be conceived of as two parallel vascular beds, one supplying blood to the intracranial and the other to the extracranial structures. Between these two vascular beds are numerous interarterial and intervenous anastomoses. The extent of the anastomoses varies in different species; they are of greater magnitude in the dog but are present even in primates (Batson, 1944; Purves, 1972; Schmidt, 1950). These anastomoses have a major functional significance in the interpretation of results of experiments designed to determine the reactivity characteristics of each of the vasculatures in parallel.

Several cerebral venous outflow techniques are currently in use, and the major advantage of these techniques is that they provide a continuous measurement of blood flow. The best known of these is the technique first used by Rapela and Green (1964) and later modified by Traystman and Rapela (1975). Venous outflow is measured because the cephalic venous vasculature lends itself to an easier functional isolation of the two parallel vascular beds than does the arterial vasculature (Rapela and Green, 1964). In the Rapela–Green technique the functional isolation of the intra- from the extracranial venous circulations can be tested efficiently and simply by measuring the rise in venous outflow pressure when the venous outflow is occluded. Testing such functional isolation is essential in any preparation designed to study the reactivity characteristics of the two vascular beds in parallel by measuring either venous outflow or arterial inflow. This testing is particularly crucial when one is studying the cerebral circulation, because it reacts to nervous, pharmacologic, or humoral stimuli differently than the extracranial circulation. The technique involves the measurement of cerebral blood flow from the confluence of the sinuses after the lateral sinuses and occipital emissary veins are occluded to prevent communication between the intracranial and extracranial venous circulations. With this technique approximately 50–70% of the mass of the brain is drained at the confluence of the sagittal and straight sinus (Rapela et al., 1967). The verification of the measurement of cerebral blood flow utilizing the technique has been described in detail elsewhere (Traystman and Rapela, 1975). O'Neill and Traystman (1977) and Wilson et al. (1981) demonstrated good agreement between this venous outflow technique and the radiolabeled microsphere technique when both techniques are used simultaneously in the same preparation. Finally, the viability and responsiveness of the cerebral vasculature to hypercapnia (Traystman and Rapela, 1975) and hypoxia (Pitt et al., 1979; Traystman et al., 1978; Traystman and Fitzgerald, 1981) and the capacity of the cerebral vessels to autoregulate (Rapela and Green, 1964) as determined using this technique has been demonstrated.

Another venous outflow technique is that used by D'Alecy and Feigl (1972). In this technique an electromagnetic flow probe is placed around the retroglenoid vein. The technique has two major difficulties. First, it has been demonstrated that extracranial contamination is likely to be present (Traystman and Rapela, 1975). Extracranial contamination with this technique may have been facilitated by the surgery involved, which included ligation or blockade of numerous extracranial venous channels. With the presence of anastomotic channels the ligation of extracranial drainage routes would increase extracranial venous pressure and contaminate the measured outflow with extracranial blood via persistent functional intervenous anastomoses; the greater number of vessels ligated, the greater the diversion of extracranial venous blood. Second, it has been demonstrated that the retroglenoid vein itself exhibits vasomotor reactivity (Pearce and Bevan, 1981). Thus, when flow changes in the D'Alecy–Feigl preparation, it may result from retroglenoid reactivity rather than from changes in reactivity of the cerebral vasculature.

One may also measure blood flow draining from the superior sagittal sinus. This method probably measures only one-third of the total mass of brain tissue but is reliable only if there is no reflux flow from the confluence of the sinuses, which would add extracranial contamination.

Problems in the determination of changes in cerebral blood flow are also encountered when arterial inflow is measured. The multiplicity of arteries supplying the brain and the efficiency of the circle of Willis restrict the value of flow measurements made through any one artery as an index of cerebral blood flow. In studies of arterial inflow all arteries bringing blood to the head have been ligated except one, and the flow in this remaining channel has been measured and called cerebral blood flow. However, it has been shown that the effects of ligating one cephalic artery in the dog are compensated for by the shunting of blood from the remaining intra- or extracranial arteries (Rein, 1929; Schneider and Schneider, 1934). It has also been shown that compensation can occur in man when one of the carotid arteries is ligated (Kristiansen and Krog, 1962). Thus, because of the presence of numerous interarterial anastomoses, the cephalic arterial circulation should be left as undisturbed as possile when arterial inflow is being measured. In addition, in many experimental animal models (i.e., sheep and goat) the carotid artery system is separated from the brain by a rete mirable system. The effect of the rete system on cerebral blood flow is unknown; however, some investigators have postulated that the rete may produce major alterations in the nature of blood flow to the brain (Nagel et al., 1968). It is also likely that the rete vessels respond to vascular stimuli (e.g., O_2, CO_2, and pharmacologic agents), as does any other network of arteries, but whether these responses are the same or different from the responses of cerebral vessels is not at all clear. Thus, the flow changes measured with a flow probe around an artery may occur not because of any change in caliber of intracranial vessels, but from changes in the rete vessels. The rete may also act as a capacitance structure, which may lead to even further difficulties and interference with the flow measurement.

Finally, with respect to measurement of arterial inflow, a number of investigators have utilized the isolated perfused brain technique. Although this technique provides complete isolation of the brain from systemic influences, the preparation has been shown to be completely inadequate. Sagawa and Guyton (1961) demonstrated that the cerebral vessels do not exhibit autoregulation with this technique. This is most likely explained by damage (hypoxic insult) to the vessels during preparation. The difficulties of the preparation also involve cerebral microembolization, platelet aggregation, and release of a variety of metabolic agents from red blood cells resulting from the pump perfusion. It is difficult to see how the cerebral circulation could be artificially perfused so that the normal cerebral vascular reactivity were preserved.

IV. Regulation of Cerebral Blood Flow

Because of the rigid nature of the skull and the incompressibility of the brain, Monro (1783) concluded that expansion of cranial contents was severely limited and that active changes in cerebral vessel caliber were unlikely. This concept was later confirmed by Kellie (1824), and it became known as the Monro–Kellie doctrine. This notion was not tested for about 75 years, and as a result reports of alterations in cerebral vascular caliber and vascular volume did not appear in the literature until the late nineteenth and early twentieth centuries. In 1890 Roy and Sherrington elucidated probably the two most important concepts concerning the regulation of the cerebral circulation, namely, (a) that the brain has an intrinsic mechanism to control its blood supply in accordance with cerebral activity and (b) that chemical by-products of cerebral metabolism can lead to alterations in the caliber of cerebral blood vessels. Although Hill (1896) and Bayliss (1902) challenged these concepts, the ideas of Roy and Sherrington (1890) actually are the basis of our current concepts of cerebral vascular regulation. Many reviews of the control of the cerebral vasculature have appeared during the past decade (Betz, 1972; Edvinsson and MacKenzie, 1977; Kuschinsky and Wahl, 1978; Lassen, 1974; Mchedlishvili, 1972; Purves, 1972). The purpose of this section is to describe briefly the accepted and some of the controversial mechanisms regulating cerebral blood flow (Fig. 1).

A. Neurogenic Control

The question of neurogenic control of cerebral vessels has been raised continually for over 100 years. Both the peripheral sympathetic and parasympathetic nervous systems have been implicated; however, much less

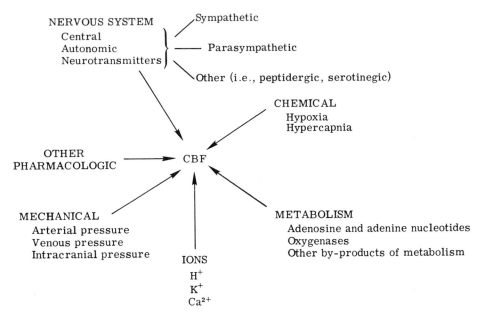

Fig. 1. Factors controling cerebral blood flow (CBF). (From Traystman, 1981.)

work has been done on the involvement of the latter. To consider effective sympathetic and parasympathetic neurogenic control of cerebral blood vessels, several prerequisites must be satisfied: (*a*) adrenergic and cholinergic innervation must be established; (*b*) vessel diameter or blood flow must change upon stimulation of the sympathetic or parasympathetic nerves; and (*c*) the vessels should have the capacity to respond to adrenergic and cholinergic transmitter substances in appropriate concentrations, and these responses should be blocked by adrenergic and cholinergic blocking agents. Unfortunately, none of these prerequisites is supported by unequivocal data, and many questions remain unanswered.

1. Sympathetic Nervous System

a. Innervation. Thomas Willis (1664) has been credited with writing the earliest description of nerves accompanying cerebral arteries, which have come to be known as the circle of Willis. It was not until the end of the nineteenth century that techniques became more refined for other investigators to describe these nerves further. Gulland (1898), Huber (1899), and Clark (1929) all demonstrated, via light microscopy, the presence of nerves on or near cerebral vessels. In the classic studies of Penfield (1932) the arteries of the pia mater and their continuations into brain parenchyma in the cat, dog, monkey, chimpanzee, and man were examined. No morphologic differences were found among species, and nerve plexuses that accompanied pia mater and that were continuous with nerves on intracerebral intraparenchymal arteries were described. Penfield (1932) described nerve endings on intraparenchymal arteries to be small with "grapelike" clusters 5 μm in diameter. These endings were found near the medial–adventitial border of vessels (arteries) as small as 40 μm in diameter. Further characterization of cerebral vascular nerves was not possible until the development of electron microscopic and histochemical techniques.

The electron microscope allowed for a much more detailed examination of the nerves identified with cerebral blood vessels. Pease and Molinari (1960) described nerves ending in the adventitia of pial arteries in cat and monkey. Since the nerves did not actually contact the smooth muscles, they concluded that pial vascular innervation was probably of no significance. Sato (1966) found nerves accompanying only large major arteries of the brain (i.e., internal carotid, vertebral, and basilar). He also observed that the richness of innervation diminished as the vessels diminished in size. Furthermore, Sato (1966) observed that many pial arteries were completely devoid of innervation. Samarasinghe (1965) found no nerves on small cerebral arteries and thus concluded that nerves were not important in the regulation of cerebral vessels. On the other hand, Dahl and Nelson (1964) and Nelson and Rennels (1970) described nerves on cerebral vessels. Dahl and Nelson (1964) also described vesicles at the ends of the nerve fibers, and these were thought to contain the neurotransmitter norepinephrine. More recently, Cervos–Navarro and Matakas (1977) concluded that nearly all cerebral vessels are innervated, and Rennels and Nelson (1975) have described small nerve terminals near cerebral capillaries. The interesting hypothesis that cerebral capillaries may be innervated has been confirmed by Itakura *et al.* (1977). This group of investigators described noradrenergic nerve terminals near cerebral parenchymal vessels beyond the fusion of the meninges, but this investigation pattern was confined to capillaries.

The important discovery of a technique for transforming intracellular catecholamines into fluorescent products by treatment with formaldehyde and the establishment of the specificity of this reaction for primary catecholamines (epinephrine, norepinephrine, and dopamine) made it possible to identify a nerve as adrenergic (Falck *et al.*, 1962). Dahlström and Fuxe (1964) discussed the histochemical and parapharmacologic criteria for specificity of the fluorescent reaction, demonstrating convincingly that the different fluorescing amines can be accurately separated from one another. With the use of this histochemical–fluorescent technique, a number of investigators demonstrated the presence of a rich adrenergic nerve supply to the main arteries at the base of the brain, especially the internal carotid, posterior communicating, and anterior cerebral arteries (Falck *et al.*, 1965; Edvinsson and Owman, 1975; Nielsen and Owmann, 1967; Owman *et al.*, 1966). Fewer nerves were present in distal branches, but pial arteries as small as 15–20 μm in diameter possessed adrenergic nerves. Few fibers were found to occur in relation to the arterial branches radiating into the brain parenchyma. Evidence was also presented that these nerves contain norepinephrine because they showed an increase in fluorescence after the injection of nialamide, a monoamine oxidase inhibitor, and the complete disappearance of fluorescence after the injection of reserpine (Nielsen and Owman, 1967). This histofluorescent technique has also enabled investigators to determine the origin of the innervation. Nielsen and Owman (1967) demonstrated a total loss of fluorescence of all vascular nerves following bilateral cervical sympathectomy. Other investigators confirmed this finding (Edvinsson and Owman, 1974; Iwayama, 1970; Sercombe *et al.*, 1975). The pial innervation has been found to be strictly unilateral, and the ascending nerves accompany the internal carotid artery and have a characteristic distribution in the vessels of the circle of Willis (Edvinsson and MacKenzie, 1977). However, the origin of the vertebral and basilar plexus is still a matter of some debate. Kajikawa (1968) showed the disappearance of fluorescence from caudal arteries following superior cervical ganglionectomy, and Ohgushi (1968) observed the degeneration of this plexus following removal of the stellate ganglion. Finally, Sercombe *et al.* (1975) demonstrated that the number of sympathetic nerves to intracerebral vessels is related to the density of adrenergic innervation of the pial artery supplying those intracerebral vessels. For example, in the caudate nucleus, which receives blood primarily from the richly innervated middle cerebral artery, at least half of the arterioles have sympathetic nerves, whereas in the lateral geniculate body, which is supplied from the poorly innervated posterior cerebral artery, few of the arterioles are accompanied by sympathetic fibers.

In summary, current experimental evidence supports the concept that cerebral blood vessels and pial vessels are plentifully supplied with adrenergic innervation. It has been shown, however, that the intracranial intraparenchymal arteries and arterioles have only a scanty adrenergic innervation compared with the rich innervation of the extraparenchymal vessels. This innervation has been well documented by light microscopy, electron microscopy, and fluorescent histochemistry.

   b. Effects of the Sympathetic Nervous System on the Cerebral Vasculature.   Although the cerebral vessels have been shown to possess sympathetic innervation, the question of the functional significance of these nerves remains controversial. This controversy over the effects of the sympathetic nerves on cerebral vessels is not new. More than 100 years ago, Brachet (1837), Callenfels (1855), Ackermann (1858), and Donders (1859) all concluded that the sympathetic nerves were responsible for vasoconstriction of the cerebral vessels. Over the next 50 years, numerous similar observations were made, particularly concerning the pial vessels. Forbes and Wolff (1928) observed pial arteries via a window placed in the cranium of cats and demonstrated that arteries $100-354$ μm in diameter constricted with sympathetic nerve stimulation. Subsequently, Forbes and Cobb (1938) observed that sympathetic nerve stimulation resulted in an 8% reduction in diameter of arteries greater than 50 μm in diameter. These studies were confirmed much more recently by Kuschinsky and Wahl (1975), who found that pial arteries ($40-221$ μm diameter) constricted by 12% in response to cervical sympathetic stimulation. On the other hand, a number of workers using similar methodology could not confirm these findings (Riegal and Jolly, 1871). Florey (1925) later demonstrated that pial artery diameter was unchanged with cervical sympathetic nerve stimulation. More recently, Raper et al. (1972) demonstrated that pial vessels ($20-85$ μm diameter) were unresponsive to sympathetic nerve stimulation, and Wei et al. (1975) showed that, whereas arteries smaller than 100 μm in diameter were unresponsive to sympathetic stimulation, vessels larger than 100 μm constricted in a frequency-dependent fashion.

The classic study of Roy and Sherrington (1890) was among the first to attempt to evaluate the role of the nervous system in the regulation of the cerebral circulation using a blood flow type of methodology. These authors measured cerebral blood volume changes via a trephine hole in the skull and concluded that vagosympathetic stimulation did not affect cerebral blood flow. These conclusions were confirmed by Bayliss and Hill (1895). Wiggers (1914) did not confirm these conclusions, however, and in fact, using a venous outflow technique, demonstrated that sympathetic nerve stimulation caused cerebral vasoconstriction. Although techniques for the measurement of cerebral blood flow have improved tremendously during the last 40 years, the controversy concerning the role of the sympathetic nervous system in the control of brain blood flow still exists. However, the predominating view until relatively recent times seemed to be, as Schmidt (1950) concluded, that the sympathetic nervous system was of only small or no physiologic importance in the regulation of the cerebral vasculature.

On the other hand, within the past 15 years, a number of investigators have reported that sympathetic stimulation can result in significant cerebral vasoconstriction. Meyer *et al.* (1967) placed electromagnetic flow probes around vertebral and common carotid arteries in baboons and found that stimulation of the superior cervial ganglion decreased blood flow in the external carotid, internal carotid, and vertebral arteries by 68, 30, and 18% respectively. James *et al.* (1969), using ^{133}Xe clearance in baboons, measured decreases in cerebral blood flow of 10–40% with cervical sympathetic stimulation. They also found that the decrease in flow was more pronounced when the arterial CO_2 tension was above 45 mm Hg. These findings were later verified by Harper *et al.* (1972), who found a 12% reduction in cerebral blood flow with sympathetic stimulation and a 25% reduction with stimulation when arterial CO_2 tension was elevated. In other experiments, using a cerebral venous outflow technique (retroglenoid vein), D'Alecy and Feigl (1972) reported an 80% decrease in cerebral blood flow with stellate ganglion stimulation, the largest change in cerebral flow with nerve stimulation reported in the literature. The usefulness of this technique depends on the careful separation of the intracranial and extracranial venous circulations. This was discussed in detail by Traystman and Rapela (1975), who also measured cerebral venous outflow but from the confluence of the sinuses with the transverse sinuses occluded to eliminate contamination from extracranial sources. They demonstrated that stellate ganglion stimulation produced an 11% reduction in venous outflow only before elimination of extracranial influences. In addition, they were able to produce further decreases in venous outflow (35% reduction) by allowing more extracranial contamination. However, when all extracerebral anastomoses were eliminated by occlusion of the lateral sinuses and occipital emissary veins, sympathetic stimulation produced no change in cerebral blood flow. This was also true with sympathetic stimulation during hypercapnia. The usually large decreases in cerebral blood flow found by D'Alecy and Feigl (1972) could be explained by the presence of extracerebral anastomoses in their preparation and/or the fact that the retroglenoid vein may itself constrict with sympathetic nerve stimulation (Pearce and Bevan, 1981). Further evidence that sympathetic stimulation results in little or no change in cerebral blood flow is provided by studies utilizing the radiolabeled microsphere technique. Alm and Bill (1973) demonstrated no regional cerebral blood flow change during sympathetic stimulation, whereas blood flow to extracranial tissues decreased by 99%. They also did not observe changes in regional cerebral blood flow with sympathetic stimulation during hypercapnia. These data were essentially confirmed by Meyer *et al.* (1977) and Heistad *et al.* (1977). Heistad *et al.* (1977) also tested the hypothesis that the sympathetic nerves affected only large cerebral vessels. They used the technique of Rapela and Martin (1975), by which the pressure gradient is measured between the carotid arteries and the circle of Willis, and found that the large-vessel resistance was not altered by sympathetic nerve stimulation.

The prevailing opinion is that under normoxic, normocapnic, normotensive conditions, the sympathetic nerves probably play little, if any, role in the regulation of the cerebral vasculature. However, this role may be more important in hypertensive conditions in the regulation of cerebral blood flow and in the protection of the blood–brain barrier. Bill and Linder (1976) observed decreases in regional cerebral blood flow with sympathetic nerve stimulation during hypertension. These decreases, however, were measured only in areas of the brain where breakdown of the blood–brain barrier had occurred. In areas with no damage to the blood–brain barrier, sympathetic stimulation had no effect on blood flow during hypertension. The authors hypothesized that the main function of the sympathetic nerves was to protect the brain from extravasation of substances during hypertension. In addition, the possibility of a species difference in response to sympathetic nerve stimulation has also been raised. Heistad *et al.* (1978) showed that vasoconstrictor responses to sympathetic stimulation occurred in cats, dogs, and monkeys when the mean arterial blood pressure was initially elevated to about 200 mm Hg. This effect was greatest in cats, less so in dogs, and essentially absent in monkeys. Under normotensive conditions, sympathetic stimulation produces significant cerebral vasoconstriction in monkeys but no reduction in cerebral blood flow in cats or dogs (Heistad *et al.*, 1977). Furthermore, Duckles *et al.* (1977) observed differences in responses of cerebral vessels *in vitro* to electrical field stimulation in dogs, cats, and monkeys. The combination of many different cerebral blood flow techniques and the species surely must add significantly to the controversial nature of the effects of sympathetic nerve stimulation on the cerebral vasculature. Tables I and II list those studies in which stimulation of the sympathetic nerves has no effect or results in cerebral vasoconstriction, respectively (only a partial listing).

2. *Parasympathetic Nervous Systems*

a. Innervation. Pial vessels, but not intracerebral vessels, are innervated by cholinergic nerve fibers (Florence and Bevan, 1979; Owman and Edvinsson, 1977). Whereas the adrenergic innervation to cerebral blood vessels has been convincingly demonstrated by the Falck histofluoresence technique (Falck *et al.*, 1965) and supportive evidence provided by electron microscopy and biochemical techniques, the cholinergic innervation has been much more difficult to demonstrate due to a lack of specific methods. Most investigators have utilized the histochemical

TABLE I

Studies Showing No Change in Cerebral Blood Flow with Sympathetic Nerve Stimulation

Species	Method	Reference
Rabbit	Pial window	Shultz (1866)
Rabbit	Pial window	Riegal and Jolly (1871)
Cat, rabbit	Pial window	Florey (1925)
Dog	Pial window	Roy and Sherrington (1890)
Dog, cat, monkey	Brain volume	Bayliss and Hill (1895)
Cat	Electromagnetic flow probe	Waltz et al. (1971)
Cat	Radiolabeled microspheres	Alm and Bill (1973)
Dog	Radiolabeled microspheres	Meyer et al. (1977)
Dog	Venous outflow	Traystman and Rapela (1975)
Cat	Radiolabeled microspheres	Bill and Linder (1976)
Dog	Radiolabeled microspheres	Heistad et al. (1977)
Dog	Radiolabeled microspheres	Mueller et al. (1977)
Dog	Venous outflow	Barber et al. (1978)
Dog, cat	Radiolabeled microspheres	Heistad et al. (1978)
Cat	Pial window	Raper et al. (1972)
Monkey	^{133}Xe	Eklof et al. (1971)
Monkey, dog, cat	Pial window	Hill and MacLeod (1900)
Baboon	^{133}Xe	Fitch et al. (1975)
Monkey	Pial window	Gurdjian et al. (1958)

technique of staining for acetylcholinesterase to localize cholinergic nerve fibers (Borodulya and Pletchkova, 1976; Denn and Stone, 1976; Edvinsson et al., 1972; Florence and Bevan, 1979) or electron microscopy (Edvinsson et al., 1972; Iwayama et al., 1970).

Florence and Bevan (1979), utilizing biochemical techniques, demonstrated that arteries at the base of the brain in the cat and rabbit possessed high choline acetyltransferase activity and [^{3}H]choline levels of uptake. Lesser activity and levels were found in cerebral arteries in the dog. Edvinsson et al. (1972) demonstrated that the extent and distribution of the cholinergic nerves are essentially similar to the arrangement of the adrenergic nerves. This group of investigators also demonstrated that cholinergic nerve fibers were present in cerebral vessels with diameters as small as 15 μm and were of greater density in arteries than veins. No cholinergic fibers have been found in intracerebral vessels by either histochemistry (Owman et al., 1974) or electron microscopy (Lindvall et al., 1975).

The origin of the cholinergic nerves is still unknown. However, Chorobski and Penfield (1932) claimed that the major supply of parasympathetic nerves to the cerebral vessels are in the facial nerve, course off in

TABLE II

Studies Showing Decreases in Cerebral Blood Flow with Sympathetic
Nerve Stimulation

Species	Method	Reference
Dog	Isolated brain	Wiggers (1914)
Dog	Isolated brain	Krog (1974)
Monkey	Electromagnetic flow probe	Yoshida et al. (1966)
Baboon	Electromagnetic flow probe	Meyer et al. (1967)
Baboon	^{133}Xe clearance	James et al. (1969)
Baboon	^{133}Xe clearance	Millar (1969)
Mouse	Blood volume	Edvinsson et al. (1971)
Cat	^{85}Kr clearance	Kobayashi et al. (1971)
Baboon	^{133}Xe clearance	Harper et al. (1972)
Mouse	Blood volume	Edvinsson et al. (1972)
Dog	Venous outflow	D'Alecy and Feigl (1972)
Dog	Isolated brain	Lang and Zimmer (1974)
Rabbit	Thermoclearance	Sercombe et al. (1975)
Rabbit	^{133}Xe clearance	Rosendorff et al. (1976)
Rabbit	[^{14}C]Ethanol	Lacombe et al. (1977)
Monkey, cat	Radiolabeled microspheres	Heistad et al. (1978)

the area of the geniculate ganglion, and continue in the greater superficial
petrosal nerve to the plexus in the internal carotid artery, where they form
ganglia. These cholinergic fibers are almost abolished by cervical sympathetic ganglionectomy (Denn and Stone, 1976; Edvinsson et al., 1972;
Iwayama et al., 1970).

*b. Effect of the Parasympathetic Nervous System on the Cerebral
Vasculature.* That the parasympathetic nervous system is involved with
the regulation of cerebral circulation was shown by Chorobski and Penfield (1932) in a morphologic study and by Cobb and Finesinger (1932).
Cobb and Finesinger (1932) reported that electrical stimulation of the petrosal nerve resulted in an increase in diameter of pial arteries. The conclusion of these early studies that the petrosal nerve can cause cerebral
vasodilation was more recently confirmed by James et al. (1969), Salanga
and Waltz (1973), D'Alecy and Rose (1977), Ponte and Purves (1974), and
Pinard et al. (1979). These groups of investigators found that electrical
stimulation of the facial or petrosal nerves can cause cerebral vasodilation. However, D'Alecy and Rose (1977) pointed out that there is a discrepancy between the degree of this vasodilation when acetylcholine is
injected into the cerebral circulation and when both petrosal nerves are
stimulated.

On the other hand, several investigators have stimulated cholinergic nerves and have observed no alteration in the cerebral circulation. Bates and Sundt (1976) transected both the seventh and eighth cranial nerves and showed no significant change in cerebral blood flow. Hoff *et al.* (1977) transected the seventh cranial nerve and found no change in cerebral blood flow. Busija and Heistad (1981) demonstrated that section or electrical stimulation of the greater superficial petrosal nerve did not alter cerebral blood flow. Ponte and Purves (1974) suggested that these cholinergic fibers were responsible for cerebral vasodilation during hypoxia or hypercapnia. However, Bates and Sundt (1976), Hoff *et al.* (1977), and Busija and Heistad (1981) showed that section of the seventh cranial nerve did not interfere with cerebral autoregulation or the responsiveness of the cerebral vessels to hypoxia or hypercapnia.

3. Central Nervous System

a. Innervation.   In addition to the potential role of the peripheral nervous system in the regulation of the cerebral vasculature, the possibility that higher centers in the brain also participate in regulating cerebral blood flow must be considered. It is conceivable that the plentiful innervation that surrounds extraparenchymal cerebral vessels originates, at least in part, from these higher neurogenic centers. Hartman *et al.* (1972) and Swanson and Hartman (1975) suggested that the central noradrenergic system directly innervates brain blood vessels and thus could participate in the control and modulation of cerebral blood flow. Many of these fibers are associated with cerebral vessels, do not disappear with sympathectomy, and appear to originate in the locus coeruleus and adjacent regions (Hartman *et al.*, 1972). That these fibers make synaptic contact with cerebral vascular smooth muscle is not clear, and in fact Owman and Edvinsson (1977) have shown that in many cases the nerve fibers are separated from the vessels by a thick basement membrane. Thus, there is some question as to whether these brainstem-originating fibers do indeed innervate the vessel. Rennels and Nelson (1975), however, demonstrated that nonmyelinated fibers of unknown origin innervate capillary pericytes and endothelial cells in the hypothalamus, and Owman *et al.* (1977) demonstrated that fibers contain actin and myocin. Thus, these fibers may be of importance not only in regulating cerebral blood flow but also in controlling the permeability of the blood–brain barrier.

b. Effect of the Central Nervous System on the Cerebral Vasculature. Electrical stimulation of the pontobulbar pressor area and the hypothalmic pressor area in the brain of cats and rabbits has been reported to decrease cerebral blood flow (Molnar and Szanto, 1964). Stimulation of the posterior region of the hypothalamus causes, in addition to other sympathetic responses, pupillary dilation, piloerection, increases in blood pressure, and bilateral vasoconstriction of the pial vessels (Stavraky, 1936). It has been shown that this pial vasoconstriction is rapid in onset and occurs before any changes in blood gas tensions. These vasoconstrictor responses are unaffected by cervical sympathectomy (Molnar and Szanto, 1964). Ingvar and Soderberg (1958) showed that regional cerebral blood flow increased when the reticular formation was stimulated and that this stimulation led to desynchronization of the electroencelographic pattern. Langfitt and Kassell (1968) also demonstrated significant increases in cerebral blood flow with electrical stimulation of the brainstem. Finally, the pons and mesencephalon may play an important role in mediating the cerebral vasodilation caused by increases in CO_2 tension. Shalit *et al.* (1967) showed that high medullary, pontine, and mesencephalic lesions decreased cerebral blood flow and diminished or abolished the responsiveness of the cerebral blood vessels to hypercapnia. More destructive lesions in the hemispheres, medulla, or cervical cord did not produce these changes.

Thus, it is clear that central neurogenic stimulation may have an influence on the regulation of cerebral circulation; however, the mechanism by which this occurs is still unclear. The question is, does the stimulation of certain central brain areas alter cerebral blood flow by direct neurogenic influence, or can the response be completely accounted for by an alteration in brain metabolism.

B. Chemical, Metabolic, and Blood Gas Control

1. Hypoxia

A tremendous amount of information concerning the effects of alterations in arterial O_2 tension on the cerebral circulation has been reported. The relatively sparse capillarity and high resting O_2 consumption of the brain indicate that the brain relies on a continuous supply of O_2 (McIlwain and Bachelard, 1971). It is generally agreed that if arterial O_2 tension is lowered sufficiently, cerebral blood flow will increase (for reviews see Betz, 1972; Fieschi and Bozzao, 1972; Purves, 1972). The increase in cerebral blood flow during hypoxemia has been observed in different animal species, with different anesthetics, with different cerebral blood flow techniques, and regardless of any accompanying alterations in CO_2 tension. Inhalation of low-O_2 mixtures results in an increase in pial vessel diameter in the dog whether or not the arterial partial pressure of CO_2 is controlled (Wolff and Lennox, 1930). Noell and Schneider (1941) reported an increase in cerebral blood flow during hypoxemia while cerebral blood flow was measured with thermocouples inserted into cerebral vessels. By measuring the arteriovenous O_2 content difference across the brain and assuming a constant cerebral O_2 consumption, Courtice (1941) reported an increase in cerebral blood flow while the animal breathed a 15% O_2 mixture. Kety and Schmidt (1948a,b), using the nitrous oxide technique in human beings, showed that inhalation of 10% O_2 in nitrogen resulted in a 32% increase in cerebral blood flow despite the accompanying hypocapnia. Also, in human subjects cerebral blood flow was shown to increase from 45 to 77 ml/min per 100 g as arterial O_2 tension decreased from 89 to 35 mm Hg (Cohen et al., 1967). These investigators used the inhaled [85]Kr technique and maintained the arterial CO_2 tension at 40 mm Hg. Johannsson and Siesjo (1974), using the ^{133}Xe clearance technique to measure cerebral blood flow, found that cerebral blood flow in anesthetized rats increased to 400% of control as arterial O_2 tension was reduced to 24 mm Hg. Using the radiolabeled microsphere technique in monkeys, Heistad et al. (1976) reported an increase in brain flow from 35 to 66 ml/min per 100 g as arterial O_2 tension decreased to 29 mm Hg, and Traystman et al. (1978) reported an increase in cerebral blood flow to 276% of control with arterial O_2 tension reduced to 18 mm Hg. These investigators used a cerebral venous outflow technique in dogs.

Several investigators have dealt with whether there is a threshold arterial O_2 tension for alterations in cerebral blood flow. McDowall (1966) reported a threshold arterial O_2 tension of 50 mm Hg in anesthetized dogs. In these experiments the animals were ventilated and normocapnic. Cerebral blood flow began to increase as arterial O_2 tension approached 50 mm Hg and, at 30 mm Hg, cerebral blood flow had increased to 220% of control. Kogure et al. (1970) confirmed McDowall's findings using a venous outflow technique. However, Borgstrom et al. (1975) reported a significant increase in cerebral blood flow at arterial O_2 tensions as high as 85 mm Hg. The latter studies were done in rats using the arteriovenous O_2 difference technique to estimate blood flow. Thus, it is a most consistent finding that if arterial O_2 tension is sufficiently reduced, an increase in cerebral blood flow is observed. This is illustrated in Fig. 2.

The increase in cerebral blood flow during hypoxemia maintains a normal cerebral O_2 consumption up to a limit. Kety and Schmidt (1948a,b) showed that cerebral O_2 consumption was maintained constant when the inspired O_2 content was reduced from 20 to 10 vol % (reducing arterial O_2 tension to 40 mm Hg) in human subjects. Cohen et al. (1967) and Shimojyo et al. (1968) confirmed these findings but at an arterial O_2 tension of 35 and less than 30 mm Hg, respectively. Grote (1975) and Traystman et al.

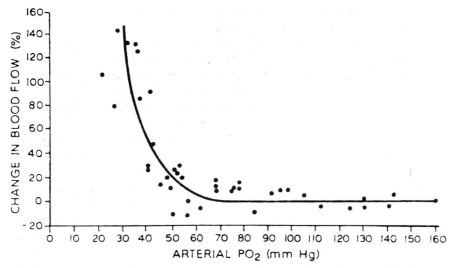

Fig. 2. Effect of alterations in arterial PO_2 on cortical blood flow in dogs. (From McDowall, 1966.)

(1978) reported that in anesthetized dogs cerebral O_2 consumption remained constant at an arterial O_2 tension of 35 and 26 mm Hg, respectively. Johannsson and Siesjo (1974) and Nilsson *et al.* (1976) found cerebral O_2 consumption in anesthetized cats to be unchanged at arterial O_2 tensions of 22 and 25 mm Hg, respectively. In addition to the maintenance of cerebral O_2 consumption, animal studies have shown that tissue concentrations of ATP, AMP, and ADP are unaltered at lower O_2 tension (MacMillan and Siesjo, 1972; Siesjo *et al.*, 1974). Duffy *et al.* (1972) showed no decrease in cerebral ATP in mice breathing only 4% O_2.

There is evidence that changes in carbohydrate and amino acid metabolism take place within the range of arterial O_2 tensions in which cerebral energy production is unilateral (McIlwain and Bachelard, 1971; Siesjo *et al.*, 1974). Cerebral glucose consumption has been reported to increase during hypoxemia in human beings (Cohen *et al.*, 1967), mice (Duffy *et al.*, 1972), dogs (Grote, 1975), and rats (Norberg and Siesjo, 1975). When the supply of oxygen to tissue fails, the acceptance of electrons, removed by dehydrogentation and transported in the electron transport chain, is slowed. Consequently, the various oxidation–reduction systems shift to a more reduced state, and protons accumulate. The reaction

$$\text{pyruvate} + \text{NADH} + \text{H}^+ \longrightarrow \text{lactate} + \text{NAD}^+$$

is driven to the right when H^+ accumulates by the production of two protons for each molecule of glucose broken down and during ATP hydrolysis. The relative value of lactate and pyruvate in blood, urine, and cerebrospinal fluid in determining tissue hypoxia has been proposed (Huckabee, 1958) and discussed by others (Posner and Plum, 1967). Cerebral lactate/pyruvate ratios do increase during hypoxemia (Gurdjian *et al.*, 1949; Miller, 1967). The increase in cerebral lactate production is indicative of an increased cellular reduction state (Chance *et al.*, 1962). The latter authors directly measured, spectrofluorometrically and *in vivo*, a 50% reduction of NAD in the cortex of rats that inspired 3% O_2.

In addition to the carbohydrate alterations, hypoxemia has been shown to decrease the concentration of the excitatory amino acids glutamate and aspartate (Norberg and Siesjo, 1975), increase that of the inhibitory transmitter γ-aminobutyric acid (Duffy *et al.*, 1972), and reduce the rate of synthesis of catechol and indole transmitters (Davis *et al.*, 1973). These metabolic alterations may be the mechanism of altered cerebral electrical activity (Meyer *et al.*, 1965) and altered central nervous system function (Cohen, 1972) with hypoxemia.

The consistent findings of a maintenance of cerebral energy production up to severe levels of hypoxemia have led to the conclusions that (*a*) the functional symptoms accompanying hypoxemia are not due to energy failure, but depend on other metabolic perturbations (Siesjo *et al.*, 1974), and (*b*) powerful homeostatic mechanisms come into play to prevent energy failure, and presumably this compensatory response is predominantly the increase in cerebral blood flow (Lewis *et al.*, 1973).

Although it is clear that hypoxemia produces cerebral vasodilation and an increase in cerebral blood flow, the precise mechanism by which hypoxia produces this vasodilation is not. Hypothesis to explain this mechanism include direct effects of O_2, neurogenic, and chemical or metabolic theories. Little experimental evidence exists concerning the direct effects of O_2 on the cerebral resistance vessels. However, there is some evidence that O_2 may act directly on the smooth muscle of cerebral vessels, with a high arterial O_2 tension resulting in vasoconstriction and a low arterial O_2 tension leading to vasodilation. In an early study Garry (1928) demonstrated that spirals of carotid artery of sheep contract with high O_2 tension. This response was confirmed by Smith and Vane (1966) and Detar and Bohr (1968), and in addition Detar and Bohr (1968) showed that isolated rabbit aortas dilated when perfused with blood or saline of low O_2 tension. A decrease in the arterial O_2 tension to less than 100 mm Hg in the perfusate caused the contractile response to epinephrine to decrease. The dependence of the contractile response to O_2 tension is explained if one assumes that O_2 plays a metabolic role within the mitochondria of smooth muscle cells. Although it has been documented that the mechanical tension of some vascular smooth muscle is sensitive to altered O_2 tension (*in vitro*), Pittman and Duling (1973) have calculated that arterioles 10 μm in diameter would be unaffected by O_2 tensions greater than 2 mm Hg. They suggested that the large-artery *in vitro* experiments showing a direct relationship between smooth muscle tension and O_2 tension may be misleading because of the high O_2 consumption and large diffusion gradients of the strips. Coburn (1977) suggested the possibility that receptors sensitive to O_2 tension could exist in vascular smooth muscle but indicated that these receptors do not appear to work through a cytochrome a_3–ATP model. Finally, in a study of pial vessels *in vivo*, Kontos *et al.* (1978) demonstrated that local hypoxia administered by application of cerebrospinal fluid containing no O_2 on the surface of the brain produced only slight arteriolar vasodilation. This group postulated that the effects of hypoxemia on cerebral arterioles is mediated via local mechanisms because the vasodilation was completely reversed by supplying O_2 via topical application of fluorocarbons to the brain surface.

It has been suggested that the mechanism of cerebral vasodilation with hypoxia is mediated chemically by extracellular acidosis secondary to cerebral lactate production (Betz, 1972; Skinhoj, 1966). Reducing the arterial O_2 tension to less than 50 mm Hg increases cerebral blood flow and the concentration of intracellular and extracellular cerebral lactate (Siesjo and Nilsson, 1971). Wahl *et al.* (1973) suggested that cerebral metabolic acidosis affects the cerebral vascular smooth muscle by altering the pH within the cell. Kogure *et al.* (1970) reported that cerebral vasodilation with hypoxemia correlated well with cerebral cortical acidosis and concluded that hypoxemia exerted its effects on the cerebral vessels secondary to the formation of parenchymal lactate from anaerobic glycolysis. However, other results have challenged this hypothesis (Borgstrom *et al.*, 1975; Nilsson *et al.*, 1976; Norberg and Siesjo, 1975). These reports demonstrated that during the initial, rapid, non-steady-state increases in cerebral blood flow during hypoxemia, there is only a slight increase in lactate, or none at all. Also, this increase in blood flow leads to a reduction in tissue CO_2 tension and a subsequent increase in pH. The actual measurements of cerebral parenchymal pH show a transient alkalotic shift of 0.02 pH unit at a time when the cerebral blood flow increase has reached its maximal level. Thus, Nilsson *et al.* (1976) concluded that the increased blood flow must be related to some aspect of cellular metabolism less sluggish than lactate formation.

The relationship between organ blood flow and the metabolism of that organ is an old physiologic issue (Pfluger, 1875), and a close relationship between blood flow to the brain and the concentration of metabolic by-products in the interstitial fluid was proposed a century ago (Gaskell, 1880; Roy and Brown, 1879). One such metabolic by-product, adenosine, has been proposed to be the means by which metabolic demands of the myocardium are transformed into the stimulus to increase coronary blood flow (Rubio and Berne, 1969). Berne *et al.* (1974) postulated that some aspect of adenosine metabolism may be involved in controlling cerebral blood vessels in hypoxemia. Berne *et al.* (1974) reported that brain adenosine levels increase rapidly (2–3 sec), and this results in cerebral vasodilation with cerebral ischemia. Hypoxemia (10.7 and 5.5% O_2 for 5 min) increases brain adenosine levels three- and sixfold, respectively (Rubio *et al.*, 1975). More recently, Winn *et al.* (1980) reported that within 30 sec of onset of hypoxemia, brain adenosine levels increase by approximately 500%. In addition, adenosine is a strong dilator of pial arterioles when applied to the perivascular space (Wahl and Kuschinsky, 1976). These alterations in adenosine levels with hypoxemia, and the fact that adenosine can cause cerebral vasodilation when presented to the cerebral circulation, support the potential role of adenosine as a chemical link between metabolism and cerebral blood flow during hypoxemia; however, Wahl and Kuschinsky (1979) point out the speculative nature of the role of this metabolite.

Other metabolic substrates such as oxygenases also may play a role in hypoxic vasodilation since oxygenase inhibitors (metyrapone and imipramine) can attenuate the cerebral vasodilation that occurs with hypoxemia (Traystman *et al.*, 1981). Enzyme systems may play an important role in O_2 delivery to brain tissue through alterations in cerebral blood flow (Harik *et al.*, 1979; Jobsis and Rosenthal, 1978; Sokoloff, 1978). The precise nature and location of these oxygenases is unclear, although Traystman *et al.* (1981) suggested that these ''receptors'' for hypoxemia are located close to the cerebrospinal fluid. The idea of a special O_2 sensor is not new. Opitz and Schneider (1950) proposed the existence of O_2 receptors in cerebral parenchyma. Other investigators (Bicher *et al.*, 1973; Burgess and Bean, 1970; Mchedlishvili *et al.*, 1976) hypothesized that tissue O_2 receptors participate in a neural feedback loop originating within cerebral tissue to produce the vasodilation associated with hypoxemia. In addition to the already mentioned adenosine and oxygenases, other vasoactive mediators of blood flow in other vascular beds are bradykinin, histamine, prostaglandin, and serotonin (Haddy and Scott, 1968).

It was pointed out some years ago that neurogenic mechanisms may be involved in the cerebral vasodilator response to hypoxemia (Sokoloff, 1959). More recently, Ponte and Purves (1974) suggested that the carotid chemoreceptors acting through neurogenic mechanisms are responsible for virtually all of the cerebral vasodilation in response to hypoxemia. James and MacDonell (1975) also showed that carotid chemoreceptor and baroreceptor denervation abolished the cerebral vascular response to stimulation of carotid chemoreceptors and barorecptors. On the other hand, a number of investigators have found that the cerebral blood vessels are not affected by reflex stimuli. Traystman *et al.* (1978) showed that the carotid chemoreceptors were not important in the cerebral vasodilation to hypoxemia because the vasodilation persisted following bilateral carotid sinus nerve section. These investigators also found that the cerebral vasodilation (increase in cerebral blood flow) with hypoxemia was not different from that induced by elevating carboxyhemoglobin concentration, so that the arterial O_2 content was reduced equally with both types of hypoxemia. More recently, the same group of investigators found that the aortic chemoreceptors were also not involved in the mechanism for the increase in cerebral blood flow with hypoxemia (either hypoxic or carbon monoxide hypoxia) and that this blood flow response is not modified by the carotid or aortic baroreceptors (Fitzgerald and Traystman, 1980; Traystman and Fitzgerald, 1981). These conclusions are in general agreement with those of Heistad and Marcus (1976), Heistad *et al.* (1976), and Bates and Sundt (1976). Heistad *et al.* (1976), using a technique to measure cerebral blood flow that was completely different from that of Traystman's group (radiolabeled microspheres), demonstrated that the cerebral vasodilation response to hypoxia was unaffected by carotid chemodenervation. Bates and Sundt (1976) showed that the hypoxic vasodilator response was not affected by section of the glassopharyngeal and vagus nerves. The early findings of Fog (1938), Heymans and Bouckaert (1932), and later Rapela *et al.* (1967) all showed that cerebral vascular responsiveness was not affected by the peripheral nervous system, that is, carotid sinus nerves, vagus, and aortic nerves. We believe strongly that the results of experiments suggesting that the chemo- and baroreceptors do affect cerebral blood flow may perhaps be explained on the basis of extracranial contamination of the measured flow. The erroneous conclusions that can be drawn concerning the regulation of cerebral blood flow when the responses of two distinctly different vascular beds, intracranial and extracranial, are not carefully and completely separated have been discussed elsewhere (Traystman and Rapela, 1975; Traystman *et al.*, 1978).

In summary, although cerebral blood flow increases markedly with hypoxemia, the precise mechanism of action of this response is unclear. The most likely explanation involves some aspect of cerebral metabolism or a by-product of metabolism, whereas the least likely explanation involves a peripheral neurogenic reflex. Although most data would be compatible with the notion that cerebral vascular control during hypoxemia is locally mediated, the possibility still exists the central (brainstem) mechanisms are involved. The importance of the pons and mesencephalon in mediating the cerebral vasodilator response to hypercapnia has been demonstrated (Shalit *et al.*, 1967). A number of other studies have demonstrated the possibility of the involvement of higher brain centers in the regulation of cerebral blood flow (Langfitt and Kassell, 1968; Molnar and Szanto, 1964; Stavraky, 1936), and it remains possible that these central neurogenic centers may also be involved in the cerebral vasodilator response to hypoxemia. In fact, the idea of a central chemoreceptor that regulates cerebral blood flow in hypoxemia has been revived (Traystman *et al.*, 1981).

2. Carbon Dioxide

Many studies in animals and man, involving the use of many different techniques, have shown that CO_2 exerts a profound influence on cerebral blood flow. An increase in arterial CO_2 tension produces the most marked vasodilation of the cerebral vasculature of any known agent and has been discussed in many studies (Gibbs *et al.*, 1935; Kety and Schmidt, 1948a,b; Novack *et al.*, 1954; Reivich, 1964) and reviews (Betz, 1972; Kuschinsky and Wahl, 1978; Purves, 1972). Thus, it is not the intent here to discuss and review all the literature on CO_2, but only to give an indication of the type of work that has been done with CO_2 and the purported mechanism of its action. In man, inhalation of 5% CO_2 raises cerebral blood flow by approximately 50%, and 7% CO_2 by 100% (Kety and Schmidt, 1948b; Patterson *et al.*, 1955). Reivich (1964) varied arterial CO_2 tension from 5 to over 400 mm Hg in monkeys and found the maximal increase in blood flow to be at about 150 mm Hg (Fig. 3). Hyperventilation to reduce arterial CO_2 tension from 45 to 26 mm Hg resulted in a 35% reduction in cerebral blood flow in human subjects (Kety and Schmidt, 1948b).

Patterson *et al.* (1955) and Wasserman and Patterson (1961) proposed that the response of cerebral blood flow to changes in arterial CO_2 tension is a threshold phenomenon. On the other hand, Reivich (1964) showed that the process was a continuous one. To demonstrate a threshold effect, cerebral blood flow was measured by the nitrous oxide technique during inhalation of 2.5 and 3.5% CO_2 mixtures (Patterson *et al.*, 1955; Wasserman and Patterson, 1961). The results of these experiments indicated that arterial CO_2 tension had to exceed a rise of 4 mm Hg before any change in cerebrovascular resistance was produced. A decrease in arterial CO_2 tension of 2 mm Hg was required before cerebral blood flow decreased during hyperventilation. Other studies, however, demonstrated that cerebral blood flow changes when arterial CO_2 tension was altered minimally (Meyer *et al.*, 1966; Noell and Schneider, 1944). Noell and Schneider (1944) showed that a change of only 2 mm Hg in arterial CO_2 tension was

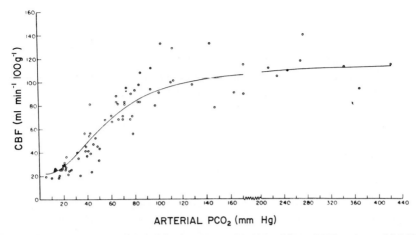

Fig. 3. Curve describing relationship between cerebral blood flow (CBF) and arterial PCO_2, $y = 20.9 + 92.8/[1 + 10{,}570 \exp(-5.251 \log x)]$, where y = CBF and x = PCO_2. The circles represent individual data points for each of the eight monkeys. (From Reivich, 1964.)

required for an 8–10% increase in cerebral blood flow, but a change in arterial CO_2 tension of 4 mm Hg might be within the range of variability for the nitrous oxide technique. Current concepts maintain that the cerebral blood flow relationship may be described by an S-shaped curve and that the relationship is a continuous one (Grubb *et al.*, 1974; Harper and Glass, 1965; Lassen, 1959; Reivich, 1964).

The question of whether alterations in arterial CO_2 tension change cerebral blood flow equally in all parts of the brain is somewhat controversial. Olesen *et al.* (1971), using a ^{133}Xe technique, found no differences in CO_2 reactivity measured in 35 regional brain areas. Animal studies involving the use of a variety of different techniques have shown that blood flow to the hemispheres, brainstem, cerebellum, and medulla is altered in the same percentage per mm Hg change in arterial CO_2 tension (Flohr *et al.*, 1971; Kindt *et al.*, 1971). On the other hand, it should not be assumed that brain vessels in different brain areas respond equally to alterations in arterial CO_2 tension. Hoedt-Rasmussen and Skinhoj (1966) found that both gray and white matter blood flow increased with increasing arterial CO_2 tension; however, the white matter increase was less than the gray matter increase. These results confirmed those of Hansen *et al.* (1957), who found that changes in gray matter blood flow with hypercapnia were proportionately greater than those in white matter blood flow. James *et al.* (1969) also showed that gray matter blood flow increased to a greater degree than that of white matter. Changes in pial vessel diameter probably occur in all intracerebral arteries in response to arterial CO_2 changes.

However, Wei *et al.* (1980a) demonstrated that the smaller arterioles are more dilated than the larger arterioles.

The potent vasoactive effect of CO_2 on cerebral blood flow is due to a local action on cerebral arteries (Kontos *et al.*, 1977b) and appears to be mediated mainly by the [H^+] of the extracellular fluid (Kontos *et al.*, 1977a). Kontos *et al.* (1977b) found that marked changes in arterial CO_2 tension and bicarbonate ion concentration of the cerebrospinal fluid do not affect pial arteriolar caliber unless a change in pH occurs. Thus, they concluded that molecular CO_2 and bicarbonate ion are not vasoactive. This pH hypothesis has been discussed in detail by Betz (1972), and more recently a number of investigators have demonstrated the vaso-active effect of H^+ at a more local level. Kuchinsky *et al.* (1972) and Wahl *et al.* (1970) showed that pial arteries constrict or dilate when they are exposed by microapplication of mock cerebrospinal fluid to alkaline or acidic solutions to the outside of the pial arteries. Pannier *et al.* (1972) demonstrated that perfusion of the ventricular system with various bicarbonate concentrations resulted in corresponding changes in caudate nucleus blood flow, and Cameron and Caronna (1976) obtained similar results for the hypothalamus during intraparenchymal injection of mock cerebrospinal fluid. Lassen (1968) compared the cerebral arteriole to a PCO_2 electrode, for, like the electrode, the H^+-sensitive apparatus of the arteriole appears to be effectively isolated from the action of plasma pH by a barrier that is relatively impermeable to charged ions. According to the extracellular pH hypothesis, the hyodrogen ion content of the extracellular fluid [ECF (H^+)] is determined by the ratio of the con-centration of bicarbonate ion in the surrounding ECF to the intraluminal PCO_2 according to the equilibrium equation

$$CO_2 + H_2O \rightleftharpoons H_2CO_3 \rightleftharpoons H^+ + HCO_3^-$$

Because CO_2 is unchanged and lipophilic, it is readily diffusible across the ion-permeable barrier, and any alteration in either the rate of endogenous CO_2 production by tissue metabolism or the PCO_2 of arterial blood is ex-pected to influence ECF (H^+) directly.

In addition to this hyothesis of pH control of cerebral blood flow with hypercapnia, it has also been proposed that the cerebral blood flow re-sponses to changes in CO_2 are mediated, at least in part, by neurogenic mechanisms. James *et al.* (1969) proposed that the carotid chemorecep-tors are responsible for some of the cerebral vasodilation with hypercap-nia. Others, however, have found unchanged responses of the cerebral vessels to changes in arterial CO_2 tension after sympathectomy and fol-lowing the administration propranolol (Waltz *et al.*, 1971). Shalit *et al.* (1967) proposed that CO_2 worked through a brainstem center. However, this idea was refuted by Kindt *et al.* (1971), who showed that medullary blood flow responses to hypercapnia were not affected by section of the medulla. It is improbable that these neurogenic mechanisms play a major role in the control of the cerebral circulation in hypercapnia.

C. Mechanical Control of Cerebral Blood Flow (Autoregulation)

1. Arterial Pressure

For many years it was thought that cerebral blood flow responded passively to alterations in arterial blood pressure. This notion can be traced to the hypothesis of Monro and Kellie formulated around 1800 that since the brain is incompressible and housed in a rigid cranium, the amount of blood within the head cannot be altered. This concept that cerebral blood flow responds passively to changes in arterial blood pressure was not seriously challenged until the late 1930s. Fog (1937, 1938, 1939a,b) showed in a series of articles that pial arteries dilated and constricted with decreases and increases in arterial blood pressure. He showed that these pial artery responses occurred regardless of how the arterial pressure was altered. To reduce blood pressure he either stimulated the central end of the cut vagus nerve or the carotid sinus nerve, or hemorrhaged the animal. In all cases the vessels dilated. To increase blood pressure he stimulated the splanchnic nerve, constricted the aorta, or administered epinephrine. In all cases the vessels constricted. Fog (1937, 1938, 1939a,b) also demonstrated that the changes in pial artery diameter with alterations in blood pressure persisted whether or not the vagus, aortic depressor, cervical sympathetic, or carotid sinus nerves were intact. Finally, in these classic studies he observed that if systemic arterial pressure was below 40 mm Hg, the pial vessels could no longer respond to changes in pressure and that they passively followed the changes in pressure. Fog interpreted his observations as evidence of an intrinsic regulatory mechanism designed to maintain cerebral blood flow constant in spite of variations in blood pressure. This concept subsequently became known as cerebral autoregulation. Forbes *et al.* (1937) confirmed the work of Fog (1937) and showed that stimulation of the vagus or carotid sinus nerves produced no change in pial artery diameter, as long as the arterial blood pressure remained constant.

Many studies using a variety of different techniques in man and animals have shown the remarkable stability of cerebral blood flow despite large alterations in arterial blood pressure (Fig. 4). In many of these experiments alterations in arterial blood pressure were produced by pharmaco-

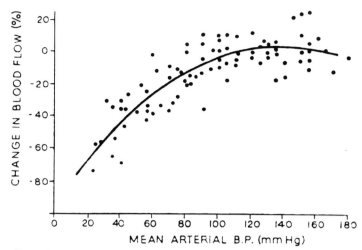

Fig. 4. Effect of lowering mean arterial blood pressure (B.P.) on cortical blood flow in a series of normocapnic dogs. Flow results are expressed as a percentage of the control value. (From Harper, 1966.)

logic means, and cerebral blood flow remained unchanged (Agnoli *et al.,* 1968; Hafkenschiel *et al.,* 1950; Olesen, 1972; Smith *et al.,* 1970). In studies on man, blood pressure was altered by means other than drugs, that is, sympathectomy (Shenkin *et al.,* 1950), spinal sympathetic blockade (Kety *et al.,* 1950), high spinal anesthesia (Kleinerman *et al.,* 1958), and tilting patients on a tilt table (Finnerty *et al.,* 1954). Cerebral autoregulation remained intact in all these studies.

The limits of autoregulation have also been studied extensively, and it is clear that this range is generally accepted to be between 60 and 160 mm Hg under normal conditions. This may vary, however, in any given animal preparation. Fitch *et al.* (1976), Olesen (1973), and Symon *et al.* (1973) found the lower limit of autoregulation at a blood pressure of 70 mm Hg during hemorrhagic hypotension, whereas a lower limit of 40 mm Hg was observed during drug-induced hypotension (Fitch *et al.,* 1976). At blood pressures above approximately 150 mm Hg a break-through phenomenon occurs, and again cerebral blood flow becomes dependent on blood pressure changes (MacKenzie *et al.,* 1976a,b; Strandgaard *et al.,* 1974). It is probable that the cerebral arterioles cannot withstand these high perfusion pressures and that the blood–brain barrier is damaged (Johansson, 1974). If the arterial blood pressure is acutely increased or decreased, there is an immediate rise and fall in cerebral blood flow before it returns to its control level (Rapela and Green, 1964). It may take as long as 2 min (Rapela and Green, 1964) or as little as 30 sec (Fog, 1938) or less

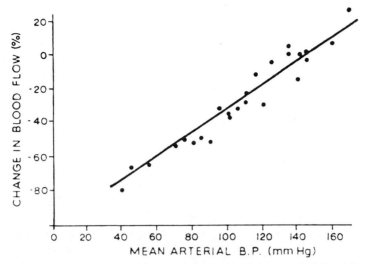

Fig. 5. Effect of lowering mean arterial blood pressure (B.P.) on cortical blood flow in hypercapnic dogs. (From Harper, 1966.)

for the vessels to dilate or constrict and for flow to be reestablished. Symon *et al.* (1972) reported that autoregulation begins within 2 sec of the blood pressure change. There are a variety of situations in which cerebral autoregulation is impaired. Sagawa and Guyton (1961) described a system in which cerebral blood flow varied linearly with changes in blood pressure. These findings were explained on the basis of the extensive surgery, cerebral trauma, pump perfusion, and deep barbiturate anesthesia utilized (Rapela and Green, 1964). High arterial CO_2 tensions have also been shown to result in impaired autoregulation (Ekstrom-Jodal *et al.*, 1972; Haggendal and Johansson, 1965; Harper, 1966; Rapela and Green, 1964). Harper (1966) demonstrated that at an arterial CO_2 tension of between 68 and 86 mm Hg the normal autoregulation curve was completely abolished (Fig. 5). Although the precise mechanism for the loss of autoregulation with CO_2 is not known, it has been suggested that since the cerebral blood vessels are essentially maximally dilated with CO_2, no further dilation can occur in response to a reduction in perfusion pressure. Rapela and Green (1968) confirmed the findings of Harper (1966) and in addition showed that the loss of autoregulation was related to the hypercapnia resulting in the loss of cerebral autoregulation (Haggendal and Johansson, 1965).

Several theories, which include myogenic, metabolic, and neurogenic, have been proposed to account for the mechanism of autoregulation. The myogenic theory proposes that changes in vessel diameter are mediated by a direct effect of variations in blood pressure on the myogenic tone of vessel walls, as postulated by Bayliss (1902). The metabolic theory argues that some metabolic factor, such as CO_2 or adenosine, is the regulating factor. A reduction in arterial blood pressure could result in a transient fall in blood flow, resulting in the buildup of tissue metabolites, which could then cause vasodilation and thus return the blood flow and the levels of metabolites to their original values. The neurogenic notion proposes that autoregulation is mediated by the adventitial nerves located on the cerebral blood vessels. Vasomotor nerves may have secondary effects on autoregulation; however, a number of investigators have found autoregulation to be absolutely independent of neurogenic mechanisms (Eklof *et al.*, 1971; Rapela *et al.*, 1967; Waltz *et al.*, 1971).

In summary, it is clear that cerebral blood flow is not dependent on arterial blood pressure within the range of pressures of from about 60 to 160 mm Hg. Blood flow does change passively below 60 mm Hg and above 160 mm Hg. The precise mechanism of cerebral autoregulation is not clear; however, the myogenic or metabolic mechanism seems to be the most significant, whereas the neurogenic mechanism is probably not of great significance.

2. *Intracranial Pressure*

The effects of elevations in intracranial pressure on cerebral blood flow have been studied extensively, and it has been suggested that intracranial pressure, or cerebrospinal fluid pressure, provides the downstream pressure for cerebral perfusion. Despite the obvious importance of intracranial pressure in clinical situations, the effects of increased intracranial pressure on cerebral blood flow are somewhat unclear. Cerebral blood flow has been reported to decrease with elevated cerebrospinal fluid pressure ranging from 30 to 100 mm Hg. However, the method of elevation of intracranial pressure, the region where cerebrospinal fluid pressure is altered, the level of intracranial pressure, and the state of the vasomotor activity of the cerebral arterioles may account for these differences. In studies on the effects of increased intracranial pressure on cerebral blood flow, Zwetnow (1970) and Miller *et al.* (1972) showed that cerebral blood flow was maintained constant until cerebral perfusion pressure was reduced to 30–50 mm Hg. Thus, it has been demonstrated that cerebral autoregulation compensates for cerebrospinal fluid pressure changes just as effectively as for alterations in systemic arterial pressure (Haggendal *et al.*, 1970; Zwetnow, 1970). If autoregulation is disturbed, the response to elevated cerebrospinal fluid pressure is affected (Miller *et al.*, 1972). It was also shown that the destruction of brainstem or spinal cord pathways may interfere with the autoregulation mechanism that maintains cerebral blood flow in the face of increasing cerebrospinal fluid pressure, whereas autoregulation to changes in blood pressure may remain intact (Rowan and Johnston, 1975). If intracranial pressure is elevated to very high levels, blood pressure will also increase, but full compensation to maintain cerebral blood flow does not occur. This increase in blood pressure in response to elevated intracranial pressures is referred to as the Cushing response. Under these conditions, cerebral perfusion pressure is not maintained, and cerebral blood flow falls as intracranial pressure is increased further (Haggendal et al., 1970; Matakas et al., 1972). When cerebral perfusion pressure was reduced to below 60 mm Hg by means of increasing cerebrospinal fluid pressure, Kjallquist et al. (1969) found an increase in glycolysis in brain tissue and a high lactate/pyruvate ratio combined with increasing cerebrovenous lactate concentrations. However, Siesjo and Zwetnow (1969) found only small changes in brain lactate concentration and no changes in phosphocreatine.

3. Venous Pressure

If cerebrospinal fluid pressure provides the back pressure (or downstream pressure) to cerebral perfusion, the importance of cerebral venous pressure in the regulation of cerebral blood flow must be minimal. This concept may or may not be correct and may involve the notion of critical downstream pressures and "vascular waterfalls," as has been proposed for the lung (Permutt et al., 1962; Permutt and Riley, 1963). In this respect the lung and the brain are analogous. Both have an arterial inflow and venous outflow pressure, and both possess a unique surrounding pressure of their vessels. In the lung, pulmonary vessels are exposed to the surrounding pressure of the alveolar pressure, whereas in the brain, cerebral vessels are exposed to the surrounding pressure of intracranial (cerebrospinal fluid) pressure. Figure 6 is a diagramatic sketch representing the pressures of concern in the lung and the brain. In the lung the distribution of pressures results in the distribution of pulmonary blood flow to essentially three major regions (zones I, II, III) depending on the magnitude of these pressures. In zone I of the lung, the alveolar pressure is greater than or at least equal to pulmonary artery pressure; thus, there is no blood flow. In zone II, pulmonary artery pressure is greater than alveolar pressure, which is greater than pulmonary venous pressure. Thus, the pressure gradient for blood flow is pulmonary artery pressure minus alveolar pressure, and under these conditions (zone II) pulmonary venous pressure has no influence on blood flow in this zone. In zone III, pulmonary arterial pressure is greater than pulmonary venous pressure, which is greater than alveolar pressure. The pressure gradient for blood flow is pulmonary artery

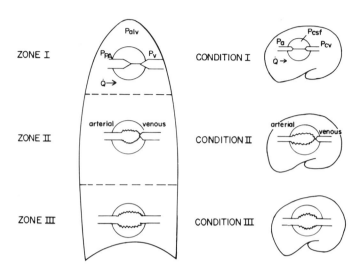

Fig. 6. Diagramatic sketch showing pressure gradients that determine blood flow in the lung and the brain. P_{alv}, Alveolar pressure; P_{PA}, pulmonary artery pressure; P_v, venous pressure; P, cerebrospinal fluid pressure; P, arterial blood pressure; P_{cv}, cerebral venous pressure; $\dot{Q}$, blood flow.

	Lung		Brain	
Zone/Condition	Pressures	Flow gradient	Pressures	Flow gradient
I	$P_{alv} > P_{PA} > P_v$	No flow	$P_{csf} > P_a > P_{cv}$	No flow
II	$P_{PA} > P_{alv} > P_v$	$P_{PA} - P_{alv}$	$P_a > P_{csf} > P_{cv}$	$P_a - P_{csf}$
III	$P_{PA} > P_v > P_{alv}$	$P_{PA} - P_v$	$P_a > P_{cv} > P_{csf}$	$P_a - P_{cv}$

pressure minus pulmonary venous pressure, and under these conditions alveolar pressure has no influence on blood flow in this zone. This analysis is also applicable to the pressures in the brain (Fig. 6). In this case the pressures involved are systemic arterial blood pressure or cerebrospinal fluid pressure. If one considers the theoretically different conditions in the brain as has been done for the lung, the following sequence is obvious. In condition I (of the brain), cerebrospinal fluid pressure is greater than or at least equal to arterial blood pressure; thus, there is no blood flow in this region. This condition is somewhat difficult to visualize in the brain because of the potent Cushing reflex so that, whenever cerebrospinal fluid pressure approaches arterial pressure, the reflex allows for an increase in blood pressure. Nevertheless, it is conceivable that this condition I situation could occur in the brain under certain clinical situations or when the

Cushing reflex is inoperable. In condition II of the brain, systemic arterial pressure is greater than cerebrospinal fluid pressure, which is greater than cerebral venous pressure. Thus, the perfusion gradient for cerebral blood flow is arterial pressure minus cerebrospinal fluid pressure, and under these conditions (condition II) cerebral venous pressure has no influence on blood flow. In condition III, systemic arterial pressure is greater than cerebral venous pressure, which is greater than cerebrospinal fluid pressure. The pressure gradient for cerebral blood flow is arterial pressure minus cerebral venous pressure, and under these conditions cerebrospinal fluid pressure has no influence on blood flow in this region.

Whereas the relationship between intracranial pressure and cerebral blood flow has been examined extensively, the relationship between cerebral blood flow and cerebral venous pressure is less well studied and the data available are controversial. In human subjects, increases in internal jugular venous pressure to 23 or 30 cm H_2O produced no changes in cerebral blood flow (Kety, 1950; Moyer *et al.*, 1954). Cerebral blood flow was not affected at this level of cerebral venous pressure, whereas cerebral O_2 uptake was slightly increased (Moyer *et al.*, 1954). Raisis *et al.* (1979) raised cerebral venous pressure to 75 mm Hg and showed that cerebral blood flow remained constant; however, with a more pronounced elevation there was a marked reduction in cerebral blood flow. These studies suggest that the cerebral vessels can autoregulate when perfusion pressure is reduced to moderate levels by elevating cerebral venous pressure. Only when cerebral venous pressure is increased to reduce cerebral perfusion below the lower limit of autoregulation does cerebral blood flow fall. However, early clincial reports indicated that cerebral blood flow is reduced when central venous pressure increases in patients with right heart failure (Kety, 1950). In other studies (Ekstrom-Jodal, 1970; Emerson and Parker, 1975) demonstrating reductions in cerebral blood flow with elevations in venous pressure, the blood supply to the brain was compromised even though perfusion pressure (arterial pressure minus cerebral venous pressure) was well within the autoregulatory range.

Although the mechanical interrelationships between cerebrospinal fluid pressure, cerebral venous pressure, systemic arterial pressure, and cerebral blood flow are complex, results from our laboratory have elucidated some of these relationships. Wagner and Traystman (1981) examined the effects of altering cerebrospinal fluid pressure, arterial pressure, and cerebral venous pressure, independent of each other, on cerebral blood flow. As cerebral venous pressure was elevated to 35 mm Hg, cerebral blood flow remained unchanged as long as the perfusion pressure gradient (arterial pressure minus cerebral venous pressure) remained greater than 60 mm Hg. As this pressure gradient was further decreased to 45 mm Hg, cerebral blood flow fell by 32%. Likewise, when cerebrospinal fluid pressure was elevated to 35 mm Hg, cerebral blood flow remained unchanged as long as the perfusion pressure gradient (arterial pressure minus cerebrospinal fluid pressure) remained greater than 60 mm Hg. As this pressure gradient was further decreased to 45 mm Hg, cerebral blood flow fell by 27%. Similar results were found when arterial pressure was reduced in order to reduce the pressure gradient. These data suggest that cerebral autoregulation fails when the perfusion pressure gradient falls below 60 mm Hg. This pressure gradient can be either arterial pressure minus cerebral venous pressure, or arterial pressure minus cerebrospinal fluid pressure, depending on whether cerebrospinal fluid pressure is greater or less than cerebral venous pressure. These findings are also consistent with the model (Starling resistor) presented previously.

D. Pharmacologic Control

Even a brief discussion of the effects of pharmacologic agents on the cerebral circulation would require the review of volumes of literature involving many methodologies. Thus, the discussion in this section is confined to a short summary of that which is known regarding sympathomimetic agents, parasympathomimetic agents, other neurotransmitters, and anesthetic agents. Most drugs that affect the cerebral circulation do so by altering cerebrovascular tone. Their effects have been studied by local application, intraarterial injection, or intravenous injection in a wide range of dosages in animals and man. In many cases the conclusions have been highly controversial, probably as a result of the different methodologies, dosages, and routes of administration used.

1. Sympathomimetic Agents

a. Norepinephrine. The cerebral circulatory response to catecholamines, in general, is a matter of some controversy. Most investigators who have observed the effects of intravenous or intraarterial injections of norepinephrine have demonstrated reduction either in cerebral blood flow or in the diameter of cerebral blood vessels (Haggendal, 1965; Lluch *et al.*, 1973; Rosenblum, 1974; Rosendorff *et al.*, 1973; Von Essen, 1972). Other investigators have observed no change in cerebral blood flow with norepinephrine injection (Greenfield and Tindall, 1968; Olesen, 1972), and still others have observed increases in blood flow (MacKenzie *et al.*, 1976a,b). Observations concerning effects on pial vessels are similarly controversial (Wei *et al.*, 1975). Most human studies have demonstrated that no change in cerebral blood flow occurs with norepinephrine aside

from that which is dependent on the hyperventilation that often follows
the injection of norepinephrine. It is generally accepted that the cerebral
vessels are much less sensitive to norepinephrine (and other catecholamines) than other peripheral vessels. There is considerable question as to
whether noepinephrine can cross the blood–brain barrier (Oldendorf,
1971). MacKenzie *et al.* (1976b) found norepinephrine to increase cerebral blood flow only after disruption of the blood–brain barrier. These increases in blood flow could not be dissociated from increases in O_2 and
glucose consumption of the brain. Thus, these authors concluded that the
increase in cerebral blood flow with norepinephrine is secondary to an increase in cerebral metabolism.

The results of a variety of studies using isolated cerebral strips of vessels (Duckles and Bevan, 1976; Edvinsson and Owman, 1974) and of pial
vessel studies (Wahl *et al.,* 1972) show that cerebral vessels appear to be
responsive to norepinephrine (contraction) but only when given in very
high doses. This constriction has been attributed to α-receptor stimulation. However, the mode of α-receptor stimulation is probably different
from that seen in other vascular beds and may be different in different
species.

b. Epinephrine. Animal studies concerning the effects of epinephrine
on the cerebral circulation are conflicting. Topical application of epinephrine on pial vessels has most often resulted in pial constriction (Fog,
1939a,b; Forbes and Wolff, 1928). In some studies intracarotid injection
constricted pial vessels (Forbes and Wolff, 1928; Wolff, 1936) and decreased blood flow in the arterial supply of the isolated cerebral circulation (Dumke and Schmidt, 1943); in others it resulted in pial dilation
(Forbes *et al.,* 1933). Greenfield and Tindall (1968) and Olesen (1972)
found no changes in cerebral blood flow when intracarotid injections of
epinephrine were administered. Large doses of epinephrine injected intravenously have been seen to increase cerebral blood flow and cerebral O_2
consumption (King *et al.,* 1952). These remarkable differences in reported
responses may be explained by differences in dose, means of administration, and effects on blood pressure. When blood pressure is unchanged,
topical or intraarterial injection of epinephrine results in slight vasoconstriction. Studies in unanesthetized man have failed to demonstrate any
cerebral vasoconstrictor action of epinephrine. Olesen (1972) reviewed
the literature concerning cerebral effects of epinephrine, and the general
opinion is that epinephrine has only a slight vasoconstrictor effect, if any,
and that this action is easily overcome by the passive dilation that occurs
in response to an increased blood pressure or the vasodilation due to an
increased cerebral metabolic rate (King *et al.,* 1952). It is well known that

epinephrine passes only slowly from the blood to the brain parenchyma (Oldendorf, 1971). Thus, if the blood–brain barrier lies in the endothelium, which has been suggested, epinephrine would not reach the vascular smooth muscle from the bloodstream, but it still might have some action if applied outside the vessel. As with norepinephrine, high doses of the drug are required to provoke any response in the cerebral vessels.

2. Parasympathomimetic Agents

a. Acetylcholine. Despite the report by Gottstein (1962) that acetylcholine was without effect on the cerebral vasculature, most investigators in a variety of preparations have shown a vasodilatory effect. Intravenous injections of acetylcholine dilate pial vessels (Wolff, 1936), increase brain blood volume (Koopmans, 1939), and raise intracranial pressure (Norcross, 1939). Kuschinsky *et al.* (1974) showed that microapplication of acetylcholine and carbamylcholine into the perivascular space results in a dose-dependent dilation. This dilation can be blocked with atropine. Infusion of acetylcholine intraarterially (carotid) increases cerebral blood flow, especially in gray matter (Heistad *et al.*, 1980). *In vitro,* acetylcholine has consistently been found to constrict vascular smooth muscle from carotid artery strips (Keatinge, 1966) and in segments of middle cerebral artery (Nielsen and Owman, 1967).

b. Methacholine. Methacoline appears to have actions that are similar to those of acetylcholine. When injected intraarterially, methacholine seems to be a more potent cerebral vasodilator than acetylcholine (Schmidt and Hendrix, 1937); however, both drugs are more potent vasodilators of extracranial vessels than intracranial vessels. Thus, the choline esters are capable of dilating cerebral vessels, and their action can be blocked by atropine.

3. Other Neurotransmitters

a. Vasoactive Intestinal Polypeptide. In the central nervous system, vasoactive intestinal polypeptide (VIP) occurs in high concentration in cortical, hypothalamic, and limbic areas, with lower concentrations in the cerebellum, brainstem, and thalamic areas (Besson *et al.*, 1979; Said and Rosenberg, 1976). Its presence in bipolar cortical neurons localized to molecular layers II–IV (Fuxe *et al.*, 1977) and the fact that it can be released from synaptosomes by calcium-dependent potassium depolarization (Emson *et al.*, 1978) suggest that VIP may perform a neurotransmitter function. Immunohistochemical methods have demonstrated the presence of VIP in nerve fibers in the aventitia and aventitial–medial border of pial arteries (Larsson *et al.*, 1976). VIP-Containing nerves have also been observed in intracerebral vessels (Larsson *et al.*, 1976).

Most investigators have shown that VIP administration results in cerebral vasodilation and an increase in cerebral blood flow. This substance has been shown to relax cerebral arterial smooth muscle *in vitro* (Larsson *et al.*, 1976) and to produce dose-dependent vasodilation in pial vessels (McCulloch and Edvinsson, 1980; Wei *et al.*, 1980b, 1981). The vasodilatory action of VIP has been proposed to be due to alterations in prostaglandin synthesis because the response is inhibited by indomethacin adminstration. Intracarotid infusion of VIP has demonstrated different responses. In dogs cerebral blood flow did not change with VIP administration (Wilson *et al.*, 1981), but it increased in rabbits (Heistad *et al.*, 1980) and baboons (McCullough and Edvinsson, 1980). Intraventricular administration (cerebrospinal fluid) of VIP resulted in increases in cerebral blood flow; however, with continued long-term infusion of VIP (60 min) these increases in flow were reduced (Wilson *et al.*, 1981). Thus, an "escape" phenomenon may be operational. Because the increases in cerebral blood flow are paralleled by an increase in cerebral O_2 consumption (McCullough and Edvinsson, 1980), the mechanism of vasodilation may be mediated by increases in metabolism.

The functional significance of the cerebral vasodilation with VIP administration is unknown. Wilson *et al.* (1981) were unable to show any change in VIP concentration in arterial or cerebral venous plasma, or in cerebrospinal fluid during hypercapnia or hypoxemia, despite the fact that cerebral blood flow increased markedly in both conditions.

b. Histamine. There is considerable evidence to suggest that histamine is stored in intracerebral neurons in the brain. Ronnberg *et al.* (1973) demonstrated with fluorescence–histochemical and chemistry studies that histamine is present in cerebral mast cells. Thus, the possibility that histamine acts as a neurotransmitter or acts by local action on cerebral vessels is a real one. There is ample evidence that histamine is a potent cerebral vasodilator. Early studies on the intravenous administration of histamine showed uniformly vasodilation of the cerebral vasculature (Sokoloff, 1959). Intraarterial administration of histamine in human beings produces immediate cerebral vasodilation (Tindall and Greenfield, 1973); however, Olesen and Skinhoj (1971) failed to observe any increase in regional cerebral blood flow with histamine. Some studies of isolated cerebral vessels (*in vitro*) have shown that histamine contracts smooth muscle (Edvinsson and Owman, 1975). The vasodilator effect of histamine appears to be mediated by stimulation of histamine$_2$ receptors (Wahl and Kuschinsky, 1979), whereas the contractile effects are nonspecific. Finally, it should be noted that *in vitro* the potency of histamine is substantially less than that of epinephrine (Purves, 1972).

  c. Serotonin (5-Hydroxytryptamine). Serotonin has been implicated frequently in the pathogenesis of several cerebral vascular diseases, that is, stroke, trauma, cold injury lesions, cerebral vasospasm, migraine, and ischemia (see Edvinsson and MacKenzie, 1977). In the body serotonin is located mainly in blood platelets, central neuronal systems, and cerebral mast cells (see Edvinsson and MacKenzie, 1977). The reported effects of serotonin on the cerebral vessels are somewhat contradictory. Swank and Hissen (1964) showed a 20% increase in internal carotid blood flow, whereas Karlsburg *et al.* (1963) found that cerebral vascular resistance increased with serotonin administration. Grimson *et al.* (1969) observed a marked reduction in internal carotid blood flow, and these findings were confirmed by Deshmukh and Harper (1973) and Welch *et al.* (1973). On the other hand, Olesen and Skinhoj (1971) were unable to demonstrate cerebral blood flow changes in man with serotonin injection into the carotid artery. When serotonin is applied directly to isolated cerebral vessels vasoconstriction results, and this response can be inhibited by the serotonin antagonist methysergide (Edvinsson and Hardebo, 1976). Injection of serotonin into the hypothalamus increased local hypothalamic flow (Rosendorff and Cranston, 1971), whereas cisternal injection provoked intracerebral vasospasm (Chow *et al.*, 1968). Thus, the cerebral circulatory effects of serotonin are complex; however, the overall action would appear to be a vasoconstriction and a reduction in cerebral perfusion.

  d. Dopamine. Apomorphine, the specific dopamine agonist, has been shown to increase cerebral blood flow markedly, and this effect could be blocked by pimozide (Von Essen and Roos, 1974). *In vitro* experiments have shown dopamine administration to result in constriction of cerebral arteries (Zervas *et al.*, 1975), which can be antagonized by phenoxybenzamine. Intracisternal administration of dopamine results in cerebral vasoconstriction in the basilar artery (White *et al.*, 1976). The mechanism of action of dopamine may take place through its effect of altering cerebral metabolism and neuronal function, thus increasing cerebral blood flow. It should also be considered that dopamine may have different effects in different brain regions, which may be dependent on regional differences in cerebral dopaminergic innervation.

  e. Prostaglandins. This large group of vasoactive substances and their effects on cerebral blood flow and metabolism have not yet been studied extensively. Topical application of PGG_2, PGH_2, PGE_2, PGI_2,

PGD_2, and arachidonic acid on the brain surface produced a dose-dependent cerebral vasodilation (Ellis *et al.*, 1979, 1980; Wei *et al.*, 1980a), whereas intraarterial administration of PGI_2 resulted in increased cerebral blood flow in baboons (Pickard *et al.*, 1980). The most potent agents were PGG_2, PGE_2, and PGH_2. Wei *et al.* (1980a) showed that the vasodilator effect of arachidonic acid could be inhibited by pretreatment with the cyclooxygenase inhibitors indomethacin and sodium amfenac (AHR-5850). Thus, this group of investigators concluded that the effect of arachidonic acid was mediated through its stimulation of prostaglandin synthesis. The only prostaglandin to show cerebral vasoconstrictor effects is $PGF_{2\alpha}$. The administration of $PGF_{2\alpha}$ resulted in pial artery vasoconstriction (Rosenblum, 1975) and has been shown to decrease cerebral blood flow and increase cerebral vascular resistance in monkeys and dogs (Denton *et al.*, 1972). The role of the prostaglandins in mediating cerebral blood flow responses to hypoxia and hypercapnia is unclear. Indomethacin or sodium amfenac was shown not to alter the cerebral vasodilator response to hypoxia (Sakabe and Siesjo, 1979; Wei *et al.*, 1980b). On the other hand, it was reported that indomethacin depressed the cerebral vasodilator response to hypercapnia (Pickard and MacKenzie, 1973; Sakabe and Siejso, 1979). In other experiments however, indomethacin did not affect cerebral vascular responses to hypercapnia or hypocapnia (Cuypers *et al.*, 1978). It is clear that further experiments are required to resolve the role of prostaglandins in the cerebral response to hypercapnia.

4. Anesthetics

a. General Anesthetics. Data concerning the effects of general anesthetics are sparse, and their interpretation is sometimes difficult. Animal experiments are generally performed under anesthesia so that comparison with the unanesthetized state is difficult, or one anesthetic is tested in the presence of another. It has also been difficult to distinguish between a direct effect of the anesthetic agent and secondary effects related to changes in cerebral metabolism, arterial blood pressure, and ventilatory changes that alter blood gas concentrations.

i. Halothane. Of all the inhalation anesthetics, halothane has the most potent effect on cerebral blood flow and metabolism. McDowall *et al.* (1963) found that halothane reduced cortical blood flow by 46% and cerebral O_2 consumption by 49% in the dog under conditions in which CO_2 tension was controlled. The level of halothane was 0.5%, to reduce hypotension. However, exactly opposite results were obtained by Wollman *et al.* (1964) in human subjects anesthetized with 1.2% halothane. In these studies cerebral blood flow increased by 15% and cerebral O_2 consumption decreased between 9 and 21%. These differences were resolved in a subsequent article by McDowall (1967) in which it was shown that halothane does increase cerebral blood flow, and because there is also a fall in blood pressure cerebral vascular resistance falls markedly. The mechanism of action of halothane is unclear, and it is not likely that the rise in cerebral blood flow is a result of catcholamine release from the adrenal medulla. A direct effect of halothane on cerebral vascular smooth muscle is a possibility that must still be confirmed by experimental evidence.

ii. Nitrous Oxide. By contrast with other anesthetics, nitrous oxide appears to have only slight effects on cerebral blood flow and metabolism. Similar cerebral blood flows have been found in studies using the Kety–Schmidt technique, which involves inhalation of 15% nitrous oxide as in studies using ^{133}Xe techniques (Lassen, 1959). Gotoh *et al.* (1966) found nitrous oxide to have no effect on cerebral blood flow and cerebral O_2 consumption. On the other hand, Wollman *et al.* (1965) observed a reduced cerebral O_2 consumption with inhalation of 70% nitrous oxide. Theye and Michenfelder (1968), however, showed a mild increase in O_2 consumption. Thus, nitrous oxide is probably without effect on the cerebral circulation, or at most its effects are minimal.

iii. Barbiturates. A number of studies using the Kety–Schmidt method to measure cerebral blood flow have shown that the administration of all barbiturates results in a dose-dependent reduction in cerebral blood flow and metabolism (see Lassen, 1959; Sokoloff, 1959). In some experiments, however, barbiturates have been reported to cause an increase in cerebral blood flow (Wechsler *et al.,* 1951) or no change in flow (Fazekas and Bessman, 1953). Most of the descrepant results in these studies can be explained by the fact that important variables such as blood gas tension, arterial pressure, and dosage of the drug were not controlled. The effects of barbiturate anesthesia are not uniform throughout the brain. Landau *et al.* (1955) reported that reduction in blood flow was limited to gray matter of the cortex, and the reduction in flow was greatest in areas in which the blood flow was highest in the unanesthetized animal. Thus, it is possible that local changes in flow can occur before a decrease in total blood flow is observed. It is most likely that general anesthetics can influence cerebral blood flow and metabolism similarly. There is little evidence that any general anesthetic has greater effects on the brain than barbiturates. Their influence may be due to direct effects on cerebral vascular smooth muscle, but also their effects on blood pressure, cerebral metabolism, and respiratory gas tensions cannot be ignored.

b. Local Anesthetics. Little information is available concerning local anesthetic agents and cerebral blood flow. Scheinberg *et al.* (1952) found that intravenous infusions of procaine failed to alter arterial blood pressure, cerebral blood flow, or cerebral O_2 consumption. The results of this study are in question, however, because it is possible that adequate blood levels of procaine were not achieved since procaine is inactivated rapidly.

5. Narcotics

Narcotic drugs appear to exert only minor influences on the cerebral circulation and, when they do have effects, they are probably secondary to their respiratory effects. Opium, morphine, and codeine have been reported to dilate cerebral vessels (Schmidt, 1950), reduce cerebral blood flow (Schmidt, 1945), or have no effect (Cobb, 1937). Morphine has been observed to exert minimal effects on pial arteries except when blood pressure is reduced; then, slight vasodilation occurs (Finesinger and Cobb, 1935). Fentanyl has been reported to increase cerebral blood flow (Freeman and Ingvar, 1967), but other authors have found a reduction in cerebral blood flow and O_2 consumption (Michenfelder and Theye, 1971). More recently, McPherson and Traystman (1981) showed that fentanyl did not affect cerebral blood flow and, more interestingly, did not interfere with the cerebral reactivity to hypoxia, hypercapnia, or the capacity of the vasculature to autoregulate.

V. Regulation of Cerebral Blood Flow in the Fetus and Neonate

The physiology of cerebral circulation in the newborn and fetus is poorly understood, with most of the information available having been collected in anesthetized, exteriorized fetuses. Although some information is available concerning the newborn, there are essentially no data within the same species that would allow comparative responses to be made concerning cerebral vascular regulation during the course of development. Because major physiologic differences exist among adult, neonate, and fetus, it might be expected that additional factors or differing values of arterial O_2 tension (P_aO_2), arterial CO_2 tension (P_aCO_2), and cerebral perfusion pressure may influence the regulation of cerebral circulation in these different age groups. Although many factors are involved in the regulation of cerebral blood flow in adults, as seen in Section III, this discussion is limited to three major factors for the fetus and neonate: P_aO_2, P_aCO_2, and cerebral perfusion pressure (CPP).

A. P_aO_2

Barker (1966) made the first direct examination of fetal cerebral blood flow and found that it was twice that of adult and newborn cerebral blood flow. She was also the first to show that the cerebral vasculature of the newborn and fetus was responsive to alterations in respiratory gas concentrations. Whereas the healthy neonate can normally meet the minimum requirements for oxygenation as it influences cerebral circulation, the margin of safety that exists is as yet unclear. The normal fetus or infants with cyanosis from respiratory distress or congenital heart disease cannot meet the minimum P_aO_2 requirements for maintenance of constant cerebral blood flow (P_aO_2 = 60 mm Hg) found in the adult. The normal neonate and especially the premature infant may be relatively hypoxic compared with the adult. The normal P_aO_2 in neonates is 65–70 mm Hg (Duc, 1971); thus, the normal P_aO_2 set point of the neonate differs from that of the adult. Independent of P_aO_2, the delivery of O_2 is a function of the binding capacity of hemoglobin, and significant differences exist between the O_2 affinity of neonate and adult red blood cells (Oski, 1979). Hence, there is reason to be concerned that the smaller infant and especially the premature and ill neonate are at risk for problems related to cerebral blood flow and its regulation through even small changes in P_aO_2.

It is known that the fetus is perfused by blood with a P_aO_2 of only 25 mm Hg, and it has been shown that cerebral circulation in the fetus is critically dependent on P_aO_2 (Cohn et al., 1974; Kjellner et al., 1974). Purves and James (1969) showed that a decrease in P_aO_2 of only 7–11 mm Hg in the fetal lamb, at constant P_aCO_2, increased cerebral blood flow. Similar changes in P_aO_2 in normal adults would not be expected to produce this change. The relationships between cerebral blood flow and hypoxia in the fetus have also been shown by Kjellner et al. (1974) and Cohn et al. (1974). This is not surprising because the cerebral circulation in the fetus and neonate is perfused by blood with lower glucose concentrations and at lower perfusion pressures when compared to the adult. Hence, when adequate delivery of metabolic substrates is to be assessed, it is critical that the fetal cerebral circulation be very responsive to small changes in P_aO_2.

Jones et al. (1977) studied cerebral arteriovenous oxygen differences and metabolic substrates in the fetal lamb and showed a correlation between arterial O_2 content and cerebral arteriovenous O_2 difference. This phenomenon could be explained either by a reduction in fetal cerebral O_2 consumption or by an increase in blood flow. Jones et al. (1977) clearly showed that cerebral O_2 consumption was not affected by hypoxia. As long as sagittal sinus P_aO_2 remained above 9 mm Hg, a decrease in arterial O_2 content produced an increase in cerebral blood flow. It is apparent that major concerns must exist about the effect of small changes in P_aO_2 on the cerebral circulation in the fetus and neonate because of the critically low values of P_aO_2 in these patients.

B. P_aCO_2

Purves and James (1969) studied the control of cerebral blood flow in the sheep fetus and newborn lamb and examined the effect of increases in P_aCO_2. In both the fetus and the lamb, as P_aCO_2 rose above 40–50 mm Hg, gray matter blood flow increased in a linear fashion, whereas below 40 mm Hg there was little change in gray matter blood flow. Changes in P_aCO_2 above 40 mm Hg were accompanied by elevations in mean arterial blood pressure so that cerebral vascular resistance fell even more so as P_aCO_2 rose. The difference in the flow/P_aCO_2 ratio was higher in the lamb than in the fetus. In addition, the authors demonstrated that the cerebral vasodilator response to CO_2 in the fetus and neonate was attenuated or completely abolished with hypotension or after vagotomy and was enhanced after sympathectomy. Precisely how these CO_2 responses differ from those in adult animals with similar hypotension, vagotomy, or sympathectomy remains unclear. Barker (1966) concluded that the responses of the cerebral vessels to P_aCO_2 changes were similar both in the neonatal rat and in man. On the contrary, Reivich et al. (1971) showed that the sensitivity of the neonatal cerebral vasculature of the monkey to alterations in P_aCO_2 was significantly reduced compared with the adult. They suggested that the cerebral vascular response to P_aCO_2 is not completely developed at birth. Reivich's data were subsequently confirmed in the dog (Hernandez et al., 1978; Shapiro et al., 1977). Thus, there is reason to doubt the ability of the fetus or neonate to respond to changes in P_aCO_2 in a manner identical to that observed in the adult.

C. Cerebral Perfusion Pressure

The capacity of cerebral blood flow to remain constant despite changes in blood pressure is commonly referred to as cerebral autoregulation. Autoregulation has been well demonstrated in both animals (Rapela and Green, 1964) and human subjects (Lassen, 1959). It has also been shown that cerebral autoregulation can be impaired or completely abolished during hypoxemia (Haggendal and Johnansson, 1965) or hypercapnia (Harper, 1966). In experimental animals and in human studies, it has been shown that CPP of approximately 60 mm Hg is necessary to maintain cerebral blood flow within the autoregulatory range. This is true over normal ranges of intracranial pressure at normal ranges of blood pressure and with the combination of increased intracranial pressure and increased blood pressure. In neonates and infants, however, there is some question regarding the determination of the value for CPP to maintain autoregulation because mean arterial blood pressure in this age group is below 60 mm Hg. Systolic pressures of from 41 to 70 mm Hg have been reported for normal newborns (Ashworth and Neligan, 1959), and these values have been corroborated by other investigators (Moss *et al.,* 1958; Woodbury *et al.,* 1938). These values are close to the lower limit of autoregulation in adults (60 mm Hg), even assuming intracranial pressure to be zero. Furthermore, a mean arterial pressure above 60 mm Hg does not appear to be common until the end of the first year of life (Moss *et al.,* 1958). Finally, in the premature infant the arterial blood pressure has been reported to be in the range of 64/39 mm Hg in a group of otherwise stable prematures. These values (Moss *et al.,* 1958) also are inconsistent with adequate cerebral blood flow and CPP using adult criteria. With arterial blood gas values held constant, Purves and James (1969) showed that fetal cerebral blood flow did not fall until mean arterial blood pressure fell below 40 mm Hg. Cerebral blood flow was independent of arterial blood pressure over the range 40–80 mm Hg. Similarly, lamb cerebral blood flow did not fall significantly until mean blood pressure fell below 40 mm Hg. This was true for both white and gray matter blood flow and appeared to be independent of elevated P_aCO_2. These observations support the concept that the fetus and neonate cerebral vasculature exhibits autoregulation; however, the critical CPP (lower limit for autoregulation) is 40 mm Hg instead of 60 mm Hg as in adults.

Whereas concern about CPP generally focuses on hypotension, it has also been shown that with hypertension there is an "escape" (upper limit) from autoregulation such that cerebral blood flow again varies directly with perfusion pressure. In the adult it has been demonstrated that the level of hypertension (mean arterial blood pressure) above which there is escape from autoregulation is in the range 150–170 mm Hg (Agnoli *et al.,* 1968). Whether this is the level of pressure that must be reached in fetuses or neonates before autoregulation is impaired is unclear.

VI. Future Directions

Although a great deal is known and accepted with regard to the cerebral vasculature, still, much is unclear and controversy exists in several areas.

Anatomic aspects of cerebral arteries, and to a lesser extent cerebral veins, are well known; however, information is sparce with respect to cerebral capillaries. The role of the blood–brain barrier and its involvement with cerebral capillaries and epithelium remain unclear. Whereas much is known about the blood–brain barrier, the hows and whys of barrier function are not so simple.

During the past 50 years an enormous number of techniques have been put forth to measure cerebral blood flow and the reactivity of the cerebral vascular bed. However, most of these techniques have certain limitations that may make the interpretation of acquired data difficult. In addition, failure to control certain experimental variables also contributes to misinterpretations. New techniques are consistently being developed, and these must be validated by experiments the results of which are already known and accepted. Systematic comparisons of one technique with another have not yet been carried out, and this must be done to ascertain what each technique measures. Finally, many of the new techniques are prohibitively expensive and can be used by only a few groups of investigators, and in addition many suffer from flaws that are similar to those of the older techniques.

With regard to neurogenic control of the cerebral circulation, much recent evidence has added to our understanding of the function of the sympathetic nerves under a variety of conditions (hypertension, hypercapnia). The sympathetic nerves may also affect cerebral capillaries and the capacity of the blood–brain barrier to remain functional. Concerning the parasympathetic and central nervous systems, there clearly is an incomplete understanding of these neural pathways themselves without considering their effects on the vasculature. For example the origin and course of the dilator pathways are obscure; the origin of certain central fibers is unknown. Although some investigators maintain that central fibers indeed can alter the control mechanisms of the cerebral vasculature, there are many skeptics. Much more work is needed in this area.

All investigators would agree that the cerebral vasculature reponds markedly to hypoxia and hypercapnia and that the capacity of the cerebral vessels to autoregulate is unequaled. However, the mechanisms of actions of these responses are unclear, except perhaps for the mechanism of action of CO_2, which has to do with the H^+ concentration of the brain extracellular fluid. For mechanisms involving hypoxia, direct effects of O_2 tension on cerebral vascular smooth muscle, by-products of metabolism, and neurogenic aspects have been proposed. Which mechanism is most important is unclear. The mechanism of cerebral autoregulation has also been hotly debated, with neurogenic, myogenic, and metabolic mechanisms being proposed.

   In this regard the relationships between cerebral blood flow, arterial blood pressure, cerebral venous blood pressure, and intracranial pressure are unclear. Is the pressure gradient for cerebral blood flow arterial minus intracranial pressure, or arterial minus cerebral venous pressure? Do the cerebral vessels care about absolute levels of arterial, venous, or intracranial pressure, or are they interested only in the pressure gradient across the vascular bed? At present the answers to these questions are unknown.

   Finally, whether the responses to O_2, to CO_2, and to changes in perfusion pressure in the adult are similar to those in the fetus and neonate is not clearly defined. There has been some work in this area, but much more must be done in order for even a preliminary understanding of the mechanisms of responses with age to be appreciated.

   Thus, I have reviewed a number of areas of importance in the cerebral vasculature, pointing out many controversies, and I hope I have made it easier for the reader to appreciate the many difficulties involved in studying the cerebral circulation.

Acknowledgment

The author would like to thank Candace Berryman for her flawless typing of this manuscript.

References

Ackermann, T. (1858). *Virchows Arch. A Pathol. Anat. Histol.* **15,** 401–464.
Agnoli, A., Fiechi, C., Bozzao, L., Battistini, N., and Prencipe, M. (1968). *Circulation* **38,** 800–812.
Alm, A., and Bill, A. (1973). *Acta Physiol. Scand.* **88,** 84–94.
Ashworth, A. M., and Neligan, G. A. (1959). *Lancet* **1,** 804.
Baez, S. (1966). *J. Appl. Physiol.* **21,** 299–301.
Baker, M. A., and Chapman, L. W. (1977). *Science (Washington, D.C.)* **195,** 781–783.
Barber, B. J., Martin, J. S., and Rapela, C. E. (1978). *Stroke* **9,** 29–34.
Barker, J. N. (1966). *Am. J. Physiol.* **210,** 897–902.
Bates, D., and Sundt, T. M. (1976). *Circ. Res.* **38,** 488–493.
Batson, O. (1944). *Fed. Proc. Fed. Am. Soc. Exp. Biol.* **3,** 139–144.
Bauer, K. F. R., and Leonhardt, H. (1956). *J. Comp. Neurol.* **106,** 363–370.
Bayliss, W. M. (1902). *J. Physiol. (London)* **28,** 220–231.
Bayliss, W. M., and Hill, L. (1895). *J. Physiol. (London)* **18,** 334–360.
Berne, R. M., Rubio, R., and Curnish, R. R. (1974). *Circ. Res.* **35,** 262–271.
Besson, J., Rotsztejn, W., Laburthe, M., Epelbaum, J., Beaudet, A., Kordon, C., and Rosselin, G. (1979). *Brain Res.* **165,** 79–85.
Betz, E. (1972). *Physiol. Rev.* **52,** 595–630.

Bicher, H. I., Bruley, D. F., Reneau, D. D., and Knisely, M. H. (1973). *Bibl. Anat.* **11,** 526–531.

Bill, A., and Linder, J. (1976). *Acta Physiol. Scand.* **96,** 114–121.

Blackwood, W., McMenemy, W. H., and Meyer, A. (1963). "Greenfield's Neuropathology." Williams & Wilkins, Baltimore, Maryland.

Borgstrom, L., Johnannsson, H., and Siesjo, B. K. (1975). *Acta Physiol. Scand.* **93,** 423–432.

Borodulya, A. V., and Pletchkova, E. K. (1976). *Acta Anat.* **96,** 135–147.

Brachet, J. L. (1837). "Recherches Experimentales sur les Fonctions due Systeme Nerveux Ganglionnaire et Son Application a la Pathologie." Bailliére, Paris.

Bradbury, M. (1979). "The Concept of a Blood Brain Barrier." Wiley, New York.

Brightman, M. W., and Reese, T. S. (1969). *J. Cell Biol.* **40,** 648–677.

Broman, T. (1949). "The Permeability of the Cerebrospinal Vessels in Normal and Pathological Conditions." Munksgaard, Copenhagen.

Buckberg, G. D., Luck, J. C., Payne, D. B., Hoffman, J. F. E., Archie, J. P., and Fixler, D. E. (1971). *J. Appl. Physiol.* **31,** 598–604.

Burgess, D. W., and Bean, J. W. (1970). *In* "Brain and Blood Flow" (R. W. R. Russell, ed.), pp. 120–124. Pitman, London.

Busija, D. W., and Heistad, D. D. (1981). *Circ. Res.* **48,** 62–69.

Callenfels, J. B. (1855). *Z. Rationelle Med.* **7,** 157–207.

Cameron, I. R., and Caronna, J. (1976). *J. Physiol. (London)* **262,** 415–430.

Cervos–Navarro, J., and Matakas, F. (1977). *Neurology* **24,** 282–286.

Chance, B., Cohen, P., Jobsis, F., and Schoener, B. (1962). *Science (Washington, D.C.)* **137,** 499–508.

Chorobski, J., and Penfield, W. (1932). *Arch. Neurol. Psychiatry* **28,** 1257–1289.

Chow, R. W., Newton, T. H., Smith, M. C., and Adams, J. E. (1968). *Invest. Radiol.* **3,** 402–407.

Clark, S. L. (1929). *J. Comp. Neurol.* **48,** 247–265.

Clemedson, C. J., Hartelius, H., and Holmberg, G. (1958). *Acta Pathol. Microbiol. Scand.* **42,** 137–149.

Cobb, S. (1937). *Res. Publ. Assoc. Nerv. Ment. Dis.* **18,** 719–752.

Cobb, S., and Finesinger, J. E. (1932). *Arch. Neurol. Psychiatry* **28,** 1243–1256.

Coburn, R. F. (1977). *Adv. Exp. Med. Biol.* **78,** 101–115.

Cohen, P. J. (1972). *Anesthesiology* **37,** 148–177.

Cohen, P. J., Alexander, S. C., Smith, T. C., Reivich, M., and Wollman, H. (1967). *J. Appl. Physiol.* **23,** 183–189.

Cohn, P. J., Alexander, S. C., and Smith, T. C. (1974). *Am. J. Obstet. Gynecol.* **120,** 817–824.

Courtice, F. C. (1941). *J. Physiol. (London)* **100,** 198–211.

Craigie, E. H. (1920). *J. Comp. Neurol.* **31,** 429–464.

Cuypers, J., Cuevas, A., and Duisberg, R. (1978). *Neurochirurgia* **21,** 62–66.

Dahl, E., and Nelson, E. (1964). *Arch. Neurol. (Chicago)* **10,** 158–164.

Dahlström, A., and Fuxe, K. (1964). *Acta Physiol. Scand.* (Suppl. 62), 485–486.

D'Alecy, L. G., and Feigl, E. O. (1972). *Circ. Res.* **31,** 267–283.

D'Alecy, L. G., and Rose, C. J. (1977). *Circ. Res.* **41,** 324–331.

Davis, J. N., Carlsson, A., MacMillan, V., and Siesjo, B. K. (1973). *Science (Washington, D.C.)* **182,** 72–74.

Denn, M. J., and Stone, H. L. (1976). *Brain Res.* **113,** 394–399.

Denton, I. C., Jr., White, R. P., and Robertson, J. T. (1972). *J. Neurosurg.* **36,** 34–42.

Deshmukh, V. D., and Harper, A. M. (1973). *Acta Neurol. Scand.* **49,** 649–658.

Detar, R., and Bohr, D. (1968). *Am. J. Physiol.* **214,** 241–244.

Diemer, K. (1968). *In* "Oxygen Transport in Blood and Tissue" (D. W. Lubbers, V. C. Luft, G. Thews, and E. Witzleb, eds.), pp. 118–123. Thieme, Stuttgart.

Donders, F. C. (1859). "Physiologie des Menschen." Hutzel, Leipzig.

Duc, G. (1971). *Pediatrics* **48,** 469–481.

Duckles, S. P., and Bevan, J. A. (1976). *J. Pharmacol. Exp. Ther.* **197,** 371–378.

Duckles, S. P., Lee, T. J. F., and Bevan, J. A. (1977). *In* "Neurogenic Control of Brain Circulation" (Ch. Owman, and L. Edvinsson, eds.), pp. 133–141. Pergamon, New York.

Duffy, T., Nelson, S. R., and Lowry, O. H. (1972). *J. Neurochem.* **19,** 959–977.

Dumke, P. R., and Schmidt, C. F. (1943). *Am. J. Physiol.* **138,** 421–431.

Dunning, H. S., and Wolff, H. G. (1937). *J. Comp. Neurol.* **67,** 433–450.

Edvinsson, L., and Hardebo, J. E. (1976). *Acta Physiol. Scand.* **97,** 523–525.

Edvinsson, L., and MacKenzie, E. T. (1977). *Pharmacol. Rev.* **28,** 275–348.

Edvinsson, L., and Owman, Ch. (1974). *Circ. Res.* **35,** 835–849.

Edvinsson, L., and Owman, Ch. (1975). *Neurology* **25,** 271–276.

Edvinsson, L., and Owman, Ch., and West, K. A. (1971). *Acta Physiol. Scand.* **82,** 521–526.

Edvinsson, L., Nielsen, K. C., Owman Ch., and Sporrong, B. (1972). *Z. Zellforsch. Mikrosk. Anat.* **134,** 311–325.

Eklof, B., Ingvar, D. H., Kagstrom, E., and Olin, T. (1971). *Acta Physiol. Scand.* **82,** 172–176.

Ekstrom-Jodal, B. (1970). *Acta Physiol. Scand.* **350,** 51–61.

Ekstrom-Jodal, B., Haggendal, E., Linder, L., and Nilsson, N. J. (1972). *Eur. Neurol.* **6,** 6–10.

Ellis, E. F., Wei, E. P., and Kontos, H. A. (1979). *Am. J. Physiol.* **237,** H381–H385.

Ellis, E. F., Kontos, H. A., and Oates, J. A. (1980). *In* "Prostaglandins in Cardiovascular and Renal Function" (A. Scriabine, A. M. Lefer, and F. A. Kuehl, Jr., eds.), pp. 209–222. Spectrum, New York.

Emerson, T. E., and Parker, J. L. (1975). *In* "Cerebral Circulation and Metabolism" (T. W. Langfitt, L. C. McHenry, Jr., M. Reivich, and H. Wollman, eds.), pp. 10–13. Springer-Verlag, Berlin and New York.

Emson, P. C., Fahrenkrug, J., DeMuckadell, O. B. S., Jessel, T. M., and Iversen, J. L. (1978). *Brain Res.* **143,** 174–178.

Falck, B., Hillarp, N. A., Thieme, G., and Torp, A. (1962). *J. Histochem. Cytochem.* **10,** 348–354.

Falck, B., Mchedlishvili, G. I., and Owman, Ch. (1965). *Acta Pharmacol. Toxicol.* **23,** 133–142.

Fazekas, J. F., and Bessman, A. N. (1953). *Am. J. Med.* **15,** 804–812.

Fedoruk, S., and Feindel, W. (1960). *Can. J. Surg.* **3,** 312–318.

Fieschi, C., and Bozzao, L. (1972). *In* "International Encyclopedia of Pharmacology and Therapeutics," pp. 1–34.

Finesinger, J. E., and Cobb, S. (1935). *J. Pharmacol. Exp. Ther.* **53,** 1–33.

Finnerty, F. A., Jr., Witkin, L., and Fazekas, J. F. (1954). *J. Clin. Invest.* **33,** 1227–1232.

Fitch, W., MacKenzie, E. T., and Harper, A. M. (1975). *Circ. Res.* **37,** 550–557.

Fitch, W., Ferguson, G. G., Sengupta, J., Garibi, D., and Harper, A. M. (1976). *J. Neurol. Neurosurg. Psychiatry* **39,** 1014–1022.

Fitzgerald, R. S., and Traystman, R. J. (1980). *Fed. Proc. Fed. Am. Soc. Exp. Biol.* **39,** 2674–2677.

Flohr, H., Poll, W., and Brock, M. (1971). *In* "Brain and Blood Flow" (R. W. R. Russell, ed.), pp. 406–409. Pitman, London.
Florence, V. M., and Bevan, J. A. (1979). *Circ. Res.* **45**, 212–218.
Florey, H. (1925). *Brain* **48**, 43–64.
Fog, M. (1937). *Arch. Neurol. Psychiatry* **37**, 351–364.
Fog, M. (1938). *J. Neurol. Neurosurg. Psychiatry* **1**, 187–197.
Fog, M. (1939a). *Arch. Neurol. Psychiatry* **41**, 109–118.
Fog, M. (1939b). *Arch. Neurol. Psychiatry* **41**, 260–268.
Forbes, H. S., and Cobb, S. S. (1938). *Brain* **61**, 221–233.
Forbes, H. S., and Wolff, H. G. (1928). *Arch. Neurol. Psychiatry* **19**, 1057–1086.
Forbes, H. S., Finley, K. H., and Nason, G. I. (1933). *Arch. Neurol. Psychiatry* **30**, 957–979.
Forbes, H. S., Nason, G. L., and Sengupta, J. (1936). *J. Neurol. Psychiatry* **39**, 1014–1022.
Forbes, H. S., Nason, G. L., and Wortman, R. C. (1937). *Arch. Neurol. Psychiatry* **37**, 334–350.
Freeman, J., and Ingvar, D. H. (1967). *Acta Anesthesiol. Scand.* **11**, 381–391.
Fuxe, K., Hokfelt, T., Said, S. I., and Mutt, V. (1977). *Neurosci. Lett.* **5**, 241–246.
Garry, R. C. (1928). *J. Phsyiol. (London)* **66**, 235–248.
Gaskell, T. W. H. (1880). *J. Physiol. (London)* **3**, 48–75.
Gibbs, F. A., Gibbs, E. L., and Lennox, W. G. (1935). *Am. J. Physiol.* **111**, 557–563.
Goldberg, M. A., Barlow, C. F., and Roth, L. J. (1961). *J. Pharmacol. Exp. Ther.* **131**, 308–318.
Goodale, R. L., Goetzman, B., and Visscher, M. B. (1970). *Am. J. Physiol.* **219**, 1226–1230.
Gotoh, F., Meyer, J. S., and Tomita, M. (1966). *Arch. Neurol. (Chicago)* **15**, 549–559.
Gottstein, V. (1962). "Der Hirnkreislauf unter dem Einfluss vasoaktiver Substanzen." Huthig, Heidelberg.
Green, H. D., and Denison, A. B., Jr. (1956). *Circ. Res.* **4**, 565–573.
Greenfield, J. C., and Tindall, G. T. (1968). *J. Clin. Invest.* **47**, 1672–1684.
Grimson, B. S., Robinson, S. C., Danford, E. T., Tindall, G. T., and Greenfield, J. C. (1969). *Am. J. Physiol.* **216**, 50–55.
Grote, J. (1975). *Arzneim. Forsch.* **25**, 1673–1674.
Grubb, R. L., Jr., Raichle, M. E., and Eichling, J. O. (1974). *Stroke* **5**, 630–637.
Gulland, G. L. (1898). *Br. Med. J.* **2**, 781–782.
Gurdjian, E. S., Stone, W. E., and Webster, J. E. (1949). *Arch. Neurol. Psychiatry* **51**, 472–477.
Gurdjian, E. S., Webster, J. E., Martin, F. A., and Thomas, L. M. (1958). *Arch. Neurol. Psychiatry* **80**, 418–435.
Haddy, F. J., and Scott, J. B. (1968). *Physiol. Rev.* **48**, 688–707.
Hafkenschiel, J. H., Crumpton, C. W. Moyer, J. H., and Jeffers, W. A. (1950). *J. Clin. Invest.* **29**, 408–411.
Haggendal, E. (1965). *Acta Physiol. Scand.* **66**, (Suppl. 258), 55–79.
Haggendal, E., and Johansson, B. (1965). *Acta Physiol. Scand.* **66**, 27–53.
Haggendal, E., Lofgren, J., Nilsson, N. J., and Zwetnow, N. N. (1970). *Acta Physiol. Scand.* **79**, 262–271.
Hansen, D. B., Sultzer, M. R., Freygang, W. H., and Sokoloff, L. (1957). *Fed. Proc. Fed. Am. Soc. Exp. Biol.* **16**, 54.
Harik, S. I., LaManna, J. C., Light, A. I., and Rosenthal, M. (1979). *Science (Washington, D. C.)* **206**, 69–71.
Harper, A. M. (1966). *J. Neurol. Neurosurg. Psychiatry* **29**, 398–403.

Harper, A. M., and Glass, H. I. (1965). *J. Neurol. Psychiatry* **28**, 449–452.

Harper, A. M., Rowan, J. O., and Jennett, W. B. (1968). *Scand. J. Clin. Lab. Invest.* **11** (Suppl. 102), XI:B.

Harper, A. M., Deshmukh, V. D., Rowan, J. O., and Jennett, W. B. (1972). *Arch. Neurol. (Chicago)* **27**, 1–6.

Hartman, B. K., Zide, D., and Udenfriend, S. (1972). *Proc. Natl. Acad. Sci. USA* **69**, 2722–2726.

Heistad, D. D., and Marcus, M. L. (1976). *Stroke* **7**, 239–243.

Heistad, D. D., Marcus, M., Ehrhardt, J., and Abboud, F. M. (1976). *Circ. Res.* **38**, 20–25.

Heistad, D. D., Marcus, M. L., Sandberg, S., and Abboud, F. M. (1977). *Cir. Res.* **41**, 342–350.

Heistad, D. D., Marcus, M. L., and Gross, P. M. (1978). *Am. J. Physiol.* **235**, H544–H552.

Heistad, D. D., Marcus, M. L., Said, S. I., and Gross, P. M. (1980). *Am. J. Physiol.* **8**, H73–H80.

Hernandez, M. J., Brennan, R. W., Vannucci, R. C., and Bowman, G. S. (1978). *Am. J. Physiol.* **234**, R209–R215.

Heymans, C., and Bouchkaert, J. J. (1932). *C. R. Seances Soc. Biol. Ses Fil.* **110**, 996–999.

Hill, L. (1896). ''The Physiology and Pathology of the Cerebral Circulation: An Experimental Research.'' Churchill, London.

Hill, L., and MacLeod, J. J. R. (1900). *J. Physiol. (London)* **26**, 394–404.

Hoedt-Rasmussen, K., and Skinhoj, E. (1966). *Neurology* **16**, 515–520.

Hoedt-Rasmussen, K., Sveinsdottir, E., and Lassen, N. A. (1966). *Circ. Res.* **18**, 237–247.

Hoff, J. F., MacKenzie, E. T., and Harper, A. M. (1977). *Circ. Res.* **40**, 258–262.

Hossman, K. A., and Olsson, Y. (1970). *Brain Res.* **22**, 313–325.

Huber, G. C. (1899). *J. Comp. Neurol.* **9**, 1–25.

Huckabee, W. (1958). *J. Clin. Invest.* **37**, 264–271.

Ingvar, D. H., and Lassen, N. A. (1962). *Acta Physiol. Scand.* **54**, 325–338.

Ingvar, D. H., and Soderberg, U. (1958). *Acta Physiol. Scand.* **42**, 130–143.

Itakura, T., Yamamoto, K., Tohyama, M., and Shimizu, N. (1977). *Stroke* **8**, 360–365.

Iwayama, T. (1970). *Z. Zellforsch. Mikrosk. Anat.* **109**, 465–480.

Iwayama, T., Furness, J. B., and Burnstock, G. (1970). *Circ. Res.* **26**, 635–646.

James, I. M., and MacDonell, L. (1975). *Clin. Sci.* **49**, 465–471.

James, I. M., Millar, R. A., and Purves, M. J. (1969). *Circ. Res.* **25**, 77–93.

Jewell, P. A. (1952). *J. Anat.* **86**, 83–94.

Jobsis, F. F., and Rosenthal, M. (1978). *Ciba Found. Symp.* **56**, 129–148.

Johannsson, H., and Siesjo, B. K. (1974). *Acta Physiol. Scand.* **90**, 281–282.

Johansson, B. (1974). *Acta Neurol. Scand.* **50**, 366–372.

Johansson, B., Li, C. I., and Olsson, Y. (1970). *Acta Neuropathol.* **16**, 117–124.

Jones, M. D., Jr., Sheldon, R. E., Peeters, L. L., Meschia, G., Battaglia, F. C., and Makowski, E. L. (1977). *J. Appl. Physiol.* **43**, 1080–1084.

Kajikawa, H. (1968). *Arch. Jpn. Chir.* **37**, 473–482.

Kaplan, H. A., and Ford, D. H. (1966). ''The Brain Vascular System.'' Elsevier, Amsterdam.

Karlsburg, P., Elliot, H. W., and Adams, J. E. (1963). *Neurology* **13**, 772–778.

Keatinge, W. R. (1966). *Circ. Res.* **18**, 641–649.

Kellie, G. (1824). *Trans. Edinburgh Med. Chirurg. Soc.* **1**, 123–169.

Kety, S. S. (1950). *Am. J. Med.* **8**, 205–217.

Kety, S. S., and Schmidt, C. F. (1948a). *J. Clin. Invest.* **27**, 476–483.

Kety, S. S., and Schmidt, C. F. (1948b). *J. Clin. Invest.* **27**, 484–492.

Kety, S. S., King, B. D., Horvath, S. M., Jeffers, W. A., and Hafkenschiel, J. H. (1950). *J. Clin. Invest.* **29,** 402–407.

Kindt, G. W., Ducker, T. B., and Huddlestone, J. (1971). In "Brain and Blood Flow" (R. W. R. Russell, ed.), pp. 401–405. Pitman, London.

King, B. D., Sokoloff, L., and Wechsler, R. L. (1952). *J. Clin. Invest.* **31,** 273–279.

Kjallquist, A., Siesjo, B. K., and Zwetnow, N. (1969). *Acta Physiol. Scand.* **75,** 267–275.

Kjellner, I., Karlsson, K., Olsson, T., and Rosen, K. G. (1974). *Pediatr. Res.* **8,** 50–57.

Kleinerman, J., Sancetta, S. M., and Hackel, D. B. (1958). *J. Clin. Invest.* **37,** 285–293.

Kobayashi, S., Waltz, A. G., and Rhoton, A. L. (1971). *Neurology* **21,** 297–302.

Kogure, K., Scheinberg, P., and Reinmuth, O. (1970). *J. Appl. Physiol.* **29,** 223–229.

Kontos, H. A., Raper, A. J., and Patterson, J. L. (1977a). *Stroke* **8,** 358–360.

Kontos, H. A., Wei, E. P., Raper, A. J., and Patterson, J. L., Jr. (1977b). *Stroke* **8,** 226–229.

Kontos, H. A., Wei, E. P., Raper, A. J., Rosenblum, W. I., Navari, R. M., and Patterson, J. L., Jr. (1978). *Am. J. Physiol.* **234,** H582–H591.

Koopmans, S. (1939). *Arch. Neerl. Physiol.* **24,** 250–266.

Kristiansen, K., and Krog, J. (1962). *Neurology* **12,** 20–22.

Krog, J. (1974). *J. Oslo City Hosp.* **14,** 3–15.

Kuschinsky, W., and Wahl, M. (1975). *Circ. Res.* **37,** 168–174.

Kuschinsky, W., and Wahl, M. (1978). *Physiol. Rev.* **58,** 656–689.

Kuschinsky, W., Wahl, M., Bosse, O., and Thurau, K. (1972). *Circ. Res.* **31,** 240–247.

Kuschinsky, W., Wahl, M., and Neiss, A. (1974). *Pfluegers Arch.* **347,** 199–208.

Lacombe, P., Reynier-Rebuffel, A. M., Mamo, H., and Seylaz, J. (1977). *Brain Res.* **129,** 129–140.

Landau, W. M., Freygang, W. H., Jr., Rowland, L. P., Sokoloff, L., and Kety, S. S. (1955). *Trans. Am. Neurol. Assoc.* **80,** 125–129.

Lang, R., and Zimmer, R. (1974). *Exp. Neurol.* **43,** 143–161.

Langfitt, T. W., and Kassell, N. F. (1968). *Am. J. Physiol.* **215,** 90–97.

Larsson, L. I., Edvinsson, L., Fahrenkrug, J., Hakansen, R., Owman, Ch., DeMuckadell, O. B. S., and Sundler, F. (1976). *Brain Res.* **113,** 400–404.

Lassen, N. A. (1959). *Physiol. Rev.* **39,** 183–238.

Lassen, N. A. (1968). *Scand. J. Clin. Lab. Invest.* **22,** 247–251.

Lassen, N. A. (1974). *Circ. Res.* **34,** 749–760.

Lennox, W. G., and Gibbs, E. L. (1932). *J. Clin. Invest.* **11,** 1155–1177.

Lewis, L. D., Ponten, V., and Siesjo, B. K. (1973). *Acta Physiol. Scand.* **88,** 284–286.

Lindvall, M., Cervos-Navarro, J., Edvinsson, L., Owman, Ch., and Stenevi, V. (1975). In "Blood Flow and Metabolish in the Brain" (A. M. Harper, W. B. Jennett, J. D. Miller, and J. O. Rowan, eds.), pp. 1.7–1.9. Livingstone, Edinburgh.

Lluch, S., Reimann, C., and Glick, G. (1973). *Stroke* **4,** 50–56.

MacKenzie, E. T., McCulloch, J., O'Keane, M., Pickard, J. D., and Harper, A. M. (1976a). *Am. J. Physiol.* **231,** 483–488.

MacKenzie, E. T., Strandgaard, S., Graham, D. I., Jones, J. V., Harper, A. M., and Farrar, K. K. (1976b). *Circ. Res.* **39,** 33–41.

MacMillan, V., and Siesjo, B. K. (1972). *Scand. J. Clin. Lab. Invest.* **30,** 127–136.

Marcus, M. L., Heistad, D. D., Ehrhardt, J. C., and Abboud, F. M. (1976). *J. Appl. Physiol.* **40,** 501–507.

Marcus, M. L., Busija, D. W., Bischof, C. J., and Heistad, D. D. (1981). *Fed. Proc. Fed. Am. Soc. Exp. Biol.* **40,** 2306–2310.

Matakas, F., Ebhardt, G., and Cervos-Navarro, J. (1972). *Eur. Neurol.* **8,** 62–68.

McCulloch, J., and Edvinsson, L. (1980). *Am. J. Physiol.* **238,** H449–H456.

McDowall, D. G. (1966). *In* "Oxygen Measurements in Blood and Tissues (J. P. Payne, and D. W. Hill, eds.), pp. 205–214. Churchill, London.

McDowall, D. G. (1967). *Br. J. Anaesth.* **39,** 186–196.

McDowall, D. G., Harper, A. M., and Jacobsen, I. (1963). *Br. J. Anaesth.* **35,** 394–402.

Mchedlishvili, G. I. (1972). "Vascular Mechanisms of the Brain." Plenum, New York.

Mchedlishvili, G., Nikolaishvili, L., and Antia, R. (1976). *Microvasc. Res.* **10,** 298–311.

McIlwain, H., and Bachelard, H. S. (1971). "Biochemistry and the Central Nervous System," 4th ed. Williams & Wilkins, Baltimore, Maryland.

McPherson, R. W., and Traystman, R. J. (1981). *Fed. Proc. Fed. Am. Soc. Exp. Biol.* **40,** 456.

Meyer, J. S., Gotoh, F., Ebihara, S., and Tomita, M. (1965). *Neurology* **15,** 892–901.

Meyer, J. S., Gotoh, F., and Takagi, Y. (1966). *Circulation* **33,** 35–48.

Meyer, J. S., Yoshida, K., and Sakamoto, K. (1967). *Neurology* **17,** 638–648.

Meyer, M. W., Smith, K. A., and Klassen, A. C. (1977). *Stroke* **8,** 197–201.

Michenfelder, J. D., and Theye, R. A. (1971). *Br. J. Anaesth.* **43,** 630–636.

Millar, R. A. (1969). *Int. Anesthesiol. Clin.* **7,** 539–556.

Miller, A. T. (1967). *In* "Quantitative Biology of Metabolism" (A. Locker, ed.), pp. 185–189. Springer-Verlag, Berlin and New York.

Miller, J. D., Stanek, A., and Langfitt, T. W. (1972). *Prog. Brain Res.* **35,** 411–432.

Molnar, L., and Szanto, J. (1964). *Q. J. Exp. Physiol.* **49,** 184–193.

Monro, A. (1783). "Observations on the Structure and Functions of the Nervous System." Creech, Edinburgh.

Moss, A. J., Liebling, W., and Adams, F. H. (1958). *Pediatrics* **21,** 950–957.

Moyer, J. H., Miller, S. I., and Snyder, H. (1954). *J. Appl. Physiol.* **7,** 245–247.

Mueller, S. M., Heistad, D. D., and Marcus, M. L. (1977). *Circ. Res.* **41,** 350–356.

Nagel, E. L., Morgane, P. J., McFarland, W. L., and Galliano, R. E. (1968). *Science (Washington, D.C.),* **161,** 898–900.

Nelson, E., and Rennels, M. (1970). *Brain* **93,** 475–490.

Nielsen, K. C., and Owman, Ch. (1967). *Brain Res.* **6,** 773–776.

Nilsson, B., Norberg, K., Nordstrom, C., and Siesjo, B. K. (1976). *In* "Blood Flow and Metabolism of the Brain" (A. M. Harper, W. B. Jennett, J. D. Miller, and J. O. Rowan, eds.), pp. 9.19–9.23. Livingstone, Edinburgh.

Noell, W., and Schneider, M. (1941). *Luftfahrtmedizin* **5,** 234–250.

Noell, W., and Schneider, M. (1944). *Pfluegers Arch. Gesamte Physiol. Menschen Tiere* **247,** 514–527.

Norberg, K., and Siesjo, B. K. (1975). *Brain Res.* **86,** 31–44.

Norcross, N. C. (1939). *Arch. Neurol. Psychiatry* **40,** 291–299.

Novack, P., Shenkin, H. A., Bortin, B., Goluboff, B., and Soffe, A. M. (1954). *J. Clin. Invest.* **32,** 696–702.

Nylin, G. (1958). *Conf. Cereb. Vasc. Dis. Ind,* pp. 40–52.

Ohgushi, N. (1968). *Arch. Jpn. Chir.* **37,** 294–303.

Oldendorf, W. H. (1962). *J. Nucl. Med.* **3,** 382–398.

Oldendorf, W. H. (1971). *Am. J. Physiol.* **221,** 1629–1639.

Olesen, J. (1972). *Neurology* **22,** 978–987.

Olesen, J. (1973). *Arch. Neurol. (Chicago)* **28,** 143–149.

Olesen, J. (1974). *Acta Neurol. Scand.* **50,** (Suppl. 57), 1–134.

Olesen, J., and Skinhoj, E. (1971). *Int. Headache Symp.,* pp. 145–152.

Olesen, J., Paulson, O. B., and Lassen, N. A. (1971). *Stroke* **2,** 519–540.

O'Neill, J. T., and Traystman, R. J. (1977). *In* "Neurogenic Control of the Brain Circulation" (C. Owman, and L. Edvinsson, eds.), pp. 254–260. Pergamon, New York.

Opitz, E., and Schneider, M. (1950). *Ergeb. Physiol. Biol. Chem. Exp.* **46,** 126–260.
Oski, F. (1979). *Crit. Care Med.* **7,** 412–418.
Owman, Ch., and Edvinsson, L. (1977). *In* '''Neurogenic Control of the Brain Circulation'' (Ch. Owman, and L. Edvinsson, eds.), pp. 15–38. Pergamon, New York.
Owman, Ch., Falck, B., and Mchedlishvili, G. I. (1966). *Fed. Proc. Fed. Am. Soc. Exp. Biol.* **25,** 612–614.
Owman, Ch., Edvinsson, L., Falck, B., and Nielsen K. C. (1974). *In* "Pathology of Cerebral Microcirculation" (J. Cervos-Navarro, ed.), pp. 184–199. de Gruyter, Berlin.
Owman, Ch., Edvinsson, L., and Hardebo, J.E. (1977). *Acta Neurol. Scand.* **56,** 384–385.
Pannier, J. L., Weyne, J., Demeester, G., and Leusen, I. (1972). *Pfluegers Arch.* **333,** 337–351.
Patterson, J. L., Jr., Heyman, A., Battey, A. L. and Ferguson, R. W. (1955). *J. Clin. Invest.* **34,** 1857–1864.
Pearce, W. J., and Bevan, J. A. (1980). *J. Cereb. Blood Flow Metab.* 1(Suppl.), S325–S326.
Pearce, W. J., and Bevan, J. A. (1980). *Adv. Physiol. Sci.* **9,** 269–278.
Pease, D. C., and Molinari, G. (1960). *J. Ultrastruct. Res.* **3,** 447–468.
Penfield, W. (1932). *Arch. Neurol. Psychiatry* **27,** 30–44.
Permutt, S., and Riley, R. L. (1963). *J. Appl. Physiol.* **18,** 924–932.
Permutt, S., Bromberger-Barnea, B., and Bane, H. N. (1962). *Med. Thorac.* **19,** 239–260.
Peters, A., Palay, S. L., and Webster, H. D. F. (1976). "The Fine Structure of the Nervous System," 2nd ed., pp. 295–305. Saunders, Philadelphia, Pennsylvania.
Pfluger, E. (1875). *Pfluegers Arch. Gesamte Physiol. Menschen Tiere* **10,** 251–367.
Pickard, J. D., and MacKenzie, E. T. (1973). *Nature New Biol.* **245,** 187–188.
Pickard, J. D., Tamura, A., and Stewart, M. (1980). *Brain Res.* **197,** 425–431.
Pinard, E., Purves, M. J., Seylaz, J., and Vasquez, J. V. (1979). *Pfluegers Arch.* **379,** 165–172.
Pitt, B. R., Radford, E. P., Jr., Gurtner, G. H., and Traystman, R. J. (1979). *Arch. Environ. Health* **34,** 354–359.
Pittman, R. N., and Duling, B. R. (1973). *Microvasc. Res.* **6,** 202–211.
Ponte, J., and Purves, M. J. (1974). *J. Physiol. (London)* **237,** 315–340.
Posner, J., and Plum, F. (1967). *Arch. Neurol. (Chicago)* **16,** 492–496.
Purves, M. J. (1972). "The Physiology of the Cerebral Circulation." Univ. of London Press, London.
Purves, M. J., and James, I. M. (1969). *Circ. Res.* **25,** 651–667.
Raisis, J. E., Kindt, G. W., and McGillicuddy, J. E. (1979). *J. Surg. Res.* **26,** 101–107.
Rapela, C. E., and Green, H. D. (1964). *Circ. Res.* **15,** 205–211.
Rapela, C. E., and Green, H. D. (1968). *Scand. J. Clin. Lab. Invest.* 5:C (Suppl. 102).
Rapela, C. E., and Martin, J. B. (1975). *In* "Blood Flow and Metabolism in the Brain" (A. M. Harper, W. B. Jennett, and J. D. Miller, eds.), pp. 4.5–4.9. Livingstone, Edinburgh.
Rapela, C. E., Green, H. D., and Denison, A. B., Jr. (1967). *Circ. Res.* **21,** 559–568.
Raper, A. J., Kontos, H. A., Wei, E. P., and Patterson, J. L., Jr. (1972). *Circ. Res.* **31,** 257–266.
Rapoport, S. I. (1976). "Blood Brain Barrier in Physiology and Medicine." Raven, New York.
Rapoport, S. I., Hari, M., and Klatzo, I. (1972). *Am. J. Physiol.* **223,** 323–331.
Reese, T. S., and Karnovsky, M. J. (1967). *J. Cell. Biol.* **34,** 207–217.
Rein, H. (1929). *Z. Biol. (Munich)* **89,** 307–318.
Reivich, M. (1964). *Am. J. Physiol.* **206,** 25–35.
Reivich, M., Brann, A. W., and Shapiro, H. (1971). *Eur. Neurol.* **6,** 132–136.

Rennels, M., and Nelson, E. (1975). *Am. J. Anat.* **144**, 233–242.

Riegal, F., and Jolly, F. (1871). *Virchows Arch. A Pathol. Anat. Histol.* **52**, 218–230.

Ronnberg, A. L., Edvinsson, L., Larsson, L. I., Nielsen, K. C., and Owman, Ch. (1973). *Agents Actions* **3**, 191–192.

Rosenblum, W. I. (1974). *Arch. Neurol. (Chicago)* **31**, 197–199.

Rosenblum, W. I. (1975). *Stroke* **6**, 293–297.

Rosendorff, C., and Cranston, W. I. (1971). *Circ. Res.* **28**, 492–502.

Rosendorff, C., Mitchell, G., and Scriven, D. R. L. (1973). *Stroke* **4**, 368.

Rosendorff, C., Mitchell, G., Scriven, D. R. L., and Shapiro, C. (1976). *Circ. Res.* **38**, 140–145.

Rowan, J. O., and Johnston, I. H. (1975). *In* "Intracranial Pressure" (N. Lundburg, V. Ponten, and M. Brock, eds.), Vol. 2, pp. 263–267. Springer-Verlag, Berlin and New York.

Roy, C. S., and Brown, J. G. (1879). *J. Physiol. (London)* **2**, 323–359.

Roy, C. S., and Sherrington, C. S. (1890). *J. Physiol. (London)* **2**, 85–108.

Rubio, R., and Berne, R. M. (1969). *Circ. Res.* **25**, 407–415.

Rubio, R., Berne, R. M., Bockman, E. L., and Curnish, R. R. (1975). *Am. J. Physiol.* **228**, 1896–1902.

Rudolph, A. M., and Heymann, M. A. (1972). *Acta Endocrinol. (Copenhagen)* (Suppl. 158), 112–127.

Sagawa, K., and Guyton, A. C. (1961). *Am. J. Physiol.* **200**, 711–714.

Said, S. I., and Rosenberg, R. N. (1976). *Science (Washington, D.C.)* **192**, 907–908.

Sakabe, T., and Siesjo, B. K. (1979). *Acta Physiol. Scand.* **107**, 283–284.

Salanga, V. D., and Waltz, A. G. (1973). *Stroke* **4**, 213–217.

Samarasinghe, D. D. (1965). *J. Anat.* **99**, 815–828.

Sapirstein, L. (1962). *J. Clin. Invest.* **41**, 1429–1435.

Sato, S. (1966). *Am. J. Anat.* **118**, 873–890.

Scheinberg, P. (1965). *Conf. Cereb. Vasc. Dis. 4th,* pp. 87–101.

Scheinberg, P., Jayne, H. W., and Blackburn, L. I. (1952). *Arch. Neurol. Psychiatry* **68**, 815–818.

Schmidt, C. F. (1945). *Anesthesiology* **6**, 113–123.

Schmidt, C. F. (1950). "The Cerebral Circulation in Health and Disease." Thomas, Springfield, Illinois.

Schmidt, C. F., and Hendrix, J. P. (1937). *Res. Publ. Assoc. Nerv. Ment. Dis.* **18**, 229–276.

Schneider, M., and Schneider, D. (1934). *Arch. Exp. Pathol. Pharmakol.* **175**, 640–664.

Sercombe, R., Aubineau, P., Edvinsson, L., Mamo, H., Owman, Ch., Pinard, E., and Seylaz, J. (1975). *Neurology* **25**, 954–963.

Shalit, M. N., Reinmuth, O. M., Shimojyo, S., and Scheinberg, P. (1967). *Arch. Neurol. (Chicago)* **17**, 342–353.

Shapiro, H. M., Greenberg, J. H., and Naughton, K. U. H. (1977). *Acta Neurol. Scand.* (Suppl. 64), 426–428.

Shenkin, H. A., Hafkenschiel, J. H., and Kety, S. S. (1950). *Arch. Surg. (Chicago)* 319–324.

Shimojyo, S., Scheinberg, P., Kogure, K., and Reinmuth, O. M. (1968). *Neurology* **18**, 127–133.

Shultz, A. (1866). *St. Peterburgs Med. Z.* **2**, 122–128.

Siesjo, B. K., and Ljundggren, B. (1973). *Arch. Neurol. (Chicago)* **29**, 400–407.

Siesjo, B. K., and Nilsson, L. (1971). *Scand. J. Clin. Lab. Invest.* **27**, 83–96.

Siesjo, B. K., and Zwetnow, N. (1969). *Acta Physiol. Scand.* **48**, 187–196.

Siesjo, B. K., Johannsson, H., Norberg, K., and Salford, L. G. (1974). *In* "Brain Work: The Coupling of Function, Metabolism, and Blood Flow in the Brain" (D. H. Ingvar, and N. A. Lassen, eds.), pp. 101–125. Munksgaard, Copenhagen.

Sjostrand, T. (1935). *Skand. Arch. Physiol.* (Suppl. 71), 1–150.

Skinhoj, E. (1966). *Acta Neurol. Scand.* **42,** 604–607.

Smith, A. L., Neigh, J. L., Hoffman, J. C., and Wollman, H. (1970). *J. Appl. Physiol.* **29,** 665–669.

Smith, D. J., and Vane, J. R. (1966). *J. Physiol.* (*London*) **186,** 284–294.

Sokoloff, L. (1959). *Pharmacol. Rev.* **11,** 1–85.

Sokoloff, L. (1977). *J. Neurochem.* **29,** 13–26.

Sokoloff, L. (1978). *Ciba Found. Symp.* **56,** 171–179.

Stavraky, G. W. (1936). *Arch. Neurol. Psychiatry* **35,** 1002–1028.

Strandgaard, S., MacKenzie, E. T., Sengupta, D., Rowan, J. O., Lassen, N. A., and Harper, A. M. (1974). *Circ. Res.* **34,** 435–440.

Swank, R. L., and Hissen, W. (1964). *Arch. Neurol.* (*Chicago*) **10,** 468–472.

Swanson, L. W., and Hartman, B. K. (1975). *J. Comp. Neurol.* **163,** 467–506.

Symon, L., Held, K., and Dorsch, N. W. C. (1972). *Eur. Neurol.* **6,** 11–18.

Symon, L., Pasztor, E., Dorsch, N. W. C., and Branston, N. M. (1973). *Stroke* **4,** 632–642.

Theye, R. A., and Michenfelder, J. D. (1968). *Anesthesiology* **29,** 1119–1124.

Tindall, G., and Greenfield, J. C. (1973). *Stroke* **4,** 46–49.

Traystman, R. J. (1981). *In* "Vasodilation" (P. Vanhoutte and I. Leusen, eds.), pp. 39–48. Raven, New York.

Traystman, R. J., and Fitzgerald, R. S. (1981). *Am. J. Physiol.* **241,** H724–H731.

Traystman, R. J., and Rapela, C. E. (1975). *Circ. Res.* **36,** 620–630.

Traystman, R. J., Fitzgerald, R. S., and Loscutoff, S. C. (1978). *Circ. Res.* **42,** 649–657.

Traystman, R. J., Gurtner, G. H., Rogers, M. D., Jones, M. D., Jr., and Koehler, R. C. (1981). *Adv. Physiol. Sci.* **9,** 167–177.

Von Essen, C. (1972). *J. Pharm. Pharmacol.* **24,** 668.

Von Essen, C., and Roos, B. E. (1974). *Acta Pharmacol. Toxicol.* **35,** 433–435.

Wagner, E. M., and Traystman, R. J. (1981). *Fed. Proc. Fed. Am. Soc. Exp. Biol.* **40,** 454.

Wahl, M., and Kuschinsky, W. (1976). *Pfluegers Arch.* **362,** 55–59.

Wahl, M., and Kuschinsky, W. (1979). *Circ. Res.* **44,** 161–165.

Wahl, M., Detjen, P., Thurau, K., Ingvar, D. H., and Lassen, N. A. (1970). *Pfluegers Arch.* **316,** 152–163.

Wahl, M., Kuschinsky, W., Bosse, O., Olesen, J., Lassen, N. A., Ingvar, D. H., Michaelis, J., and Thurau, K. (1972). *Circ. Res.* **31,** 248–256.

Wahl, M., Kuschinsky, W., Bosse, O., and Thurau, K. (1973). *Circ. Res.* **32,** 162–169.

Waltz, A. G., Yamaguchi, T., and Regli, F. (1971). *Am. J. Physiol.* **221,** 298–302.

Wasserman, A. J., and Patterson, J. L., Jr. (1961). *J. Clin. Invest.* **40,** 1297–1303.

Wechsler, R., Dripps, R. L., and Kety, S. S. (1951). *Anesthesiology* **12,** 308–314.

Wei, E. P., Raper, A. J., Kontos, H. A., and Patterson, J. L., Jr. (1975). *Stroke* **6,** 654–658.

Wei, E. P., Ellis, E. F., and Kontos, H. A. (1980a). *Am. J. Physiol.* **238,** H226–H230.

Wei, E. P., Kontos, H. A., and Patterson, J. L., Jr. (1980b). *Am. J. Physiol.* **238,** H697–H703.

Wei, E. P., Kontos, H. A., and Said, S. I. (1981). *Am. J. Physiol.* **8,** H765–H768.

Wei, E. P., Raper, A. J., Kontos, H. A., and Patterson, J. L., Jr. (1975). *Stroke* **6,** 654–659.

Welch, K. M., Hashi, K., and Meyer, J. S. (1973). *J. Neurol. Neurosurg. Psychiatry* **36,** 724–735.

Wellens, D. L., Wouters, L. J., Dereese, R. J., Beirnaert, P., and Reneman, R. S. (1975). *Brain Res.* **86,** 429–438.

Westergaard, E. (1977). *Acta Neuropathol.* **39,** 181–187.

White, R. P., Hagen, A., and Robertson, J. T. (1976). *J. Neurosurg.* **44,** 45–49.

Wiggers, C. F. (1914). *J. Physiol.* (*London*) **48,** 109–233.

Willis, T. (1664). "Cerebri Anatome." Martin & Allestry, London.

Wilson, D. A., O'Neill, J. T., Said, S. I., and Traystman, R. J. (1981). *Circ. Res.* **48,** 138–148.

Winn, H. R., Berne, R. M., and Rubio, R. (1980). *Blood Vessels* **17,** 168–169.

Wolff, H. G. (1936). *Physiol. Rev.* **16,** 545–596.

Wolff, H. G., and Lennox, W. G. (1930). *Arch. Neurol. Psychiatry* **23,** 1097–1120.

Wollman, H., Alexander, S. C., Cohen, P. J., Chase, P. E., Melman, E., and Behar, M. G. (1964). *Anesthesiology* **25,** 180–184.

Wollman, H., Alexander, S. C., and Cohen, P. J. (1965). *Anesthesiology* **26,** 329–334.

Woodbury, R. A., Robinow, M., and Hamilton, W. F. (1938). *Am. J. Physiol.* **122,** 472–479.

Yoshida, K., Meyer, J. S., Sakamoto, K., and Handa, J. (1966). *Circ. Res.* **19,** 726–738.

Zervas, N. T., Lavyne, M. H., and Negoro, M. (1975). *N. Engl. J. Med.* **293,** 812–816.

Zwetnow, N. N. (1970). *Acta Physiol. Scand.* (Suppl. 339), 1–31.

7 Microcirculation of the Eye

Albert Alm

I. Introduction

In the following presentation of the microcirculation of the eye all the different vascular beds of the eye are discussed to some extent, but the discussion deals mainly with the parts of the circulation that are responsible for the nutrition of the retina, that is, the retinal and the choroidal circulations. In this respect the retina is unique, because its functional survival depends on two vascular beds that could be said to represent two extremes from practically all points of view with regard to anatomy, physiol-

THE PHYSIOLOGY AND PHARMACOLOGY
OF THE MICROCIRCULATION, VOLUME 1

ogy, and pharmacology. Thus, studies on the microcirculation of the eye permit one to make recordings of the response of highly different vascular beds to various identical physiologic or pharmacologic stimuli. Therefore, the microcirculation of the eye should be a topic of some interest not only to ophthalmologists but also to students and investigators in various fields of circulatory research.

The fact that we lack a clinical method for the quantitative determination of blood flow through the various vascular beds of the eye makes it necessary to rely chiefly on studies with experimental animals. The ocular vascular anatomy in lower mammals differs from that in primates. Therefore, data obtained in studies on primates are used as far as possible. Various aspects of the microcirculation are dealt with, including exchange of fluids and metabolic substrates within the eye. My intention is to make a clinically oriented presentation. Information of clinical interest will be discussed in some detail. It should be kept in mind, however, that clinical conclusions based on results from experiments on healthy animals are always to some extent speculations.

Recently, three major reviews of the ocular circulation have been published (Henkind et al., 1979; Bill, 1981, 1983), where the reader may find further information and references.

II. Anatomic Considerations

A. Gross Anatomy of Ocular Vessels

In most higher mammals the eye is supplied by two separate vascular systems: the retinal and the uveal vessels. The uveal vessels include the choroid and the vessels of the anterior uvea, that is, the iris and the ciliary body. With the exception of the eel (Michaelson, 1954) all vertebrates have a choroid, but the pattern of retinal vascularization varies. Leber (1903) classified the various patterns of retinal vascularization into four groups.

1. Holangiotic. The entire retina is vascularized. Several higher mammals, including all primates, belong to this group.
2. Merangiotic. Retinal vessels are present only where the optic nerve extends into the retina as two wing-shaped areas of medullated nerve fibers. This pattern is found in rabbits.
3. Paurangiotic. Retinal vessels are found only within a narrow ring around the optic disc, as seen in guinea pigs.
4. Anangiotic. The retina is completely avascular, as, for example, in chinchillas.

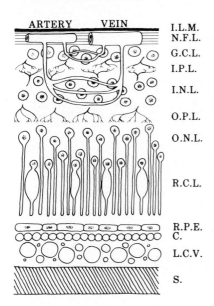

Fig. 1. Schematic representation of retinal and choroidal vessels in relation to the layers of the retina. I.L.M., Inner limiting membrane; N.F.L., nerve fiber layer; G.C.L., ganglion cell layer; I.P.L., inner plexiform layer; I.N.L., inner nuclear layer; O.P.L., outer plexiform layer; O.N.L., outer nuclear layer; R.C.L., rod and cone layer; R.P.E., retinal pigment epithelium; C., choriocapillaries; L.C.V., large choroidal vessels; S., sclera.

The following presentation deals with the holangiotic retina. In primates, including man, both vascular systems are derived from the ophthalmic artery, which is a branch of the internal carotid. Within the orbit the ophthalmic artery divides into several branches, among them the central retinal artery and, as a rule, two posterior ciliary arteries (Hayreh, 1962) and several anterior ciliary arteries. The retinal and the uveal vascular systems are strictly separate, apart from anastomoses at the capillary level within the optic nerve head (ONH). There are no lymph vessels within the eye.

1. Retina

The central retinal artery enters the optic nerve 7–10 mm behind the globe and appears in the retina at the optic disc. From the disc the retinal vessels are distributed within the retina in four major branches (see Fig. 8, Section III,B,1). Studies on ink-injected (Michaelson, 1954) and trypsin-digested (Toussaint et al., 1961) specimens revealed the following vascular pattern. The arteries and veins are located in the optic nerve fiber layer, whereas the capillaries in a large part of the retina are distributed as two essentially flat, two-dimensional, interconnecting networks, one located mainly in the ganglion cell layer and one in the inner nuclear layer (Fig. 1). Nowhere does the capillary network extend beyond the inner nuclear layer, and the photo-receptors and their nuclei are thus situated in a

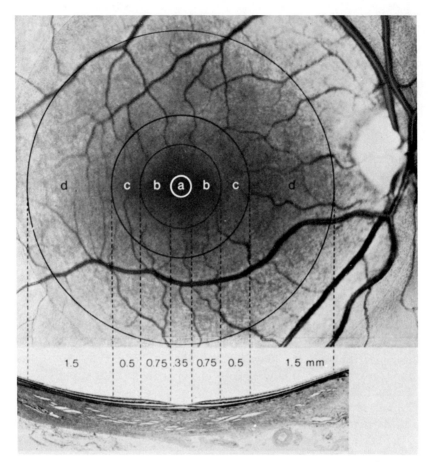

Fig. 2. Photograph of the fundus matched with a meridonial light micrograph of the macular region. The central, avascular zone is represented by a. There are no superficial retinal layers within this zone in the corresponding micrograph. (From Hogan *et al.*, 1971.)

completely avascular part of the retina. Aligned to the optical axis of the eye is the fovea, the central part of the macula. In the fovea the number of photoreceptors per area is higher than anywhere else in the retina, which results in a high visual acuity. Furthermore, the central beam of light reaches the cones of the fovea without interference from blood vessels or superficial retinal layers because these are displayed peripherally (Fig. 2), which results in an avascular central zone in the fovea (Fig. 3). Capillary-free zones can be seen close to the arterioles (Fig. 4) as a result of secondary vascular remodeling during maturation (Henkind and Oliveira, 1967), probably caused by high local oxygen tension. Except for the fovea, the

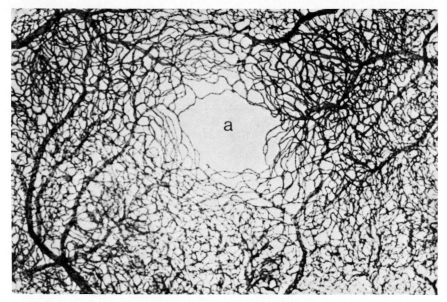

Fig. 3. Capillary bed of the macular region. The central, avascular zone (a) corresponds to region a in Fig. 2. (From Hogan *et al.*, 1971.)

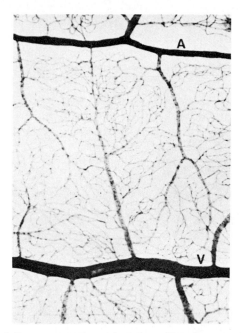

Fig. 4. Human retinal digest preparation. A broad, capillary-free zone is present around the artery (A), and a much narrower zone is seen around the vein (V). PAS and hematoxylin; magnification 9×. (From Wise *et al.*, 1971.)

general arrangement of the capillaries favors the central part of the retina, where the dense two-layered network may become three- or four-layered. In the periphery the network becomes less dense, and the basic two-layered pattern is gradually reduced to one layer and finally disappears completely in the extreme periphery. A special part of the capillary network is the radial peripapillary capillaries, which extend from the optic disc mainly in the upper and lower temporal directions, thus resembling a glaucomatous visual field defect. Their possible role in glaucoma has been discussed (Henkind, 1967).

A cilioretinal artery may be found in one-third of carefully examined eyes (Justice and Lehmann, 1976). Its ciliary origin can be verified with fluorescein angiography, which demonstrates its rapid filling before the true retinal arteries. Nutrition from this artery may save useful vision if the central retinal artery is occluded (Brown and Shields, 1979).

The veins of the retina leave the eye through the optic disc as a central retinal vein, which drains in the cavernous sinus.

2. Uvea

The posterior ciliary arteries give off a large number of small arteries, which supply the various parts of the uvea (Fig. 5). Ten to twenty short posterior ciliary arteries pierce the sclera at the posterior pole to form the choroid. The choroid is a pigmented vascular tissue with its capillaries arranged in one single layer, the choriocapillaris, adjacent to Bruch's membrane and the retinal pigment epithelium (RPE) (Hogan *et al.*, 1971). Some of the short posterior ciliary arteries may form a complete or partial circle within the sclera around the optic nerve, the circle of Zinn-Haller. Sectors of the choroid in the nasal and temporal periphery are supplied by one long posterior ciliary artery each (Hayreh, 1974a). The choriocapillaris is denser in the central regions than in the periphery, but the pattern of the submacular choroid is not different from that of other areas equidistant from the optic disc (Wybar, 1954; Ring and Fujino, 1967). A characteristic of the choroid is the sudden transition from large choroidal arterioles into the choriocapillaris.

The peripheral choroid receives additional blood supply from recurrent branches of the major arterial circle of the iris. This is formed by the long posterior ciliary arteries and the anterior ciliary arteries. The latter arrive at the anterior segment with the extraocular muscles. The iris and the ciliary body are supplied by radial vessels from the major arterial circle and by direct vessels from the anterior ciliary and the long posterior ciliary arteries. The venous blood from the anterior uvea drains mainly into the choroid and leaves the eye via the vortex veins (Fig. 5), of which there are usually four, one in each quadrant of the eye.

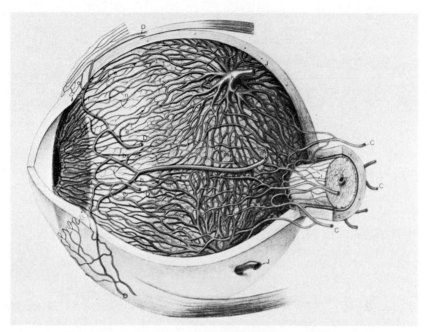

Fig. 5. The uveal blood vessels. A, Long posterior ciliary artery; b, branches of the long posterior ciliary artery; c, short posterior ciliary artery; D, anterior ciliary arteries; e, branches of the anterior ciliary arteries; f, major circle of the iris; g, branches into the ciliary body and iris from the major circle of the iris; h, circle of Zinn-Haller; i, pial arteries; J, vortex veins; k, ampulla of the vortex veins; l, m, uveal veins forming the vortex veins; n, veins draining the iris and the ciliary body; o, veins entering the episcleral venous system. (From Hogan *et al.*, 1971.)

In the pericorneal region of the sclera one can see the aqueous veins that drain aqueous humor from the anterior chamber of the eye. They were first recognized as such by Ascher (1942), although they had already been described by Herman Boerhaave early in the eighteenth century (Knutson and Sears, 1973).

3. Optic Nerve Head

The axons of the retina leave the eye as the optic nerve through a sieve-like hole in the posterior part of the sclera. This hole is bridged by numerous fibrous strands, the lamina cribrosa. The surface of the ONH can be observed ophthalmoscopically as the papilla or the optic disc. The circulation of the ONH has attracted a great deal of attention in recent years because of the possibility that a disturbed circulation within this small piece of tissue might be the cause of the axonal damage observed in glaucoma. The ONH is traditionally divided into the superficial nerve fiber layer, the prelaminar part, and the lamina cribrosa. Meticulous studies of the angioarchitecture of the ONH have been performed with various techniques (Henkind and Levitsky, 1969; Levitsky and Henkind, 1969; Anderson, 1974; Lieberman *et al.,* 1976; Hayreh, 1978). Although there are large interindividual variations the main bulk of evidence suggests the following pattern (Fig. 6). The superficial nerve fiber layer is supplied with capillaries from the retinal arterioles, mainly branches from the peripapillary retina. The prelaminar part of the ONH receives no branches from the central retinal artery. Its main supply is from the ciliary circulation, either by branches from the choroidal arteries or directly from the short posterior ciliary arteries. It is important to note that communications between the choriocapillaris and the capillary network of the ONH probably are of minor importance. The lamina cribrosa, which is richly vascularized, receives its blood supply from intrascleral branches of the short posterior ciliary arteries. Geijer and Bill (1979) have convincingly shown that all of these three regions are supplied by branches that are under the influence of the intraocular pressure (IOP), unlike the retrolaminar region, which is supplied by branches from the central retinal artery and by pial vessels.

B. Fine Structure of the Ocular Microvessels

A meaningful discussion of the exchange of fluid and metabolites in the eye requires an understanding of the construction of the microvasculature, because there is a close correlation between ultrastructure and permeability of the exchange microvessels. Microvessels can be classified into four main types (Majno, 1966), and this classification is used in this presentation of the microvessels of the eye.

1. Microvessels in which nonfenestrated endothelial cells are connected by tight junctions. This is the type of vessel that constitutes the blood–brain barrier (BBB), and a similar ultrastructure is found in the retinal microvessels (Cunha-Vaz *et al.,* 1966) and in the monkey iris (Vegge, 1972). The capillaries of the retina are narrow, with a mean diameter ranging from 3.5 to 6 μm (Ishikawa, 1963).

2. Microvessels in which nonfenestrated endothelial cells are connected by junctions of various widths, as seen in skeletal muscle. This type is found in the iris of several lower mammals (Saari, 1975).

3. Microvessels with fenestrated endothelial cells in which the fenestrae may be covered by a thin membrane. Such capillaries are usually associated with large fluid movements between the intra- and extravascular

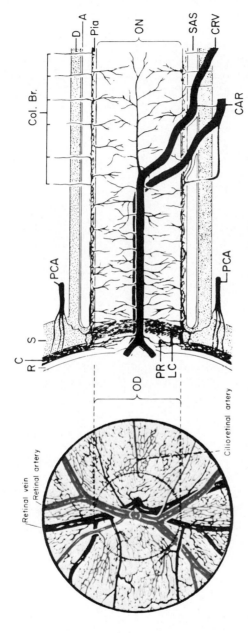

Fig. 6. Diagrammatic representation of blood supply of the optic nerve head and intraorbital optic nerve. A, Arachnoid; C, choroid; CAR, central retinal artery; Col. Br., collateral branches; CRV, central retinal vein; D, dura; LC, lamina cribrosa; OD, optic disc; ON, optic nerve; PCA, posterior ciliary arteries; PR, prelaminar region; R, retina; S, sclera; SAS, subarachnoid space. (From Hayreh, 1974.)

spaces, and they are found in the kidney, the small intestine, and various glands. In the eye they can be found in the ciliary processes (Holmberg, 1959), where rapid net movement of fluid is required to provide for the formation of aqueous humor. Fenestrations can also be found in the choriocapillaris (Bernstein and Hollenberg, 1965), particularly on the retinal side. A need for a large fluid movement through the walls of the choriocapillaris is probably not the reason for these fenestrations (see Section VII,A). In histologic sections the width of the choriocapillaris and the capillaries of the ciliary processes is unusually large, 15–50 μm (Hogan *et al.*, 1971). However, in this respect a difference exists between the anterior uvea and the choroid. In rabbits (Alm *et al.*, 1977) and pigs (P. Törnquist, personal communication) 50% of 8- to 10-μm radiolabeled microspheres pass through the vascular beds of the anterior uvea, whereas only about 5% pass through the choroid. The reason for this difference seems to be that most choriocapillaris have at least one narrow part preventing the passage of 8- to 10-μm microspheres (A. Bill, personal communication).

4. Microvessels with a discontinuous endothelial lining with large openings, as seen in the liver. Such vessels are not found within the eye.

C. Blood–Ocular Barriers

A continuous, nonfenestrated endothelium connected by tight junctions, as seen in the brain, retina, and the monkey iris, constitutes a barrier that limits free diffusion of water-soluble molecules between blood and tissue. In the brain this barrier, the BBB, provides protection from blood-borne toxins, prevents escape of neurotransmitters, and provides homeostasis for several ions (Bradbury, 1979). The existence of continuous, nonfenestrated capillaries with tight junctions between the endothelial cells in the retina and the iris would obviously be meaningless if substances passing out through the fenestrae of the choriocapillaris and the capillaries of the ciliary processes had free access to the retina. However, epithelial barriers complete the endothelial blood–ocular barriers and give the retina the same protection from noxious blood-borne substances as the brain. The blood–ocular barriers can be divided into two parts: an anterior part, the blood–aqueous barrier, and a posterior part, the blood–retinal barrier (BRB). The epithelial part of the blood–aqueous barrier is constituted by the nonpigmented epithelium covering the ciliary processes (Hogan *et al.*, 1971) and that of the BRB by the retinal pigment epithelium (Hudspeth and Yee, 1973). Both these epithelial layers have tight junctions connect-

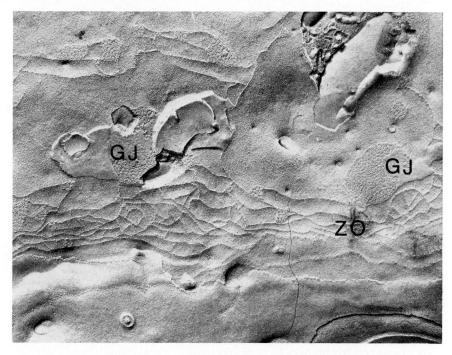

Fig. 7. Freeze–fracture view of a membrane cleavage face at the junctional complexes of the frog pigment epithelial cells. The apex of the cell lies toward the top of the figure. GJ, Gap junction; ZO, zonula occludens. [From Hudspeth and Yee, (1973). *Invest. Ophthalmol.* **12**, 354–365.]

ing the epithelial cells (Fig. 7). In the BRB there is a defect at the level of the ONH where small water-soluble substances, such as sodium fluorescein, may enter the optic nerve from the choroid (Grayson and Laties, 1971).

III. Methods Used in Studies of Ocular Blood Flow

The problems inherent in studies on blood flow through the various tissues of the eye have inspired the application of many markedly different techniques, some of them unique for the eye. A brief presentation of some of them may serve as a background for the following presentation of data obtained in studies utilizing these techniques.

A. Methods Used on Experimental Animals

1. Cannulation of Venous Outflow Channels

Quantitative determinations of total uveal blood flow, without undue disturbance of the venous pressure, have been possible in several species. Thus, Bill (1962a) found that total uveal blood flow in rabbits could be calculated from the flow through one opened vortex vein as long as the IOP was 10–15 mm Hg or higher. In cats (Bill, 1962b) and dogs (Elgin, 1964) a large intrascleral venous plexus permits the determination of total uveal blood flow by cannulating the large superior anterior ciliary vein and ligating the vortex veins and the remaining ciliary veins. It is possible to cannulate venous channels in this plexus that drain mainly choroidal blood or blood from the anterior uvea, respectively. This has been utilized in studies on the arteriovenous differences for oxygen (Alm and Bill, 1970) and glucose (Törnquist, 1979a). In the pig the retinal veins form a ring-shaped plexus surrounding the optic nerve as it leaves the globe, and it has been possible to cannulate this plexus and sample pure retinal venous blood (Törnquist *et al.*, 1979).

2. Calorimetric Methods

The temperature of a heated thermocouple introduced into a tissue is determined by the heating current, the blood flow rate in the tissue adjacent to the thermocouple, and, if the thermocouple is placed on the surface of the tissue, the heat loss to the environment. If heating current and environment temperature are kept constant, changes in temperature of the thermocouple can be assumed to be due to changes in blood flow. The disadvantage of the method is that only semiquantitative data can be obtained if there is no quantitative method at hand for calibration in each experiment. The main advantage is that the temperature of the probe is influenced only by blood flow in the tissue within 1–2 mm from the probe. This has permitted separate studies to be carried out on blood flow through the choroid and through the anterior uvea in rabbits (Bill, 1962c; Niesel, 1962; Rodenhäuser, 1963; Namba and Takase, 1978). A similar separation of the various parts of the uvea in cats and dogs is not possible due to the large intrascleral venous plexus.

3. Tissue Clearance of Inert Gases

In many tissues blood flow has been determined by external monitoring of the clearance rate of a radioactive inert gas, such as ^{133}Xe or ^{85}Kr (Lassen and Perl, 1979). Friedman *et al.* (1964b) used this technique in studies on blood flow through the posterior pole of the eye in cats, rabbits, dogs, and monkeys. They found that the decay curve could be separated into four exponential curves with different rate constants. Exchange of tracer with the vitreous body influences the washout, but the exponential rate constant of the initial slope seems to be related only to the choroidal blood flow (Strang *et al.*, 1977). Interruption of retinal blood flow does not affect the washout curves (Friedman and Smith, 1965).

4. Oxygen Tension Measurements

Semiquantitative determinations of changes in retinal blood flow can be obtained by recording the oxygen tension in the vitreous body, close to the retina, by inserting an oxygen-sensitive electrode into the eye (Jacobi and Driest, 1965; Alm and Bill, 1972a; Tsacopoulos *et al.*, 1973). The retina, with the adjacent vitreous body, is unusually well suited for such studies, because continuous recording of the oxygen tension can be obtained without damage to the tissue or disturbance of retinal circulation. One advantage of this method is its comparatively good spatial resolution, and it has been used in studies on the oxygen tension of the surface of the optic disc (Ernest, 1974).

5. Radioactively Labeled Microspheres

There is no doubt that the introduction of commercially available, radioactively labeled microspheres has resulted in a breakthrough in studies on the ocular microcirculation, because this method, for the first time, enables us to make quantitative determinations of blood flow through all the tissues of the eye (O'Day *et al.*, 1971; Alm and Bill, 1972b). The labeled microspheres are injected into the left ventricle of the heart. They follow the bloodstream of the various tissues in proportion to blood flow and become trapped in the capillary beds. Thus, the radioactivity of the tissue is proportional to blood flow. The main advantage of using this technique is that blood flow can be determined without any previous surgical trauma to the eye. One disadvantage is that only a limited number of measurements can be made in the same animal.

6. Various Methods

Blood flowing through the ciliary processes is efficiently cleared of ascorbic acid at low plasma concentrations. This was utilized by Linnér (1952) to determine the effect of unilateral carotid ligation on blood flow through the anterior uvea in rabbits. Bettman and Fellows (1956) measured the change in blood volume of the choroid by external monitoring of

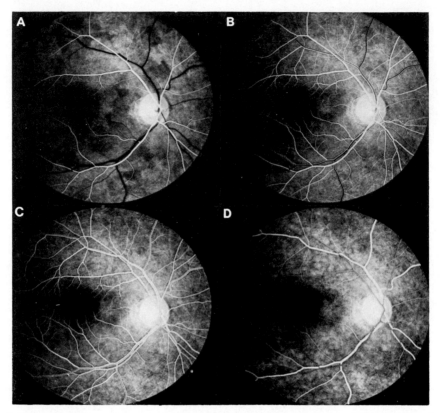

Fig. 8. Fluorescein angiograms. (A) Arterial phase, observe the uneven filling of the background choroidal fluorescens. (B) Early venous phase with laminar filling of the veins. (C) Both arteries and veins are filled with fluorescein. (D) Late venous phase; the arteries are no longer fluorescent.

the radioactivity due to ^{32}P-labeled red blood cells, and they were able to demonstrate a marked increase in blood volume when 10% carbon dioxide in air was inhaled. Trokel (1964) calculated the blood volume and blood flow for the rabbit choroid by determining the light reflected by the fundus after an intravenous (iv) injection of a light-absorbing dye. Direct observations of the choroid and retinal microvasculature through scleral windows at high magnification have shown a continuous flow of blood through all capillaries without evidence of precapillary sphincters or arteriovenous shunts (Wudka and Leopold, 1956; Friedman *et al.*, 1964a). Ernest and Goldstick (1979) determined choroidal blood flow by continuously recording the concentration of a nondiffusible tracer (indocyanin-labeled albumin) in the vortex vein after a bolus injection.

B. Clinical Methods

1. Angiography

Since its first application in human beings (Novotny and Alvis, 1961) fluorescein angiography (Fig. 8) has provided an impressive amount of clinical information on retinal blood flow, and studies of fluorescein angiograms have increased our knowledge of the etiology and pathology of several retinal diseases (Schatz *et al.*, 1978). Fluorescein angiography can also be used in studies on iridial blood flow (Vannas, 1969). Fluorescein angiograms are not suitable for the evaluation of the choroidal circulation because the RPE absorbs most light with wavelength below 700 nm and the light emitted by sodium fluorescein has a peak at 520 nm. Other dyes have a more favorable spectrum. Kogure *et al.* (1970) presented infrared absorption angiograms after intracarotid injections of indocyanid green (ICG), which has an absorption peak at 800 nm. In these angiograms the large choroidal vessels were clearly visualized. An added advantage of using ICG in the interpretation of choroidal blood flow is that, unlike sodium fluorescein, ICG is almost completely bound to albumin and therefore remains within the vascular space of the choriocapillaris. Flower and Hochheimer (1973) found that ICG fluorescence angiograms may give better visualization of the choriocapillaris than absorption angiograms, and for this purpose other dyes, with a better fluorescent yield, have been used in experimental animals (Fig. 9).

2. Blood Flow Velocity Measurements

Flocks *et al.* (1959) and Hickam and Frayser (1965) developed methods to determine the mean retinal circulation time from fluorescein angiograms. If it were possible to calculate the volume of the vascular bed, one would be able to calculate blood flow. Absolute values for the retinal vascular volume cannot be obtained with present techniques. Attempts have been made, however, to estimate the volume from the diameters of large arteries and veins, resulting in retinal blood flow values in arbitrary units (Bulpitt and Dollery, 1971; Hill and Young, 1976). Determinations of blood flow velocity from angiograms require densitometric determinations of a large number of frames, and direct fluorophotometric determinations at two points of the retinal vascular tree seem to be an important improvement (Niesel and Gassman, 1972). Laser doppler velocimetry is another technique utilized in determinations of retinal blood flow velocity (Riva *et al.*, 1972).

The main drawback of making determinations of blood flow on the basis of mean retinal circulation time is the difficulty of observing changes in

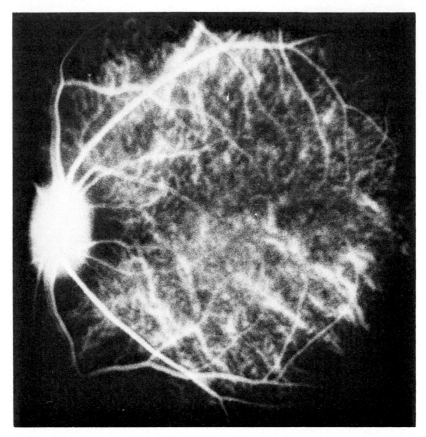

Fig. 9. Fluorescent angiogram from a monkey eye. The dye used in this angiogram (NK 1841) has a peak fluorescence at 720 nm, which results in a better visualization of the choroidal vessels than angiograms obtained with sodium fluorescein. (From Hochheimer, 1979.)

the diameter of small vessels, where a major part of the vascular flow resistance is situated. Thus, delayed appearance of fluorescein in the veins may be due to increased volume in the parts of the vascular bed that cannot be determined from angiograms rather than due to reduced blood flow. An attempt to avoid this difficulty consists of measuring the velocity of blood flow through a short segment of an artery, where measurements of the diameter are more reliable. This is particularly important because the volume is determined by the square of the radius. With present techniques the combined errors of velocity and volume determinations have been reported to result in an error of volume flow of about 30% (Vilser *et al.*, 1979).

3. Various Methods

Measurements of changes in the reflectance of the fundus for orange light, fundus oximetry (Gloster, 1967), during the breathing of oxygen or nitrogen give information on choroidal blood oxygenation. It is possible to observe leukocytes flowing in one's own parafoveal capillaries, particularly against a background illuminated by a diffuse blue light. This entoptic phenomenon has been utilized to observe the effect of increased IOP on the speed of the leukocytes (Riva and Loebl, 1977). Because the diameter of the actual microvessels can be assumed to be constant, flow velocity should be related to volume flow. Thus, this technique enables one to make semiquantitative measurements of changes in blood flow through the parafoveal part of the retina.

IV. Normal Blood Flow

A. Blood Flow Rates and Regional Distribution

Blood flow values in undisturbed eyes have been obtained with the labeled microsphere technique in anesthetized monkeys. The mean values for iris, ciliary body, retina, and choroid were 8, 81, 34, and 677 mg/min, respectively (Alm et al., 1973). Blood flow through the ciliary processes was somewhat higher than that through the ciliary muscle: 227 and 163 g/min per 100 g tissue, respectively. Thus, only about 4% of the total ocular blood flow goes to the retina and 85% to the choroid. Similar relationships between retina and choroid have been demonstrated in cats (Alm and Bill, 1972b), rabbits (O'Day et al., 1971), and pigs (Malik et al., 1976; Törnquist et al., 1979). Figure 10 shows blood flow through the various tissues of the eye in comparison with other tissues. Blood flow through the choroid is three to four times that through the kidney. Blood flow through the retina lies between the values for white and gray matter of the brain. Because both retinal and choroidal blood aid in nourishing the retina, the true nutritional blood flow of the retina may be expressed as the sum of retinal and choroidal blood flow per weight retina. As seen in Fig. 10 this value, about 1000 ml/min per 100 g retina, is about 10 times that of the brain. The reason for this extremely high choroidal blood flow rate is not clear, but it is obvious that a high choroidal blood flow aids in maintaining high concentrations of oxygen and glucose at the RPE, which may be necessary for adequate nutrition of the retina. An additional advantage of the extremely high blood flow rate in the submacular choroid may be the prevention of a harmful increase in the temperature of the mac-

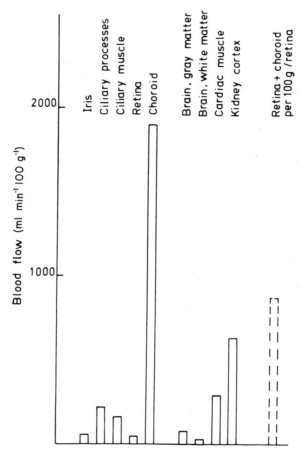

Fig. 10. Blood flow through tissues of the monkey eye. Flow through other tissues is included for comparison. (Values for extraocular tissues are taken from Folkow and Neil, 1971.)

ula. When light is focused on the macula, the heat produced by light absorbance in the RPE increases the temperature of the macula, and this increase becomes more marked at reduced choroidal blood flow (Parver *et al.*, 1980).

In primates there are marked regional differences in blood flow rates within the retina and the choroid (Fig. 11 and Table I). This finding corresponds to the observations on the angioarchitecture presented above and to the fact that the number of photoreceptors per square millimeter is higher in the central retina than in the periphery (Österberg, 1935). No marked regional differences in choroidal or retinal blood flow was ob-

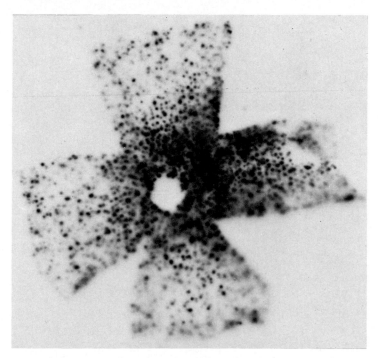

Fig. 11. Autoradiograph of a flat-mount choroid from the left eye of a monkey. The hole in the middle is due to the removed optic nerve head. The black spots represent trapped microspheres, and the number of black spots is a measure of the blood flow rate. Maximal blood flow is seen in the submacular area at two o'clock. (From Alm and Bill, 1973a.)

served in cats (Alm and Bill, 1972b) or pigs (Törnquist *et al.*, 1979). On the other hand, high-speed cineangiography has revealed that moderate regional differences also exist in the cat retina (Laatikainen, 1976).

Although the choriocapillaris constitutes a two-dimensional, dense anastomotic vascular network with anatomically free communications, it has been shown that blood flow through the choroid is lobular and segmental (Hayreh, 1974a, 1975). This has been supported by anatomic studies (Torczynski and Tso, 1976). Thus, a precapillary arteriole feeds the central part of a small lobule, and the draining postcapillary venules constitute the borders of the two-dimensional lobule (Fig. 12). This filling pattern was convincingly demonstrated by fluorescein angiography in monkeys in which the bolus was improved by making the injection into the internal carotid (Hayreh, 1974a). In human beings this pattern can be seen now and then (Fig. 13). Usually, however, the bolus, which is injected into the cubital vein, becomes too diluted. Furthermore, the extreme ra-

TABLE I

Blood Flow through Regions of the Choroid
and Retina[a]

Region	Choroid (mg/min/mm²)	Retina (mg/min/mm²)
Peripapillary	4.53 ± 0.52 (17)	0.18 ± 0.02 (16)
Foveal	6.49 ± 0.62 (17)	0.28 ± 0.03 (16)
Intermediary	2.38 ± 0.35 (17)	0.08 ± 0.01 (16)
Peripheral	0.76 ± 0.14 (17)	0.04 ± 0.01 (16)

[a] Values are mean $\pm$ SE. Numbers in parentheses indicate number of animals. (From Alm and Bill, 1973a.)

pidity of the choroidal blood flow renders it difficult to register each phase of the filling of the choroid.

In addition, the larger choroidal arterioles act as terminal arterioles, resulting in segmental filling of the choroid with watershed zones in the borderline between the areas supplied by two adjacent larger arterioles (Fig. 14).

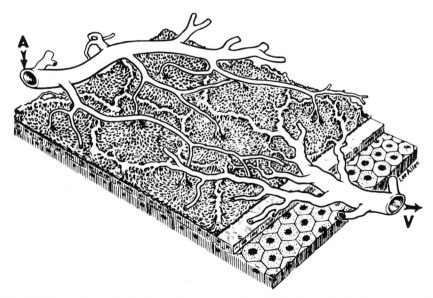

Fig. 12. Three-dimensional schematic representation of choriocapillaris flow pattern. A, Choroidal artery; V, choroidal vein. (From Hayreh, 1975.)

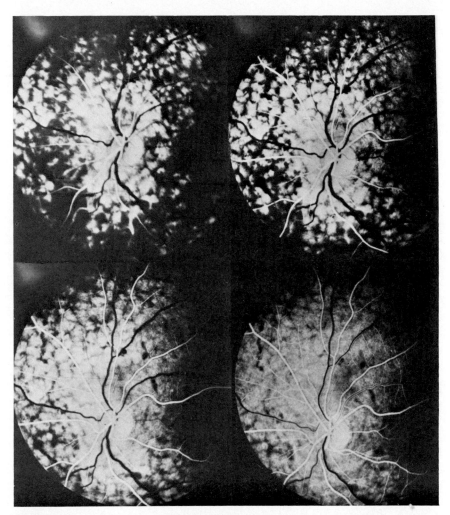

Fig. 13. Fluorescein angiograms from a human eye with reduced blood flow rate. The lobular choroidal filling can easily be observed and is still obvious even in the early venous phase of the retinal angiogram (bottom right).

B. Oxygen and Glucose Supply to the Retina

It is well known that the retina is a metabolically very active tissue and that a large part of the glucose consumed by the retina under *in vitro* conditions is converted to lactate (Graymore, 1969). The possibility of sampling uveal and retinal venous blood in pigs was utilized to study the me-

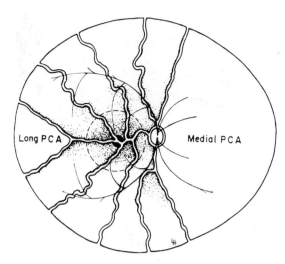

Fig. 14. Diagrammatic representation of areas supplied by various temporal short posterior ciliary arteries and their water-shed zones in the posterior part of the fundus. Stippled circle represents the macular region. PCA, Posterior ciliary artery. (From Hayreh, 1975.)

tabolism of the retina *in vivo* (Törnquist and Alm, 1979). The uveal arteriovenous differences for oxygen and glucose were very low: 0.11 and 0.07 mmol/liter, respectively, corresponding to a net extraction of less than 2%. Similar figures for the uveal arteriovenous difference for oxygen was observed in cats (Alm and Bill, 1970) and dogs (Cohan and Cohan, 1963). The arteriovenous differences for retinal blood were 2.15 and 0.44 mmol/liter for oxygen and glucose respectively, corresponding to net extractions of 35 and 12%, respectively. The oxygen saturation of retinal venous blood obtained in the study on pigs, 56% agrees with values estimated for human retinal venous blood by photometric methods, 59% (Hickam and Frayser, 1966). In the same study on pigs a negative arteriovenous difference for lactate was observed, indicating that the high degree of anaerobic glycolysis obtained under *in vitro* conditions exists also *in vivo*. The results are summarized in Table II, where values for the retina *in vitro* and for the brain are included for comparison. Glucose consumption in the retina is of the same order as that in the cerebral cortex of rats, whereas the oxygen consumption is only about half of that in the rat brain. This results in complete oxidation of less than 40% of the glucose extracted by the retina.

Despite the low arteriovenous differences for the choroid, the extremely high choroidal blood flow results in a larger contribution of retinal metabolism from choroidal than from retinal blood. In the study on pigs

TABLE II
Glucose and Oxygen Consumption of the Pig Retina *in Vivo*[a]

	Present study	Rat retina *in vitro*[b]	Young men brain[c]	Rat cerebral cortex[d]
Glucose consumed	110	187	31	91
Oxygen consumed	224	226	156	491
Fraction of glucose not oxidized[e]	0.63	0.80	0.16	0.10

[a] Values for the retina *in vitro* and the brain obtained by other investigators are included for comparison. (From Törnquist and Alm, 1979.)
[b] Reading and Sorsby (1962).
[c] Sokoloff (1960).
[d] Norberg and Siesjö (1974).
[e] Calculated for oxygen and glucose consumption on the assumption that (1) all oxygen is used for glucose oxidation, (2) 6 mol oxygen is used for oxidation of 1 mol glucose.

about 60% of the oxygen and 80% of the glucose consumed by the retina were delivered by the choroid. In cats it was estimated that about 60% of the oxygen consumed by the retina is delivered by the choroid (Alm and Bill, 1972b).

C. Clinical Implications

1. Collaborative Nutrition of the Retina

The dual nutrition of the retina makes it vulnerable, because occlusion of either vascular bed is enough to cause irreparable damage. Thus, embolization of the retinal vessels (Shakib and Ashton, 1966) or the choroid (Collier, 1967) destroys the inner or outer layers of the retina, respectively. Generally, the choroid seems to be responsible for the photoreceptors, their nuclei, and synapses, whereas the retinal circulation is responsible for the ganglion cells and retinal nerve fibers. Embolization of the retinal arteries in pigs (Dollery *et al.*, 1966) clearly shows that the retinal arterioles are end arteries without anastomoses, except at the capillary level. The slow, recurrent blood flow through these capillary anastomoses is insufficient to prevent retinal damage after arterial occlusion. The retina can withstand complete occlusion of the central retinal artery for about 90 min without irreparable damage. This is considerably longer than the time that the brain can withstand occluded circulation. Possible explanations for this difference have been discussed by Hayreh and Weingast (1980a). An intact choroidal circulation does not seem to be an adequate explanation, because the retina seems to tolerate an IOP above the systolic blood pressure for at least 1 h (Fujino and Hamasaki, 1967). The possibility that the vitreous body is an important metabolite reserve seems unlikely. Anaerobic glycolysis yields only about 5% of the amount of ATP obtained with complete oxidation of glucose (Lehninger, 1975). Thus, oxygen seems to be the limiting factor, and the content of oxygen in the vitreous body is probably too low to sustain the high metabolic demands of the retina for any prolonged time. If we assume a solubility of oxygen in vitreous humor of the same order as that in plasma, 0.03 μl/ml per mm Hg (Guyton, 1966), 4 ml vitreous at a mean oxygen tension of about 20 mm Hg (Alm and Bill, 1972a) would contain a total of about 2.4 μl oxygen, that is, about 100 nmol. This is only about one-third of the amount of oxygen consumed by the pig retina in 1 min *in vivo* (Törnquist and Alm, 1979).

As discussed by Hayreh and Weingast (1980a) one probably very important difference between the retina and the brain that might explain their different reactions to vascular occlusion is the difference in capacity to tolerate edema. In the brain marked edema leads to prolonged occlusion of the intracerebral vascular bed by compression, because the brain is enclosed in a rigid compartment and unable to expand. Thus, even though the original cause of the occlusion is overcome, edema prevents restoration of cerebral blood flow, and the true period of ischemia will be much longer. The edematous retina, on the other hand, can easily expand, and retinal circulation is restored shortly after removal of the occlusion (Hayreh and Weingast, 1980b).

2. Choroidal Filling Pattern

a. Lobular Filling. Occlusion of one terminal choroidal arteriole results in nonperfusion of that lobule. One cannot expect adjacent, perfused lobules to take over the blood supply. This may seem odd when each lobule shares common venous draining channels with adjacent lobules (Fig. 12). However, these venous channels cannot act as feeding vessels and recipient vessels at the same time, because the pressure promoting blood flow through the occluded lobule would then be zero. Thus, occlusion of terminal choroidal arterioles may be expected to result in retinal changes and the well-defined rounded retinal lesions observed in paving-stone degeneration, and acute posterior multifocal plaquoid pigment epitheliopathy may well be due to the involvement of single or grouped choroidal lobules (O'Malley *et al.*, 1965; Deutman *et al.*, 1972).

b. Segmental Filling. Senile macular degeneration has generally been assumed to be caused by circulatory disturbance. One explanation, based on the physiology of the choroidal circulation, has been put forward by Hayreh (1975), who suggests that senile macular degeneration is due to a generalized, chronic, ischemic disorder of the choroid. Underperfusion of the choroid, due to sclerotic choroidal arterioles, would affect principally the periphery of the area of the supply for each short posterior ciliary artery, that is, the watershed zones. The macula seems to be the meeting place of several such watershed zones (Fig. 14), which could explain the disproportionate localization of severe degenerative changes to the macula. However, alternative explanations to senile macular degeneration, based on atrophic changes of the RPE and Bruch's membrane as the primary event, also merit consideration (Green and Key, 1977).

V. Physiologic Regulation of Ocular Blood Flow

A. Arterial and Intraocular Pressures

1. Ocular Perfusion Pressure

In the eye, as elsewhere, the amount of blood flowing (BF) through a vascular bed is determined by the perfusion pressure and the vascular resistance (R), where the perfusion pressure is defined as the difference between the mean arterial pressure and the venous pressure ($P_a - P_v$):

$$BF = (P_a - P_v)/R.$$

The ocular perfusion pressure is then the difference between the pressure in the arteries entering the eye and the veins just leaving it. Presently there is no adequate clinical method for determining the pressure in the ocular arteries. Existing methods are based on the appearance of pulsations and cessation of blood flow in the central retinal artery at increased IOP (Weigelin and Lobstein, 1962; Stepanik, 1977). Because such increments in IOP cause marked reductions in total ocular blood flow and thus in flow through the ophthalmic artery, the pressure fall through the ophthalmic artery is proportionately reduced. Consequently, the IOP at which the blood flow through the retina stops is close to the pressure in the internal carotid artery. There is probably a fall in pressure of 5–10 mm Hg between the internal carotid and the arteries just entering the eye. In normal clinical practice the P_a of the eye is estimated from the mean arterial pressure in the brachial artery. With a pressure in the brachial artery of 140/80 mm Hg the mean pressure is 100 mm Hg (diastolic pressure plus one-third of the pulse pressure). Because the eye is located some 40 cm above the heart, corresponding to a mercury column of about

30 mm, the arterial pressure in the internal carotid at the level of the ophthalmic artery will then be about 70 mm Hg in the upright position. With a further reduction in pressure of 5–10 mm Hg along the ophthalmic artery, the remaining pressure at the globe is 60–65 mm Hg.

Unlike P_a, the P_v of the eye can be determined with great accuracy because it equals IOP, at least at an IOP of 10 mm Hg or more (Bill, 1963). Thus, in the example given above, the remaining ocular perfusion pressure at an IOP of 15 mm Hg will be about 50 mm Hg, and an increase in IOP will cause a corresponding reduction in the perfusion pressure. It is interesting that, at least in young individuals, normal functioning of the eye seems to be consistent with perfusion pressures even of the order of 30 mm Hg or lower (blood pressure 90/60 and IOP 10 mm Hg).

2. Effects of Reductions in Perfusion Pressure on Ocular Blood Flow

In general ophthalmologic practice some 20% of the patients are controlled and treated for glaucoma, a disease that, untreated, is characterized by increased IOP. The effect of a reduced ocular perfusion pressure due to an increased IOP has received much attention both in clinical discussions and in experimental work. It is possible that reductions in perfusion pressure due to low arterial blood pressure may damage the eye as well, because glaucomatous visual field defects have been observed in some eyes with normal or even low IOP, so-called low-tension glaucoma (Drance, 1972). Experimentally the effects on blood flow of blood pressure reductions are less well documented than are those of IOP increments, but in one study in which both methods of reducing the ocular perfusion pressure were utilized the effects on the retinal oxygen tension were similar (Alm and Bill, 1972a). The results discussed below, however, were obtained in studies in which changes in perfusion pressure were induced by changes in IOP.

In most vascular beds blood flow is autoregulated, which means that moderate reductions in perfusion pressure induce a dilation of the resistance vessels. As a result of this local regulation of the vascular resistance, blood flow is largely unchanged within a rather wide range of perfusion pressures (Fig. 15). When there is no autoregulation each reduction in perfusion pressure is followed by a corresponding reduction in blood flow. The local regulation of the vacular resistance is induced by myogenic and metabolic mechanisms (Folkow and Neil, 1971). The stimulus for the myogenic mechanism is the transmural pressure, that is, the difference between the intravascular pressure and the tissue pressure. The stimuli for the metabolic mechanism are a local accumulation of vasodilatory metabolites and a local anoxia.

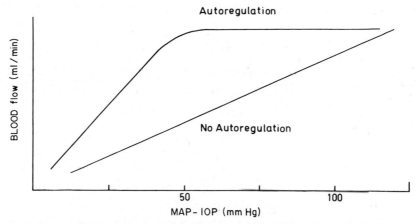

Fig. 15. Diagram illustrating the relationship between blood flow and ocular perfusion pressure in tissues with and without autoregulation. MAP, Mean arterial blood pressure; IOP, intraocular pressure.

a. Uvea. Moderate increments in IOP do not reduce blood flow through the iris or the ciliary body in cats or monkeys (Alm and Bill, 1972b, 1973a); that is, blood flow is autoregulated in the anterior uvea in these species. There is no obvious difference in autoregulatory capacity between the ciliary processes and the ciliary muscle. In rabbits the anterior uvea does not autoregulate (Bill, 1974).

Unlike the anterior uvea the choroid shows no autoregulatory capacity at moderate increments in IOP in either cats or monkeys (Alm and Bill, 1972b, 1973a). In this respect the choroid is rather unique because most tissues show autoregulation. The lack of autoregulation in the choroid implies that a myogenic stimulus has no effect on choroidal blood flow. However, responsiveness to metabolic stimuli cannot be ruled out. The arteriovenous differences in the choroid for metabolic vasodilators, such as carbon dioxide and lactate, are very low (Alm and Bill, 1970; Törnquist and Alm, 1979). Thus, even though choroidal blood flow is reduced by 50% and as a consequence the choroidal arteriovenous difference for, say, carbon dioxide is doubled, the increase in choroidal carbon dioxide tension, in absolute terms, is too small to cause a measurable reduction in choroidal vascular resistance. The existence of an operating metabolic mechanism in the choroid is suggested by studies on the effect of carbon dioxide on choroidal blood flow (see Section V,B,2).

b. Retina and Optic Nerve Head. Several studies have shown that there is efficient autoregulation of retinal blood flow in monkeys, cats, pigs, and rabbits (Alm and Bill, 1972a,b, 1973a; Bill, 1974; ffytche *et al.*,

1974). The fact that the ONH is supplied by branches from the ciliary circulation and not from the central retinal artery has raised the question of whether a defective autoregulation of blood flow in the prelaminar part of the optic nerve is responsible for the damage to the ONH observed in glaucoma. In a study on monkeys Geijer and Bill (1979) determined blood flow through the retina and the various parts of the optic nerve at various levels of IOP. No difference in autoregulation between the peripapillary retina and the prelaminar part of the optic nerve was observed. When IOP was raised above the autoregulatory range of retinal blood flow, flow decreased in the retina and the prelaminar part of the optic nerve, whereas blood flow in the immediate retrolaminar part of the optic nerve tended to increase. This suggests that vasodilatory metabolites diffused from the prelaminar part into the retrolaminar part of the optic nerve.

   c. *Clinical Studies.*   Dobree (1956) found that retinal arteries and veins were dilated when the IOP was increased in glaucoma patients compared to the vessel width when IOP was normalized. This observation suggests autoregulation of blood flow also in human beings. Studies on the bluefield entoptic phenomenon (see Section III,B,3) have also given results that indicate autoregulation of retinal blood flow in human beings (Riva and Loebl, 1977).

3. Effects of Increments in Intraocular Pressure on Retinal Oxygen and Glucose Supply

   The supply of oxygen and glucose from the retinal vessels is probably unchanged within the autoregulatory range of retinal blood flow. Fortunately, the same seems to be true for the supply from choroidal blood. As mentioned above the choroidal arteriovenous differences for oxygen and glucose are about 2%, which, of course, favors a large concentration gradient for diffusion (passive or facilitated) into the retina from the extravascular space of the choroid. A moderate increment in IOP with a subsequent corresponding reduction in choroidal blood flow does not cause any marked changes in the choroidal supply of glucose and oxygen to the retina (Alm and Bill, 1970; Törnquist and Alm, 1979). Thus, a moderate reduction in choroidal blood flow, up to about one-half, is compensated for by an increased extraction of oxygen and glucose from each milliliter of choroidal blood, and the lack of choroidal autoregulation will not have any obvious effect on the metabolic situation of the retina (Fig. 16). This observation supports the assumption that normal choroidal blood flow is in excess of the metabolic demands of the retina and that other factors may determine the level of choroidal blood flow.

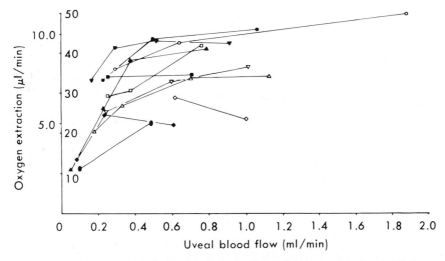

Fig. 16. Oxygen extraction at different levels of uveal blood flow. Uveal blood flow was varied by changing the intraocular pressure. The numbers on the right side of the ordinate indicate oxygen extraction in units of 10^{-5} mmol/l. (From Alm and Bill, 1970.)

4. Clinical Implications

What, then, are the relevant conclusions that can be drawn from these animal experiments in a discussion on the etiology of glaucomatous damage to the ONH? Apparently, no obvious relationship between ocular circulation and glaucomatous damage can be found in these studies. The crucial aspect is the circulation through the prelaminar part of the ONH, where extraretinal vessels are responsible for the supply of capillaries and where the vascular bed is under the full influence of the IOP. The autoregulation in that part of the optic nerve, however, seems to be just as efficient as it is in the retina. Furthermore, neither the stop in anterograde or retrograde axoplasmic flow observed in eyes with increased IOP (Quigley and Anderson, 1976; Minckler *et al.*, 1977) nor early histologic lesions in glaucoma (Vrabec, 1976) indicate that the initial effect is in the prelaminar part of the optic nerve. In fact, accumulation of axoplasmic flow and early histologic lesions are found in the posterior part of the lamina cribrosa and the adjacent part of the retrolaminar optic nerve. At this level blood flow is, if anything, increased when IOP is increased (Geijer and Bill, 1979). Before we dismiss the ocular circulation as a possible etiologic factor in glaucoma damage, however, it should be kept in mind that acute experiments performed in young, healthy monkeys are not a very good model for a chronic disease in elderly patients in whom sclerotic vessels may reduce the autoregulatory capacity. Several clinical studies, based on fluorescein angiography, have indicated a disturbed circulation in the ONH in glaucomatously damaged eyes, with persisting hypoperfusion of the optic disc as a characteristic finding in subjects with glaucoma (Spaeth, 1977). The extent to which such changes are etiologic or secondary is not clear. Explanations not based on the circulation must also be considered. Thus, one may speculate on the effect of a defective BRB at the level of the ONH (Grayson and Laties, 1971) and on the possibility that fibrous strands of the lamina cribrosa compress axons through a shearing stress (Emery *et al.*, 1974; Quigley *et al.*, 1980), which might explain the blockade of axoplasmic flow observed at increased IOP. This theory has received support from the demonstration of regional differences in the structure of the lamina cribrosa, which might explain the selective destruction of axons that gives rise to the characteristic Bjerrum scotoma (Quigley and Addicks, 1981).

B. Arterial Oxygen and Carbon Dioxide Contents

It is well known that changes in the arterial concentration of oxygen and carbon dioxide have marked effects on the cerebral circulation (Folkow and Neil, 1971). A similar sensitivity for the retinal circulation, at least in the case of oxygen, could be inferred from the observations of Cusick *et al.* (1940) on the effect of various levels of oxygen in the arterial blood on the diameters of the retinal vessels. Since then a large number of studies on this subject have been performed and, despite the great variation in techniques and species utilized in these studies, there is a general agreement on the effect of various blood gases on the ocular circulation.

1. Oxygen

Hyperoxia constricts retinal vessels, whereas hypoxia dilates them (Cusick *et al.*, 1940; Frayser and Hickam, 1964; Eperon *et al.*, 1975). Despite the retinal vasoconstriction during oxygen breathing, there is a tendency for oxygen tension to increase in the vitreous body close to the retina (Fig. 17). In monkeys the estimated reduction in retinal blood flow during oxygen breathing is only about 12% (Eperon *et al.*, 1975), which may explain the increase in tissue oxygen tension. Increased diffusion of oxygen from the choroid also tends to increase retinal oxygen tension.

In addition, the retinal vasodilation obtained in hypoxia seems to be inadequate to prevent a fall in retinal oxygen tension (Alm and Bill, 1972a) despite a marked increase in the estimated retinal blood flow (Eperon *et al.*, 1975).

Neither hyperoxia nor hypoxia has any marked effect on blood flow through the uvea (Bill, 1962d; Friedman and Chandra, 1972).

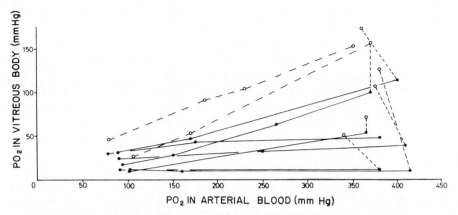

Fig. 17. Effect on the oxygen tension in the vitreous body close to the retina of changes in arterial oxygen tension. In seven experiments the arterial oxygen tension was first increased at a normal arterial carbon dioxide tension (—, PCO_2 = 21–34 mm Hg); then the arterial carbon dioxide tension was also increased, (---, PCO_2 = 60–100 mm Hg). In two experiments (— —) the arterial carbon dioxide tension was increased to levels above 75 mm Hg from the beginning of the experiment, and the arterial oxygen tension then changed in steps. (From Alm Bill, 1972a.)

2. Carbon Dioxide

Carbon dioxide is a very potent vasodilator, and increments in arterial PCO_2 cause marked increments in the retinal oxygen tension in cats (Alm and Bill, 1972a) and monkeys (Tsacopoulos *et al.*, 1973). Retinal blood flow is markedly increased (Table III), and there is a linear relationship between arterial PCO_2 and retinal blood flow (Fig. 18). Increased arterial PCO_2 relieves experimental spasm of the retinal vessels (Elllis and Lende,

TABLE III

Blood Flow through Tissues of the Eye in Normocapnic and Hypercapnic Cats[a]

Tissue	Normocapnia (PCO_2, 26 ± 1 mm Hg)	Hypercapnia (PCO_2, 81 ± 4 mm Hg)
Retina	19 ± 3 (10)	66 ± 17 (4)
Iris	97 ± 21 (12)	245 ± 37 (7)
Ciliary body	223 ± 27 (10)	537 ± 77 (7)
Choroid	1382 ± 185 (10)	3504 ± 371 (4)
Optic nerve	14 ± 2 (12)	93 ± 14 (6)

[a] Blood flow is expressed as grams per 100 g tissue each minute. The values are mean ± SE. Numbers in parentheses indicate number of animals. (Values adapted from Alm and Bill, 1972b.)

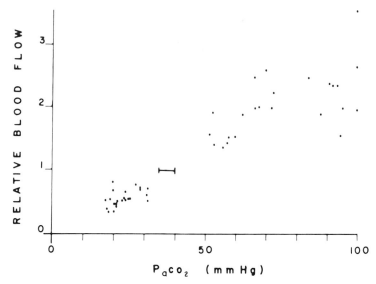

Fig. 18. Graph illustrating the linear relationship between retinal blood flow and arterial carbon dioxide tension in monkeys. Relative retinal blood flow was calculated from fluorescein angiograms. (From Tsacopoulos and David, (1973). *Invest. Ophthalmol.* **12,** 335–347.)

1964), and it seems to release much of the arterial spasm induced by oxygen breathing, because a combination of carbon dioxide and oxygen increases retinal oxygen tension more than oxygen alone (Fig. 17).

Increased arterial PCO_2 increases the blood flow through the uvea in cats (Table III) and rabbits (Bill, 1962d; Alm and Bill, 1972b; Friedman and Chandra, 1972). In baboons Wilson *et al.* (1977) found a linear relationship between arterial PCO_2 and choroidal blood flow similar to that observed for the retina and the brain.

3. Clinical Implications

One may speculate on the possibility of enhancing the chances of retinal survival after occlusion of the central retinal artery by utilizing the choroidal circulation. As discussed by Dollery *et al.* (1969) breathing high concentrations of oxygen may be sufficient for the choroid to take over the entire supply of oxygen to the retina. The possible clinical merits of oxygen therapy were evaluated in cases of retinal vein occlusion in which a mixture of carbon dioxide and oxygen was administered to counteract the vasoconstrictive effect of oxygen (Sedney, 1976). This investigator concluded that in selective cases such therapy might be of some value. In premature infants increased arterial oxygen tension may inhibit the normal

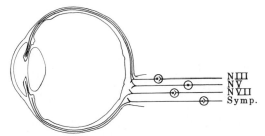

Fig. 19. Summary of current information on the innervation of ocular blood vessels based on anatomic and/or stimulation experiments. The ganglions illustrated are the ciliary ganglion (NIII), the trigeminal ganglion (NV), the pterygopalatine ganglion (NVII) and the superior cervical sympathetic ganglion (Symp.).

development of retinal vessels, which later may cause retrolental fibroplasia (Ashton, 1968).

C. Neural Tone

1. Innervation

The effect of sympathetic stimulation on ocular blood flow has been the subject of several studies during the last 20 years. It has been discovered that stimulation of some of the parasympathetic cranial nerves also causes marked changes in ocular blood flow. Figure 19 summarizes the current information on ocular vascular innervation. Adrenergic nerves to the eye are supplied by the roots of the lower cervical and upper thoracic sympathetic segments, almost exclusively through the ipsilateral superior cervical ganglion. The vessels of the iris, ciliary body, and choroid receive adrenergic innervation, whereas the central retinal artery has a normal adrenergic innervation only up to the point where it passes through the lamina cribrosa (Ehinger, 1966a; Laties and Jacobowitz, 1966). Beyond this point the retinal arteries receive no adrenergic nerves, which means that the main resistance vessels are noninnervated.

A few cholinesterase-positive vascular nerve fibers in the uvea of albino rabbits, rats, and quinea pigs have been described by Ehinger (1966b). Ruskell (1971) described parasympathetic vascular nerve terminals in the primate choroid that are derived from the facial nerve via the pterygopalatine ganglion. Ocular nerve fibers of trigeminal origin running with a maxillary nerve were described in monkeys (Ruskell, 1974). It was concluded that these nerve fibers were sensory, but stimulation experiments, presented below, have indicated that some vasoactive nerve fibers may be included in the maxillary nerve.

2. Sympathetic Nerves

Stimulation of the cervical sympathetic chain causes marked reductions in blood flow through all parts of the uvea in cats, rabbits, and monkeys (Bill, 1962e; Alm, 1977), whereas there is no effect on retinal blood flow. Prolonged stimulation in cats showed a persistent reduction in blood flow through the choroid and the ciliary body, whereas there was a tendency toward escape of the vasoconstriction in the iris (Alm and Bill, 1973b). The lack of effect observed for retinal blood flow is similar to the effect on the brain, in which sympathetic stimulation has no effect or only minimal effect on normal blood flow (Lassen, 1974). The physiologic role of the vascular sympathetic nerves in the eye, as well as in the brain, has only recently been clarified (Bill and Linder, 1976; Bill *et al.*, 1977). Thus, in sympathectomized animals a sudden, marked increase in blood pressure will break through the autoregulatory mechanisms and cause a marked increase in blood flow through the eye and the brain. This overperfusion and pressure increase will also break down the blood–aqueous barrier and the BBB. The same increase in blood pressure during sympathetic stimulation will not cause these effects. Because sudden blood pressure increments, as observed in daily life (Bevan *et al.*, 1969), are the result of increased sympathetic activity, the concomitant cerebral and ocular vasoconstriction will prevent the eye and the brain from overperfusion and breakdown of the barriers.

3. The Oculomotor Nerve

Stimulation of the oculomotor nerve has very complex effects on the ocular blood vessels (Stjernschantz *et al.*, 1976, 1977; Bill *et al.*, 1976; Alm *et al.*, 1976; Stjernschantz and Bill, 1979; Bill and Stjernschantz, 1980).

a. Iris. A marked vasoconstriction takes place in the iris in rabbits, cats, and monkeys when the oculomotor nerve is stimulated stereotactically. Such stimulation is preganglionic since hexamethonium abolishes the effect. The effect can be divided into two parts: one aminergic and one cholinergic. In rabbits, at least, the aminergic component can be blocked by either the α-adrenergic blocker phentolamine or the serotoninergic blocker methysergide. However, the transmitter seems to be neither norepinephrine nor serotonin, since the vasoconstrictor effect is essentially unchanged by sympathectomy, norepinephrine depletion, and serotonin depletion.

The cholinergic effect observed in anesthetized animals seems to represent a normal cholingeric vasoconstrictor tone because marked vasodilation is obtained in conscious rabbits by cholinergic blockade. This is not observed in anesthetized rabbits because pentobarbital anesthesia completely abolishes the spontaneous cholinergic vasoconstrictor tone. Part of the cholinergic vasoconstrictor tone can be induced by light stimulation.

Although most of these results have been obtained in rabbits, it is clear that a combined cholinergic and aminergic constriction of the iris vessels also takes place in monkeys. This is a surprising observation because topically applied cholinergic agonists cause a marked vasodilation in the monkey iris (Alm *et al.*, 1973). Different concentrations of the transmitter at the receptor level may explain this discrepancy. Acetylcholine may constrict or dilate pial vessels *in vitro* depending on its concentration (Edvinsson and Owman, 1975).

b. Ciliary Body.   The effect of oculomotor nerve stimulation on blood flow through the ciliary body shows marked species differences. In rabbits there is a vasoconstriction that is less intense than in the iris and seems to be mainly aminergic. In cats and monkeys there is a vasodilation. Part of this vasodilation may be due to muscular contraction and subsequent release of vasodilatory metabolites.

c. Choroid.   Stimulation of the oculomotor nerve probably has no effect on choroidal blood flow. Although a significant vasodilation was noted in rabbits, it seems likely that this is due to costimulation of the adjacent trigeminal nerve (Stjernschantz *et al.*, 1979).

4. The Facial Nerve

Stimulation of the facial nerve in rabbits (Stjernschantz and Bill, 1980) and monkeys (Nilsson *et al.*, 1980) has marked effects on uveal blood flow. There is a marked vasodilation in the choroid and a less intense vasodilation in the anterior uvea. Cholinergic blockade has no effect on the response. It seems likely that the nerves mediating the vasodilation are the nonadrenergic nerves described by Ruskell (1971). These nerves go with the facial nerve via the pterygopalatine ganglion in monkeys. In cats "peptidergic" nerves with a similar distribution have been found containing vasoactive intestinal peptide (VIP) (Uddman *et al.*, 1980). The assumption that the uveal vasodilation induced by facial nerve stimulation is transmitted by VIP is supported by the observation that VIP injected iv or into the anterior chamber of the eye also causes marked vasodilation in the uvea (Nilsson *et al.*, 1980).

5. The Trigeminal Nerve

Electrical stimulation of the ophthalmic–maxillary trunk of the trigeminal nerve in rabbits induces miosis, vasodilation in the whole uvea, increased

IOP, and breakdown of the blood–aqueous barrier (Stjernschantz *et al.,* 1979). The transmitter mediating this response seems to be substance P, an undecapeptide found in primary sensory neurons (Hökfelt *et al.,* 1975). Thus, trigeminal nerve stimulation releases substance P into the aqueous humor (Bill *et al.,* 1979), and injections of substance P into the anterior chamber produce an effect that is similar to that of trigeminal stimulation (Mandahl and Bill, 1981). It is well known that these effects can also be seen after topical application of a chemical irritant, such as nitrogen mustard (Davson and Huber, 1950), or mechanical stimulation of the rabbit iris (Ambache *et al.,* 1965) and that the response induced by chemical and mechanical stimulation, respectively, is mediated by different transmitters. It seems likely that the transmitter released by chemical stimulation is the same as the transmitter released by electrical stimulation of the nerve, that is, substance P, whereas the substances mediating the effect of mechanical stimulation seem to be prostaglandins. Ambache (1957) isolated a substance from iris extracts, irin, that was subsequently shown to consist of a mixture of prostaglandins. Aspirin, an inhibitor of prostaglandin synthesis, prevents the breakdown of the blood–aqueous barrier after mechanical stimulation, but not after topical application of nitrogen mustard (Neufeld *et al.,* 1972). Topical application of prostaglandins also produces vasodilation, increased IOP, and breakdown of the blood–aqueous barrier (Eakins, 1977). Thus, both prostaglandin and substance P may induce an inflammatory response in the eye, and studies suggest that there is some interaction between these two substances. Low doses of prostaglandin are ineffective if the trigeminal nerve has been sectioned previously (Butler and Hammond, 1980) or if nerve conduction has been blocked by pretreatment with tetrodotoxin (Mandahl and Bill, 1981). These observations suggest that part of the prostaglandin effect in mediated by substance P. Miosis, in particular, seems to be due to substance P, because large doses of prostaglandin produce vasodilation, increased IOP, and breakdown of the blood–aqueous barrier but not miosis in tetrodotoxin-treated eyes. It is also possible that prostaglandins are involved in the response to substance P, because indomethacin pretreatment reduces the response of substance P injected into the anterior chamber (Mandahl and Bill, 1981).

VI. Pharmacologic Regulation of Ocular Blood Flow

The effects of vasoactive drugs on blood flow through the tissues of the eye are of particular interest from two points of view. One is that several ocular diseases are suspected to be caused, at least partially, by a vascular insufficiency. This possibility has been discussed in relation to glaucomatous damage to the optic disc and degenerative changes of the retina, including the macula, and the lens. The other is that characteristics other than the vascular effects are utilized for some vasoactive drugs in normal clinical practice, and the vascular effects will be included whether or not they may be considered beneficial. Thus, both adrenergic agonists (epinephrine) and antagonists (β blockers) and cholinergic agonists (pilocarpine) are used chronically in glaucoma, and long-term therapy with cholinergic antagonists (atropine) is common in various ocular inflammations.

Before we discuss the effects of individual drugs, it is important to stress that two factors are of utmost importance for the effect on ocular blood flow: the mode of administration and the BRB. Topical application of eye drops has an effect mainly on the anterior uvea, and active substance probably does not reach therapeutic concentrations in the posterior pole. In aphakic eyes, however, there is an increased diffusion into the posterior segment of the eye (Kramer, 1976), and repeated administration may have effects on the retina. The cystic macular edema observed after epinephrine therapy in aphakic eyes (Kolker and Becker, 1968) may be such an effect. Retrobulbar injections of vasoactive agents may result in high local concentrations without systemic side effects, whereas systemically administered drugs affect other vascular beds as well. A general vasodilation reduces blood pressure and thus eliminates the benefit of local vasodilation. A reduced intraocular blood volume has been observed after systemic administration of vasodilators (Bettman and Fellows, 1962), and Chandra and Friedman (1972) found different effects on choroidal blood flow when vasoactive agents were given in close-arterial or iv injections, respectively. Dilation or constriction of retinal vessels after systemic administration of vasoactive drugs may thus be due to an autoregulatory response to a change in blood pressure rather than to a pharmacologic effect on the retinal vessels. For this reason only results obtained in studies with topical application, retrobulbar injections, or close-arterial injections are discussed here.

The BRB prevents small water-soluble molecules from entering the retina (see Section VII,A). An analogous situation exists in the brain, and vasoactive drugs usually have only small or inconsistent effects on the cerebral circulation (Sokoloff, 1959). A similar lack of response to many blood-borne vasoactive drugs can be expected in the retina, because the BRB prevents the drug from reaching the receptor on the vascular smooth muscle. For amines an additional BBB mechanism exists, because the endothelial cells contain the catabolic enzyme monoamine oxidase (Bertler

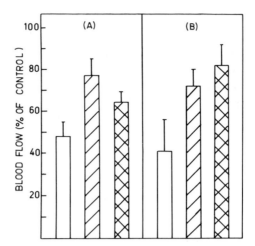

Fig. 20. Effects of blood flow through the anterior uvea in monkeys of stimulation of the cervical sympathetic chain at 10 Hz (A) and with 25 μl 1% *l*-epinephrine applied on the cornea (B), respectively. Blood flow through the treated side is expressed as percentage of blood flow through the control side. Key: □, iris; ▨, ciliary processes; ⊠, ciliary muscle. (Data from Alm, 1977, 1980.)

et al., 1966). A similar mechanism also seems likely for the retinal blood vessels.

A. Vasoconstrictors

1. Uvea

The long posterior ciliary artery from bovine eyes responds to serotonin, norepinephrine, and histamine by contraction *in vitro* with a rank of sensitivities in that order (Dalske, 1974). Close-arterial injections of norepinephrine reduce choroidal blood flow in cats (Chandra and Friedman, 1972). Topical application of epinephrine on the cornea reduces blood flow through the anterior uvea in rabbits (Namba and Takase, 1978) and monkeys (Alm, 1980). In monkeys the effects on the iris and the ciliary body was similar to those obtained by stimulation of the cervical sympathetic chain at 10 Hz (Fig. 20), whereas there was no effect on choroidal blood flow, presumably due to a failure to reach significant concentrations of epinephrine in the posterior pole. Close-arterial injections of dihydroergotamine increase the uveal vascular resistance in both cats and rabbits (Bill, 1962d).

2. Retina

Norepinephrine, angiotensin, and dihydroergotamine injected into the thyroid artery in cats have no effect on retinal oxygen tension, which indicates unchanged retinal blood flow (Alm, 1972). At least for norepinephrine and angiotensin the BRB may be a sufficient explanation for the lack of effect, and these studies do not rule out the existence of retinal vascular receptors. However, direct application of norepinephrine on the exposed retinal vessels in cats did not constrict the vessels (Ellis and Lende, 1964), which makes the existence of α-adrenergic receptors in the vessels of the retina doubtful.

B. Vasodilators

1. Uvea

Isoproterenol has no effect on the isolated long posterior ciliary artery from bovine eyes *in vitro* (Dalske, 1974), and intraarterial injections in cats and rabbits do not induce vasodilation (Bill, 1962e; Chandra and Friedman, 1972). These observations indicate that there are no vascular β-adrenergic receptors in the uvea. A marked uveal vasodilation in cats and rabbits was observed after intraarterial injections of acetylcholine (Bill, 1962e; Chandra and Friedman, 1972), aminophylline, and papaverine (Bill, 1962d). Topical application of pilocarpine or neostigmine eye drops more than doubled blood flow through the iris and the ciliary body in monkeys, whereas there was no effect on choroidal or retinal blood flow (Alm et al., 1973).

2. Retina

Direct application of papaverine, tolazoline hydrochloride and a mixture of caffein and sodium benzoate dilates retinal vessels in cats, whereas nicotin amide, histamine, neostigmine, phenoxybenzamine, and phentolamine have no effect (Ellis and Lende, 1964). Papaverine, tolazoline hydrochloride, and phentolamine also relieve experimental spasm of the retinal arterioles. The effect of various vasodilators on the retinal oxygen tension in cats has been determined (Alm, 1972). Isoproterenol, histamine, nicotinic acid, and xanthinol nicotinate were ineffective, whereas papaverine markedly increased retinal oxygen tension whether administered intraarterially or iv (Fig. 21). Papaverine has also been found to increase retinal blood flow in pigs and monkeys (ffytche et al., 1973). Thus, papaverine is the only vasoactive drug that has been shown consistently to affect retinal blood flow. Normally, papaverine is a comparatively

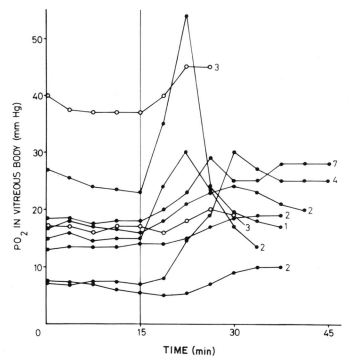

Fig. 21. Oxygen tension in the vitreous body close to the retina was continuously determined while papaverine was injected into the homolateral carotid artery in seven cats and into the femoral vein in two cats. The vertical line at 15 min represents the starting time of the injections. The total dose in milligrams per kilogram body weight is given in each experiment. Key: ○, intravenous injections; ●, intraarterial injections. (From Alm, 1972.)

weak vasodilator (Nickerson, 1970), but it is one of the few drugs that also increase cerebral blood flow (Häggendal, 1965). One obvious explanation is that, unlike most other drugs tested in the studies described above, it is very lipid soluble and therefore easily passes through the BRB and the BBB.

C. Clinical Implications

As far as I know the only possible use of a vasoactive agent in clinical ophthalmology would be the rare case of a recent retinal emboli in which a retrobulbar injection of papaverine, at least theoretically, could be of some value in aiding to release the spasm. With the exception of this rare situation recent textbooks on ocular therapy mention no indications for the use of vasodilators in clinical ophthalmology (Havener, 1978; Fraunfelder and Roy, 1980). The lack of a clinically useful effect on retinal blood flow is due mainly to the efficient autoregulation. This will induce any vasodilation possible in conditions with reduced retinal blood flow, because there will be a local accumulation of carbon dioxide, which is one of the most potent vasodilators known. In fact, nature succeeds in achieving what medical therapy so far has not been able to achieve: a high concentration of a potent agent only at the exact localization where it is most needed.

The fact that the retina, and particularly the fovea, depends on the choroidal circulation, which lacks autoregulation and responds to many vasodilators, is probably the rationale for the previous wide-spread use of vasodilators in, for example, senile macular degeneration. To my knowledge, however, there is no controlled clinical study that shows any beneficial effect of vasodilators in this condition. As pointed out above, systemic administration of vasodilators causes a general vasodilation and a fall in blood pressure, which eliminates the benefit of the drug. For the retina it may even make the situation worse. Vasodilation in the choroid increases blood flow through the ophthalmic artery, which causes a larger pressure drop along this artery. The effect is a reduction of the intravascular pressure in the ophthalmic artery at the point of origin of the central retinal artery and thus a reduced perfusion pressure for retinal blood flow. In a condition with reduced retinal blood flow through a maximally dilated vascular bed, this reduction in perfusion pressure will reduce retinal blood flow even more, and something that might be called an "intraocular steal syndrome" may be created.

VII. Fluid Exchange within the Eye

As discussed in Section II,B there are large structural differences among various microvessels within the eye. Thus, fenestrated capillaries are present within the ciliary processes and the choroid, whereas the retinal and iridial capillaries, together with the nonpigmented epithelium of the ciliary processes and the RPE, constitute the blood–ocular barriers without fenestrations and with the intracellular clefts closed by tight junctions. For the fenestrated capillaries one can expect a relatively high permeability even to large substances, such as proteins. In relation to the retina, lens, vitreous body, and aqueous humor these fenestrated capillaries are situated outside the blood–ocular barriers, and a large permeability of the fenestrated vessels will therefore not have a direct influence on the concentration of large molecules in these tissues and fluids. However, as discussed below, the effect of this high permeability on the colloid osmotic pressure in the various tissues of the eye has important implications for the functioning of the eye, and detailed knowledge of hydrostatic and colloid osmotic pressures is important for discussions on fluid movement within the eye.

The largest and most important ocular fluid movement is the production and drainage of aqueous humor. However, this subject is beyond the scope of this presentation, and the reader is referred to some recent reviews (Bill, 1975, 1981b; Stamper, 1979; Sears, 1981).

A. Permeability of Ocular Blood Vessels

Studies with the single-injection technique have provided valuable information on the permeability of the choroidal and retinal vessels and the RPE (Törnquist, 1979a; Törnquist et al., 1979). Figure 22 illustrates the method. A close-arterial injection is made of a mixture of a labeled test substance and an intravascular reference substance, as a rule [125I]iodoalbumin. The passage of these two substances through the vascular bed is followed by analysis of the radioactivity of repeated venous samples, and the concentration of the test substance, in relation to that of the reference substance, is plotted against time. This plot will show one of three possible patterns.

1.   Test and reference tracers pass through the vascular bed in parallel. This pattern is obtained if the test substance remains within the vascular bed during the entire passage, that is, if the vessels are as impermeable to the test substance as to the reference substance (Fig. 23).

2.   The test substance is delayed, but there is no loss of test substance. The result is a low relative concentration of the test substance in initial venous samples, compensated for by a high relative concentration in the later venous samples. This pattern is obtained if, for example, the test substance passes out into the extravascular space but is then prevented from diffusing any farther by another barrier and rapidly returns to the vascular bed. Passage through the walls or fenestrations of the choriocapillaris but not through the RPE would give such a pattern (Fig. 24).

3.   The test substance is delayed, and there is an incomplete recovery of the test substance. This results in a low relative concentration of the test substance in the initial venous samples, which is not adequately compensated for by high concentrations in the later samples. This pattern could be expected for a test substance that passes through both the walls of the choriocapillaris and the RPE.

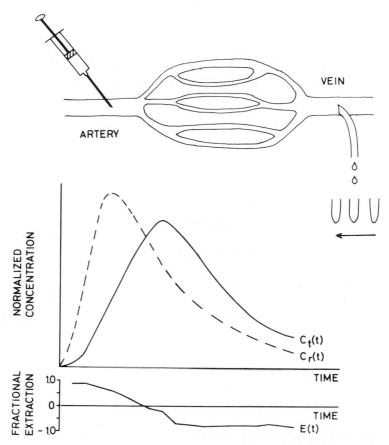

Fig. 22. Schematic illustration of the single-injection technique. The concentrations of the test substance (C_t) and the reference substance (C_r) are determined in repeated venous samples after an arterial bolus injection and plotted against time. The concentrations are normalized with respect to the concentrations in the injectate. For each sample the fractional extraction of the test substance is calculated from the difference between the outflow curves for test and reference substances, respectively. In this example the normalized concentration of test substance is considerably lower than that of the reference substance in the initial samples, whereas the relationship is reversed in later samples. The calculated fractional extraction of the test substance (lower curve) shows an initial extraction that is almost complete, but later it is reduced and even becomes negative. The late negative "extraction" indicates that previously extracted test substance now is returning to the vascular bed. See also Fig. 24. (From Törnquist, 1979b.)

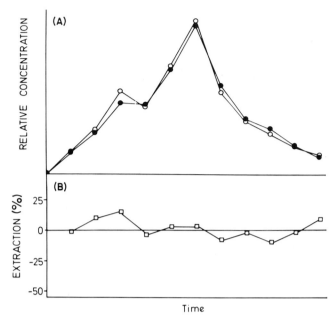

Fig. 23. Venous outflow curves for ²²Na (●) and [¹²⁵I]iodoalbumin (○) from a single-injection experiment on the pig retina. The parallel curves (A) indicate a negligible extraction of ²²Na compared with the intravascular reference tracer [¹²⁵I]iodoalbumin. (From Bill *et al.*, 1980.)

1. Uvea

The iris stroma is in direct contact with the aqueous humor, and there is no complete endothelial layer between the iridial vessels and the aqueous (Inomata *et al.*, 1972). Thus, the iridial microvessels constitute part of the blood–aqueous barrier. Because normally aqueous humor is practically free of proteins, we can assume that the iris vessels are impermeable to such large molecules. It has been shown that they are also largely impermeable to smaller molecules, such as horseradish peroxidase (MW about 40,000) (Smith and Rudt, 1975) and microperoxidase (MW about 2000) (Smith and Rudt, 1973). For even smaller molecules, such as sodium fluorescein (MW about 350), species differences have been reported that correspond to the species differences in structure presented above. Thus, the iridial microvessels are impermeable to sodium fluorescein in monkeys and human beings (McMahon *et al.*, 1975; Laties and Rapoport, 1976) but not in cats (Bellhorn, 1980). Cunha-Vaz *et al.* (1966) found that the iridial microvessels in rats, rabbits, and cats allowed the passage of Trypan blue (MW about 960). The permeability of the iris vessels in rats is

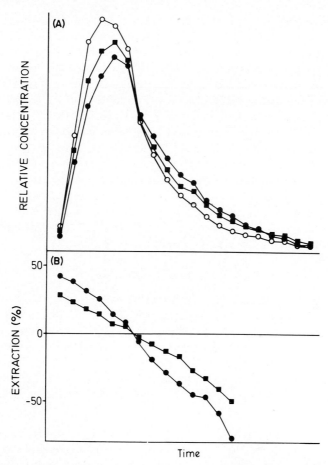

Fig. 24. Venous outflow curves for ^{22}Na (●), ^{51}Cr-EDTA (■), and [^{131}I]iodoalbumin (○) from a single-injection experiment of the cat choroid. The ^{22}Na and ^{51}Cr-EDTA both show an initial positive extraction and a late return into the vascular bed. See also Fig. 22. (From Bill *et al.,* 1981.)

increased by paracentesis, prostaglandins, and histamine (Szalay *et al.,* 1976) and by isoproterenol (Szalay, 1980).

The permeability to proteins of the fenestrated microvessels of the ciliary processes and the choroid has been determined in rabbits (Bill, 1968a). From these data it has been possible to calculate the permeability to albumin, expressed as a permeability coefficient. This coefficient is about 30×10^{-8} cm/sec for these vessels (Bill *et al.,* 1981). This figure is considerably higher than the figures calculated for the nonfenestrated capillaries in skeletal muscle (1.1×10^{-8} cm/sec) and the fenestrated capillaries in the kidney cortex (5.7×10^{-8} cm/sec). For small molecules, such as sodium and Cr-EDTA, the permeability of the choroid is 50–80 times that in skeletal muscle (Törnquist, 1979a). The choroidal venous outflow curves from a single-injection experiment are shown in Fig. 24. This difference between the permeabilities to small molecules for fenestrated and nonfenestrated capillaries in unexpectedly large. Previously, the permeability to, say, sodium in fenestrated capillaries had been assumed to be about 5 times that in skeletal muscle (Renkin, 1978). However, a more recent study found values for the permeability to sodium and Cr-EDTA of the fenestrated capillaries in the salivary glands (Mann *et al.*, 1979) that were similar to those of the choroid. As pointed out by Bill *et al.* (1981) this large permeability of the choriocapillaris is probably necessary to maintain a high concentration of glucose at the RPE and to permit passage of the (retinol-binding protein)–prealbumin complex.

2. Retina and Retinal Pigment Epithelium

As expected the permeability of the retinal vessels is very low (Törnquist *et al.*, 1979). Single-injection experiments (Fig. 23) indicate that the retinal microvessels are as impermeable as those of the brain. Figure 24 illustrates a single-injection experiment on the cat choroid. As mentioned above this pattern indicates that sodium and Cr-EDTA pass through the walls of the choriocapillaris but not through the RPE. Thus, the RPE seems to be as impermeable to sodium as the retinal and cerebral microvessels.

B. Intraocular Pressure Gradients

1. Flow of Fluids and Solutes

Two types of pressure are responsible for the net movement of fluids between different adjacent compartments in the body. One is the hydrostatic pressure, and the other is the osmotic pressure. It is practical to separate the osmotic pressure into the colloid osmotic pressure, due to large molecules such as plasma proteins, and the crystalloid osmotic pressure, due to small molecules such as ions and metabolites.

Solutes are moved by convection, passive diffusion, or transport mechanisms. Convection, or solvent drag, means that solutes are carried along with the flow of water, for example, through large pores. If these pores are large enough to permit the unrestricted passage even of large proteins, one speaks of bulk flow. The drainage of aqueous humor through the trabecular meshwork is an example of bulk flow. Another important example is the flow through the sclera, which permits unrestricted passage even of proteins (Bill, 1971). Convection is determined only by the hydrostatic pressure gradient and osmotic pressures have little influence. One might expect convection to be important for the movement of glucose through the large pores of the choriocapillaris. However, calculations on pore area and hydrostatic and colloid osmotic pressure gradients suggest that the major part of glucose leaves the choriocapillaris by passive diffusion (P. Törnquist, personal communication). Passive diffusion is determined only by the concentration gradient. The movement of solutes via transport mechanisms is dealt with in Section VIII.

Fluid movement through membranes that have very low permeability to proteins is influenced not only by the hydrostatic pressure but also by the colloid osmotic pressure difference. This situation exists for fluid movement between the intra- and extravascular spaces of the choroid and the ciliary processes. If the membrane is impermeable even to small molecules, the crystalloid osmotic pressure is also important. Thus, for fluid movement through the RPE, for example, hydrostatic, colloid osmotic, and crystalloid osmotic pressure gradients are all important.

2. Osmotic Pressures

The crystalloid osmotic pressure in all the tissues and fluids of the eye can normally be assumed to be very close to that of plasma. Normal fluid movements within the eye are thus due to hydrostatic and colloid osmotic pressures. The protein content in the stroma of the ciliary processes and the choroid is 60–70% of that in plasma (Bill, 1968a,b). The colloid osmotic pressure in plasma is about 25 mm Hg (Folkow and Neil, 1971), and that in choroid and ciliary processes is thus about 16 mm Hg. This leaves a colloid osmotic pressure gradient over the vessel wall of about 9 mm Hg. The colloid osmotic pressure in the retina and the iris stroma is close to zero.

3. Hydrostatic Pressures

The hydrostatic pressure in the tissues of the eye is unusually high due to the IOP. There are no large hydrostatic pressure gradients within the eye, but a few probably rather important ones exist. Fatt and Shantinath (1971) determined the hydraulic conductivity of the retina, and from these data they calculated a small pressure difference across the retina of the order of 4×10^{-4} mm Hg. The hydrostatic pressure in the suprachoroid is probably a few millimeters mercury lower than the IOP (van Alphen, 1961; Bill, 1980). This leaves an important hydrostatic pressure difference

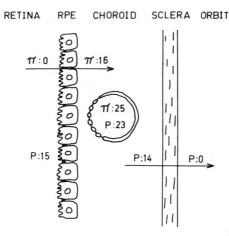

RETINA   RPE   CHOROID   SCLERA   ORBIT

Fig. 25. Schematic illustration of estimated hydrostatic pressure (P) and colloid osmotic (π) pressure differences across the RPE, the walls of the choriocapillaris, and the sclera. See text for explanation.

across the sclera, because the tissue pressure in the orbit is around zero. The hydrostatic pressure in the microvessels is not known. A value for the choriocapillaris can be estimated since it is likely that colloid osmotic and hydrostatic pressure gradients more or less balance each other. As discussed above the colloid osmotic pressure gradient is about 9 mm Hg, tending to absorb fluid into the choroidal vessels. With an IOP of 15 mm Hg and a slightly lower hydrostatic pressure in the choroidal extravascular space, about 14 mm Hg, a mean hydrostatic pressure in the choriocapillaris of 23 mm Hg would balance the colloid osmotic pressure gradient (Fig. 25). A larger hydrostatic pressure would result in a net flow of fluid into the choroidal extravascular space, which would have to be drained through the sclera. Kleinstein and Fatt (1977) determined the transscleral outflow in rabbits and found a value corresponding to 1.1 μl/min for the whole sclera. The true figure is probably somewhat higher, because flow through the transscleral perivascular spaces was not included in these experiments. Still, it is obvious that the capacity to remove fluid through the sclera is limited, and it is clear that a large net filtration from the choroid would create a problem because choroidal edema is obtained as soon as the net filtration exceeds the transscleral outflow. Thus, the highly permeable choriocapillaris makes it unlikely that the hydrostatic pressure gradient exceeds the colloid osmotic pressure gradient by more than a few millimeters mercury. The unusually abrupt transition of large arterioles into choriocapillaris might suggest an unusually high pressure in the choriocapillaris. However, pressure reduction along a vascular bed is related to resistance and flow, and the large choroidal blood flow will cause a large pressure drop along the precapillary arterioles.

In the ciliary processes we may expect a capillary hydrostatic pressure a few millimeters of mercury larger than in the choroid because the Starling equilibrium does not apply. There has to be a net outward filtration corresponding to the aqueous humor production and the outward flow through the sclera.

4. Interaction between Hydrostatic and Colloid Osmotic Pressures

It is important to remember that the colloid osmotic pressure in the tissue to some extent is influenced by the hydrostatic pressure in the capillaries. This is probably very fortunate for the functioning of the eye. If the colloid osmotic pressures were stable, the net movement of fluid into or out of the fenestrated capillaries in the choroid and the ciliary processes would be very sensitive to changes in the hydrostatic pressure in the capillaries. In a tissue with highly permeable microvessels and limited means of removing tissue fluid, this would lead to edema even with small increments in the capillary pressure. However, changes in the hydrostatic pressure gradient induce changes in the colloid osmotic pressure gradient. For example, if the pressure in the choriocapillaris is Fig. 25 were increased by 5 mm Hg, there would suddenly be a net outward filtrating pressure of 5 mm Hg. This would force protein-free fluid into the stroma, dilute the tissue proteins, and consequently reduce the cholloid osmotic pressure in the stroma. The result would be an increased colloid osmotic pressure gradient that would, at least partly, balance the increase in the hydrostatic pressure gradient. A reduction in the hydrostatic pressure gradient would correspondingly reduce the colloid osmotic pressure gradient by reabsorption of tissue fluid.

C. Pressure-Induced Fluid Movement

The net movements of fluid in the eye have already been touched on in the previous section and will only be summarized here. A small net movement of fluid from the vitreous body through the retina and into the choroid is likely to take place, mainly due to the pressure gradient caused by differences in colloid osmotic pressure. Ion pumps in the RPE may aid in maintaining this flow (Marmor et al., 1980a). A hydrostatic pressure gradient slightly larger than the colloid osmotic pressure gradient results in a net outward filtration in the ciliary processes, whereas the net movement of fluid through the walls of the choriocapillaris probably is very small and might just as well be inward as outward. The hydrostatic pressure in the suprachoroid causes a net outward flow of protein-rich fluid through the sclera. This flow is important because the eye lacks lymph vessels, and a transscleral flow is the only available means of disposing of the small amount of proteins that leak through the fenestrated capillaries of the choroid and the ciliary processes.

D. Clinical Implications

1. Increased Permeability of Blood–Ocular Barriers

The concentration of sodium fluorescein in the vitreous body can be determined *in vivo* by vitreous fluorophotometry (Cunha-Vaz and Maurice, 1967). This technique has been utilized in studies of diseases in which an increased permeability of the blood–ocular barriers is suspected. Thus, an increased fluorescence of the vitreous body, 1 h after an iv injection of sodium fluorescein, has been demonstrated in early diabetes (Cunha-Vaz *et al.*, 1975), in experimental arterial hypertension in rats (Dutton *et al.*, 1980), and in female carriers of X-linked, recessive retinitis pigmentosa (Gieser *et al.*, 1980).

2. Net Flow from the Vitreous to the Choroid

The small net flow of fluid from the vitreous body through the retina and into the choroid is probably important for the attachment of the retina (Fatt and Shantinath, 1971). Studies on the effect of the osmolarity of the vitreous body support this assumption. Thus, intravitreal injections of hypertonic solutions detach the retina in rabbits and monkeys (Marmor, 1979; Marmor *et al.*, 1980b). The slight ocular hypotoni observed in eyes with retinal ruptures and detachment may be due to an increase in the flow from the vitreous body. Also, the reduction in IOP observed after scatter photocoagulation of the retina (Schiödte *et al.*, 1980) may have a similar etiology.

3. Net Filtration in the Ciliary Processes

Aqueous humor production is considered to result from active secretion through the ciliary epithelium. A certain fraction due to ultrafiltration has been proposed by several investigators, and it has even been suggested that a major fraction, about 70%, is due to ultrafiltration (Green and Pederson, 1972; Pederson and Green, 1973). As discussed by Bill (1975) the pressure gradients needed to support this hypothesis are of some interest. The hypothesis requires a positive pressure gradient across the ciliary epithelium with the highest pressure in the ciliary stroma. The colloid osmotic pressure in the stroma of the ciliary processes is around 16 mm Hg (see Section VII,B,2), whereas that in the protein-free aqueous humor is zero. Thus, to balance the colloid osmotic pressure gradient we need a hydrostatic pressure in the stroma that is 16 mm Hg above the IOP. To obtain ultrafiltration through the ciliary epithelium even higher pressures are needed. Because a hydrostatic tissue pressure only a few millimeters mercury higher than the surrounding pressure creates a marked edema in most tissues (Guyton, 1966), it is difficult to understand how a tissue pressure at least 16 mm Hg above the IOP can exist in the ciliary processes without any sign of edema. Another consequence of a high tissue pressure in the ciliary processes would be that protein-rich fluid would be forced out through the ciliary muscle and the iris stroma into the anterior chamber (Bill, 1975).

Still, there is no doubt that ultrafiltration is involved in aqueous humor production since there has to be a net filtration from the capillaries into the stroma of the ciliary processes. Because several vasoactive drugs are used in the treatment of glaucoma, the question is often raised as to whether the effect on IOP can partly be explained by a reduced aqueous humor production secondary to a reduced filtration for the blood vessels. Studies on the effect on blood flow and on aqueous humor production of pilocarpine, epinephrine, and sympathetic stimulation do not support this assumption. The important parameter in this connection, the pressure in the capillaries, can be expected to be increased by the vasodilator pilocarpine and decreased by the vasoconstrictor epinephrine and by sympathetic stimulation. This would lead to increased and decreased net filtration, respectively. However, the effects on aqueous humor production in monkeys is quite opposite to the expected effects on the net filtration. Thus, pilocarpine reduces aqueous humor production (Bill and Wålinder, 1966), whereas epinephrine and sympathetic stimulation have no effect or cause a slight increase (Bill, 1969, 1970). This indicates that aqueous humor production normally is independent of the pressure in the capillaries of the ciliary processes. It seems likely that this is a consequence of secondary compensatory adjustments of the colloid osmotic pressure in the ciliary processes by changes in the volume of the tissue fluid, as discussed above. *In vitro* studies on the rabbit ciliary processes have shown marked volume changes during secretion (Berggren, 1964).

4. Choroidal Edema

Obviously, there is an upper limit to the increments in transmural hydrostatic pressure gradients that can be compensated for by small, clinically unnoticed adjustments in tissue volume. When this limit is surpassed,

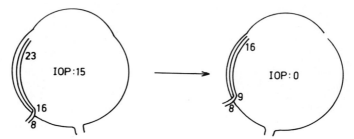

Fig. 26. Effect of surgical opening of the eye on the estimated hydrostatic pressures. Opening of the eye (right) reduces the IOP to zero while the hydrostatic pressure in the veins leaving the eye has to remain slightly above the pressure in the extraocular recipient veins in order to ensure blood flow. In this example the transmural hydrostatic pressure difference at the capillary level is thus increased from 8 (23 minus 15) to 16 mm Hg. See text.

there is an edema. Choroidal edema, or choroidal detachment (which is an unfortunate term since it tends to worry the patient and gives no information concerning the etiology), is a common clinical diagnosis. When the eye is surgically opened, the IOP is suddenly reduced to zero. The pressure in the ocular veins is also reduced, but not to the same extent. As pointed out above the IOP and the venous pressure in the eye are practically equal as long as the IOP is 10 mm Hg or higher. At lower levels of IOP the venous pressure becomes higher than the IOP. The reason for

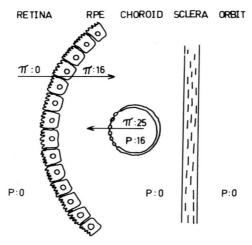

Fig. 27. Effect of a reduction of the IOP to zero on the estimated hydrostatic and colloid osmotic pressure differences across the RPE, the walls of the choriocapillaris, and the sclera. In comparison with Fig. 25 there is now a net outward flow from the choriocapillaris and no flow through the sclera, which results in a choroidal edema. See text.

this is that it must always be higher than the pressure in the recipient extraocular veins. Thus, when the IOP becomes zero the transmural hydrostatic pressure gradient for the ocular blood vessels increases with a value corresponding to the pressure in the extraocular veins (Fig. 26). This pressure gradient moves a large amount of fluid into the choroidal stroma. Since the transscleral hydrostatic pressure gradient now is zero, this fluid cannot be disposed of, and a choroidal edema will arise (Fig. 27). Such a choroidal edema can be observed in 90% of all eyes immediately after a lens extraction (Swyers, 1972). The loss of a transscleral hydrostatic pressure gradient is probably the most important etiologic factor in postsurgical choroidal edema, but sometimes an increased intravascular pressure may be enough to create a "spontaneous" choroidal edema. One example may be the choroidal edema reported in connection with arteriovenous fistulas in the cavernous sinus (Klein *et al.*, 1978).

VIII. Exchange of Metabolites between Blood and Retina

The impermeability of the BRB to small water-soluble molecules means that metabolic substrates are also prevented from reaching the retina in adequate amounts by passive diffusion only. In the brain, where a similar situation exists because of the BBB, this problem is solved by the existence of carriers for various metabolic substrates (Rapoport, 1976; Bradbury, 1979). Studies indicate that metabolic substrates pass the BRB by carrier-mediated transport systems very similar to those present in the BBB.

Monosaccharides, such as glucose, pass the BRB by a stereospecific, carrier-mediated transport (Dollery *et al.*, 1971; Törnquist, 1979a). The carrier has characteristics that are similar to those of the hexose carrier that transports monosaccharides across the BBB, and several hexoses, besides D-glucose, can be transported across the BRB by this carrier (Alm *et al.*, 1981). A saturable transport through the BRB has also been demonstrated for lactic acid (P. Törnquist and A. Alm, unpublished observation).

Since various metabolic substrates can diffuse freely from the posterior chamber to the retina, transport through the ciliary epithelium also may be of some importance for the retina. Both glucose and amino acids pass the ciliary epithelium into the posterior chamber (Reddy, 1979; Bito and DeRousseau, 1980). Reddy *et al.* (1977a,b) have suggested that amino acids are transported by active, energy-dependent transport systems into the posterior chamber and then, after having passed through the vitreous body by passive diffusion, out of the eye by active transport through the RPE. An active transport of amino acids through the RPE, in the retina-to-choroid direction, has also been found in studies on the isolated RPE of the frog *in vitro* (Miller and Steinberg, 1976). An outward transport of anions, such as sodium fluorescein, through the BRB *in vivo* has been proposed by Cunha-Vaz and Maurice (1967). Active transport mechanisms are, as a rule, unidirectional. However, *in vivo* studies on rats suggest that there are also carriers in the BRB that can transport amino acids in the blood-to-retina direction (Crockett *et al.*, 1978). Other studies on rats have shown the existence of at least three different carriers, one for neutral amino acids, one for basic amino acids, and one for taurine (Törnquist and Alm, 1982). A similar arrangement is found in the BBB. These seemingly contradictory observations on the transport of amino acids through the BRB make it clear that further studies are needed to elucidate this subject.

IX. Concluding Remarks

A recapitulation of our present knowledge of the ocular microcirculation emphasizes the large amount of information that has appeared during the last 10 years, mainly as a consequence of new techniques for the determination of ocular blood flow. The value of a quantitative technique is indisputable, and for studies on experimental animals the labeled microsphere technique has proved very valuable. The main drawback with studies on experimental animals is that they seldom provide a good model for human ocular diseases, such as glaucoma, senile macular degeneration, and diabetic proliferative retinopathy. Therefore, there is an urgent need for a nontraumatic technique that is also applicable to human beings. Improvements in the techniques for the determination of vascular diameters and flow velocity in the retina may eventually make these valuable tools in studies on the circulation of the diseased retina, particularly if they are combined with known techniques for estimating the oxygen saturation of retinal venous blood. A complete evaluation of the metabolic situation of the retina, however, requires quantitative information on choroidal blood flow as well. At present there is no technique that promises to provide such information, but it is hoped that choroidal angiography may expand our knowledge of the involvement of the choroidal circulation in various diseases. Vitreous fluorophotometry is another clinical technique that promises to become a valuable tool, particularly in the management and evaluation of diabetic retinopathy. Its main advantage seems to be the possibility of detecting small changes in the permeability of the BRB. This may give early information on the effect of various treatments of diabetes and diabetic retinopathy.

For studies on the physiology of ocular blood flow in experimental animals the most interesting recent development is the information on previously unknown, marked vasoactive effects of stimulation of some of the parasympathetic cranial nerves. The clinical implications of these findings are difficult to evaluate, but further studies to reveal their physiologic role will be of considerable interest.

Acknowledgment

This work was supported in part by research grant B80-04X-05655-02 from the Swedish Medical Research Council.

References

Alm, A. (1972). *Acta Ophthalmol.* **50,** 707–719.
Alm, A. (1977). *Exp. Eye Res.* **25,** 19–24.
Alm, A. (1980). *Invest. Ophthalmol. Visual Sci.* **19,** 487–491.
Alm, A., and Bill, A. (1970). *Acta Physiol. Scand.* **80,** 19–28.
Alm, A., and Bill, A. (1972a). *Acta Physiol. Scand.* **84,** 261–274.
Alm, A., and Bill, A. (1972b). *Acta Physiol. Scand.* **84,** 306–319.
Alm, A., and Bill, A. (1973a). *Exp. Eye Res.* **15,** 15–29.
Alm, A., and Bill, A. (1973b). *Acta Physiol. Scand.* **88,** 84–94.
Alm, A., Bill, A., and Young, F. A. (1973). *Exp. Eye Res.* **15,** 31–36.
Alm, A., Stjernschantz, J., and Bill, A. (1976). *Exp. Eye Res.* **23,** 609–613.
Alm, A., Törnquist, P., and Stjernschantz, J. (1977). *Bibl. Anat.* **16,** 24–29.
Alm, A., Törnquist, P., and Mäepea, O. (1981). *Acta Physiol. Scand.* **113,** 81–84.
Ambache, N. (1957). *J. Physiol. (London)* **135,** 114–132.
Ambache, N., Kavanagh, L., and Whiting, J. M. C. (1965). *J. Physiol. (London)* **176,** 378–408.
Anderson, D. R. (1974). *Int. Glaucoma Symp. Albi 1974,* pp. 15–20.
Ascher, K. W. (1942). *Am. J. Ophthalmol.* **25,** 31–38.
Ashton, N. (1968). *Br. J. Ophthalmol.* **52,** 505–531.
Bellhorn, R. (1980). *Invest. Ophthalmol. Visual Sci.* **19,** 870–877.
Berggren, L. (1964). *Invest. Ophthalmol.* **3,** 266–272.
Bernstein, M. H., and Hollenberg, M. J. (1965). *Invest. Ophthalmol.* **4,** 1016–1025.
Bertler, Å., Falck, B., Owman, Ch., and Rosengren, E. (1966). *Pharmacol. Rev.* **18,** 369–385.
Bettman, J. W., and Fellows, V. G. (1956). *Am. J. Ophthalmol.* **42,** 161–167.
Bettman, J. W., and Fellows, V. (1962). *Trans. Am. Acad. Ophthalmol. Otolaryngol.* **66,** 480–487.

Bevan, A. T., Honour, A. J., and Stott, F. H. (1969). *Clin. Sci.* **36**, 329–344.
Bill, A. (1962a). *Acta Physiol. Scand.* **55**, 101–110.
Bill, A. (1962b). *Arch. Ophthalmol. (Chicago)* **67**, 156–162.
Bill, A. (1962c). *Acta Ophthalmol.* **40**, 1–18.
Bill, A. (1962d). *Acta Soc. Med. Ups.* **67**, 122–134.
Bill, A. (1962e). *Acta Physiol. Scand.* **56**, 70–81.
Bill, A. (1963). *Arch. Ophthalmol. (Chicago)* **69**, 780–782.
Bill, A. (1968a). *Acta Physiol. Scand.* **73**, 204–219.
Bill, A. (1968b). *Acta Physiol. Scand.* **75**, 511–522.
Bill, A. (1969). *Exp. Eye Res.* **8**, 35–43.
Bill, A. (1970). *Exp. Eye Res.* **10**, 31–46.
Bill, A. (1971). *Exp. Eye Res.* **11**, 195–206.
Bill, A. (1974). *Invest. Ophthalmol.* **13**, 954–958.
Bill, A. (1975). *Physiol. Rev.* **55**, 383–417.
Bill, A. (1980). *In* "The Blood-Retinal Barriers" (J. G. Cunha–Vaz, ed.), pp. 179–193. Plenum, New York.
Bill, A. (1981). *In* "Adler's Physiology of the Eye: Clinical Application" (R. A. Moses, ed.), 7th ed., pp. 184–203. Mosby, St. Louis, Missouri.
Bill, A. (1983). *Handb. Physiol. Sect. 2 Cardiovasc. Sys.* (in press).
Bill, A., and Linder, J. (1976). *Acta Physiol. Scand.* **96**, 114–121.
Bill, A., and Stjernschantz, J. (1980). *Acta Physiol. Scand.* **108**, 419–424.
Bill, A., and Wålinder, P.-E. (1966). *Invest. Ophthalmol.* **5**, 170–175.
Bill, A., Stjernschantz, J., and Alm, A. (1976). *Exp. Eye Res.* **23**, 615–622.
Bill, A., Linder, M., and Linder, J. (1977). *Bibl. Anat.* **16**, 30–35.
Bill, A., Stjernschantz, J., Mandahl, A., Brodin, E., and Nilsson, G. (1979). *Acta Physiol. Scand.* **106**, 371–373.
Bill, A., Törnquist, P., and Alm, A. (1980). *Trans. Opthalmol. Soc. U.K.* **100**, 332–336.
Bito, L., and DeRousseau, C. J. (1980). *In* "The Blood-Retinal Barriers" (J. G. Cunha–Vaz, ed.), pp. 133–163. Plenum, New York.
Bradbury, M. (1979). *In* "The Concept of a Blood-Brain Barrier," pp. 406–407. Wiley, Chichester.
Brown, G. C., and Shields, J. A. (1979). *Arch. Ophthalmol. (Chicago)* **97**, 84–92.
Bulpitt, C. J., and Dollery, C. T. (1971). *Cardiovasc. Res.* **5**, 406–412.
Butler, J. M., and Hammond, B. R. (1980). *Br. J. Pharmacol.* **69**, 495–502.
Chandra, S. R., and Friedman, E. (1972). *Arch. Ophthalmol. (Chicago)* **87**, 67–69.
Cohan, B. E., and Cohan, S. B. (1963). *Am. J. Physiol.* **205**, 60–66.
Collier, R. H. (1967). *Arch. Ophthalmol. (Chicago)* **77**, 683–695.
Crockett, M. E., Daniel, P. M., and Pratt, O. E. (1978). *J. Physiol. (London)* **280**, 39P.
Cunha-Vaz, J. G., and Maurice, D. M. (1967). *J. Physiol. (London)* **191**, 467–486.
Cunha-Vaz, J. G., Shakib, M., and Ashton, N. (1966). *Br. J. Ophthalmol.* **50**, 441–453.
Cunha-Vaz, J. G., Abrev, J. R. F., Campos, A. J., and Figo, G. M. (1975). *Br. J. Opthalmol.* **59**, 649–656.
Cusick, P. L., Benson, O. O., Jr., and Boothby, W. M. (1940). *Proc. Mayo Clinic,* **15**, 500–502.
Dalske, F. (1974). *Invest. Ophthalmol.* **13**, 389–392.
Davson, H., and Huber, A. (1950). *Ophthalmologica* **120**, 118–124.
Deutman, A. F., Oosterhuis, J. A., Boen-Tab, T. N., and Aan de Kerk, A. L. (1972). *Br. J. Ophthalmol.* **56**, 863–874.
Dobree, J. H. (1956). *Br. J. Ophthalmol.* **40**, 1–13.
Dollery, C. T., Henkind, P., Paterson, J. W., Ramalho, P. S., and Hill, D. W. (1966). *Br. J. Ophthalmol.* **50**, 285–324.

Dollery, C. T., Bulpitt, C. J., and Kohner, E. M. (1969). *Invest. Ophthalmol.* **6,** 588–594.
Dollery, C. T., Henkind, P., and Orme, M. (1971). *Diabetes* **20,** 519–521.
Drance, S. M. (1972). *Br. J. Ophthalmol.* **56,** 223–229.
Dutton, J. J., Krupin, T., Waltman, S. R., Koloms, B. A., and Becker, B. (1980). *Arch. Ophthalmol.* (*Chicago*) **98,** 731–733.
Eakins, K. E. (1977). *Exp. Eye Res.* **25,** (Suppl.) 483–498.
Edvinsson, L., and Owman, C. (1975). *In* "Blood Flow and Metabolism in the Brain" (A. M. Harper, J. D. Miller, and J. O. Rowan, eds), pp. 1–18. Churchill Livingstone, Edinburgh.
Ehinger, B. (1966a). *Invest. Ophthalmol.* **5,** 42–52.
Ehinger, B. (1966b). *Acta Univ. Lund. Sect. 2,* No. 2.
Elgin, S. S. (1964). *Invest. Ophthalmol.* **3,** 417–426.
Ellis, P. P., and Lende, R. A. (1964). *Arch. Ophthalmol.* (*Chicago*) **71,** 706–711.
Emery, J. M., Landis, D., Paton, D., Boniuk, M., and Craig, J. M. (1974). *Trans. Am. Ophthalmol. Soc.* **90,** 290–297.
Eperon, G., Johnson, M., and David, N. J. (1975). *Invest. Ophthalmol.* **14,** 342–352.
Ernest, J. T. (1974). *Invest. Ophthalmol.* **13,** 101–106.
Ernest, J. T., and Goldstick, T. K. (1979). *Exp. Eye Res.* **29,** 7–14.
Fatt, I., and Shantinath, K. (1971). *Exp. Eye Res.* **12,** 218–226.
ffytche, T. J., Bulpitt, C. J., Archer, D., Kohner, E. M., and Dollery, C. T. (1973). *Br. J. Ophthalmol.* **57,** 910–920.
ffytche, T. J., Bulpitt, C. J., Kohner, E. M., Archer, D., and Dollery, C. T. (1974). *Br. J. Ophthalmol.* **58,** 514–522.
Flocks, M., Miller, J., and Chad, P. (1959). *Am. J. Ophthalmol.* **48,** 3–6.
Flower, R. W., and Hochheimer, B. F. (1973). *Invest. Ophthalmol.* **12,** 248–261.
Folkow, B., and Neil, E. (1971). *In* "Circulation." Oxford Univ. Press, New York.
Fraunfelder, F. T., and Roy, F. H. (1980). *In* "Current Ocular Therapy." Saunders, Philadelphia, Pennsylvania.
Frayser, R., and Hickam, J. B. (1964). *Invest. Ophthalmol.* **3,** 427–431.
Friedman, E., and Chandra, S. R. (1972). *Arch. Ophthalmol.* (*Chicago*) **87,** 70–71.
Friedman, E., and Smith, T. R. (1965). *Invest. Ophthalmol.* **4,** 1122–1128.
Friedman, E., Smith, T. R., and Kuwabara, T. (1964a). *Invest. Ophthalmol.* **3,** 217–226.
Friedman, E., Kopald, H. H., and Smith, T. R. (1964b). *Invest. Ophthalmol.* **3,** 539–547.
Fujino, T., and Hamasaki, D. J. (1967). *Arch. Ophthalmol.* (*Chicago*) **78,** 757–765.
Geijer, C., and Bill, A. (1979). *Invest. Ophthalmol. Visual Sci.* **18,** 1030–1042.
Gieser, D. K., Fishman, G. A., and Cunha-Vaz, J. G. (1980). *Arch. Ophthalmol.* (*Chicago*) **98,** 307–310.
Gloster, J. (1967). *Exp. Eye Res.* **6,** 187–212.
Graymore, C. (1969). *In* "The Eye" (H. Davson, ed.), Vol. 1, 2nd ed., pp. 601–645. Academic Press, New York and London.
Grayson, M. C., and Laties, A. M. (1971). *Arch. Ophthalmol.* (*Chicago*) **85,** 600–609.
Green, K., and Pederson, J. E. (1972). *Am. J. Physiol.* **222,** 1218–1226.
Green, W. R., and Key, S. N. (1977). *Trans. Am. Ophthalmol. Soc.* **75,** 180–254.
Guyton, A. C. (1966). *In* "Textbook of Medical Physiology," 3rd ed., pp. 453–583. Saunders, Philadelphia, Pennsylvania.
Häggendal, E. (1965). *Acta Physiol. Scand.* **66** (Suppl. 258), 55–79.
Havener, W. H. (1978). *In* "Ocular Pharmacology," 4th ed., pp. 499–504. Mosby, St. Louis, Missouri.
Hayreh, S. S. (1962). *Br. J. Ophthalmol.* **46,** 212–247.
Hayreh, S. S. (1974a). *Albrecht von Graefes Arch. Klin. Exp. Ophthalmol.* **192,** 165–179.
Hayreh, S. S. (1974b). *Trans. Am. Acad. Ophthalmol. Otolaryngol.* **78,** 240–254.

Hayreh, S. S. (1975). *Br. J. Ophthalmol.* **59**, 631–648.
Hayreh, S. S. (1978). *In* "Glaucoma: Conceptions of a Disease" (K. Heilmann, and K. T. Richardson, eds.), pp. 78–96. Thieme, Stuttgart.
Hayreh, S. S., and Weingast, T. A. (1980a). *Br. J. Ophthalmol.* **64**, 818–825.
Hayreh, S. S., and Weingast, T. A. (1980b). *Br. J. Ophthalmol.* **64**, 896–912.
Henkind, P. (1967). *Invest. Ophthalmol.* **6**, 103–108.
Henkind, P., and Levitsky, M. (1969). *Am. J. Ophthalmol.* **68**, 979–986.
Henkind, P., and Oliveira, L. F. (1967). *Invest. Ophthalmol.* **6**, 520–530.
Henkind, P., Hansen, R. I., and Szalay, J. (1979). *In* "Physiology of the Human Eye and Visual System" (R. E. Records, ed.), pp. 98–155. Harper, Hagerstown, Maryland.
Hickam, J. B., and Frayser, R. (1965). *Invest. Ophthalmol.* **4**, 876–884.
Hickam, J. B., and Frayser, R. (1966). *Circulation* **33**, 302–325.
Hill, D. W., and Young, S. (1976). *Exp. Eye Res.* **23**, 35–45.
Hochheimer, B. F. (1979). *Exp. Eye Res.* **29**, 141–143.
Hogan, M. J., Alvarado, J. E., and Weddell, J. E. (1971). *In* "Histology of the Human Eye," pp. 320–522. Saunders, Philadelphia, Pennsylvania.
Hökfelt, T., Kellerth, J. O., Nilsson, G., and Pernow, B. (1975). *Brain Res.* **100**, 235–252.
Holmberg, Å. (1979). *Arch. Ophthalmol.* (*Chicago*) **62**, 949–951.
Hudspeth, A. J., and Yee, A. G. (1973). *Invest. Ophthalmol.* **12**, 354–365.
Inomata, H., Bill, A., and Smelser, G. K. (1972). *Am. J. Ophthalmol.* **73**, 893–907.
Ishikawa, T. (1963). *Invest. Ophthalmol.* **2**, 1–15.
Jacobi, K. W., and Driest, J. (1965). *Ber. Dtsch. Ophthalmol. Ges.* **67**, 193–198.
Justice, J., and Lehmann, R. P. (1976). *Arch. Ophthalmol.* (*Chicago*) **94**, 1355–1358.
Klein, R., Meyers, S. M., Smith, J. L., Myers, F. L., Roth, H., and Becker, B. (1978). *Arch. Ophthalmol.* (*Chicago*) **96**, 1370–1373.
Kleinstein, R. N., and Fatt, I. (1977). *Exp. Eye Res.* **24**, 335–340.
Knutson, S. L., and Sears, M. L. (1973). *Am. J. Ophthalmol.* **76**, 648–654.
Kogure, K., David, N. J., Yamanouchi, U., and Choromokos, E. (1970). *Arch. Ophthalmol.* (*Chicago*) **83**, 209–214.
Kolker, A. E., and Becker, B. (1968). *Arch. Ophthalmol.* (*Chicago*) **79**, 552–562.
Kramer, S. G. (1976). **9**, 73–86.
Laatikainen, L. (1976). *Exp. Eye Res.* **23**, 47–56.
Lassen, N. A. (1974). *Circ. Res.* **34**, 749–760.
Lassen, N. A., and Perl, W. (1979). *In* "Tracer Kinetic Methods in Medical Physiology," p. 2. Raven, New York.
Laties, A. M., and Jacobowitz, D. (1966). *Anat. Rec.* **156**, 383–396.
Laties, A. M., and Rapoport, S. (1976). *Arch. Ophthalmol.* (*Chicago*) **94**, 1086–1091.
Leber, T. (1903). *In* "Handbuch der gesamten Augenheilkunde" (A. van Graefes, and T. Saemisch, eds.), 2nd ed., Vol. 2, pp. 20–26. Engelman, Leipzig.
Lehninger, A. (1975). *In* "Biochemistry," 2nd ed., pp. 419–517. Worth, New York.
Levitsky, M., and Henkind, P. (1969). *Am. J. Ophthalmol.* **68**, 986–996.
Lieberman, M. F., Maumenee, A. E., and Green, W. R. (1976). *Am. J. Ophthalmol.* **82**, 405–423.
Linnér, E. (1952). *Acta Physiol. Scand.* **26**, 70–78.
Majno, G. (1966). *Handb. Physiol. Sect. Circ.* **3**, 2293–2359.
Malik, A. B., van Heuven, W. A. J., and Satler, L. F. (1976). *Invest. Ophthalmol.* **15**, 492–495.
Mandahl, A., and Bill, A. (1981). *Acta Physiol. Scand.* **112**, 331–338.
Mann, G. E., Smaje, L. H., and Yudilevich, D. L. (1979). *J. Physiol.* (*London*) **297**, 335–354.

Marmor, M. F. (1979). *Invest. Ophthalmol. Visual Sci.* **18**, 1237–1244.

Marmor, M. F., Abdul-Rahim, A. S., and Cohen, S. D. (1980a). *Invest. Ophthalmol. Visual Sci.* **19**, 893–903.

Marmor, M. F., Martin, L. J., and Tharpe, S. (1980b). *Invest. Ophthalmol. Visual Sci.* **19**, 1016–1029.

McMahon, R. T., Tso, M. O. M., and McLean, I. W. (1975). *Am. J. Ophthalmol.* **80**, 1058–1065.

Michaelson, I. C. (1954). *In* "Retinal Circulation in Man and Animals," pp. 4–11, 74–79. Thomas, Springfield, Illinois.

Miller, S., and Steinberg, R. H. (1976). *Exp. Eye Res.* **23**, 177–189.

Minckler, D. S., Bunt, A. H., and Johanson, G. W. (1977). *Invest. Ophthalmol. Visual Sci.* **16**, 426–441.

Namba, H., and Takase, M. (1978). *Jpn. J. Ophthalmol.* **22**, 437–448.

Neufeld, A. H., Jampol, L. M., and Sears, M. L. (1972). *Nature (London)* **238**, 158–159.

Nickerson, M. (1970). *In* "The Pharmacological Basis of Therapeutics" (L. S. Goodman, and A. Gilman, eds.), 4th ed., pp. 753–754. Macmillan, London.

Niesel, P. (1962). *In* "Messungen von experimentell erzeugten Änderungen der Aderhautdurchblutung bei Kaninchen," pp. 16–40. Karger, Basel and New York.

Niesel, P., and Gassman, H. B. (1972). *Ophthalmologica* **165**, 297–302.

Nilsson, S., Linder, J., and Bill, A. (1980). *In Abstr. Int. Cong. Eye Res. 4th,* p. 29P.

Norberg, K., and Siesjö, B. K. (1974). *J. Neurochem.* **22**, 1127–1129.

Novotny, H. R., and Alvis, D. L. (1961). *Circulation* **24**, 82–86.

O'Day, D. M., Fish, M. B., Aronson, S. B., Pollycove, M., and Coon, A. (1971). *Arch. Ophthalmol. (Chicago)* **86**, 205–209.

O'Malley, P., Allen, R. A., Straatsam, B. R., and O'Malley, C. C. (1965). *Arch. Ophthalmol. (Chicago)* **73**, 169–182.

Österberg, G. (1935). *Acta Ophthalmol.* **13**(Suppl. 6), 64–88.

Parver, L. M., Auker, C., and Carpenter, D. O. (1980). *Am. J. Ophthalmol.* **89**, 641–646.

Pederson, J. E., and Green, K. (1973). *Exp. Eye Res.* **15**, 265–276.

Quigley, H. A., and Addicks, E. M. (1981). *Arch. Ophthalmol. (Chicago)* **99**, 137–143.

Quigley, H. A., and Anderson, D. R. (1976). *Invest. Ophthalmol.* **15**, 606–616.

Quigley, H. A., Flower, R. W., Addicks, E. M., and McLeod, D. S. (1980). *Invest. Ophthalmol. Visual Sci.* **19**, 505–517.

Rapoport, S. I. (1976). *In* "Blood-Brain Barrier in Physiology and Medicine," pp. 177–206. Raven, New York.

Reading, H. W., and Sorsby, A. (1962). *Vision Res.* **2**, 315–325.

Reddy, V. N. (1979). *Invest. Ophthalmol. Visual Sci.* **18**, 1000–1018.

Reddy, V. N., Chakrapani, B., and Lim, C. P. (1977a). *Exp. Eye Res.* **25**, 543–554.

Reddy, V. N., Thompson, M. R., and Chakrapani, B. (1977b). *Exp. Eye Res.* **25**, 555–562.

Renkin, E. M. (1978). *Microvasc. Res.* **15**, 123–135.

Ring, H. J., and Fujino, T. (1967). *Arch. Ophthalmol. (Chicago)* **78**, 431–444.

Riva, C. E., and Loebl, M. (1977). *Invest. Ophthalmol. Visual Sci.* **16**, 568–571.

Riva, C., Ross, B., and Benedek, G. B. (1972). *Invest. Ophthalmol.* **11**, 936–944.

Rodenhäuser, J. H. (1963). *In* "Uveadurchblutung und Augeninnendruck." Enke, Stuttgart.

Ruskell, G. L. (1971). *Exp. Eye Res.* **12**, 166–172.

Ruskell, G. L. (1974). *J. Anat.* **118**, 195–203.

Saari, M. (1975). *Albrecht von Graefes Arch. Klin. Exp. Ophthalmol.* **194**, 87–93.

Schatz, H., Burton, T. C., Yanuzzi, L. A., and Rabb. M. F. (1978). *In* "Interpretation of Fundus Fluorescein Angiography." Mosby, St. Louis, Missouri.

Schiödte, S. N., Scherfig, E., and Nissen, O. J. (1980). *Acta Ophthalmol.* **58**, 369–376.
Sears, M. (1981). *In* "Adler's Physiology of the Eye: Clinical Application" (R. A. Moses, ed.), 7th ed., pp. 204–226. Mosby, St. Louis, Missouri.
Sedney, S. C. (1976). *In* "Photocoagulation in Retinal Vein Occlusions," pp. 100–111. Junk, The Hague.
Shakib, M., and Ashton, N. (1966). *Br. J. Ophthalmol.* **50**, 325–354.
Smith, R. S., and Rudt, L. A. (1973). *Am. J. Ophthalmol.* **76**, 937–947.
Smith, R. S., and Rudt, L. A. (1975). *Invest. Ophthalmol.* **14**, 556–560.
Sokoloff, L. (1959). *Pharmacol. Rev.* **11**, 1–86.
Sokoloff, L. (1960). *Handb. Physiol. Sect. Neurophysiol.* **3**, 1849.
Spaeth, G. L. (1977). *In* "The Pathogenesis of Nerve Damage in Glaucoma," pp. 131–132. Grune & Stratton, New York.
Stamper, R. L. (1979). *In* "Physiology of the Human Eye and Visual System" (R. E. Records, ed.), pp. 156–182. Harper, Hagerstown, Maryland.
Stepanik, J. (1977). *Arch. Ophthalmol. (Chicago)* **95**, 698–699.
Stjernschantz, J., and Bill, A. (1979). *Invest. Ophthalmol. Visual Sci.* **18**, 99–103.
Stjernschantz, J., and Bill, A. (1980). *Acta Physiol. Scand.* **109**, 45–50.
Stjernschantz, J., Alm, A., and Bill, A. (1976). *Exp. Eye Res.* **23**, 461–469.
Stjernschantz, J., Alm, A., and Bill, A. (1977). *Bibl. Anat.* **16**, 42–46.
Stjernschantz, J., Geijer, C., and Bill, A. (1979). *Exp. Eye Res.* **28**, 229–238.
Strang, R., Wilson, T. M., and MacKenzie, E. T. (1977). *Invest. Ophthalmol. Visual Sci.* **6**, 571–576.
Swyers, E. M. (1972). *Arch. Ophthalmol. (Chicago)* **88**, 632–634.
Szalay, J. (1980). *Exp. Eye Res.* **31**, 299–311.
Szalay, J., Goldberg, R., and Klug, R. (1976). *Acta Ophthalmol.* **54**, 731–742.
Torczynski, E., and Tso, M. O. (1976). *Am. J. Ophthalmol.* **81**, 428–440.
Törnquist, P. (1979a). *Acta Physiol. Scand.* **106**, 425–430.
Törnquist, P. (1979b). *Acta Univer. Ups. Abstr. Uppsala Diss. Fac. Sci.,* **326.**
Törnquist, P., and Alm, A. (1979). *Acta Physiol. Scand.* **106**, 351–357.
Törnquist, P., and Alm, A. (1982). *Invest. Ophthalmol. Visual Sci.* **22**(Suppl.), 179.
Törnquist, P., Alm, A., and Bill, A. (1979). *Acta Physiol. Scand.* **106**, 343–350.
Toussaint, D., Kuwabara, C. T., and Cogan, D. G. (1961). *Arch. Ophthalmol. (Chicago)* **65**, 575–581.
Trokel, S. (1964). *Arch. Ophthalmol. (Chicago)* **71**, 88–92.
Tsacopoulos, M., and David, N. J. (1973). *Invest. Ophthalmol.* **12**, 335–347.
Tsacopoulos, M., Baker, R., Johnson, M., Strauss, J., and David, N. J. (1973). *Invest. Ophthalmol.* **12**, 449–455.
Uddman, R., Alumets, J., Ehinger, B., Håkanson, R., Lorén, I., and Sundler, F., (1980). *Invest. Ophthalmol. Visual Sci.* **19**, 878–885.
Van Alphen, G. W. (1961). *Ophthalmologica.* **142**, (Suppl.), 1–92.
Vannas, A. (1969). *Acta. Ophthalmol.* **105**, (Suppl.), 1–75.
Vegge, T. (1972). *Z. Zellforsch. Mikrosk. Anat.* **123**, 195–208.
Vilser, W., Brabdt, H. P., Königsdörfer, E., Wittwer, B., Jütte, A., Dietze, V., and Deufrains, A. (1979). *Albrecht von Graefes Arch. Klin. Exp. Ophthalmol.* **212**, 41–47.
Vrabec, F. (1976). *Albrecht von Graefes Arch. Klin. Exp. Ophthalmol.* **198**, 223–234.
Weigelin, E., and Lobstein, A. (1962). *In* "Ophthalmodynamometrie," pp. 37–46. Karger, Basel and New York.
Wilson, T. M., Strang, R., and MacKenzie, E. T. (1977). *Invest. Ophthalmol. Visual Sci.* **16**, 576–580.

Wise, G. N., Dollery, C. T., and Henkind, P. (1971). *In* "Retinal Circulation," p. 26.
    Karger, New York.
Wudka, E., and Leopold, I. H. (1956). *Arch. Ophthalmol. (Chicago)* **55,** 857–885.
Wybar, K. C. (1954). *Br. J. Ophthalmol.* **38,** 513–527.

8 Microcirculation of the Heart

Harvey V. Sparks, Jr.
Jerry B. Scott
Mark W. Gorman

I. Functional Anatomy

The following is a brief synopsis of coronary vessel anatomy. For a more detailed treatment of the subject, the reader is referred to chapters in the *Handbook of Physiology* by Gregg and Fisher (1963) and Berne and Rubio (1979). The right and left coronary arteries originate from the aorta at the sinuses of Valsalva behind the anterior and posterior cusps of the aortic valve, respectively. The left coronary artery courses down and to the left of the anterior interventricular groove, between the pulmonary artery and the left atrial appendage. The length of the left common coronary artery is 1.0–1.5 cm in man and only 2.0–4.0 mm in the dog. The left common coronary artery bifurcates into anterior descending and circumflex branches. In many primates including man, a septal artery arises from the left anterior descending branch. It is important to note that in dogs, pigs, cattle, and small laboratory animals, a septal artery frequently arises just prior to bifurcation of the left coronary artery. The anterior descending artery courses along the anterior ventricular groove toward the apex and supplies adjacent left and right ventricular myocardium as well as a large portion of the interventricular septum. The circumflex artery follows

THE PHYSIOLOGY AND PHARMACOLOGY
OF THE MICROCIRCULATION, VOLUME 1

the auriculoventricular groove to the left and, depending on the species, terminates before, at, or beyond the posterior sulcus.

The right coronary artery courses anteriorly behind the pulmonary artery and follows the auriculoventricular groove to the right border of the heart. In many species this vessel supplies the right ventricular free wall, right atrium, and atrioventricular and sinoatrial nodes. When the right coronary artery gives rise to the posterior descending artery, it supplies a major portion of the posterior right and left ventricles, and such hearts are designated right coronary artery dominant. When the posterior right and left ventricles are supplied by the circumflex artery, the circulation is designated left coronary dominant. The dog is a good example of the latter. Anatomic studies indicate a fairly even balance between left and right coronary arteries of human hearts. However, in a perfusion study of human hearts left coronary flow was greater than right coronary flow in most hearts studied (Vasko et al., 1961). Studies in the authors' laboratory indicate that in the pig the right coronary artery supplies 50% (range 35–65%) of the heart.

Most (80–85%) blood that enters the coronary arteries passes through a capillary bed and is returned to the right atrium via the anterior cardiac veins (right coronary) or the coronary sinus (left coronary). The remainder of the blood entering the coronary system returns via direct connections between the arteries and veins and the heart chambers.

II. The Coronary Vessel Wall

Coronary arteries and arterioles contain a medium of densely packed smooth muscle cells. Berne and Rubio (1979) have estimated that smooth muscle cells from large coronary arteries of the dog have a mean cross-sectional area of $13.03 \pm 0.56 \ \mu m^2$ and a cell perimeter of $20.56 \pm 0.83 \ \mu m$. Using these data they calculated a cell thickness of $2.54 \ \mu m$. Assuming a muscle length of $150 \ \mu m$ this yields a calculated cell volume of $2000 \ \mu m^3$. These figures are similar to those quoted for other smooth muscle.

Studies of isolated vessel strips of coronary arteries indicate that the properties of coronary smooth muscle are similar to those of most other vessels of the same size. We shall briefly mention a few characteristics of coronary smooth muscle as an introduction to our consideration of vascular control. Most details of vascular smooth muscle function are not covered here. The membrane potential of dog coronary artery smooth muscle is approximately -55 mV (Harder et al., 1979). Dog coronary artery smooth muscle does not exhibit spontaneous action potentials, but other species, including man, may do so (Ross *et al.*, 1980).

Activation of contraction in vascular smooth muscle apparently starts with a rise in intracellular Ca^{2+} concentration. There are four determinants of intracellular Ca^{2+} concentration at any given time: (*a*) passive influx across the plasma membrane down its concentration and electrical gradient; (*b*) release from cellular sources including sarcoplasmic reticulum, mitochondria, surface vesicles, and the plasma membrane; (*c*) active efflux across the plasma membrane; and (*d*) intracellular sequestration, including active transport into cell organelles (mitochondria, sarcoplasmic reticulum, and surface vesicles) and passive binding to membranes. Intracellular Ca^{2+} concentration is then determined by the rates of each of these processes (Bohr and Webb, 1978).

The removal of Ca^{2+} from the bathing solution or the use of Ca^{2+} antagonists (e.g., verapamil or nifedipine) demonstrates that the development of coronary smooth muscle active tension is very sensitive to the influx of extracellular Ca^{2+} (Fleckenstein, 1977).

At least three classes of potent coronary vasodilators seem to act by reducing Ca^{2+} influx: adenosine (Harder *et al.*, 1979), nitroglycerin, (Harder *et al.*, 1979), and calcium antagonists (Fleckenstein, 1977). α-Receptor-mediated contraction of coronary smooth muscle appears to be initiated by increased influx of extracellular Ca^{2+} (Van Breeman and Siegel, 1980).

Agents that modify the activity of the Na^+–K^+ pump alter intracellular Ca^{2+} concentration (Bohr and Webb, 1978). Two mechanisms account for this. First, changing intracellular Na^+ concentration results in parallel changes in Ca^{2+} concentration. This is because Ca^{2+} is extruded from smooth muscle cells via a tightly coupled cotransport with Na^+ in which the electrochemical gradient for Na^+ entry serves as a source of energy for Ca^{2+} exit. Also, Ca^{2+} and Na^+ compete for carrier sites. If intracellular Na^+ concentration rises, this inhibits the efflux of Ca^{2+}. Thus, agents such as ouabain that inhibit the Na^+–K^+ pump can cause contraction by raising intracellular Na^+ concentration, which in turn raises Ca^{2+} concentration. (Ouabain may cause coronary constriction for other reasons as well. It stimulates Ca^{2+} influx and, in addition, has distant actions that may lead to coronary constriction. See Section IV,D.) The second mechanism is related to the fact that the Na^+–K^+ pump is electrogenic. Its inhibition causes membrane depolarization and this increases Ca^{2+} concentration.

The coronary vessel wall is the main site of prostaglandin (PG) biosynthesis within the heart (Sivakoff *et al.*, 1979). At least two cellular elements, endothelium and smooth muscle, are sites of PG synthesis (Alexander and Gimbrone, 1976; Gimbrone and Alexander, 1975). The primary vasoactive metabolite of arachidonic acid produced by coronary vessels appears to be PGI_2, although other PGs, such as $PGF_{2\alpha}$ and PGE_2, are also produced. Prostaglandin I_2 is a vasodilator, whereas $PGF_{2\alpha}$ and thromboxane A_2 (TxA_2) are vasoconstrictors (Needleman and Isakson, 1980). Prostaglandin E_2 contracts some isolated preparations but causes vasodilation *in vivo* (Nutter and Crumley, 1972). Constrictor PGs may well act by enhancing the influx of Ca^{2+}. Vasodilators may act by stimulating the $Na^+ - K^+$ pump (Lockette *et al.*, 1980) and/or by elevating cyclic AMP. Stimuli for endogenous synthesis of PGs as well as their role in vascular regulation are discussed in Section IV,D.

III. Microcirculatory Exchange

Coronary capillary endothelium is characterized anatomically as nonfenestrated endothelium. There is approximately one capillary for every muscle fiber and an intercapillary distance of approximately 15–20 μm (Bassingthwaighte *et al.*, 1973). Capillary density (≈ 3500/mm²) of the capillary bed appears to be uniform from subepicardium to subendocardium, but interendothelial clefts may be larger in subendocardial capillaries (Giacomelli *et al.*, 1975). Capillary endothelial cells are richly populated with vesicles, especially at the venous end of the capillaries. It is likely that interendothelial clefts correspond to the "small-pore system." The vesicles, operating either via transcellular movement or as continuous transendothelial channels, could correspond to the "large-pore system." Alternatively, a larger set of interendothelial gaps may serve this function (Berne and Rubio, 1979). Capillaries run parallel to myocardial fibers with functional capillary lengths of approximately 500–1000 μm. Capillaries branch so that there are two to four times as many venous connections as arterial to the capillary network. Individual capillaries of canine myocardium are approximately 5.6 μm in diameter, which means that red blood cells must be deformed during their passage. Juxtaposition of arterioles and venules suggests that the arteriovenous (A–V) shunting of gases observed in functional studies may be the result of diffusion from arteries to veins. This suggests that diffusional shunting of O_2 and CO_2 is also possible (Bassingthwaighte *et al.*, 1973; Roth and Feigl, 1981).

Although there have been many intravital studies of the capillaries of other tissues, very few such studies exist for the heart because the movement of the beating heart makes such studies so difficult. Honig and coworkers have approached this problem by using a motion picture camera and studying the frames that are in focus. This group has found that systemic hypoxia and hypercapnia reduce and hyperoxia increases intercapillary distance (Honig and Bourdeau-Martini, 1974; Bourdeau-Martini, 1973).

Much of our understanding of capillary exchange in the heart results from the study of the behavior of diffusible tracers injected into the heart. This type of experiment coupled with more and more sophisticated models of capillary transport has produced a significant body of information about the overall behavior of myocardial capillaries. These studies of diffusible tracers are compatible with a model of capillary transport in which lipid-soluble substance diffuse through the entire capillary wall (in fact, even through small arterioles and venules), whereas water-soluble substances diffuse through water-filled clefts between endothelial cells (Duran et al., 1977; Duran and Yudilevich, 1978). Thus, only a very small percentage of total capillary surface area is available for diffusion of water-soluble substances. In general, these studies indicate that the capillary endothelial barrier is similar to that of skeletal muscle in its permeability characteristics but that its total surface area is several times larger. Tracer studies indicate that the number of capillaries capable of exchange increases with increased flow and that this is not the result of vasodilation, but instead of increased flow per se (Rose et al., 1980). Although the data are not yet adequate to give a complete picture, it appears that the capillary surface area available for exchange increases approximately twofold when myocardial blood flow is increased from baseline to maximum values. Other tracer studies are interpreted as indicating that, during myocardial ischemia, capillary surface area falls, but permeability increases (Harris et al., 1981). There is much to be studied on the role of the capillary wall and Starling forces across the wall in influencing the formation of myocardial edema.

IV. Determinants of Coronary Blood Flow

A. General Considerations

Under resting conditions myocardial blood flow in man is reported to range between 0.7 and 1.0 ml min^{-1} g^{-1} (for references see Marshall and Shepherd, 1968; Haddy, 1969). Left ventricular flow under similar conditions is 0.7–0.8 ml min^{-1} g^{-1} in the awake dog (Cobb et al., 1974) and 0.97 ml min^{-1} g^{-1} in the awake calf (Manohar et al., 1979). Right ventricular flow in the awake dog ranges from 0.37 ± 0.1 to 0.67 ± 0.04 ml min^{-1} g^{-1} (Murray et al., 1979a) and in the calf is reported to be 0.73 ± 0.13 ml min^{-1} g^{-1} (Manohar et al., 1979). Right ventricular flow in the anesthetized dog ranges from 0.49 ± 0.06 (Weiss *et al.*, 1978) to 0.68 ± 0.09 ml min^{-1} g^{-1} (Ely, 1979) and in the anesthetized pig is 0.89 ± 0.12 ml min^{-1} g^{-1} (Ely *et al.*, 1981). For a given weight of tissue it appears that the ratio of left ventricular flow to right ventricular flow is 1.29 for the calf (Manohar *et al.*, 1979) and 1.43 for the dog (Domenech and Ayuy, 1974).

Coronary sinus O_2 content is between 5 and 7 vol %. This gives an A–V O_2 difference of 10–12 vol. %. The above measurements of coronary blood flow combined with this A–V O_2 difference give a myocardial O_2 consumption in man at rest of between 8.5 and 11.3 ml min^{-1} 100 g^{-1} (Marshall and Shepherd, 1968; Haddy, 1969). Coronary sinus O_2 content remains relatively constant in a variety of circumstances including exercise, excitement, hyperthyroidism, and anemia. This demonstrates the remarkable capacity of the left ventricle to adjust blood flow to match its metabolism.

Oxygen consumption of the muscle supplied by the right coronary artery of pig (Ely *et al.*, 1981) and dog (Weiss *et al.*, 1978) is of the order of 5.0–7.0 ml min^{-1} 100 g^{-1}, substantially less than that of the left ventricle. Most studies indicate that right coronary flow (milliliters per gram each minute) is only slightly less than left coronary flow. This would suggest that the A–V difference for this tissue is less and that the O_2 content of the venous blood draining this muscle is higher. However, Weiss and coworkers (1978) used a microspectrophotometric method to determine venous O_2 content and found that O_2 extraction and venous O_2 content of right ventricular blood is almost identical to that of left ventricular blood in the anesthetized dog. They also found in their experiments that increased right heart O_2 needs are met by increased delivery rather than increased extraction (Weiss, 1979). When venous blood draining the right ventricle is directly sampled in the pig, the O_2 content of the venous blood is higher. In this animal modest increases in O_2 demand appear to be met primarily by increased extraction (Ely *et al.*, 1981). More data are needed before a full evaluation of the relation of flow to metabolism in the right heart can be made.

Left coronary blood flow is highest during diastole and lowest during systole (Berne and Rubio, 1979). This reversal of the pattern observed in most vascular beds is attributed to phasic alterations in tissue pressure produced by rhythmic contraction and relaxation of the myocardium. Changes in tissue pressure are larger in the left ventricle than in the right and therefore have a greater influence on this vascular bed. In the right coronary artery the ratio of systolic to diastolic flow is several times higher than in the left coronary artery (Feinberg *et al.*, 1960).

It is generally accepted that time-averaged coronary blood flow is nearly evenly distributed across the myocardial wall (Domenech *et al.*,

1969; Buckberg *et al.*, 1972; Cobb *et al.*, 1974). This even flow distribution is maintained in spite of the greater compression of subendocardial vessels by systolic extravascular pressure. This is because, when compared to subepicardium, subendocardial vascular resistance is lower and flow is higher during diastole. Although under all physiologic conditions mean subendocardial flow is maintained at a level similar to subepicardial flow, this is not true in some pathologic situations, most notably coronary artery stenosis. In this case subendocardial resistance vessels cannot dilate sufficiently to compensate for the reduced flow resulting from extravascular compressive forces during systole.

The effect of tissue pressure on coronary flow can be conceptualized in terms of a vascular waterfall. The vascular waterfall theory was first suggested by Duomarco and Rimini (1954). It was subsequently expressed in explicit terms by Permutt (Permutt *et al.*, 1962; Lopez-Muniz *et al.*, 1968). Let P_i and P_o represent the inflow and outflow pressures, respectively, through a collapsible tube and P_e represent the external (tissue) pressure. The waterfall model is represented by

$$Q = (P_i - P_o)/R \qquad \text{if} \qquad P_i > P_o > P_e, \qquad (1)$$
$$Q = (P_i - P_e)/R \qquad \text{if} \qquad P_i > P_e > P_o, \qquad (2)$$
$$Q = 0 \qquad \text{if} \qquad P_e > P_i > P_o. \qquad (3)$$

Here, Q is the flow, and R is the resistance of the fully open circular tube. The first equation holds for laminar flow and is unaffected by the smaller external pressure P_e. When P_e becomes greater than the outflow pressure P_o, partial collapse of the tube occurs. Then the flow Q, described by Eq. (2), is dependent only on the pressure difference $P_i - P_e$ and is independent of the outflow pressure P_o. This is similar to a waterfall in which the flow rate is independent of the height of the water level below the falls. The third equation shows that the flow is completely stopped by vascular collapse when the external pressure P_e is larger than the inlet pressure P_i. The waterfall model correlates well with experiments on a single tube when the Reynolds number is small, for example, the vessels in the microcirculation (Lyon *et al.*, 1980). It was subsequently applied to the coronary circulation (Scharf *et al.*, 1971), notably by Downey and Kirk (1974, 1975).

In studies designed to separate the physical factors discussed above from metabolic and neural factors, maximum vascular smooth muscle relaxation is usually obtained by inducing myocardial ischemia or by infusing vasodilators. Then coronary flow should be influenced only by the coronary arterial pressure (P_i), coronary sinus pressure (P_o), and the intramyocardial pressure (P_e), which is in turn affected by the heart rate, the ventricular systolic pressure, the ventricular diastolic pressure, and cardiac contractility. Since during systole the intramyocardial pressure increases from the epicardium toward the endocardium (although the location and the magnitude of the maximum are still controversial), the subendocardium is either not perfused or very much underperfused during systole; most of the subendocardial flow occurs during diastole (Downey and Kirk, 1974; Archie, 1975; Hess and Bache, 1976).

Downey and Kirk (1975) investigated pressure–flow relationships in the maximally dilated beating heart and arrested heart. They found a linear pressure–flow relationship for the arrested state with a positive pressure intercept at zero flow. This conforms to the waterfall model. For the beating heart the pressure–flow relationship is nonlinear at low flow rates, but this can be explained by several parallel waterfall models across the myocardium. Evidence for the waterfall phenomenon is also seen in conscious dogs (Bellamy, 1978) and in the right ventricle (Bellamy and Lowensohn, 1980). Downey and Kirk's work was confirmed and extended by Panerai et al. (1979), who obtained pressure–flow relationships at different phases of the cardiac cycle. L'Abbate et al. (1977) found that, whereas extravascular resistance (due to passive physical factors) increases toward the endocardium, the intravascular resistance is less in the subendocardium. Whether changes in intravascular resistance are due to changes in vascular smooth muscle tone or recruitment of more flow paths is still controversial (Wüsten et al., 1977).

Other research that supports the waterfall model include experiments demonstrating that increased diastolic ventricular pressure (Domenech, 1978; Ellis and Klocke, 1979) and heart rate (Bache and Cobb, 1977) reduce coronary blood flow. The effect of contractility is more controversial. L'Abbate et al. (1977) and Trimble and Downey (1979) showed a decrease in subendocardial flow with increased local contractility, which is consistent with the waterfall model. However, Klassen and Zborowska-Sluis (1979) found no effect on regional blood flow during changes in contractility. Another result incompatible with the waterfall model was obtained by Bellamy et al. (1980). They slightly raised outflow pressure by partially occluding the coronary sinus and, contrary to the results of Scharf et al. (1971), found that the flow rate was decreased instead of unaffected. If the waterfall model applies to the heart, flow rate should be unaffected by downstream pressure. They suggested that there may be some hitherto unidentified extravascular interaction between the coronary sinus pressure and intramyocardial tissue pressure.

If the waterfall model is indeed applicable to most of the coronary circulation, it should be possible to model the coronary vasculature in terms of an electrical network analog and predict its behavior. This was suggested by Downey and Kirk (1975) and implemented by Collens et al.

(1976), Horikawa *et al.* (1977), and Panerai *et al.* (1979) with very good agreements with experimental data.

Since the subendocardium is more vulnerable than the subepicardium to ischemic damage, it would be useful if its perfusion could be predicted from easily measured hemodynamic variables. Because the subendocardium is perfused mainly during diastole, it might be reasonable to use the area between the aortic pressure and left ventricular pressure in diastole (the diastolic pressure–time index, DPTI) for this purpose (Buckberg *et al.*, 1972; Hoffman and Buckberg, 1978; Hoffman, 1978). The work of the heart can be correlated with the area under the left ventricular pressure curve in systole, known as the tension–time index (TTI, Sarnoff *et al.*, 1958). Thus, the coronary O_2 supply–demand ratio may be represented by the DPTI-to-TTI ratio. Munch and Downey (1980) showed that the use of DPTI as an index of subendocardial flow is in agreement with the waterfall model.

B. Local Vascular Control

As previously pointed out coronary blood flow is adjusted so as to maintain the myocardial flow-to-metabolism ratio approximately constant in a variety of conditions. For the most part the exquisite control mechanisms responsible for these adjustments are located either in the blood vessels themselves or in the surrounding tissue. Three phenomena that are the result of these local regulatory mechanisms are autoregulation, reactive hyperemia, and functional hyperemia. *Autoregulation* refers to the capacity of an organ or vascular bed to maintain a relatively constant blood flow in the face of alterations in the pressure gradient for flow (see the preceding section on the complexities of determining the pressure gradient for the left ventricle). Figure 1 shows the transient and steady-state coronary blood flow changes following a step increase in arterial pressure. As soon as arterial pressure is increased, flow increases to a peak value, representing the increase that would occur in the steady state if autoregulation did not occur. However, flow quickly falls to just above the control value because of increased vascular resistance. When steady-state flow is plotted as a function of arterial pressure, it is relatively constant over a range of pressures from 50 to 150 mm Hg. Studies have demonstrated that both subendocardium and subepicardium exhibit autoregulation (Gallagher *et al.*, 1980). Autoregulatory adjustments can defend against changes in the perfusion pressure over a limited range; at pressures outside this range, passive forces begin to dominate the pressure–flow relationship. Consequently, either a local (clot, vessel spasm, or plaque) or

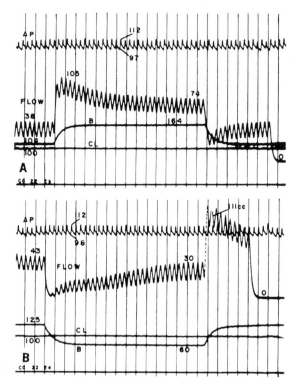

Fig. 1. Branch coronary blood flow changes in response to changes in branch coronary artery pressure (B) while common coronary artery pressure (CL) and aortic pressure (AP) remain constant. Flow in milliliters per minute; pressures in millimeters of mercury. Perfusion pressures electronically damped. Time lines 1 sec apart. (From Driscol *et al.*, 1964, by permission of the American Heart Association, Inc.)

systemic reduction in perfusion pressure below 50 mm Hg will cause a reduction in resting coronary flow. Such a reduction affects subendocardial flow more than subepicardial flow.

Figure 2 shows the relationship between perfusion pressure and flow in the right coronary circulation. The right coronary vasculature exhibits an autoregulatory response that is very similar (although not quite as efficient) to that of the left coronary circulation.

Reactive hyperemia refers to the increase in blood flow above control that follows a brief period of arterial occlusion. As the duration of occlusion of the left coronary artery increases, the magnitude of the hyperemia increases. Reactive hyperemia of the coronary circulation is pronounced when compared with that of many other organs (e.g., kidney and intestine). This is probably because of the low flow relative to metabolism in

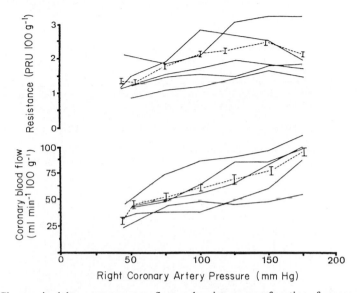

Fig. 2. Changes in right coronary artery flow and resistance as a function of coronary artery pressure. Cannulated right coronary arteries of five dogs were pump-perfused at constant pressure. Pressure was increased or decreased in gradations of 25 mm Hg. Steady-state flows were recorded and resistance calculated. Note that blood flow remains relatively constant between 50 and 150 mm Hg. (From Ely, 1979.)

the heart. This is also evident when reactive hyperemia of the left coronary bed is compared with that of the right, which serves a region of myocardium with a lower O_2 consumption and has a smaller hyperemic response (Lowensohn et al., 1976).

Functional hyperemia refers to the increase in blood flow that accompanies an increase in metabolism. Figure 3 shows the linear relationship between blood flow and O_2 consumption that exists over the entire range of metabolic activity of the left ventricle. Myocardial O_2 consumption appears to be the dominant factor determining myocardial blood flow under normal circumstances.

Several vasoactive agents appear to participate in local control of the coronary circulation. The relative importance of each of these agents probably depends on the particular condition under investigation. For example, reduced arterial wall pO_2 may be important in determining vascular conductance under conditions of systemic hypoxia but may have little influence during increased myocardial metabolism.

If the *oxygen* content of arterial blood perfusing the myocardium is sufficiently decreased, coronary vasodilation results. It appears that arterial pO_2 must fall below approximately 40 mm Hg to produce vasodilation

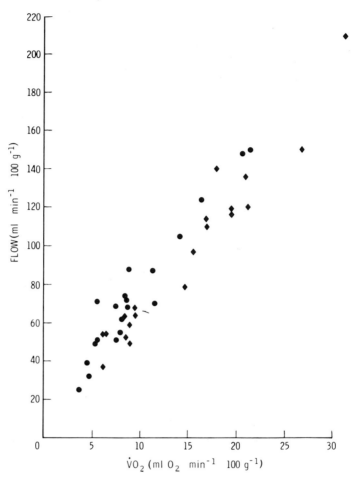

Fig. 3. Left anterior descending coronary artery flow as a function of myocardial oxygen consumption ($\dot{V}O_2$) in four dogs. Myocardial $\dot{V}O_2$ was raised by infusing isoproterenol at various rates.

(Daugherty *et al.*, 1967). This vasodilation could result from a direct effect of pO_2 in the arteriolar wall or an indirect release of a vasodilator from hypoxic myocardium. Support of the former mechanism is the finding that when the pO_2 of isolated coronary strips falls below 10–15 mm Hg, relaxation results (Gellai and Detar, 1974). This substantiates the possibility that low pO_2 could have a direct effect. On the other hand, cardiac hypoxia results in the release of several vasoactive substances, including K^+ (Gerlings *et al.*, 1969), H^+, PGs (Kalsner, 1976), and adenosine (for references see Berne and Rubio, 1979).

Oxygen may be a direct determinant of vascular caliber when O_2 delivery to the heart is reduced, for example, at the lower limits of autoregulation, in the initiation of reactive hyperemia and in any circumstance that causes severe arterial hypoxemia. We doubt that reduced vessel wall pO_2 is an important factor in functional hyperemia because (*a*) O_2 delivery increases and (*b*) venous O_2 does not fall when metabolism is raised. This combination of circumstances should maintain, or perhaps even raise, arteriolar wall pO_2 (for references see Sparks, 1980).

Increasing plasma K^+ concentration (over the range between 4 and 10 mEq/liter) results in modest, transient coronary vasodilation. This appears to be the result of a direct effect on coronary smooth muscle via stimulation of the Na^+-K^+ pump (for references see Sparks, 1980; Anderson, 1976). Potassium ions are released transiently when metabolic activity is increased and could account for a portion of the initial vasodilation (Murray *et al.*, 1979b). Potassium is also released during severe hypoxia and ischemia and so may be partially responsible for hypoxic vasodilation and reactive hyperemia (Scott and Radowski, 1971; Gerlings *et al.*, 1969). We doubt that K^+ is involved in the maintenance of any steady-state functional hyperemia because both its release and its vasoactivity are transient (Gellai and Detar, 1974; Sparks, 1980; Murray *et al.*, 1979b).

Increases in blood *carbon dioxide* concentration cause vasodilation and decreases cause vasoconstriction in both the left and right ventricles (for references see Case *et al.*, 1978; Ely, 1979; Daugherty *et al.*, 1967). The potency of CO_2 seems highly dependent on the experimental conditions, including route of administration of CO_2, constant flow or constant pressure perfusion, and direct and indirect effects on myocardial metabolism (Case *et al.*, 1978; Ely, 1979; Rooke and Sparks, 1980; Daugherty *et al.*, 1967; Ehrhart and Smith, 1980). It is likely that the vascular effect of pCO_2 is mediated by changes in extracellular H^+ concentration (Rooke and Sparks, 1981).

Ischemia results in a substantial increase in pCO_2 (decrease in pH) (Case *et al.*, 1979) and so it seems likely that pCO_2/pH participates in reactive hyperemia and perhaps at the lower end of the autoregulatory range. However, there is little evidence to suggest that myocardial pCO_2 increases enough during functional hyperemia to be an important vasodilator influence (Rooke and Sparks, 1980). Decreased pH potentiates the effect of adenosine, and this may be an important additional effect of H^+ under conditions that cause both increased H^+ and adenosine concentration (Raberger *et al.*, 1971; Degenring, 1976; Merrill *et al.*, 1978).

A *myogenic response* is defined as a contraction of smooth muscle in response to stretch or a relaxation in response to reduced length. Theoretically, the myogenic response could be involved in both reactive hyperemia and autoregulation. Because it is very difficult to test the myogenic hypothesis directly in the heart, it is always proposed after an attempt has been made to rule out other possible mechanisms. Reactive hyperemia occurs after coronary occlusion during a single cardiac cycle (Eikens and Wilcken, 1974). Because the reduction in O_2 supply is so small, this has been taken as evidence of a myogenic mechanism. There is no convincing evidence on either side of the question of whether a myogenic response is involved in coronary autoregulation.

Several *arachidonic acid metabolites* may be found in coronary sinus effluent, including the vasodilators PGE_2 and PGI_2 and the vasoconstrictors $PGF_{2\alpha}$ and TxA_2, in one circumstance or another (Needleman and Isakson, 1980; Berger *et al.*, 1977). These agents act directly on coronary vascular smooth muscle. The use of cyclooxygenase inhibitors to block the formation of these substances failed to provide convincing evidence that they are involved in hypoxic vasodilation, autoregulation, reactive hyperemia, or functional hyperemia (Hintze and Kaley, 1977; Owen *et al.*, 1975; Harlan *et al.*, 1978). Prostaglandin synthesis may modulate the vasoconstrictor effects of high levels of angiotensin II (Gunther and Cannon, 1980). The balance between the vasoconstrictor effect of TxA_2 synthesis by platelets and vasodilator effects of PGI_2 synthesis by coronary vessels may be an important determinant of coronary vessel caliber in disease states (Needleman and Isakson, 1980).

Over the past 18 years, Berne and Rubio and associates as well as other investigators have published numerous papers providing evidence that *adenosine* formed by myocardial cells causes metabolic vasodilation. Initially, the evidence was necessarily indirect because of technical limitations. However, through persistent and imaginative experiments, a large amount of data supporting the hypothesis has accumulated. Evidence favoring the adenosine hypothesis is as follows:

1. Adenosine is a potent ($ED_{50}2 \times 10^{-7} M$) dilator of coronary vessels, preferentially affecting small resistance vessels.
2. Levels of adenosine and its degradation products, inosine and hypoxanthine, are elevated in myocardium as well as in venous effluent and pericardial perfusate during ischemia and hypoxia.
3. Bioassay studies show increased coronary sinus levels of a substance that has the properties of adenosine during hypoxic and reactive dilation.
4. Adrenergic stimulation of myocardial metabolism results in increased myocardial adenosine content and the appearance of adenosine in venous effluent and pericardial perfusate.

5. Adenosine tissue levels and/or release are increased by aortic constriction and histamine.
6. The biochemical pathways necessary for the rapid formation and degradation of interstitial adenosine are present in myocardium.

A complete description of the above lines of evidence can be found in several reviews (Berne and Rubio, 1979; Belloni, 1979; Berne, 1980). Originally, Berne and Rubio suggested that a reduction in O_2 supply relative to consumption caused degradation of adenine nucleotides and adenosine formation. More recently they proposed that increased O_2 consumption is associated with adenosine release even in the absence of a relative deficiency of O_2 supply. They suggested that in this situation increased adenosine formation results from disinhibition of 5'-nucleotidase by an elevation of intracellular Mg^{2+} and diminished creatine phosphate levels.

The first serious challenge to the adenosine hypothesis was a series of studies showing that pharmacologic interventions that alter the vascular effects of exogenous adenosine have only small effects on hypoxic vasodilation, as well as functional and reactive hyperemia. In general, studies that have employed drugs to alter the metabolism of adenosine or block its action do not support the idea that adenosine is the major metabolic vasodilator (see, e.g., Bittar and Pauly, 1971; Juhran and Dietmann, 1970). However, these studies are difficult to interpret because of lack of simultaneous measurements of adenosine. For example, methylxanthines may be unable to abolish metabolic regulation because high levels of adenosine overwhelm the competitive blockade. It would be helpful to know what happens to interstitial adenosine in the presence of methylxanthines. Also, dipyridamole has been used to block cellular uptake of adenosine, but it may trap endogenous adenosine inside of myocardial cells and thereby depress interstitial adenosine concentration rather than raise it, as has been assumed in the past (see below). Thus, in the absence of measurements of adenosine content, studies using dipyridamole cannot be interpreted.

Measurements of tissue adenosine content have provided some of the most compelling evidence favoring the adenosine hypothesis. The interpretation of tissue levels has relied on the assumption that almost all adenosine is confined to the interstitial space. This assumption is based on the high affinity of intracellular adenosine deaminase and adenosine kinase for adenosine, which would prevent buildup of free intracellular adenosine. In addition, most 5'-nucleotidase activity has been shown to be located on the outer surface of the sarcolemma. Thus, adenosine formed by this enzyme should be deposited in the interstitium (Berne, 1980). However, five lines of evidence suggest that this "extracellular assumption" may not be correct. First, following infusions of radiolabeled precursor into isolated guinea pig hearts, effluent adenosine had a higher specific activity than tissue adenosine (Schrader and Gerlach, 1976). This suggests compartmentation of tissue adenosine into at least two pools.

Second, several studies suggest the existence of an intracellular or bound pool of adenosine. In particular, Olsson et al. (1978) isolated and described a protein from cow and dog heart that binds adenosine and appears to be capable of protecting adenosine from deamination. This raises the possibility of a significant intracellular content of adenosine. Such a possibility has been reinforced by the finding that the cytosolic enzyme S-adenosylhomocysteine hydrolase has the capacity to protect adenosine from metabolism. (Saebo and Ueland, 1979). Measurements of this protective binding capacity in crude tissue extracts from mouse, rat, rabbit, and bovine heart indicate that a significant amount of adenosine may exist intracellularly (Ueland and Saebo, 1979). Other reports indicate that there is an intracellular adenosine pool in vascular smooth muscle and hepatocytes (Bruttig et al., 1980; Belloni et al., 1980).

Third, the use of adenosine-methylene diphosphonate (AOPCP) to inhibit ecto-5'-nucleotidase [which has been postulated to catalyze a vectorial reaction in which AMP hydrolysis is accompanied by transfer of adenosine across the cell membrane (Frick and Lowenstein, 1978)] did not decrease adenosine production in two preparations. In isolated, perfused rat hearts AOPCP increased, rather than decreased, both the production of tissue adenosine and the release of adenosine into the effluent perfusate in response to anaerobic conditions (Frick and Lowenstein, 1976). Schrader and Shutz (1979) reported a similar inability to decrease adenosine production by hypoxic dog hearts in vivo when the hearts were treated with AOPCP. These experiments suggest that the AOPCP-inhibitable ecto-5'-nucleotidase may not be involved in the production of adenosine, which thereby raises the possibility that adenosine is formed intracellularly.

Fourth, inhibition of facilitated transport of adenosine with dipyridamole or nitrobenzylthioguanosine has yielded results suggesting that adenosine is produced intracellularly. In both dog and guinea pig Langendorff preparations, dipyridamole increased the tissue concentration of adenosine but reduced its release into the perfusate (Kubler et al., 1970; Degenring, 1976). These results constitute evidence that dipyridamole blocks the efflux of adenosine from the myocardial cell, resulting in increased intracellular adenosine levels and decreased adenosine release. Such an interpretation is consistent with the finding that dipyridamole blocks both adenosine release and the hyperemia in isolated guinea pig hearts subjected to anoxia, a condition that is known to increase adenosine production (Kukovetz and Poch, 1971). More recent evidence suggesting an intracellular site for the generation of adenosine has been obtained in dog hearts *in situ,* where Schrader and Shutz (1979) reported a decreased release of adenosine in the presence of nitrobenzylthioguanosine.

Last, Schrader and Gerlach (1976) pointed out that, if total cardiac tissue adenosine were distributed only in the interstitial fluid, the resting interstitial adenosine concentration would result in a dilation inconsistent with resting blood flow.

All the foregoing findings and considerations collectively introduce a strong element of uncertainty regarding the validity of the "extracellular assumption." It appears to us that the best explanation of available information is that measured tissue adenosine exists in the interstitial (perivascular) space and also intracellularly, perhaps in bound form, which is not metabolized. If this is true, total tissue adenosine values do not necessarily give an adequate index of perivascular adenosine.

In an attempt to estimate interstitial adenosine concentration we measured adenosine content in cardiac lymph. The concentration of adenosine in cardiac lymph was very low ($0.04 \pm 0.02 \; \mu M$) compared with that in pericardial fluid, $0.4 \pm 0.3 \; \mu M$. The low values in cardiac lymph appear to be due to a combination of degradation of adenosine in lymph by adenosine deaminase and uptake and degradation by cellular elements in the lymph channels. Thus, it does not seem likely that cardiac lymph can be used as a means of estimating interstitial adenosine content.

Two procedures have been used to estimate adenosine release: appearance of adenosine in pericardial perfusate and appearance of adenosine in venous blood. One reason that pericardial perfusate measurements have been used is that earlier studies indicated that the disappearance of adenosine from dog plasma was too rapid to allow quantitative estimate to be made of release into venous blood. The pericardial perfusate studies indicate that a wide range of stimuli of myocardial metabolism increase adenosine release (Watkinson *et al.,* 1979). However, the use of pericardial perfusate involves certain difficulties. First, it can reflect adenosine release from only a very superficial layer of myocardium. Thus, it does not provide an index of transmural interstitial adenosine concentration for comparison with transmural coronary blood flow, conductance, and myocardial O_2 consumption. Second, we do not know whether changes in perfusate concentration always reflect changes in interstitial adenosine concentration. This is because of our lack of knowledge concerning the factors responsible for transport of adenosine from the heart to pericardial fluid. For example, we do not know what influence increased stirring associated with increased rate or contractile force might have. These potential limitations may account for the relatively poor correlation between coronary blood flow and pericardial perfusate adenosine concentration in some studies.

The major objection to using the release of adenosine into venous blood as an index of interstitial adenosine concentration has been the reported rapid degradation rate in blood. However, more recent chemical and bioassay studies suggested that adenosine remains in venous plasma of dogs for a sufficient period of time to allow its measurement (Scott *et al.*, 1979; Manfredi and Sparks, 1982). Unfortunately, there have been very few studies using this approach. Also, it remains to be demonstrated that adenosine measured in coronary sinus blood is an accurate reflection of interstitial concentration. It is possible that it comes from formed elements in blood or endothelium rather than myocardial cells. The available studies show that adenosine release into venous effluent is increased by hypoxia, ischemia, and adrenergic stimulation (Berne, 1980). However, a strong indication that adenosine cannot be the sole mediator of metabolic vasodilation is the observation that the increase in myocardial metabolism caused by electrical pacing is not paralleled by an increase in adenosine release into blood (Manfredi and Sparks, 1982). Thus, the studies that provide the most direct evidence concerning interstitial adenosine favor an important, but not exclusive role for adenosine in local control.

C. Neural Control

Histochemical studies have demonstrated that the coronary vasculature is innervated by branches of both the sympathetic and parasympathetic divisions of the autonomic nervous system (see, e.g., Denn and Stone, 1976). Assessing the physiologic role of these nerves has been hampered by the fact that activation of these fibers has concomitant effects on both blood vessels and myocardium. In recent years it has been possible to separate these effects by the use of pharmacologic probes and more sophisticated experimental instrumentation. These studies have demonstrated that parasympathetic and sympathetic nerves exert direct effects on coronary vessels independent of their effects on the myocardium, even though these effects are frequently masked by the myocardial events.

If heart rate is held constant, *parasympathetic* stimulation produces vasodilation, which is blocked by cholinergic receptor blockers and mimicked by acetylcholine administration (Feigl, 1969). The physiologic importance of these fibers is unknown.

Stimulation of the *sympathetic* nerves of the heart either by direct stellate ganglion stimulation or by reflex activation results in a decrease in steady-state left coronary vascular resistance. The steady-state decrease in resistance is preceded by a transient vasoconstriction (Granata *et al.*, 1965). This biphasic response can be mimicked by the intracoronary injection of norepinephrine. The transient increase in vascular resistance is blocked by α-adrenergic receptor blockers and is potentiated by β-adrenergic blocking agents (for references see Berne and Rubio, 1979). It appears that an initial vasoconstrictor effect of sympathetic nerve stimulation is overwhelmed by increased metabolic vasodilator activity. Even in the steady state the α-adrenergic vasoconstrictor influence of sympathetic nerve stimulation decreases the vasodilator response resulting from increased metabolic activity (Mohrman and Feigl, 1978). A number of studies have demonstrated that α-adrenergic vasoconstrictor tone exists in many circumstances, including rest (Holtz *et al.*, 1977) and reactive hyperemia (Schwartz and Stone, 1977).

Coronary vascular smooth muscle has both α- and β-adrenergic receptors (Zuberbuhler and Bohr, 1965). There is some question as to whether the coronary β receptors are activated by norepinephrine released from sympathetic nerve terminals. The answer has been difficult to obtain because of controversy concerning the subtype of β receptors of coronary vascular smooth muscle. Studies on intact hearts indicate that the β_2 receptor is dominant in coronary vascular smooth muscle (Gross and Feigl, 1975). Assuming that this is true, the lack of coronary vasodilation observed in the presence of a β_1-receptor antagonist demonstrates that sympathetic nerves do not exert a direct vasodilator influence (Hamilton and Feigl, 1976). On the other hand, if β_1 receptors dominate, as has been suggested by some *in vitro* work, current information does not allow us to assess the importance of β-receptor-mediated sympathetic vasodilation. Further understanding must await the development of a highly specific β_2 blocker.

β-Receptor activation causes cyclic AMP levels to rise in coronary smooth muscle (Seidel *et al.*, 1975). Protein kinases activated by cyclic AMP may mediate relaxation by effects on Ca^{2+} sequestration and phosphorylation of myosin (Kramer and Hardman, 1980; Conti and Adelstein, 1980).

Circulating levels of catecholamines have a variable influence on coronary vascular tone. Increased norepinephrine (or epinephrine) levels appear to exert a direct α-receptor-mediated vasoconstrictor effect, which is counteracted to a variable extent by increased metabolic activity of the heart (Vatner *et al.*, 1974; Pitt *et al.*, 1967). Norepinephrine causes a slower onset of vasodilation when compared with a dose of isoproterenol giving the same increase in O_2 consumption. This may be because of the competing effects of α-receptor activation (Smith *et al.*, 1978).

D. Circulating Factors

1. Polypeptides

Intravenous infusion of *bradykinin* reduces coronary resistance and elevates coronary flow in dog, rat, primates, and cat (Haddy *et al.*, 1970; Sander and Huggins, 1972). The same responses are produced by kallidin in a variety of species (Haddy *et al.*, 1970). Because there is a concomitant increase in myocardial O_2 consumption the alterations in flow and resistance could result from direct or indirect actions of the agents. However, local infusion of bradykinin or kallidin into the coronary circulation causes vasodilation with only minimal increases in myocardial O_2 consumption. Coronary flow also increases when bradykinin is added to the perfusate of isolated heart preparations (Needleman *et al.*, 1975; Sander and Huggins, 1972). Thus, it seems quite clear that the coronary vasodilation is not secondary to increased cardiac metabolism but rather is due to the action of bradykinin on the vasculature. At least part of the vasodilation caused by high doses of bradykinin may result from increased synthesis of PGs (Needleman *et al.*, 1975; Regoli *et al.*, 1977), but lower doses may act directly on vascular smooth muscle (Rocha e Silva *et al.*, 1976).

Vasopressin is a potent coronary vasoconstrictor. It reduces coronary blood flow and elevates coronary resistance over a wide dose range during either local (Haddy and Scott, 1966) or intravenous administration (Wilson *et al.*, 1980; Heyndrickx *et al.*, 1976; Ericsson, 1972; Corliss *et al.*, 1968; Fisher *et al.*, 1974; Sirinek *et al.*, 1976). Part of the increase in coronary vascular resistance produced by vasopressin is undoubtedly related to the fact that this agent reduces myocardial contractility and heart rate. However, it has been shown that coronary constriction occurs in the conscious dog during intravenous vasopressin administration in the face of little or no change in either heart rate or contractility (Heyndrickx *et al.*, 1976). It seems likely that the vasoconstriction is due to a direct action of vasopressin on the vascular smooth muscle because the response is not blocked by denervation (Heyndrickx *et al.*, 1976) or adrenergic blockers (Beller *et al.*, 1971). Oddly enough, the effects of vasopressin on the heart and coronary vasculature are not seen in hypovolemic dogs (Ericsson, 1972).

Intravenous *angiotensin II* causes a modest coronary vasoconstriction in spite of causing increased cardiac metabolic activity (Gunther and Cannon, 1980). The increase in resistance is probably a direct effect on coronary vascular smooth muscle because angiotensin II causes contraction of isolated vascular strips (Drimal and Boska, 1973) and vasoconstriction in isolated perfused hearts (Gerlings and Gilmore, 1974). Angiotensin I causes coronary constriction of isolated hearts, but its effect is blocked by converting enzyme inhibitor, indicating that it is converted to angiotensin II before exerting its effect (Gerlings and Gilmore, 1974). The constrictor action of angiotensin II appears to be modulated by vasodilator arachidonic acid metabolites, because indomethacin enhances the vasoconstrictor effect and angiotensin II promotes the release of these metabolites from the heart (Gunther and Cannon, 1980). It is conceivable that this mechanism protects the heart against high levels of circulating angiotensin II and that administration of cyclooxygenase inhibitors could be deleterious to myocardial O_2 supply in high-renin states (Watkins et al., 1976).

2. Drugs

Mannitol passes freely through capillary pores but not through cell membranes. Because of these properties it can be used to increase extracellular fluid osmolarity and decrease intracellular fluid volume. This may prove beneficial during myocardial ischemia, when cardiac cells demonstrably swell (see below for further discussion). In addition to effects on cell volume, hyperosmotic mannitol solutions exert a direct vasodilator effect on coronary vessels that is not mediated by adrenergic receptors and does not increase intracellular cyclic AMP levels (Krishnamurty et al., 1977, 1978). The vasodilator mechanism of hyperosmotic mannitol may be due to a decrease in intracellular volume, which would increase the intracellular K^+ concentration, hyperpolarize the membrane, and result in relaxation (Haljamae et al., 1970). Vessel wall dehydration could also increase lumen diameter. Accompanying mannitol-induced vasodilation is a general loss of vascular reactivity to both vasoconstrictor and vasodilator agents (Krishnamurty et al., 1978). Hyperosmotic mannitol also has a positive inotropic effect, which appears to be independent of changes in blood flow (Willerson et al., 1974).

Several organic compounds, including verapamil, nifedipine, and compound D600, have been labeled *calcium antagonists* because they reduce the effectiveness of extracellular Ca^{2+} in excitation–contraction coupling (Fleckenstein, 1977). Probably the three listed above all inhibit the entry of Ca^{2+} via the slow channel (Kohlhardt and Fleckenstein, 1980). Although all of the agents in this class reduce net Ca^{2+} entry by definition, it is by no means apparent that all work by the same mechanism. These compounds cause coronary vasodilation and reduce cardiac metabolism by reducing afterload and cardiac contractility. The vascular effects occur at a lower concentration than the cardiac effects, allowing one to produce coronary vasodilation without undue depression of cardiac performance (Fleckenstein, 1977). The agents seem to have more effect on the coronary circulation than on total peripheral resistance. Nifedipine and other Ca^{2+} antagonists increase flow within ischemic myocardium (Jolly et al., 1981), reduce coronary artery spasm, and suppress angina pectoris (Antman et al., 1980).

There are relatively few studies that describe the effect of *morphine* on the coronary circulation despite the fact that the drug has been used for decades in the treatment both of acute pulmonary edema accompanying left heart failure and of myocardial infarction. Early studies showed that morphine produced modest coronary dilation in isolated artificially perfused hearts of various species including man (Macht, 1915; Kountz, 1932; Gruber and Robinson, 1929). It was also reported not to affect, or to relax modestly, coronary rings (Macht, 1915; Kountz, 1932). Later *in vivo* studies yielded more conflicting results. Intravenous administration of morphine sulfate to conscious dogs resulted in substantial coronary vasoconstriction, which could be blocked by an α-receptor antagonist (Vatner et al., 1975). This vasoconstrictor response was not seen in anesthetized dogs or in conscious dogs if a respiratory-depressant dose of morphine was used. In contrast, intravenous morphine has been reported to produce a substantial increase in coronary flow and decrease in coronary resistance in the conscious monkey (Miller et al., 1972). It has also been reported to decrease coronary resistance slightly in patients with coronary artery disease (Leaman et al., 1978; Sethna et al., 1981). We have found that intravenous morphine produces a modest vasoconstriction in the right coronary circulation of the anesthetized pig, whereas local intracoronary administration is without effect in this vascular bed (Ely et al., 1981). The former response can be immediately reversed by naloxone. In summary, it appears that the drug has little direct effect on the coronary vasculature. The response produced when morphine is given systemically is probably mediated through the action of the drug on various remote controling systems, which may be affected differently depending on existing physiologic conditions and perhaps species. In addition, morphine has been shown to cause the release of histamine (Thompson and Walton, 1964).

Nitroglycerin (GTN) has been used for over a century to ameliorate the pain of angina pectoris. Initially, it was postulated that the beneficial effect of GTN was due to systemic vasodilation (Brunton, 1867), but later authors attributed the effect to improved coronary blood flow (Muller and Rorrick, 1958; Kaverina and Chumburidze, 1979). However, more recent studies have shown that both of those suggestions are an oversimplification of the mechanisms of action.

Intracoronary administration of GTN elevates coronary flow and reduces coronary resistance in the normal coronary vascular bed (Frohlich and Scott, 1962; Fam and McGregor, 1968; Weiss and Winbury, 1972; Pennington *et al.*, 1979), but studies suggest that this is not the case in the presence of arterial stenosis (Santamore and Walinsky, 1980) or in atherosclerotic vascular disease (Ganz and Marcus, 1972). Intravenous administration of GTN to normal subjects has been reported to cause coronary blood flow to increase slightly, not to change (Weisse *et al.*, 1972; Howe *et al.*, 1975), or to increase and then fall below control (Vatner *et al.*, 1978; Fam and McGregor, 1968; Uchida *et al.*, 1978; Mathes and Rival, 1971). The decreased coronary flow results from a fall in perfusion pressure in the presence of a slightly reduced or in some cases an elevated coronary vascular resistance. The latter appears to be mediated by increased α activity reflexly initiated by the systemic hypotension (Vatner *et al.*, 1978) as well as reduced myocardial metabolism. It appears that in normal animals intravenous GTN increases coronary flow if blood pressure is not allowed to fall. However, most studies report a decrease in coronary blood flow during intravenous administration of GTN in patients with coronary artery disease. Thus, it seems unlikely that the capacity of GTN to relieve angina is attributable to an elevated coronary blood flow.

It is more likely that the beneficial effect of GTN in angina is related to its capacity to improve the flow-to-metabolism ratio in the ischemic zone. Several studies indicate that GTN is capable of increasing flow to the ischemic area (Kaverina and Chumburidze, 1979; Jolly and Gross, 1980; Warren and Francis, 1978; Gross *et al.*, 1980; Rudolph *et al.*, 1977). A major factor in this redistribution is attributed to the action of GTN to dilate selectively large coronary arteries including functional coronary collateral vessels (Fam and McGregor, 1968; Winbury, 1971; Schnaar and Sparks, 1972; Weisse *et al.*, 1972; Capurro *et al.*, 1977). Nitroglycerin may also increase flow by further dilating vessels within the ischemic zone (Gorman and Sparks, 1980). The drug also reduces myocardial O_2 requirements via reductions in both preload and afterload (Kaverina and Chumburidze, 1979; Warren and Francis, 1978). The former results from systemic postcapillary dilation and the latter from systemic precapillary dilation. It has also been suggested that an action of GTN on the central nervous system is responsible for its antianginal effect (Kaverina and Chumburidze, 1979).

Adrenergic blocking agents inhibit the responses to catecholamines by occupying catecholamine receptor sites of the effector cells. The observed effects of these agents depend on the prevailing level of receptor occupancy by circulating or neurogenic catecholamines. The effects of the blockers may be minimal in resting conditions but dramatic during periods of high sympathetic neuronal activity or when circulating concentrations of catecholamines are high.

The relaxation of coronary smooth muscle produced by β-adrenergic receptor activation is inhibited by *β-receptor blockers*. As discussed above, studies on isolated coronary vessels provide strong evidence that the β receptors are of subtype 1, that is, the same as myocardial β receptors (Baron *et al.,* 1972). On the other hand, most studies on *in vivo* resistance vessels lead to the opposite conclusion, that coronary β receptors are of subtype 2 (Ross, 1974; Gross and Feigl, 1975). Intravenous administration of propranalol, which blocks both receptor types, results in increased coronary resistance and reduced flow. These changes may be entirely a result of the reduction in myocardial metabolism that accompanies propranalol administration (Stein *et al.,* 1968; Downey, 1977). The contribution of direct blockade of coronary β receptors is probably quite small.

The intravenous administration of *α-receptor blockers* such as phentolamine or phenoxybenzamine causes decreased total peripheral resistance. The resulting tendency of systemic pressure to fall triggers a reflex increase in heart rate, cardiac contractility, and cardiac output. A modest increase in coronary blood flow accompanies these reflex changes. If α-adrenergic blockade is added to a previous β blockade, neither the reflex changes nor the increase in coronary blood flow are observed (Murray and Vatner, 1979). Thus, it appears that the increase in blood flow caused by α blockade in the resting dog results from a reflex increase in myocardial metabolism. Intracoronary administration of these agents (in a dose that blocks coronary vascular α receptors with little effect on the periphery) results in coronary vasodilation. The magnitude of this vasodilation is small under resting conditions but becomes much larger during periods of increased adrenergic tone such as exercise, carotid occlusion, or norepinephrine infusion (Mohrman and Feigl, 1978; Murray and Vatner, 1979). A decrease in coronary O_2 extraction accompanies the vasodilation produced by α blockade.

The two most commonly used α blockers are phentolamine and phenoxybenzamine. Phentolamine is a short-acting, competetive blocker (for references see Nickerson and Collier, 1975). The initial binding of phenoxybenzamine is also a competetive process, but this agent forms a covalent bond with the receptor and cannot subsequently by displaced by high agonist concentrations. This results in a longer duration of action (Nickerson, 1962).

In addition to α receptors of vascular smooth muscle cells (designated

α_1), there are α receptors (α_2) on adrenergic nerve endings. Stimulation of α_2 receptors causes a decreased release of norepinephrine from the nerve ending (Langer, 1977). Phentolamine and phenoxybenzamine block both α_1 and α_2 receptors, and so α blockade by these agents is accompanied by increased neuronal norepinephrine release. The α blocker prazosin blocks only α_1 receptors and so does not cause increased norepinephrine release. Prazosin therefore decreases total peripheral resistance but results in less cardiac stimulation than either phentolamine or phenoxybenzamine (for references see Cavero and Roach, 1980).

Cardiac glycosides cause constriction of coronary vessels both *in vivo* (Vatner *et al.*, 1971) and *in vitro* (Fleckenstein *et al.*, 1975). At least two separate mechanisms contribute to this vasoconstriction. The vasoconstriction observed *in vivo* is largely due to α-adrenergic receptor stimulation (Hamlin *et al.*, 1974), which may originate from an effect of ouabain on the central nervous system (Garan *et al.*, 1974). Ouabain can also elicit α-adrenergic contraction in isolated vessels (Toda, 1980), and so local norepinephrine release may be an additional source of ouabain-induced constriction. In addition to the α-adrenergic mechanism, cardiac glycosides can directly cause smooth muscle contraction by inhibition of the membrane Na^+-K^+ pump. Inhibition of the pump results in an increased intracellular Ca^{2+} concentration due to either membrane depolarization and increased Ca^{2+} permeability or an inhibition of Ca^{2+} efflux (Belardinelli *et al.*, 1979; Lang and Blaustein, 1980; Toda, 1980).

V. Coronary Circulation during Ischemia

A. Collateral Vessels

It is now firmly established that connections between coronary arteries larger than capillaries (35–500 μm) exist in many species, including dog, pig, and human being (Schaper, 1971). In human and pig hearts these anastomoses are located mainly subendocardially and intramurally, whereas in the dog heart most are subepicardial. Collateral vessels are usually more numerous and larger in the dog than in either pig or man. Thus, the canine collateral circulation should be functionally more important than either that of man or pig, at least following an acute insult. Measurement of coronary collateral flow in the dog and pig following acute ligation of a major coronary artery substantiates this conclusion (Schaper, 1971). However, it should be pointed out that regardless of the species studied or the method used to estimate collateral flow (retrograde flow, tracer microsphere distribution, radioactive inert gases, radioactive rubidium, or donor coronary inlet flow), it is rarely more than 50% of preocclusion flow to the area supplied by the occluded vessel following an acute ligation (Schaper, 1971; Cibulski *et al.*, 1973). In fact, in most cases it is substantially less than 25%. After 6 h of coronary artery ligation, collateral flow begins to rise (perhaps because of passive stretch of existing collateral vessels) and continues to increase for the next few months following ligation (due to collateral vessel growth) (Schaper, 1971; Jugdutt *et al.*, 1979; Schaper and Pasyk, 1976). Indeed, after several months collateral vessels can supply more than the basal needs of the tissue they serve (Schaper, 1971; Scheel *et al.*, 1972). The exact mechanisms involved in collateral vessel development are not clear, but tissue hypoxia and/or ischemia may be major stimulants (Scheel *et al.*, 1976; Gensini and DaCosta, 1969), as may be changes in transmural pressure (Schaper, 1971). Whatever the stimulants, collateral growth is directed toward the ischemic region and does not occur in nonischemic regions (Scheel *et al.*, 1976). If collateral vessels have no vascular smooth muscle, they must initially behave like passive tubes, responding only to alterations in transmural pressure. With time, however, their wall-to-lumen ratio increases and smooth muscle cells are present, and at this point they may very well be influenced by vasoactive agents. Chronic ventricular sympathectomy accelerates the growth of collateral vessels (Jones and Scheel, 1980).

B. Control of Resistance Vessels

Coronary resistance vessels dilate in response to ischemia. All of the mediators of local vascular control discussed earlier could be contributing to this dilation: tissue pO_2 decreases (Flaherty *et al.*, 1978), adenosine is released (Rubio *et al.*, 1969), extracellular pCO_2 and H^+ concentration increase (Case *et al.*, 1978), interstitial K^+ concentration increases (Hill and Gettes, 1980), PGE_2 and PGI_2 are released (Berger *et al.*, 1977; Needleman *et al.*, 1978), and the decrease in intravascular pressure could implicate myogenic dilation. If myocardial ischemia is maintained for longer than 2 h, however, vascular resistance begins to increase. This phenomenon has been observed in two types of ischemic preparations. In one of these a coronary artery is occluded for approximately 2 h and is then reopened (reflow preparation). In the second type of preparation a coronary artery is partially occluded, and vascular resistance in the ischemic region is observed over roughly a 3-h period (stenosis preparation).

1. Reflow Preparations

When a coronary arterial occlusion is released after 2 h, there is an initial hyperemia. However, the peak flow level is not as great as it is following a short occlusion. This suggests that the minimum vascular resistance in the ischemic area has increased as compared with the value before occlusion. Furthermore, serial blood flow measurements during the 2–4 h following release of the occlusion indicate that (a) the minimum vascular resistance (measured during the reactive hyperemia following a 90-sec occlusion) continues to increase, and (b) resting flow declines to levels significantly below the preocclusion value (Parker et al., 1975). Microsphere flow measurements indicate that the increase in vascular resistance occurs primarily in the subendocardium (Willerson et al., 1975). Histologic examination of this region reveals extensive capillary damage and swelling of myocardial cells (Kloner et al., 1974). These findings led to the hypothesis that the swollen myocardial cells (and perhaps swollen endothelial cells) compress the vasculature, decrease vascular caliber, and increase the resistance to blood flow. This hypothesis is supported by the finding that hyperosmotic mannitol (which should reduce cell swelling) administered before release of the occlusion results in higher flows during the initial reflow period (Willerson et al., 1975; Parker et al., 1979). Mannitol-treated hearts also exhibit less structural damage and swelling, together with reduced areas of necrosis following a 60-min occlusion (Powell et al., 1976). Mannitol also improves perfusion during the initial reflow period after a 120-min occlusion, but in one study after 4 h of reperfusion the beneficial hemodynamic effects of mannitol had disappeared (Parker et al., 1979). It is possible that some of the beneficial effects of hyperosmotic mannitol may be due to its vasodilator properties (which are also transient), although the beneficial hemodynamic effects of mannitol during reflow are superior to at least one known coronary vasodilator (Willerson et al., (1975).

In summary, reflow preparations demonstrate that after prolonged coronary occlusion there is an increase in vascular resistance, which appears to be caused at least in part by cell swelling. One question that reflow experiments have not answered is whether increased resistance exists without reperfusion. For example, it may be that reperfusion itself leads to the structural changes associated with increased resistance. This question has been addressed by experiments employing coronary arterial stenosis instead of occlusion.

2. Stenosis Preparations

In these preparations regional myocardial ischemia is produced by imposing an arterial stenosis so that distal coronary perfusion pressure falls
to some predetermined value. Alternatively, a coronary artery is cannulated and perfused at reduced pressure. The situation is one of relative
ischemia rather than the more severe ischemia following coronary occlusion. Some preparations also utilize cardiac pacing at an elevated rate in
order to increase the disparity between myocardial O_2 supply and demand. The advantage of this type of preparation is that vascular resistance (distal coronary pressure/ischemic bed flow) can be measured without introducing the possibility of structural damage due to reflow.
Because of the presence of collateral blood flow, accurate flow measurements in the ischemic region require the use of either radioactive microspheres or diffusible indicators.

Following flow reduction imposed by a stenosis, resistance in the ischemic area first declines and then increases during the subsequent 2–3 h
(Frame and Powell, 1976; Guyton et al., 1977; Gorman and Sparks, 1982;
Harris et al., 1981). This suggests that the increased resistance seen in reperfusion preparations is not solely due to the effects of reperfusion; some
process or processes occurring during myocardial ischemia lead(s) to increased vascular resistance. The question is whether the mechanism responsible for increased resistance in reflow preparations is the same as
that at work in stenosis preparations. The available evidence suggests that
there is at least one common mechanism: (a) the time course of the increase in resistance is roughly the same, (b) the increase in resistance is
greatest in the subendocardium, and (c) hyperosmotic mannitol greatly
reduces the increase in resistance in both preparations. Thus, swelling of
myocardial cells may contribute to the increased resistance in stenosis
preparations as well as in reflow preparations.

On the other hand, evidence from stenosis preparations suggests that
cell swelling is not the only source of increased resistance. Cell swelling
would be expected to cause a passive increase in resistance by means of
extravascular compression. Ordinarily, the resistance vessels would respond to extravascular compression with a compensatory dilation. Therefore, if cell swelling is the only cause of increased resistance during prolonged ischemia, the resistance vessels should be maximally dilated by
the time the resistance has become elevated. Results from stenosis preparations indicate that this is not the case. Infusion of adenosine or norepinephrine into myocardium that has been ischemic for 3 h decreases vascular resistance (Gorman and Sparks, 1982). Coronary vasodilators also
reduce vascular resistance in reflow preparations (Willerson et al., 1975),

and the vasodilator properties of hyperosmotic mannitol may account for some of its beneficial effects. It seems, therefore, that there must be at least one mechanism in addition to cell swelling that causes increased vascular resistance during prolonged myocardial ischemia.

Acknowledgment

The authors would like to express their appreciation to Dr. C. Y. Wang for his invaluable assistance in the preparation of the vascular waterfall section of this chapter.

References

Alexander, R. W., and Gimbrone, M. A. (1976). *Proc. Natl. Acad. Sci. USA* **73,** 1617–1620.
Anderson, D. K. (1976). *Fed. Proc. Fed. Am. Soc. Exp. Biol.* **35,** 1294–1297.
Antman, E., Muller, J., Goldberg, S., MacAlpen, R., Rubenfire, M., Tabatznek, B., Liang, C. S., Heupler, F., Achuff, S., Reichek, N., Geltman, E., Kerin, N. A., Neff, R. K., and Braunwald, E. (1980). *N. Engl. J. Med.* **302,** 1269–1273.
Archie, J. P. (1975). *Am. J. Cardiol.* **35,** 904–911.
Bache, R. J., and Cobb, F. R. (1977). *Circ. Res.* **41,** 648–653.
Baron, G. D., Speden, R. N., and Bohr, D. F. (1972). *Am. J. Physiol.* **223,** 878–881.
Bassingthwaighte, J. B., Yipintsoi, T., and Harvey, R. B. (1973). *Microvasc. Res.* **7,** 229–249.
Belardinelli, L., Harder, D., Sperelakis, N., Rubio, R., and Berne, R. M. (1979). *J. Pharmacol. Exp. Ther.* **209,** 62–66.
Bellamy, R. F. (1978). *Circ. Res.* **43,** 92–101.
Bellamy, R. F., and Lowensohn, H. S., (1980). *Am. J. Physiol.* **238,** H481–486.
Bellamy, R. F., Lowensohn, H. S., Erlich, W., and Baer, R. W. (1980). *Am. J. Physiol.* **239,** H57–64.
Beller, B. M., Trevino, A., and Urban, E. (1971). *Am. J. Med.* **51,** 675–679.
Belloni, F. L. (1979). *Cardiovasc. Res.* **13,** 63–85.
Belloni, F. L., Rubio, R., and Berne, R. M. (1980). *Fed. Proc. Fed. Am. Soc. Exp. Biol.* **39,** 270.
Berger, H. J., Zaret, B. L., Speroff, L., Cohen, L. S., and Wolfson, S. (1977). *Am. J. Cardiol.* **39,** 481–486.
Berne, R. M. (1980). *Circ. Res.* **47,** 807–813.
Berne, R. M., and Rubio, R. (1979). *Handb. Physiol. Sec-2 Cardiovasc. Sys.* **1,** 873–952.
Bittar, N., and Pauly, T. J. (1971). *Am. J. Physiol.* **220,** 812–815.
Bohr, D. F., and Webb, R. C. (1978). *In* "Mechanisms of Vasodilation" (P. M. Vanhoutte, and S. Leusen, eds.), pp. 37–47. Karger, Basel.
Bourdeau–Martini, J. (1973). *Microvasc. Res.* **6,** 286–296.

Brunton, T. B. (1867). Lancet **2**, 97.
Bruttig, S. P., Belloni, F. L., Rubio, R., and Berne, R. M. (1980). *Microvasc. Res.* **20**, 103.
Buckberg, G. D., Fixler, D. E., Archie, J. P., and Hoffman, J. I. E. (1972). *Circ. Res.* **30**, 67–81.
Capurro, N. L., Kent, K. M., and Epstein, S. E. (1977). *J. Clin. Invest.* **60**, 295–301.
Case, R. B., Felix, A., Wachter, M., Kyriabidis, G., and Castellana, F. (1978). *Circ. Res.* **42**, 410–478.
Case, R. B., Felix, A., and Castellana, F. (1979). *Circ. Res.* **45**, 324–330.
Cavero, I., and Roach, A. G. (1980). *Life Sci.* **27**, 1525–1540.
Cibulski, A. A., Lehan, P. H., and Hellems, H. H. (1973). *Am. Heart J.* **86**, 485–494.
Cobb, F. R., Bache, R. J., and Greenfield, J. C., Jr. (1974). *J. Clin. Invest.* **53**, 1618–1625.
Collens, J. C., Goatman, G. A., Utley, J. R., and Todd, E. P. (1976). *Proc. Annu. Conf. Eng. Med. Biol.* **18**, 22.
Conti, M. A., and Adelstein, R. S. (1980). *Fed. Proc. Fed. Am. Soc. Exp. Biol.* **39**, 1569–1573.
Corliss, R. J., McKenna, D. H., Sialer, S., O'Brien, G. S., and Rowe, G. G. (1968). *Am. J. Med. Sci.* **256**, 293–299.
Daugherty, R. M., Scott, J. B., Dabney, J. M., and Haddy, F. J. (1967). *Am. J. Physiol.* **213**, 1102–1110.
Degenring, F. H. (1976). *Basic Res. Cardiol.* **71**, 291–296.
Denn, J., and Stone, H. L. (1976). *J. Appl. Physiol.* **41**, 30–35.
Domenech, R. J. (1978). *Cardiovasc. Res.* **12**, 639–645.
Domenech, R. J., and Ayuy, A. H. (1974). *Cardiovasc. Res.* **8**, 611–620.
Domenech, R. J., Hoffman, J. I. E., Noble, M. I. M., Saunders, K. B., Henson, J. R., and Subijanto, S. (1969). *Circ. Res.* **25**, 581–596.
Downey, J. M. (1977). *Eur. J. Pharmacol.* **46**, 119–124.
Downey, J. M., and Kirk, E. S. (1974). *Circ. Res.* **34**, 251–257.
Downey, J. M., and Kirk, E. S. (1975). *Circ. Res.* **36**, 753–760.
Drimal, J., and Boska, D. V. (1973). *Eur. J. Pharmacol.* **20**, 130–138.
Driscol, T. E., Moir, T. W., and Eckstein, R. W. (1964). *Circ. Res.* **15**, 103–111.
Duomarco, J. L., and Rimini, R. (1954). *Am. J. Physiol.* **178**, 215–219.
Duran, W. N., Marsicano, T. H., and Anderson, R. W. (1977). *Am. J. Physiol.* **232**, H276–H281.
Duran, W. M., and Yudilevich, D. L. (1978). *Microvasc. Res.* **15**, 195–206.
Ehrhart, J. C., and Smith, C. W. (1980). *Proc. Soc. Exp. Biol. Med.* **165**, 264–270.
Eikens, E., and Wilcken, D. E. L. (1974). *Circ. Res.* **35**, 702–712.
Ellis, A. K., and Klocke, F. J. (1979). *Circ. Res.* **46**, 68–77.
Ely, S. W., (1979). "Factors Involved in the Local and Remote Control of the Right Coronary Circulation in the Dog." Thesis, Michigan State Univ., Lansing.
Ely, S. W., Sawyer, D. C., Anderson, D. L., and Scott, J. B. (1981). *Am. J. Physiol.* **241**, H149–H154.
Ericsson, B. F. (1972). *Acta Chir. Scand.* **138**, 235–238.
Fam, W. M., and McGregor, M. (1968). *Circ. Res.* **22**, 649–659.
Feigl, E. O. (1969). *Circ. Res.* **25**, 509–519.
Feinberg, H., Gerola,A., and Katz, L. N. (1960). *Am. J. Physiol.* **199**, 349–354.
Fisher, C. H., Sheff, R. N., Novak, G., and White, R. J., Jr. (1974). *Invest. Radiol.* **9**, 456–461.
Flaherty, T. T., O'Riordan, J., Khuri, S., and Gott, V. (1978). *Recent Adv. Stud. Card. Struc. Metab.* **12**, 219–226.

Fleckenstein, A. (1977). *Annu. Rev. Pharmacol. Toxicol.* **17,** 149–166.
Fleckenstein, A., Nakoyama, K., Fleckenstein, G., and Byon, Y. K. (1975). *In* "Calcium Transport in Contraction and Secretion" (E. Carafoli, ed.), pp. 555–564. North Holland, New York.
Frame, L. H., and Powell, W. J., Jr. (1976). *Circ. Res.* **39,** 269–276.
Frick, G. P., and Lowenstein, J. M. (1976). *J. Biol. Chem.* **251,** 6372–6378.
Frick, G. P., and Lowenstein, J. M. (1978). *J. Biol. Chem.* **253,** 1240–1244.
Frolich, E. D., and Scott, J. B. (1962). *Am. Heart J.* **63,** 362–366.
Gallagher, K. P., Folts, J. D., Shebuski, R. J., Rankin, J. H. G., and Rowe, G. G. (1980). *Am. J. Cardiol.* **46,** 67–73.
Ganz, W., and Marcus, H. S. (1972). *Circulation* **46,** 880–889.
Garan, H., Smith, T. W., and Powell, W. J., Jr. (1974). *J. Clin. Invest.* **54,** 1365–72.
Gellai, M., and Detar, R. (1974). *Circ. Res.* **35,** 681–691.
Gensini, G. G., and DaCosta, B. C. (1969). *Am. J. Cardiol.* **24,** 393–420.
Gerlings, E. D., and Gilmore, J. P. (1974). *Basic Res. Cardiol.* **69,** 222–227.
Gerlings, E. D., Miller, D. T., and Gilmore, J. P. (1969). *Am. J. Physiol.* **216,** 559–562.
Giacomelli, F., Anversa, P., and Weiner, J. (1975). *Microvasc. Res.* **10,** 38–42.
Gimbrone, M. A., and Alexander, R. W. (1975). *Science (Washington, D.C.)* **189,** 219–220.
Gorman, M. W., and Sparks, H. V. (1980). *Cardiovasc. Res.* **14,** 515–521.
Gorman, M. W., and Sparks, H. V. (1982). *Circ. Res.* **51,** 411–420.
Granata, L., Olsson, R. A., Huvos, A., and Gregg, D. E. (1965). *Circ. Res.* **16,** 114–120.
Gregg, D. E., and Fisher, L. C. (1963). *In* "Handbook of Physiology" (W. F. Hamilton, ed.), Sect. 2, Vol. II, pp. 1517–1584. Am. Physiol. Soc., Washington, D.C.
Gross, G. J., and Feigl, E. O. (1975). *Am. J. Physiol.* **228,** 1909–1913.
Gross, G. J., Warltier, D. C., Jolly, S. R., and Hardman, H. F. (1980). *J. Cardiovasc. Pharmacol.* **2,** 797–813.
Gruber, C. M., and Robinson, P. I. (1929). *J. Pharmacol. Exp. Ther.* **37,** 429–499.
Gunther, S., and Cannon, P. J. (1980). *Am. J. Physiol.* **238,** H895–H901.
Guyton, R. A., McClenathan, J. H., and Michaelis, L. L. (1977). *Am. J. Cardiol.* **40,** 381–392.
Haddy, F. J. (1969). *Am. J. Med.* **47,** 274–276.
Haddy, F. J., and Scott, J. B. (1966). *Annu. Rev. Pharmacol.* **6,** 49–76.
Haddy, F. J., Emerson, T. E., Jr., Scott, J. B., and Daugherty, R. M., Jr. (1970). *Handb. Exp. Pharmacol.* **25,** 362–384.
Haljamae, H., Johansson, B., Jonsson, O., and Rockert, H. (1970). *Acta Physiol. Scand.* **78,** 255–268.
Hamilton, F. N., and Feigl, E. O. (1976). *Am. J. Physiol.* **230,** 1569–1576.
Hamlin, N. P., Willerson, J. T., Garan, H., and Powell, W. J., Jr. (1974). *J. Clin. Invest.* **53,** 288–296.
Harder, D. R., Belardidnelli, L., Sperelakis, N., Rubio, R., and Berne, R. M. (1979). *Circ. Res.* **44,** 176–182.
Harlan, D. M., Rooke, T. W., Belloni, F. L., and Sparks, H. V. (1978). *Am. J. Physiol.* **235,** H372–H378.
Harris, J. R., Overholser, K. A., and Stiles, R. G. (1981). *Am. J. Physiol.* **240,** H262–H273.
Hess, D. S., and Bache, R. J. (1976). *Circ. Res.* **38,** 5–15.
Heyndricks, G. R., Boettcher, D. H., and Vatner, S. F. (1976). *Am. J. Physiol.* **231,** 1579–1587.
Hill, J. L., and Gettes, L. S. (1980). *Circulation* **61,** 768–778.
Hintze, T. H., and Kaley, G. (1977). *Circ. Res.* **40,** 313–320.

Hoffman, J. I. E. (1978). *Circulation* **58**, 381–391.

Hoffman, J. I. E., and Buckberg, G. D. (1978). *Am. J. Cardiol.* **41**, 327–332.

Holtz, J., Restorff, W., Bard, P., and Bassenge, E. (1977). *Basic. Res. Cardiol.* **72**, 286–292.

Honig, C. R., and Bourdeau-Martini, J. (1974). *Circ. Res.* **35**, (Suppl. II), 97–103.

Horikawa, M., Chino, M., Takahashi, M., and Nagoshi, H. (1977). *Jpn. Heart J.* **18**, 246–258.

Howe, B. B., Vreiss, H. R., Wilkes, S. B., and Winbury, M. M. (1975). *Clin. Exp. Pharmacol. Physiol.* **2**, 529–543.

Jolly, S. R., and Gross, G. J. (1980). *Am. J. Physiol.* **8**, H163–H171.

Jolly, S. R., Hardman, H. F., and Gross, G. J. (1981). *J. Pharmacol. Exp. Ther.* **217**, 20–25.

Jones, C. F., and Scheel, K. W. (1980). *Am. J. Physiol.* **238**, H196–H201.

Jugdutt, B. I., Becker, L. C., and Hutchins, G. M. (1979). *Am. J. Physiol.* **237**, H371–H380.

Juhran, W., and Dietmann,   (1970). *Pfluegers Arch.* **315**, 105–109.

Kalsner, S. (1976). *Blood Vessels* **13**, 155–166.

Kaverina, N. V., and Chumburidze, V. B. (1979). *Pharmacol. Ther.* **4**, 109–153.

Klassen, G. A., and Zborowska-Sluis, D. T. (1979). *Cardiovasc. Res.* **13**, 365–369.

Kloner, R. A., Ganote, C. E., and Jennings, R. B. (1974). *J. Clin. Invest.* **54**, 1496–1507.

Kohlhardt, M., and Fleckenstein, A. (1980). *Br. J. Clin. Pract.* (Suppl. 8), 3–8.

Kountz, W. B. (1932). *J. Pharmacol. Exp. Ther.* **45**, 65–76.

Kramer, G. L., and Hardman, J. G. (1980). *Handb. Physiol. Sect. 2 Cardiovasc. Sys.* **2**, 179–200.

Krishnamurty, V. S. R., Adams, H. R., Smitherman, T. C., Templeton, G. H., and Willerson, J. T. (1977). *Am. J. Physiol.* **232**, H59–H66.

Krishnamurty, V. S. R., Adams, H. R., Templeton, G. H., and Willerson, J. T. T. (1978). *Am. J. Physiol.* **235**, H728–H735.

Kubler, W., Spieckermann, P. G., and Bretschneider, H. J. (1970). *J. Mol. Cell. Cardiol.* **1**, 23–38.

Kukovetz, W. R., and Poch, G. (1971). *Cardiology* **56**, 107–113.

L'Abbate, A., Marzilli, M., Ballestra, A. M., and Camici, P. (1977). *In* "Pathogenic Mechanism of Angira Pectoris" (A. Maseri, G. A. Klassen, and M. Lesch, eds.), pp. 21–28. Grune & Stratton, New York.

Lang, S., and Blaustein, M. P. (1980). *Circ. Res.* **46**, 463–470.

Langer, S. Z. (1977). *Br. J. Pharmacol.* **60**, 481–497.

Leaman, D. M., Nellis, S. H., Zelis, R., and Field, J. M. (1978). *Am. J. Cardiol.* **41**, 324–326.

Lockette, W. E., Webb, R. C., and Bohr, D. F. (1980). *Circ. Res.* **46**, 714–720.

Lopez–Muniz, R., Stephens, N., Bromberger–Barnea, B., Permitt, S., and Riley, R. (1968). *J. Appl. Physiol.* **24**, 625–635.

Lowensohn, H. S., Khouri, E. M., Gregg, D. E., Pyle, R. L., and Patterson, R. E. (1976). *Circ. Res.* **39**, 760–765.

Lyon, C. K., Scott, J. B., and Wang, C. Y. (1980). *Circ. Res.* **47**, 68–73.

Macht, D. E. (1915). *JAMA J. Am. Med. Assoc.* **64**, 1489–1494.

Manfredi, J. P., and Sparks, H. V. (1982). *Am. J. Physiol.* **243**, H536–H545.

Manohar, M., Bisgano, G. E., Bullard, V., Will, J. A., Anderson, D., and Rankin, J. H. G. (1979). *Circ. Res.* **44**, 531–539.

Marshall, R. J., and Shepherd, J. T. (1968). "Cardiac Function in Health and Disease." Saunders, Philadelphia, Pennsylvania.

Mathes, P., and Rival, T. (1971). *Cardiovasc. Res.* **5**, 54–61.

Merrill, G. F., Haddy, F. J., and Dabney, J. M. (1978). *Circ. Res.* **42**, 255–229.
Miller, R. L., Forsyth, R. P., and Melmon, K. L. (1972). *Pharmacology* **7**, 138–148.
Mohrman, D. E., and Feigl, E. O. (1978). *Circ. Res.* **42**, 79–86.
Muller, O., and Rorrick, K. (1958). *Br. Heart J.* **20**, 302.
Munch, D. F., and Downey, J. M. (1980). *Am. J. Physiol.* **239**, H308–H315.
Murray, P. A., and Vatner, S. F. (1979). *Circ. Res.* **45**, 654–660.
Murray, P. A., Baig, H., Fishbein, M. C., and Vatner, S. F. (1979a). *J. Clin. Invest.* **64**, 421–427.
Murray, P. A., Belloni, F. L., and Sparks, H. V. (1979b). *Circ. Res.* **44**, 767–780.
Needleman, P., and Isakson, P. C. (1980). *Handb. Physiol. Sect. 2 Cardiovasc. Sys.* **2**, 613–634.
Needleman, P., Marshall, G. R., and Sobel, B. E. (1975). *Circ. Res.* **37**, 802–808.
Needleman, P., Bronson, S. D., Wycke, A., Sivakoff, M., and Nicolasu, K. C. (1978). *J. Clin. Invest.* **61**, 839–849.
Nickerson, M. (1962). *Arch. Int. Pharmacodyn. Ther.* **140**, 237–250.
Nickerson, M., and Collier, B. (1975). *In* "The Pharmacological Basis of Therapeutics" (L. S. Goodman, and A. Gilman, eds.), 5th ed., pp. 541–543. Macmillan, New York.
Nutter, D. O., and Crumley, H. J. (1972). *Cardiovasc. Res.* **6**, 217–222.
Olsson, R. A., Vomarka, R. B., and Nixon, D. C. (1978). *Fed. Proc. Fed. Am. Soc. Exp. Biol.* **37**, 418.
Owen, T. L., Ehrhart, I. C., Weidner, W. J., Scott, J. B., and Haddy, F. J. (1975). *Proc. Soc. Exp. Biol. Med.* **149**, 871–876.
Panerai, R. B., Chamberlain, J. H., and Sayers, B. McA. (1979). *Circ. Res.* **45**, 378–390.
Parker, P. E., Bashour, F. A., Downey, H. F., Kechejian, S. J., and Williams, A. G. (1975). *Am. Heart J.* **90**, 593–599.
Parker, P. E., Bashour, F. A., Downey, H. F., and Bouvros, I. S. (1979). *Am. Heart J.* **97**, 745–752.
Pennington, G. D., Vezeridis, M. P., Giffin, G., O'Keefe, D. D., Lappas, D. G., and Daggett, W. M. (1979). *Circ. Res.* **45**, 351–359.
Permutt, S., Bromberger–Barnea, B., and Bane, H. (1962). *Med. Thorac.* **19**, 239–260.
Pitt, B., Elliot, E. C., and Gregg, D. E. (1967). *Circ. Res.* **21**, 75–84.
Powell, W. J., Jr., DiBona, D. R., and Leaf, A. (1976). *Circulation* **53**, (Suppl. I), I45–I49.
Raberger, G. M., Weissel, M., and Kraup, O. (1971). *Naunyn-Schmiedebergs Arch. Pharmacol.* **271**, 302–310.
Regoli, D., Barable, T., and Theriault, B. (1977). *Can. J. Physiol. Pharmacol.* **55**, 307–310.
Rocha e Silva, M., Morato, M., de Almeida, A. P., and Antonio, A. (1976). *Adv. Exp. Med. Biol.* **70**, 117–118.
Rooke, T., and Sparks, H. V. (1980). *Circ. Res.* **47**, 217–225.
Rooke, T., and Sparks, H. V. (1981). *Experientia* **37**, 982–983.
Rose, L. P., Goresky, C. A., Belanger, P., and Chen, M. J. (1980). *Circ. Res.* **47**, 312–328.
Ross, G. (1974). *Cardiovasc. Res.* **8**, 1–7.
Ross, G., Stinson, E., Schoeder, J., and Ginsburg, R. (1980). *Cardiovasc. Res.* **14**, 613–618.
Roth, A. C., and Feigl, E. O. (1981). *Circ. Res.* **48**, 470–480.
Rubio, R., Berne, R. M., and Katori, M. (1969). *Am. J. Physiol.* **216**, 56–62.
Rudolph, W., Fleck, E., Dirschinger, J., Larachner, C., Brandt, R., Redl, A., and Hall, D. (1977). *In* "Heart Function and Metabolism" (T. Kobayashi, T. Sano, and N. S. Dhallo, eds.), Vol. 2, pp. 501–505. University Park Press, Baltimore.
Saebo, J., and Ueland, P. M. (1979). *Biochim. Biophys. Acta* **587**, 333–340.

Sander, G. E., and Huggins, C. G. (1972). *Annu. Rev. Pharmacol.* **12**, 227–264.

Santamore, W. P., and Walinsky, P. (1980). *Am. J. Cardiol.* **45**, 276–285.

Sarnoff, S. J., Braunwald, E., Welch, G. H., Case, R. B., Stainsby, W. N., and Marcruz, R. (1958). *Am. J. Physiol.* **192**, 148–156.

Schaper, W. (1971). *In* ''The Collateral Circulation of the Heart.'' North Holland, Amsterdam.

Schaper, W., and Pasyk, W. (1976). *Circulation* **53**, 157–65.

Scharf, S. M., Bernea, B. B., and Permutt, S. (1971). *J. Appl. Physiol.* **30**, 657.

Scheel, K. W., Banet, M. O., and Lehan, P. H. (1972). *Am. J. Physiol.* **222**, 687–694.

Scheel, K. W., Brody, D. A., Ingram, L. A., and Keller, F. (1976). *Circ. Res.* **38**, 553–559.

Schnaar, R. L., and Sparks, H. V. (1972). *Am. J. Physiol.* **223**, 223–228.

Schrader, J., and Gerlach, E. (1976). *Pfluegers Arch.* **367**, 129–135.

Schrader, J., and Schutz, W. (1979). *Fed. Proc. Fed. Am. Soc. Exp. Biol.* **38**, 1037.

Schwartz, P. J., and Stone, H. L. (1977). *Circ. Res.* **41**, 51–58.

Scott, J. B., and Radowski, D. (1971). *Circ. Res.* **28**, 126–32.

Scott, J. B., Chou, W. T., Swindall, B. T., Dabney, J. M., and Haddy, F. J. (1979). *Circ. Res.* **45**, 451–459.

Seidel, C. L., Schaar, R. L., and Sparks, H. V. (1975). *Am. J. Physiol.* **229**, 265–269.

Sethna, D., Moffitt, E., Gray, R., Bussell, J., Raymond, M., Conklin, C., Shell, V., Prause, J., and Matloff, J. (1981). *Clin. Res.* **29**, 19.

Sirinek, K. R., Martin, E. W., and Thomford, N. R. (1976). *J. Surg. Res.* **20**, 299–308.

Sivakoff, M. Pure, E., Hseuh, W., Needleman, P. (1979). *Fed. Proc. Fed. Am. Soc. Exp. Biol.* **38**, 78–82.

Smith, R. E., Belloni, F. L., and Sparks, H. V. (1978). *Cardiovasc. Res.* **12**, 391–400.

Sparks, H. V. (1980). *Handb. Physiol. Sect. 2 Cardiovasc. Sys.* **2**, 475–513.

Stein, P. O., Brooks, H. L., Matson, J. L., and Hyland, J. W. (1968). *Cardiovasc. Res.* **2**, 63–67.

Thompson, W. L., and Walton, R. R. (1964). *J. Pharmacol. Exp. Ther.* **143**, 131–136.

Toda, N. (1980). *Am. J. Physiol.* **239**, H199–H205.

Trimble, J., and Downey, J. (1979). *Am. J. Physiol.* **236**, H121–H126.

Uchida, Y., Yoshimoto, N., and Murao, S. (1978). *Jpn. Heart J.* **19**, 112–124.

Ueland, P. M., and Saebo, J. C. (1979). *Biochim. Biophys. Acta* **587**, 341–352.

Van Breeman, C., and Siegel, B. (1980). *Circ. Res.* **46**, 426–429.

Vasko, J. S., Gutelius, J., and Sabiston, D. C. (1961). *Am. J. Cardiol.* **8**, 379–384.

Vatner, S. F., Higgins, C. B., Franklin, D., and Braunwald, E. (1971). *Circ. Res.* **28**, 470–479.

Vatner, S. F., Higgins, C. B., and Braunwald, E. (1974). *Circ. Res* **34**, 812–823.

Vatner, S. F., Marsh, J. D., and Swain, J. A. (1975). *J. Clin. Invest.* **55**, 207–217.

Vatner, S. F., Pagani, M., Rutherford, J. D., Millard, R. N., and Manders, W. T. (1978). *Am. J. Physiol.* **234**, H244–H252.

Warren, S. E., and Francis, G. S. (1978). *Am. J. Med.* **65**, 53–62.

Watkins, L., Jr., Burton, J. A., Haber, E., Cant, J. R., Smith, F. W., and Barger, A. C. (1976). *J. Clin. Invest.* **57**, 1606–1617.

Watkinson, W. P., Foley, D. H., Rubio, R., and Berne, R. M. (1979). *Am. J. Physiol.* **236**, H13–H21.

Weiss, H. R. (1979). *Am. J. Physiol.* **236**, H231–H237.

Weiss, H. R., and Winbury, M. M. (1972). *Microvasc. Res.* **4**, 273–284.

Weiss, H. R., Neubauer, J. H., Lipp, J. A., and Sinha, A. K. (1978). *Circ. Res.* **42**, 394–401.

Weisse, A. B., Senft, A., Khan, M. I., and Regan, T. J. (1972). *Am. J. Cardiol.* **30,** 362–370.

Willerson, J. T., Weisfeldt, M. L., Sanders, C. A., and Powell, W. J., Jr. (1974). *Cardiovasc. Res.* **8,** 8–17.

Willerson, J. T., Watson, J. T., Hutton, I., Templeton, G. H., and Fixler, D. E. (1975). *Circ. Res.* **36,** 771–781.

Wilson, M. F., Brackett, D. J., Archer, L. T., and Hinshaw, L. B. (1980). *Ann. Surg.* **191,** 494–500.

Winbury, M. M. (1971). *Circ. Res.* **18,** I140–I147.

Wüsten, B., Buss, D. D., Deist, H., and Schaper, W. (1977). *Basic Res. Cardiol.* **72,** 636–650.

Zuberbuhler, R. C., and Bohr, D. F. (1965). *Circ. Res.* **16,** 431–440.

9

Microcirculation of the Kidneys

L. Gabriel Navar
Andrew P. Evan
László Rosivall

I. Introduction

The microcirculatory environment within the kidney contributes in a critical manner to the optimum achievement of the processes of ultrafiltration

THE PHYSIOLOGY AND PHARMACOLOGY
OF THE MICROCIRCULATION, VOLUME 1

across the glomerular capillaries into Bowman's space, reabsorption from
the interstitial spaces into the peritubular capillaries, and maintenance of
an appropriate medullary environment essential for the concentration of
urine. To subserve these diverse processes, the vascular structures have
developed unique characteristics that allow them to participate selectively in the regulation of blood flow and of the intrarenal pressures
directly involved in fluid and solute exchange across the capillary systems
in the kidney. Because of this intimate association between renal excretory function and intrarenal hemodynamics, it is generally recognized that
the various mechanisms involved in the regulation of the intrarenal hydraulic forces and flows are determined not so much by the nutritional requirements of the renal parenchyma, but more specifically by requirements for the achievement of optimum excretory and endocrine function.
In this chapter attention is focused on those aspects of the microcirculation that are most directly related to the unique functional requirements
for the filtration of large volumes of fluid into the tubular system and the
return of the tubular reabsorbate into the vascular system.

II. Structural Aspects of the Renal Microcirculation

A. General Features

The nonanastomotic nature of the renal arterial system provides an independent blood supply to the glomeruli of each nephrovascular unit
(Huber, 1907). As shown in Fig. 1, the arterial tree continues to branch in
an orderly manner and terminates by giving off afferent arteriolar
branches. Each afferent arteriole divides into a bundle of capillary channels that form the glomerular tuft. These glomerular capillaries coalesce
at the vascular pole to form an efferent arteriole. Although it was once
thought that there was a significant flow of blood that did not initially traverse the glomeruli (Graves, 1971), most investigators now agree that in
the normal mammalian kidney essentially all blood first passes through
the glomeruli before distribution to the postglomerular vessels. Relatively
rare exceptions have been shown to exist in some juxtamedullary units
(Ljungquist, 1975). Casellas and Mimran (1981) observed that approximately 10% of juxtamedullary glomeruli were associated with some type
of vascular bypass.

As shown in Fig. 2 the efferent arteriolar patterns are complex and different in the various layers of the cortex (Barger and Herd, 1973;
Beeuwkes and Bonventre, 1975; Evan and Dail, 1977; Weinstein and Szyjewicz, 1978). Efferent vessels of superficial nephrons ascend toward the

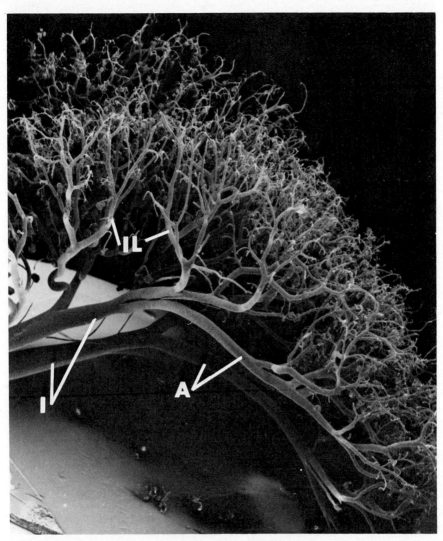

Fig. 1. Scanning electron micrograph showing a replicated cast of a part of the renal arterial vasculature of the dog kidney. The large arteries branch in an orderly fashion, as shown here, from interlobar (I) to arcuate (A) and to interlobular (IL). Magnification is 30×.

surface of the kidney and, at various positions beneath the kidney capsule, divide into numerous peritubular capillaries that are closely associated with the proximal and distal convolutions of the parent nephron unit. Some peritubular capillaries may extend to the capsule and form a "welling point" on the surface. The efferent vessels of midcortical neph-

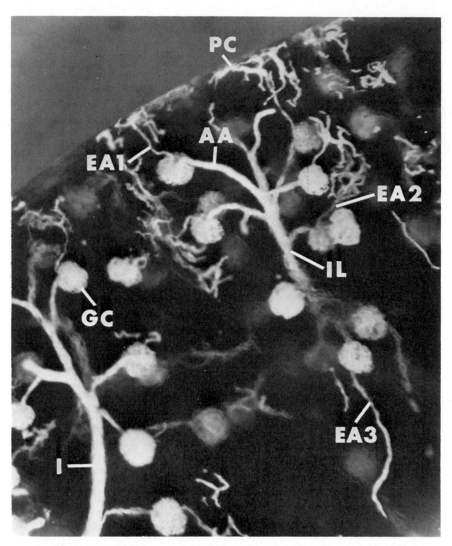

Fig. 2. Light micrograph showing the vasculature of the cortex of a rat kidney as revealed by a Microfil cast. The interlobular arteries (IL) are seen progressing toward the kidney capsule, with numerous afferent arterioles (AA) branching from these vessels. Just beneath the surface, an interlobular artery terminates in a cluster of AA. At the renal corpuscle each AA forms a tuft of glomerular capillaries (GC). An efferent arteriole (EA) emerges from each glomerulus. Each EA has a predictable location and branching pattern depending on its position within the cortex. Superficial glomeruli send their EA (EA1) toward the capsule whereas, in the midcortex, the vessel traverses laterally (EA2) or occasionally descends. In the inner cortex almost all EA (EA3) descend to form vascular bundles in the medulla. Some peritubular capillaries (PC) are noted. Magnification is 200×.

rons terminate quickly into a peritubular plexus that is only partly associated with the proximal and distal tubules of the same nephron unit.
Some of the efferent vessels arising from inner and middle cortical glomeruli descend into the outer medulla, and these branch into a dense vascular bundle. In the inner cortex the efferent arteriole has a larger diameter and often has two branches. One division branches immediately to
form peritubular capillaries, whereas the other descends to give rise to a
vascular bundle. The convoluted segments of the innermost nephrons are
completely dissociated from efferent vessels of their parent glomerulus.
In most cases the straight tubular segments and loops of Henle are surrounded by capillaries originating from efferent vessels of other nephrons.
Thus, in contrast to the discrete localization of the glomerular capillaries,
the peritubular capillaries must be considered in terms of regional local-
izations.

The venous drainage shows considerable variation among different species (Fourman and Moffat, 1971). The human and feline kidneys possess
superficial veins that drain the capillary beds near the capsule of the kidney. The rest of the venous flow from the cortex is directed to the interlobular veins. The venous return from the medulla generally enters the
arcuate veins. The larger veins follow the arterial path. In contrast to the
arterial tree the venous system is characterized by numerous anastomos-
ing channels.

B. Afferent Arteriole, Efferent Arteriole, and
Juxtaglomerular Complex

The afferent arterioles vary greatly in their length and the angle at
which they branch from the interlobular artery (Fig. 2). The tunica media
changes from two muscle cells to one in thickness as it approaches the
renal corpuscle. As shown in Fig. 3 the muscular components change in
appearance as they approach the vascular pole such that they resemble
pericytes and become the juxtaglomerular cells known to be responsible for renin secretion (Davis and Freeman, 1976). Similar cells are
occasionally found in the wall of efferent arterioles.

Efferent arterioles show even greater variation in length, diameter, and
distribution than do afferent arterioles. The muscular wall of efferent arterioles varies from one level of the cortex to the next (Fourman and Moffat, 1971). In the outer cortex these vessels possess cells that resemble
pericytes rather than typical smooth muscle cells. The pericytes continue
for variable distances along the arteriole. These cells may be seen extending onto the peritubular capillaries. The walls of the short arterioles

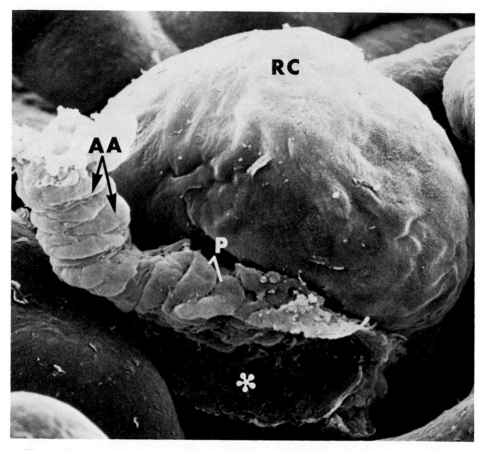

Fig. 3. Scanning electron micrograph of an isolated renal corpuscle (RC) with an attached afferent arteriole (AA). Portions of the proximal tubule are found encircling the glomerulus. The proximal portion of the AA possesses typical elongated smooth muscle cells resembling pericytes (P). As the AA approaches the glomerulus, these cells correspond to the juxtaglomerular cells. A groove is noted for the distal tubule and associated macula densa (asterisk). Magnification is 2000×.

of the midcortex appear to be similar to those of the superficial regions. The longer efferent arterioles in the deeper portions of the cortex appear to have a complete layer of smooth muscle cells surrounding the vessel (Edwards, 1956). Because the glomerular tuft is "nested" between the afferent and efferent arterioles (Fig. 4), the efferent arterioles contribute to the maintenance of glomerular capillary pressure by imposing a downstream resistance. The efferent arterioles also provide the resistance necessary to decrease the intravascular pressure to values required for opti-

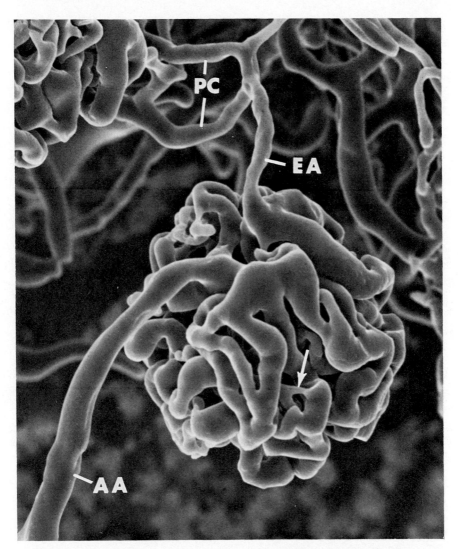

Fig. 4. Vascular cast showing a glomerular tuft and associated arterioles. The afferent arteriole (AA) is seen entering the tuft at its vascular pole. Immediately upon entering the renal corpuscle the AA divides into several large capillaries, which ultimately reunite to form an efferent arteriole (EA). Smaller capillaries (arrow) are seen interconnecting the larger loops. This is a midcortical glomerulus, and the efferent arteriole is short and quickly forms numerous peritubular capillaries (PC). Magnification is 2000×.

mum reabsorptive function of the peritubular capillaries. Because the efferent arterioles are variable in length and in degree of muscular development, the actual pressure drop between the glomerular capillaries and the peritubular capillaries may vary substantially not only among various species but also among the regions of the kidney.

The peritubular capillary pressure is maintained in part by the venous "effluent constrictions" (Koester et al., 1955). The structures are of two types. Stenoses are located at the junction of the arcuate and interlobar veins and consist of abrupt narrowings of the vascular bed, where the tributaries drain into larger channels. Sinusoidal cushions are found close to the junction of the arcuate veins with the interlobar veins and consist of cushions of connective tissue pierced by numerous large thin-walled smooth muscle fibers. These may contribute to the regulation of peritubular capillary pressure and help to maintain a functional distension of the renal parenchyma. The degree to which these venous components contribute to the actual regulation of the total renal vascular resistance remains uncertain, but it would seem to be rather minor. Accordingly, the major resistance sites of physiologic interest are the afferent and efferent resistance segments.

A unique feature associated with the afferent arterioles is the juxtaglomerular apparatus. This interesting structure consists of several types of cells and includes the macula densa cells of the ascending loop of Henle (Barajas, 1970; Hatt, 1967; Oberling and Hatt, 1960; Rouiller and Orci, 1971). The cells associated with the afferent arteriole are embedded in a delicate fibrillar network, which partially or completely surrounds the afferent arteriole and also occupies the region between the angle of the afferent and efferent arterioles. The granular epithelioid cells are associated primarily with the wall of the afferent arteriole, and the nongranular extraglomerular mesangial cells are located between the two arterioles and seem to be in continuity with the glomerular mesangial cells. As the distal tubule approaches the vascular pole of the glomerulus, it comes into direct contact with the cells of the juxtaglomerular apparatus and the arterioles. As shown in Fig. 5 the cells of the distal tubule are modified, and those in opposition to the glomerulus are columnar in shape and are densely packed. This appearance gave rise to the term *macula densa cells*. The lacis or extraglomerular mesenchymal cells are found positioned between the two arterioles and also appear to have interdigitation with the macula densa cells (Oberling and Hatt, 1960). The intimate association between the tubular and vascular elements has served as a basis for the hypothesis that feedback signals are transmitted from the macula densa cells to control the function of the afferent arteriole (Navar et al., 1980, Schnermann, 1981).

It has been suggested that the mesangial cells associated with the glomerular capillaries have some actin and myosin filaments (Ausiello et al., 1980) and have contractile capability. However, at present, few direct data exist to allow a realistic assessment to be made of the *in vivo* contrac-

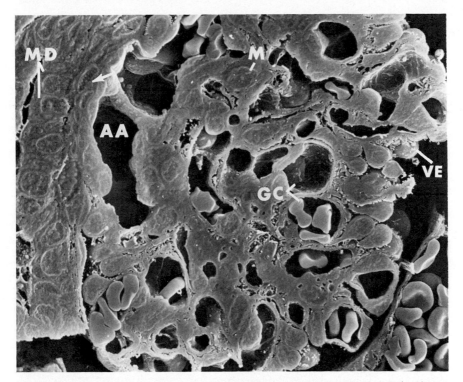

Fig. 5. Fractured renal corpuscle revealing the afferent arteriole (AA) and associated macula densa (MD) and lacis cells (arrow). In addition, one can see numerous capillary loops (GC), mesangial cells (M), and the visceral epithelium (VE). From Bell and Navar (1982). Magnification is 2500×.

tile capabilities of the mesangial cells. Because the pressure drop within the glomerular capillaries is often considered to be quite slight (Marsh *et al.*, 1974; Shea and Raskova, 1981), it might be presumed that relatively small contributions are made by intraglomerular structures to the overall renal vascular resistance.

C. Exchange Vessels of the Renal Cortex

1. Glomerular Capillaries

As the afferent arteriole enters the renal corpuscle it expands into a reservoir lined by endothelial cells. Subsequently, a series of glomerular capillary loops is formed, subdividing each tuft into several lobules (Fig. 4). From these larger capillaries smaller intercapillary channels often branch, serving to connect all lobules. The larger vessels return to the vascular pole, where they reconnect to form the efferent arteriole.

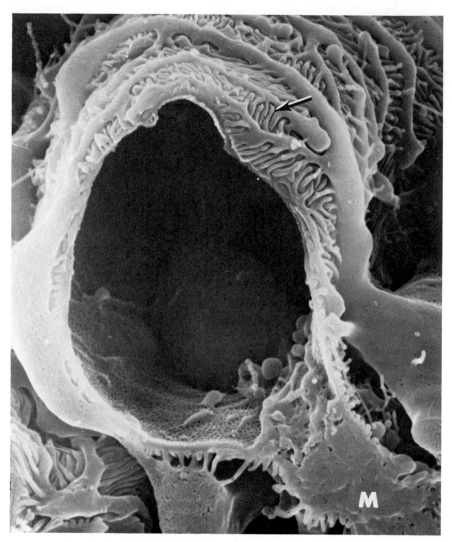

Fig. 6. Scanning electron micrograph revealing all cell types normally associated with a glomerular capillary. The luminal wall is covered by attenuated endothelial cells having abundant fenestrations. The outer surface is surrounded by numerous interdigitating foot processes (arrow). Interposed between these two layers is the glomerular basement membrane. A mesangial cell (M) is seen in its intercapillary position. Magnification is 9000×.

As shown in Fig. 6 each glomerular capillary is composed of several layers: the endothelial cells, a thick basement membrane, and visceral epithelial cells. In addition, the mesangial cells are found in intercapillary locations.

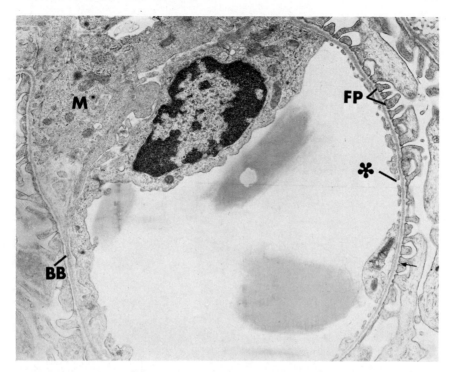

Fig. 7. Transmission electron micrograph showing the ultrastructural features of the glomerular capillaries. The endothelium possesses numerous fenestrae (asterisk) that appear to lack a diaphragm. The thick basement membrane (BB) has three layers: a central electron-dense layer and electron-lucent layers on either side. The visceral epithelium consists of interdigitating foot processes (FP) resting on the basement membrane. The narrow space between individual foot processes is termed the filtration slit. Bridging each filtration slit is a thin membrane called the filtration slit membrane (arrow). In the upper left is a mesangial cell (M). Magnification is 9700×.

The endothelial cells are characteristically attenuated, possessing numerous large fenestrae except at the cell nucleus, where the cell has a more rounded appearance. The round fenestrae are approximately 500–1000 Å in diameter and are thought to lack a diaphragm. It is generally accepted that these fenestrations provide the avenues for the bulk flow of fluid that filters across the glomerular capillaries. Interspersed between the fenestrae are cytoplasmic ridges or folds, which mark the position of the cytoplasmic organelles. Generally, the endothelial cells become irregular in shape and lose most of the fenestrae in the inner portions of the glomerular capillary that are in juxtaposition to a mesangial cell. The ultrastructural features of the glomerular capillaries are also shown Fig. 7.

The basement membrane of the human glomerulus is approximately 3000 Å in thickness and may be divided into three distinct regions (Jorgensen and Bentzon, 1968). There is a central electron-dense zone, the lamina densa, and two electron-lucent areas on either side, the lamina rara externa and the lamina rara interna. The thickness of the basement membrane is substantially less in dog and rat (1000–2000 Å). It varies greatly among species and also with age and amount of glomerular disease. The basement membrane consists of a dense network of fibrils that are composed primarily of collagen and glycoproteins. The glycoproteins are of particular importance in that they contain sialic acid, which provides these structures with a strong negative charge (Mohos and Skoza, 1970). Heparan sulfate may also confer a negative charge on the basement membrane (Kanwar and Farquhar, 1979). These anionic residues present in the basement membrane and the endothelium may contribute significant electrostatic resistance to the passage of negatively charged macromolecules (Farquhar and Kanwar, 1980).

The visceral epithelium consists of a nonsyncytial discontinuous lining of cells called podocytes, which cover the capillary loops (Latta, 1973). Extending from each cell body are a series of primary and secondary branches that terminate into numerous interdigitating foot processes. The adjacent pedicles are separated by narrow spaces of about 250 Å in width. These spaces are termed filtration slits, and a thin membrane is often seen bridging the filtration slits and interconnecting adjoining foot processes. The free surfaces of the foot processes are also covered with a thick polysaccharide coat rich in sialic acid residues.

2. Peritubular Capillaries

Peritubular capillaries are arranged in complex interconnecting networks throughout the cortex down until the tip of the papilla. These vessels are found in close apposition to the different segments of the nephron. As shown in Figs. 8 and 9 the peritubular capillary cells are characterized by their attenuated shape, numerous small fenestrae, and a thin basement membrane. The thickness of the basement membrane is only about 500 Å and is occasionally incomplete (Evan and Hay, 1981). The peritubular capillaries are lined only by the thin wall of the endothelial cells. Most of the cell cytoplasm is attenuated except at the cell nucleus. The diameters of the peritubular capillaries vary, but they are generally larger than the diameters of the glomerular capillaries. The flattened portion of the cell possesses numerous fenestrae approximately 200 Å in diameter. Each fenestra is bridged by a diaphragm. These can be observed in Fig. 10, which is a freeze–fracture micrograph showing the fenestrae and the intracytoplasmic ridges. Thus, there are two important differences between the fenestrations of the glomerular capillaries and

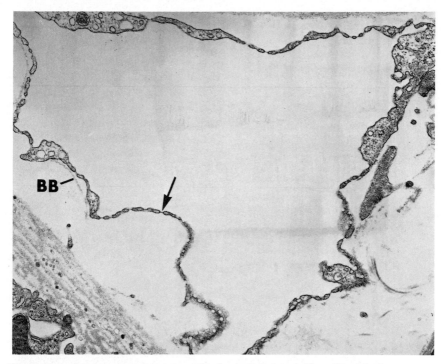

Fig. 8. Transmission electron micrograph of a peritubular capillary found in the outer cortex. The endothelial cells are characteristically flattened with many small fenestrae (arrow). Each fenestra is bridged by a diaphragm. The basement membrane (BB) is thin and at times incomplete. Magnification is 10,500×.

those of the peritubular capillaries. Those of the peritubular capillaries are much smaller, and they possess a diaphragm.

The overall density of the peritubular capillaries is impressive, being many times greater than that of the glomerular capillaries. It can be realized that the collective cross-sectional area for fluid reabsorption by the peritubular capillaries is several orders of magnitude greater than that of the glomerular capillaries. Accordingly, it can be expected that the specific permeability and hydraulic conductivity characteristics per unit of surface area could be markedly different between these two capillary beds (Table I).

D. Renal Interstitium and Lymphatics

The renal interstitial spaces and renal lymphatics have been investigated in efforts to obtain a more complete understanding of the dynamics

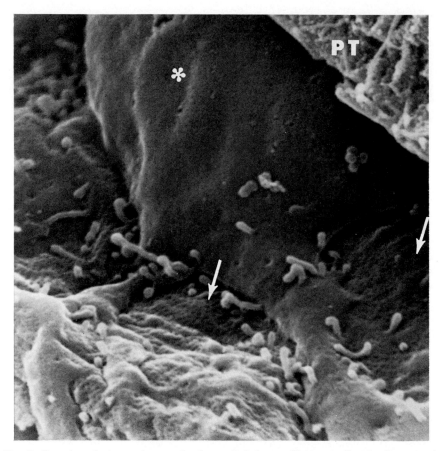

Fig. 9. Scanning electron micrograph of a peritubular capillary revealing its fenestrated nature (arrows). The cell body (asterisk) with its cytoplasmic ridges are seen. Magnification is 20,000×.

of peritubular capillary fluid exchange and solute permeation. The renal lymphatics are distributed rather densely throughout the cortex of the kidney, beneath the capsule, and around the peritubular vessels (Albertine and O'Morchoe, 1979; McIntosh and Morris, 1971; Nordquist *et al.*, 1973; Rojo-Ortega *et al.*, 1973). Medullary structures appear to have a rather limited lymphatic network. As shown in Fig. 11 the walls of the lymphatic capillaries are formed by nonfenestrated endothelial cells without a basement membrane. There are often discrete openings in the lymphatic plexus, indicating that little or no hindrance to macromolecular uptake is offered by the lymphatic terminals. In addition, bundles of fine filaments appear to be inserted in limited areas of the abluminal surface of the en-

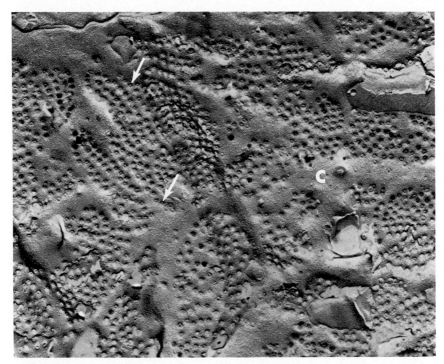

Fig. 10. Freeze–fracture micrograph of the adult peritubular capillary wall. The endothelial cells of the peritubular capillaries possess numerous small fenestrae (arrows). Areas of cytoplasmic ridges (C) are common. Magnification is 24,300×.

dothelium, and it is possible that the filaments help to maintain the terminal ends of the lymphatic channels open.

The renal interstitial spaces themselves have an abundance of microfibrils approximately 200 Å in diameter. Langer (1975) suggested that these are the ultrastructural equivalent of reticulin fibrils. In studies in which the overall volume of the renal interstitium was assessed in instantly frozen freeze-dried tissue and in which precautions were taken to avoid loss of interstitial volume, this volume was rather significant, being about 14% of the kidney cortex. Peritubular capillary volume was an additional 7% (Faarup *et al.*, 1971). The occurrence of substantive interstitial space in the functioning kidney is of importance and indicates that fluid reabsorbate traverses a finite interstitial space as it moves from tubules into capillaries. Thus, movement of the fluid into the peritubular capillaries should be influenced by the hydrostatic and colloid osmotic forces of the renal interstitium.

TABLE I

Representative Values for Various Indices of Glomerular and Peritubular Capillary Function for Dog and Rat

Index[a]	Dog		Rat	
	Glomerular	Peritubular	Glomerular	Peritubular
Hydrostatic pressure (mm Hg)				
Intraluminal	55–60	12–17	45–50	9–13
Extraluminal	20	6	14	2
ΔP (mm Hg)	35–40	6–11	31–36	7–11
Average colloid osmotic pressure pressure (mm Hg)	22	22	25	25
Effective filtration or resorption pressure (mm Hg)	12–16	7–12	6–10	3–6
GFR or PCU				
Per nephron (nl min^{-1})	50–60	50–60	25–30	25–30
Per gram of kidney wt (ml min^{-1})	0.6–0.8	0.6–0.8	0.9–1.2	0.9–1.2
K_f				
Per glomerulus [nl min^{-1} (mm Hg)$^{-1}$]	3–5	5–20	2–6	7–14
Per 100 g of kidney wt [ml min^{-1} (mm Hg)$^{-1}$]	5–6	7	8–13	15–20
S_f				
Per glomerulus (mm^2)	0.4	—	0.2	—
Per 100 g of kidney wt (mm^2)	5560	35,000	7200	40,000
L_p [nl sec^{-1} (mm Hg)$^{-1}$ cm^{-2}]	14–80	4	20–30	4

[a] GFR, Glomerular filtration rate; PCU, peritubular capillary uptake; K_f, filtration coefficient; S_f, surface area available for filtration; L_p, hydraulic conductivity of capillary membrane.

E. Vasculature of the Renal Medulla

The major blood supply to the entire renal medulla is derived from numerous vascular bundles that originate in the cortex and then traverse the medulla. Each bundle is composed of both descending (arterial) and ascending (venous) components. The descending vasa recta are formed from efferent arterioles, most of which originate from juxtamedullary efferent arterioles and a smaller number from the midcortical glomeruli. These vessels correspond to one of two types of arteriolae rectae. The arteriolae rectae supuriae (false straight arterioles) are mentioned in the older literature (Virchow, 1857). The arteriolae rectae verae, or true straight arteriole, were thought to originate directly from either an arcuate or interlobular artery without an associated glomerulus. However, Ljung-

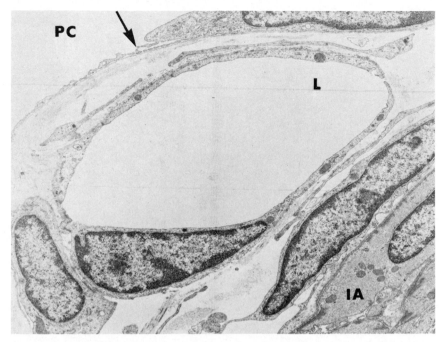

Fig. 11. Transmission electron micrograph showing a lymphatic vessel (L) and its relation to a peritubular capillary (PC) and an interlobular artery (IA). The lymphatic vessel is characterized by a nonfenestrated endothelium, whereas the peritubular capillary has numerous fenestrations (arrow). Magnification is 9700×.

quist (1963) and MacCallum (1939) showed these arterioles to be continuous with degenerated glomeruli of the inner cortex. The descending vasa recta gradually terminate into capillary beds as they proceed to the papilla tip. Thus, the vascular bundles show a gradual decrease in size.

As a single efferent arteriole enters a vascular bundle, it branches into numerous descending vasa recta, often having the same diameter as the parent vessel. These vessels form three distinct capillary plexi corresponding to the different zones of the medulla: the outer stripe of the outer medulla, the inner stripe of the outer medulla, and the inner medulla. The capillary plexus of the outer medulla is very dense compared with that of the inner medulla, thus giving the former region a "frizzled" appearance (Barger and Herd, 1973; Beeuwkes, 1971). The innermost vessels of the vascular bundles reach the papilla. The ascending (venous) vasa recta arise and are much larger than the descending vasa recta. Their density increases as they approach the corticomedullary junction. The ascending vessels from the inner medulla are positioned within the

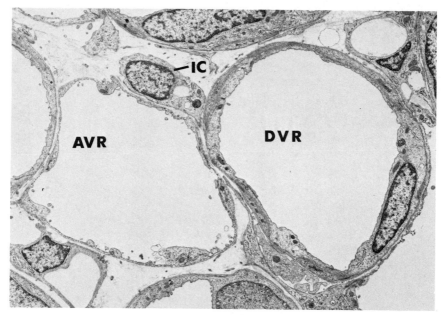

Fig. 12. Transmission electron micrograph showing both a descending and an ascending vasa recta of the inner medulla. The descending vasa recta (DVR) is characterized by a continuous endothelium, whereas the ascending vessel (AVR) possesses numerous fenestrations that are bridged by a diaphragm. A medullary interstitial cell (IC) is also seen. Magnification is 6500×.

vascular bundle, whereas those from the outer medulla are directed between bundles.

The descending and ascending vasa recta can be distinguished by their ultrastructural features (Fig. 12) (Schwartz *et al.*, 1976). The descending vessels are characterized by a thick, continuous endothelium possessing pinocytotic vesicles but lacking fenestrations and having infrequent intercellular junctions. However, the ascending vasa recta show a thin, attenuated endothelium with numerous fenestrae (500–800 Å). Each fenestra possesses a diaphragm 40 Å thick. Both vessel types have zonulae occludens, or tight junctions.

As the vascular bundles enter the outer stripe of the outer medulla, they merge with the medullary rays to establish a precise organization between the vascular and tubular structures (Kriz, 1968). The vascular bundles in the outer stripe of the outer medulla contain a few arterial and venous vasa recta intermingled with the straight proximal tubule segments and thin descending limbs of Henle loops from short-looped nephrons. At the periphery of the vascular bundle are the ascending thick limbs of short-

looped nephrons, thin descending and thick ascending loops of long nephrons, and collecting tubules. The arrangement in the inner stripe is essentially the same as that in the outer stripe. There is a transition of proximal
tubule to descending limbs at the outer–inner stripe interface and a transition of thin ascending to thick ascending limbs at the inner stripe–inner
medullary junction. In the inner medulla the vascular bundles are smaller,
and only long loops of Henle are noted. The collecting tubules are still
seen in groups of four. However, they decrease in number and increase in
size as they approach the tip of the papilla. Both the thin loops of Henle
and the vasa recta are associated with the collecting tubules.

F. Innervation of the Vascular Structures

The kidney has a dense pattern of innervation by unmyelinated nerves
(Barajas, 1978; DeMuylder, 1952). It has been suggested that the kidney is
innervated by both adrenergic and cholinergic nerves. A rich plexus of
adrenergic fibers is associated with the renal artery and its branches, including the afferent arteriole, the efferent arteriole, vasa recta, and large
veins. Cholinergic nerves have also been found associated with the same
vessels, but the pattern is not as dense. In addition, adrenergic nerves innervate the juxtaglomerular apparatus and surrounding tubules, mainly
the proximal and distal segments (Barajas and Muller, 1973). It must be
noted that a controversy exists regarding which vessels are innervated by
cholinergic nerves (Ganong, 1972). Also, some authors have not been able
to show an innervation of the efferent arteriole (Dieterich, 1974). Of particular interest is the finding of Dinerstein et al. (1979) that provided evidence for dopamine-containing neuronal elements in the dog kidney.
They found these fibers to be associated with the glomerular vascular
pole, whereas the rest of the arterial tree possessed norepinephrine histofluorescence.

Myelinated fibers have been found running in the paravasal tissue of the
interlobar and arcuate arteries (Dieterich, 1974). These afferent fibers are
few in number and have not been found associated with arteriolar vessels.

III. Fluid and Solute Exchange across the Cortical Capillaries

A. Forces Governing Filtration and Reabsorption

The renal microcirculatory structures are unique in that anatomically
separate units have developed to subserve the functions of filtration and

reabsorption. Furthermore, an epithelial barrier is interposed between the filtration and reabsorption processes. Although the forces governing the filtration of fluid from the glomerular capillaries into the tubules are not directly coupled with the forces governing the reabsorption of fluid from the renal interstitial compartment back into the peritubular capillaries, normal physiologic conditions require a close functional coupling between these processes. Thus, the crucial importance of the physiologic mechanisms that continuously adjust the determining forces is apparent (Thurau, 1981).

1. Basic Principles Governing Filtration and Reabsorption

The same basic principles govern fluid exchange in both the glomerular and peritubular capillaries. The interaction of the various forces can be described by the Starling filtration–reabsorption principle, which is based on the premise that fluid moves through extracellular water-filled channels that are relatively large with respect to the water molecules and the hydrated solute molecules and ions (Renkin and Gilmore, 1973). The larger molecules that cannot readily permeate the channels are restricted and exert a colloid osmotic pressure that counteracts the influence of the hydrostatic pressure. In essence, then, fluid flux (J_v) across the capillary membranes is determined by a complex balance between the hydraulic and colloid osmotic forces existing across the membrane and the collective hydraulic conductivity characteristics of the membrane, termed the filtration coefficient (K_f). Specifically, J_v can be quantified by the equation of Kedem and Katchalsky (1958):

$$J_v = K_f(\Delta P - \sigma \Delta \pi), \tag{1}$$

where ΔP is the transcapillary hydrostatic pressure gradient, $\Delta \pi$ is the transcapillary colloid osmotic pressure gradient, and σ is the osmotic reflection coefficient, which can have a range from 0 to 1. Under conditions in which σ is 1, the effectiveness of the net colloid osmotic pressure is equivalent to the maximal theoretical value. In contrast, capillary membranes that have very high permeabilities to the macromolecules have a low value of σ, and the colloid osmotic pressure is only partially effective. It is of importance that both the glomerular and peritubular capillary systems appear to have values for σ that closely approach 1 (Deen *et al.*, 1976; Pinter and Wilson, 1981). In particular, the normal glomerular capillaries are very effective in restricting the passage of macromolecules, and the amount of plasma proteins normally found in the proximal tubule fluid is very slight (Dirks *et al.*, 1966; Oken and Flamenbaum, 1971) so that, for the purposes of considering fluid flux across the capillaries of the renal cortex, σ can be considered to have a value of unity. Thus, for the glomerular capillaries the fluid flux is the glomerular filtration rate (GFR), and the protein concentration in Bowman's space can be disregarded, yielding the basic equation

$$\text{GFR} = K_{f(g)}(P_g - P_b - \pi_g), \tag{2}$$

where P_g is the average glomerular hydrostatic pressure, P_b is the hydrostatic pressure in Bowman's space, and π_g is the integrated value for the colloid osmotic pressure in the glomerular capillaries.

The fluid flux at the level of the peritubular capillaries is termed the peritubular capillary uptake (PCU) and is expressed as

$$\text{PCU} = K_{f(p)}[P_c - P_i - (\pi_c - \pi_i)], \tag{3}$$

where P_c is the peritubular capillary pressure, P_i is the interstitial fluid pressure, π_c is the integrated colloid osmotic pressure within the peritubular capillaries, and π_i is the average colloid osmotic pressure of the surrounding interstitial fluid. The relationship pertaining to the peritubular capillary is more involved because the interstitial colloid osmotic pressure must be taken into consideration. There is also the possiblity that σ may not be as high for the peritubular capillaries as for the glomerular capillaries.

2. Hydrostatic Pressure and Colloid Osmotic Pressure Profiles

Most portions of the arterial system of the kidney show a small degree of resistance to flow. However, it appears that the largest fall in hydrostatic pressure occurs at the level of the afferent arteriole. This may include more proximal portions of the preglomerular vessels in certain species. It has been suggested that the arterioles proximal to the afferent vessels may contribute significantly to the intrarenal arterial pressure drop in the rat (Källskog *et al.*, 1976; Ofstad *et al.*, 1975; Tonder and Aukland, 1979–1980). The degree to which this occurs in other species remains uncertain. Studies in the dog (Navar *et al.*, 1982a) have suggested that the hydrostatic pressure in the superficial cortical arterioles is within 10% of the systemic arterial pressure. Furthermore, the pressure in these superficial vessels does not exhibit autoregulation and varies directly with arterial pressure, indicating that the autoregulatory resistance adjustments occur beyond the large arterioles and probably at the level of the afferent arterioles. Estimates in the literature indicate that there is an

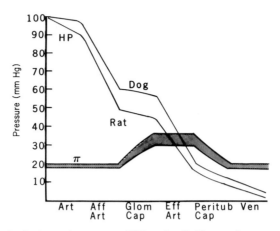

Fig. 13. Profiles for hydrostatic pressure (HP) and colloid osmotic pressure (π) at various segments of the intrarenal microcirculation. For HP, representative values for the dog and rat (Munich–Wistar strain) are depicted. The shaded area represents the ordinary range of π for rat and dog. Art, Arterial; Aff Art, afferent arteriolar, Glom Cap, glomerular capillary; Eff Art, efferent arteriolar; Peritub Cap, peritubular capillary, Ven, venous.

arterial pressure drop of some 40–60% at normal arterial pressures. The relative contribution of this segment to the total vascular resistance is also quite variable because it is capable of substantial adjustments under a variety of circumstances. The relative pressure drops that occur along the length of the renal circulation as they apply to the dog and the rat are shown in Fig. 13 (Baer and Navar, 1973; Brenner *et al.,* 1971).

As shown in the pressure profile of Fig. 13 the arterial pressure is reduced substantially by the afferent arterioles such that it enters the glomerular capillaries at a force of about 45–50 mm Hg in the rat (Brenner *et al.,* 1974). and 50–60 mm Hg in the dog (Navar, 1978b; Thomas *et al.,* 1979). This elevated hydrostatic pressure predominates throughout the length of the glomerular capillaries because the large number of effective parallel channels offer a relatively small resistance to blood flow (Shea and Raskova, 1981). The maintenance of this unusually high hydrostatic pressure (P_g) is of critical importance because this serves as the major positive force for filtration and is counteracted by the proximal tubule pressure (P_t) and the plasma colloid osmotic pressure (π_g) as it rises along the length of the glomerular capillary due to the unidirectional movement of fluid across the glomerular capillaries and the increase in the plasma protein concentration. The progressive increase in the plasma proteins during filtration leads to proportionally greater increases in colloid osmotic pressure (Navar, 1978b), and in certain strains of rats or under certain specific conditions the magnitude of the increase in colloid osmotic pressure is sufficient for an equilibrium of the Starling forces to occur (Brenner et al., 1974; Deen et al., 1974). The latter condition has been termed *filtration equilibrium* and has been shown to occur under normal conditions in the Munich–Wistar rat. In other rats where glomerular capillary pressure is somewhat greater (Källskog et al., 1975b) and in the dog (Navar et al., 1977a; Ott et al., 1976) it appears that the usual case in these species is continued filtration throughout the length of the glomerular capillary. This issue of filtration equilibrium has remained highly controversial (Navar, 1978b) and is largely dependent on the actual magnitude of the glomerular pressure measurements and the filtration fraction. Using a corticotomy technique, Aukland et al., (1977) observed values of 58–63 mm Hg for glomerular pressure in deep and superficial nephrons. Also, Arendshorst and Gottschalk (1980) observed significant differences in the characteristics of glomerular filtration dynamics in a different colony of Munich–Wistar rats. Thus, this remains a topic of major controversy in the field. Representative values for the hydrostatic pressures and colloid osmotic pressures along the length of renal microcirculatory vessels are shown in Fig. 13.

Following the filtration process, blood having an elevated hematocrit and an elevated plasma protein concentration flows out of the glomeruli, through the efferent arterioles, and is distributed to either the cortical peritubular capillaries or the medullary capillary network. The cortical blood flow is many times greater than the medullary blood flow and constitutes approximately 85–90% of the total postglomerular blood flow (Thurau and Levine, 1971). The major role of the postglomerular vessels is to return to the vascular compartment the volume of fluid (99% of the GFR) that has been reabsorbed by the tubular components and transported into the interstitial spaces. Whereas the reabsorption of fluid and solute from the tubules involves a complex interaction of active and passive processes across epithelial barriers having selective permeability characteristics, it is generally recognized that the movement across the peritubular capillary segments back into the vascular volume is dependent entirely on the balance of the Starling forces and the reabsorption coefficient of the peritubular capillary system.

Because of the substantial resistance of the efferent arterioles, the hydrostatic pressure within the blood vessels decreases to the relatively low values existing in the peritubular capillaries. As shown in Fig. 13 this marked hydrostatic pressure drop is of major importance because it lowers the peritubular capillary pressure (P_c) to values that are below the colloid osmotic pressure of the blood flowing into the peritubular capillaries. Although there is still a significant hydrostatic pressure gradient favoring filtration out of the peritubular capillaries, this outward gradient is exceeded by the rather striking colloid osmotic pressure gradient, which allows the predominance of this reabsorptive force. As reabsorbate enters the peritubular capillaries, the plasma proteins are diluted and the net reabsorptive force is dissipated.

The quantification of the transcapillary forces across the peritubular capillaries is complicated because of the uncertainties associated with the hydrostatic pressure and colloid osmotic pressure of the interstitial fluid compartment and the magnitude of the protein permeability of the peritubular capillaries. These issues are discussed in greater detail in Sections III,C and D.

B. Filtration and Reabsorption Coefficients of the Glomerular and Peritubular Capillaries

The filtration coefficient (K_f) is a lumped constant that represents the hydraulic conductivity of the capillary membrane (L_p) expressed per unit of surface area and the total available surface area available for filtration (S_f). The total-surface-area term can be subdivided in terms of the number of functioning capillaries and the average surface area per capillary. Alterations in any of these factors could contribute to changes in transcapillary fluid movement even without associated changes in the Starling forces. In addition, the actual L_p term represents the collective hydraulic conductivity of the membrane segments. In the case of the glomerular membrane, several barriers to hydraulic flow exist. These include the size and number of the endothelial fenestrations, since these contribute to the total cross-sectional area available for fluid flow; the specific hydraulic conductivity characteristics of the basement membrane; and the structural configuration of the slit pores between the foot processes of the visceral epithelium. At present, the quantitative contribution of each of these factors to the overall hydraulic conductivity has not been analyzed rigorously. In fact, it has been difficult to obtain a definitive quantitative appreciation of the actual L_p of the glomerular membrane because of the uncertainty associated with estimates of the filtering surface area of glomerular capillaries (Table I). It has been estimated that the surface area per glomerulus is about 0.4 mm² in the dog and 0.2 mm² in the rat (Navar, 1978b). However, because of the greater than twofold difference in the number of glomeruli per gram of kidney, the total surface area per 100 g of kidney is greater in the rat. Calculations of L_p based on these surface-area estimates indicated that L_p values are about 17 nl sec^{-1} (mm Hg)$^{-1}$ cm^{-2} in the dog and perhaps as high as 30 nl sec^{-1} (mm Hg)$^{-1}$ cm^{-2} in some rat strains. These values are more than one order of magnitude greater than those that have been obtained in any other capillary beds (Deen *et al.*, 1973; Renkin, 1977; Renkin and Gilmore, 1973).

Actual K_f values have varied substantially in the rat, ranging from as high as 6 nl min^{-1} (mm Hg)$^{-1}$ per glomerulus (Brenner *et al.*, 1972) to about 2 nl min^{-1} (mm Hg)$^{-1}$ per glomerulus (Arendshorst and Gottschalk, 1980). Studies in the dog have yielded K_f values ranging from around 3 to 5 nl min^{-1} (mm Hg)$^{-1}$ per glomerulus (Navar, 1978b; Thomas *et al.*, 1979; Ott and Marehand, 1976).

Because the fluid flux across the peritubular capillaries is unidirectional into the vascular compartment, the membrane filtration coefficient $K_{f(p)}$ is primarily a barrier to reabsorption. On the basis of morphologic considerations, the factors contributing to this parameter would appear to be less complicated because fluid has to traverse only a thin fenestrated endothelial barrier having a thin adjoining basement membrane. Nevertheless, the quantitative evaluation of the K_f of the peritubular capillary network is particularly difficult because of its dense and nonlocalized nature. From the basic distribution of the peritubular capillaries it is apparent that the total surface area of the cortical peritubular capillary network is several times that of the glomerular capillaries and has been estimated to be 350 cm^2 per milliliter cortex compared with 10–50 cm^2 per milliliter cortex for the surface area of glomerular capillaries (Kugelgen and Braunger, 1962). Using the value of 50×10^{-6} ml sec^{-1} cm^{-2} for fluid flux, Schnermann *et al.* (1972) calculated a minimal hydraulic conductivity (L_p) of about 4 nl sec^{-1} (mm Hg)$^{-1}$ cm^{-2}. This approximation is useful for comparison with the values of 15–30 nl sec^{-1} (mm Hg)$^{-1}$ cm^{-2} for the glomerular capillaries (Navar, 1978b). In other regards, however, it would seem more practical to consider the overall K_f or the lumped coefficient for transmembrane reabsorption of fluid. Viewed in this manner it would appear that this constant is as great or perhaps greater than the filtration coefficient of the glomerular capillaries (Blantz and Tucker, 1975; Ott, 1981). However, this would seem to be due primarily to the very large surface area available, and it is not necessary to postulate unusually high hydraulic conductivity for the peritubular capillaries.

C. Permeability of the Cortical Capillaries
to Macromolecules

It is generally acknowledged that essentially all of the fluid flow across the glomerular and peritubular capillaries occurs through extracellular channels that do not restrict the passage of the many dissolved constituents having molecular dimensions considerably smaller than the channels. In terms of the normal constituents of the plasma, the capacity of the glomerular and peritubular capillaries to restrict passage of the plasma proteins effectively is of substantial importance. One major reason is related to the relatively low capacity of the tubules to reabsorb filtered proteins such that even slight excesses in the amount of proteins passing across the glomerular capillaries lead to a loss of plasma proteins in the urine (Oken and Flamenbaum, 1971; Von Baeyer *et al.*, 1976). In addition, the major factor responsible for reabsorption of fluid into the peritubular capillaries is the effectiveness of the high plasma colloid osmotic pressure. This suggests that the efficiency of the peritubular capillaries in restricting the passage of plasma proteins is also quite high. Originally, this was not thought to be the case because of the relatively higher protein concentration in the renal lymph and the observations that there could be substantial accumulation of electron-dense macromolecules in the renal interstitium (Renkin and Gilmore, 1973; Venkatachalam and Karnovsky, 1972). However, it now appears that, because of the very low lymph flow, only a very small protein leak can lead to substantial accumulation within the interstitium (Pinter and Wilson, 1981).

For both the glomerular and peritubular capillaries, the transport of protein (J_p) is determined by the rate of fluid filtration (J_v), the average protein concentration ($\bar{C}_p$), and the transcapillary protein concentration difference between plasma and tissue fluid (ΔC). These variables can be related by the equation of Kedem and Katchalsky (1958):

$$J_p = J_v(1 - \sigma)\bar{C}_p \times PS\ \Delta C. \tag{4}$$

The parameters of the membrane that must be considered are the solvent-drag reflection coefficient (σ) and the permeability surface-area product (PS). The two terms that determine J_p are related to the amount of protein that flows as a consequence of the volume flow, the convective component, and the amount of protein that diffuses across as a result of the concentration gradient, the diffusion component (Parker *et al.*, 1981; Taylor and Granger, 1983). In the glomerular capillaries the effects of the convective and diffusion components are additive so that both of these tend to move protein out of the capillaries into the tubules. For the peritubular capillaries these two components oppose each other because the bulk flow movement is into the capillaries whereas the concentration gradient favors outward movement of protein. The J_v term is essentially the same because essentially all the volume filtered is reabsorbed and returned to the intravascular compartment.

Simple considerations of the maximum protein flux occurring at the glomerular and peritubular capillaries indicates that both σ and the PS parameter must be extremely low as compared with other organ systems. If one uses a relatively high value of 8 mg dl^{-1} (milligrams per deciliter) (Von Baeyer *et al.*, 1976; Dirks *et al.*, 1966; Oken and Flamenbaum, 1971) for proximal tubule albumin concentration, then the normal ratio of tubular fluid albumin concentration to plasma albumin concentration would be in the range 0.002–0.004. If one uses the arithmetic average for mean albumin concentration and a J_v of 1 ml min^{-1} per gram of kidney weight, the value for σ is 0.995 even if one assumes that all the albumin passage occurred by convection. If one assumes that all of the albumin passage occurred by diffusion, the PS value is about 0.0027 ml min^{-1} per gram kidney weight. This PS value is expressed as a flow term and represents the equivalent clearance of protein from the filtered amount. Thus, the 0.0027 can be related to the total filtrate of 1 ml min^{-1}, indicating that more than 99.8% of the protein in the plasma being filtered was restricted from passage. These are both the maximal values possible but still demonstrate the remarkably low permeability of the glomerular membrane structures to proteins.

For the peritubular capillary system the amount of protein lost by convection can be considered to be negligible because fluid flows into the capillaries. Thus, if one neglects the convective component, then

$$J_p = PS \, \Delta C. \tag{5}$$

Assuming that the lymph protein concentration is an adequate reflection of the interstitial fluid protein concentration, then the amount of protein movement (J_p) is expressed as the product of lymph flow [$J_{v(l)}$] and lymph protein concentration (C_l) and the transmembrane protein concentration gradient ($C_p - C_l$). In the case of the peritubular capillary system it can be considered that lymph flow does not represent net capillary outflow as it does in other capillary beds (Parker *et al.*, 1981) but rather fluid reabsorbed from the tubules that was not reabsorbed by the capillaries. Accordingly, the J_v term relative to lymph flow is not equivalent to the J_v term of the standard equation defined earlier. Thus, the protein flux equation can be rearranged to

$$PS = J_{v(l)}C_l/(C_p - C_l). \tag{6}$$

As discussed in Section III,D,2 there is considerable variation in the data regarding the interstitial fluid protein concentrations. However, for analysis a relatively high lymph-to-plasma protein ratio of 0.5 and a lymph flow of 0.3 ml min^{-1} per gram kidney weight can be utilized. Assuming a plasma albumin concentration of 30 mg ml^{-1}, one can calculate a PS value of about 0.03 ml min^{-1}. In terms of the amount of protein flow along the peritubular capillary, the amount that diffuses out into the cortical interstitial spaces is in the range 0.5–0.8%. Thus, it can be concluded that, although more permeable, peritubular capillaries still have a remarkable capacity to restrict protein passage into the interstitial spaces. It should be recognized, however, that the interstitial spaces are washed away very slowly by the lymph flow, and proteins can accumulate within the interstitial fluid compartment even when the leak component is very low (Deen *et al.*, 1976).

The prior analysis assumes that the reflection coefficient involved in convective movement of protein is very close to 1 and that little protein is returned to the circulation by the peritubular capillary reabsorbate. There is a theoretical inconsistency, however, that has been pointed out by Taylor and Granger (1983). Even if one assumes a σ value of 0.99 for albumin and a net reabsorption rate of 60 ml min^{-1} 100 g^{-1}, the net transcapillary flux of albumin due to convection would be in the range of three to six times the net loss of albumin calculated as the product of lymph flow and lymph albumin concentration. Thus, to the extent that there is a substantial reentry of albumin accompanying the reabsorbate, then the true PS is substantially greater than generally considered. However, regardless of the actual unidirectional flow of protein across the peritubular capillaries, it can be considered that the osmotic reflection coefficient is still in the range of 0.99 and that the plasma proteins exert near maximum colloid osmotic pressure effects. Pinter and Wilson (1981) calculated a lower bound for σ of albumin in the peritubular capillaries of 0.996 based on unidirectional flux of labeled albumin.

Studies evaluating macromolecular passage across the glomerular and peritubular capillaries have also been undertaken to obtain a more complete understanding of the restrictive characteristics of the membrane channels. This has been a particularly useful approach with regard to the glomerular capillary system because the tracer macromolecules can be readily recovered in the urine. The relative amount of tracer filtered can be determined from the quotient of the urine-to-plasma ratio for tracer molecule and the urine-to-plasma ratio of a glomerular marker such as inulin. Conceptually, this has developed into a very complicated arena, and numerous factors including molecular size, molecular shape and rigidity, molecular charge, and the prevailing hemodynamic environment have been implicated as influencing transport across the glomerulus (Bohrer *et al.*, 1979; Chang *et al.*, 1975a; Deen *et al.*, 1980; Rennke and Venkatachalam, 1977).

Although initial studies attempted to evaluate permeability characteristics using various proteins of different sizes (Pappenheimer *et al.*, 1951; Pappenheimer, 1955; Renkin and Gilmore, 1973), later studies generally incorporated the use of sized neutral macromolecules such as dextran or

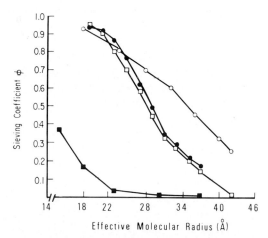

Fig. 14. Representative relationships between effective molecular radius and the sieving coefficient for glomerular and peritubular capillaries. The sources of the data are explained in text. Key: □, ^{125}I-PVP, glomerular capillaries; ●, neutral dextran, glomerular capillaries; ■, dextran sulfate, glomerular capillaries; ○, neutral dextran, peritubular capillaries.

polyvinylpyrrolidone (PVP). This allowed the precise delineation of complete "sieving curves" such as those depicted in Fig. 14, generally plotted as a function of molecular size or estimated radius (Lambert *et al.*, 1975; Vanrenterghem *et al.*, 1980). Also plotted in this figure is the sieving relationship obtained from dog studies when dextran sulfate was used (Vanrenterghem *et al.*, 1980). This general effect related to the electrostatic nature of the tracer molecule has been demonstrated in several studies (Bohrer *et al.*, 1978; Chang *et al.*, 1975a; Rennke *et al.*, 1978). In essence, for any given molecular size or effective radius, polyanions of various types are markedly restricted in their passage across the glomerular membrane, whereas polycations appear to undergo accelerated transport. These differences have been attributed, in large part, to the characteristic polyanionic constituents of the glomerular basement membrane. These glycoproteins are rich in sialic acid and dicarboxylic amino acids and set up a negative electrostatic field that repels polyanions and accelerates the passage of polycations (Rennke and Venkatachalam, 1977).

In addition to the size and the molecular charge, the specific molecular configuration may also directly influence the ease of passage across the glomerular membrane (Bohrer *et al.*, 1979; Rennke and Venkatachalam, 1979). Rennke and Venkatachalam evaluated the glomerular permeability of neutral horseradish peroxidase and neutral dextran having the same effective molecular radius. There was a marked difference in their fractional clearances, the dextran having a clearance of 0.483 and the neutral horseradish peroxidase having a clearance of 0.068. It was suggested that such factors as shape, flexibility, and deformability play important roles in the transport of macromolecules across the extracellular matrix of the glomerular membrane. It has also been reported that the highly cross-linked polymer Ficoll has a lower fractional clearance than dextran molecules having the same effective molecular radius (Bohrer *et al.*, 1979).

Although studies involving the transglomerular passage of macromolecules have contributed to our understanding of the glomerular membrane, there remains substantial uncertainty regarding the quantitative aspects of this issue. The actual determination of true molecular radius is a problem because the gel permeabilities of different types of macromolecules are variable (Jorgensen and Moller, 1979). In addition, several factors other than the idealized or effective molecular radius influence the permeability of a specific molecule. Thus, the true dimensions of the extracellular channels can only be approximated. Nevertheless, the current data available from the transport of noncharged molecules would indicate that the channel half-width of the glomerular membrane is in the range 45–60 Å depending on the specific test molecules used for this determination. The sophisticated analysis based on pore theory that attempts to relate the sieving data to glomerular dynamics (Gassee *et al.*, 1976; Lambert *et al.*, 1975; Renkin and Gilmore, 1973) provides an additional means of estimating the glomerular hemodynamics and how these are altered during various types of manipulations.

Studies evaluating the passage of macromolecules across the peritubular capillaries have been more limited (Deen *et al.*, 1976; Le Brie, 1967; Pinter and Wilson, 1981). As mentioned earlier the interpretation of data is compromised by the dependence on the relative lymph-to-plasma ratios, which can be influenced by numerous factors. Nevertheless, if it is assumed that the tubular reabsorbate is in free communication with the lymph as it flows along the lymphatic channels, then the use of lymph protein concentrations as estimates of the interstitial fluid protein concentration appears to be valid. Although this assumption remains somewhat controversial (Taylor and Granger, 1983), in the absence of alternative approaches, sieving data based on the renal lymph-to-plasma concentrations can be used to estimate the restrictive properties of the cortical peritubular capillaries (D. R. Bell *et al.*, 1978; Deen *et al.*, 1976; Hargens *et al.*, 1977; Le Brie, 1967; Pinter and Wilson, 1981). Studies related to the native endogenous proteins have already been reviewed. A more complete evaluation of the passage of macromolecules of various sizes has indicated that the relationship between molecular radius and the lymph-to-plasma ratio is more gradual, such that dextran molecules having a radius of 42 Å still have a sieving coefficient of about 0.25 as compared with a value of about 0.01 for the glomerular capillaries. A representative curve from the study of Deen *et al.* (1976) is also shown in Fig. 14. Earlier data from the dog (Le Brie, 1967) suggested that the peritubular capillary membrane may have both small and large pores. As in the case of the glomerular capillaries, neutral dextran molecules seem to permeate peritubular capillaries more readily than protein molecules of equivalent size, indicating that other factors such as charge, deformability, and overall configuration also influence passage across the peritubular capillaries. As emphasized earlier many aspects related to macromolecular passage across peritubular capillaries remain uncertain because the convective and diffusive forces operate against each other, and there is a tremendous flow of fluid into the peritubular capillaries. Some of the fluid may not traverse the interstitial compartment but may go directly from the lateral spaces across the basement membranes into the capillaries. However, the amount of fluid that must traverse the interstitial environment is still very great, and it is possible that, even with a very high reflection coefficient, substantial reentry of macromolecules could occur. Thus, only net transport can be deduced from the lymph-to-plasma ratios, and the unidirectional permeability characteristics of the peritubular capillary remain largely unknown.

D. Starling Forces within the Renal Interstitium

The dynamics of fluid and solute exchange across the peritubular capillaries remain incompletely understood because of the uncertainties associated with the magnitude of the Starling forces within the renal interstitium. Specifically, interstitial fluid composition has usually been assessed on the basis of renal lymph composition, and renal interstitial fluid pressure has been estimated using various techniques that have yielded somewhat variable results.

1. Renal Interstitial Fluid Pressure

Numerous earlier studies attempted to evaluate renal interstitial fluid pressure (RIFP) on the basis of the pressures obtained from needles or pipettes inserted into the renal parenchyma. This procedure was refined and minitiarized by Gottschalk (1952), who inserted small glass micropipettes and evaluated the pressure necessary to produce a slight inflow. It is likely, however, that these techniques tended to cause substantial tissue distortion and damage and thus did not provide a measure of true renal tissue pressure. In more recent studies RIFP has been measured with hollow "Guyton" capsules (Ott *et al.*, 1971), polyethylene matrix capsules (Ott *et al.*, 1975; Ott and Knox, 1976), or catheters inserted into the subcapsular interstitial space (Källskog and Wolgast, 1975; Wunderlich et al., 1971). In dogs, RIFP averaged 6.1 ± 0.5 mm Hg (Ott et al., 1971, 1975) and was highly responsive to increases in ureteral pressure and renal venous pressure (Ott et al., 1971). In contrast, decreases in renal arterial pressure to values of 65–75 mm Hg did not lead to steady-state decreases in RIFP, indicating effective autoregulation of RIFP (Ott et al., 1971). The RIFP has also been shown to be highly responsive to intraarterial infusion of vasodilators (Ott et al., 1975) and to extracellular volume expansion with saline solutions (Navar and Guyton, 1975). Because of the constraints imposed by the size of the capsule, RIFP in rats has been measured primarily by the subcapsular catheter method (Källskog and Wolgast, 1975; Schnermann et al., 1972; Wunderlich et al., 1971). By the use of this technique much lower RIFP values have been found in the rat than in the dog, averaging only 1–3 mm Hg above atmospheric pressure. Similar experiments in dogs yielded values of about 8 mm Hg. As with the studies using implanted capsules, RIFP increased with renal venous constrictions and elevation in ureteral pressure. Thus, it seems likely that the renal interstitial fluid compartment has a free fluid pressure that is substantially lower than that occurring in surrounding tubules and peritubular capillaries. These results also indicate that RIFP values are much lower in the rat than in the dog.

2. Interstitial Fluid Colloid Osmotic Pressure

The interstitial fluid composition has been studied by numerous investigators, but most studies have assumed that the composition of interstitial fluid is identical to that of lymph fluid (Gartner et al., 1973; Wolgast et al., 1973). However, there is substantial variation in the reported values for the plasma protein concentration of renal lymph fluid. Samples taken from dog lymphatic vessels have yielded protein concentrations of from relatively low values of 2 g dl⁻¹ to as high as 5 g dl⁻¹. The calculated lymph-to-protein ratios have been reported to be in the range of 0.3–0.5 (Henry et al., 1967). O'Morchoe et al. (1978) compared the protein concentrations in plasma with hilar lymphatic fluid and thoracic duct lymphatic fluid. The averge control value of 2.1 ± 0.14 g dl⁻¹ during conditions in which plasma protein concentration was 5.5 ± 0.12 g dl⁻¹ yields a lymph-to-plasma ratio of 0.38 and is representative of most reported studies. These values suggest an interstitial fluid colloid osmotic pressure of 8–10 mm Hg. Various situations such as expansion of extracellular fluid volume, water diuresis, and mannitol infusions have been shown to elicit an increase in lymph flow with a corresponding decrease in the lymph protein concentration (O'Morchoe et al., 1977). This is not necessarily related to a simple increase in lymph flow because in other circumstances, such as renal vasodilation (Bell, 1971; Bell *et al.,* 1974), ureteral obstruction (Heney *et al.,* 1971), and furosemide administration (Stowe and Hook, 1976), the lymph-to-plasma protein concentration may remain unchanged. In studies in the sheep McIntosh and Morris (1971) investigated the anatomy of renal lymphatics and the flow and composition of renal lymph. The lymph-to-plasma ratio was found to be 0.43, with a greater percentage of albumin present in lymph fluid than in plasma. There was no correlation between the rate of lymph flow and urine flow, and the composition of the lymph indicated that there was little contribution from medullary structures.

The studies in the rat have yielded somewhat lower values for lymph protein concentration, in the range $1-2$ g dl^{-1} (Deen *et al.,* 1976; Hargens *et al.,* 1977; Wolgast *et al.,* 1973). Plasma volume expansion and extracellular volume expansion resulted in marked decreases in lymph protein concentration to below 1 g dl^{-1}, indicating that renal interstitial colloid osmotic pressure in the rat may be substantially lower under these conditions. Hargens *et al.* (1977) suggested that the higher values obtained in earlier studies were probably contaminated and that "pure renal lymph" may have a protein concentration of about 1 g dl^{-1} with a calculated colloid osmotic pressure of 2.5 mm Hg. These more recent findings suggest that the renal interstitial fluid colloid osmotic pressure may be lower than previously estimated and is probably no higher than 8 mm Hg for the dog and as low as $2-3$ mm Hg for the rat. Nevertheless, because of the overall variation that seems to exist, one should be cautious in interpreting specific values for the reabsorption coefficient of the peritubular capillary system when renal lymph or interstitial fluid protein concentration is not determined in the same experiments.

E. Capillary and Interstitial Hydrostatic and Colloid Osmotic Forces across the Medullary Capillaries

Those efferent arterioles from juxtamedullary and midcortical nephrons destined to branch into medullary capillaries are generally larger than other arterioles, and it is justifiable to expect that they might have higher pressures and greater flows (Prong *et al.,* 1969). However, direct data regarding the transcapillary forces of these medullary structures are rather meager. Likewise, the actual fraction of the flow from the efferent arterioles that is distributed to the medullary structures is not known, and the specific mechanisms and elements responsible for regulating the relative distribution of flow to the medullary segments have remained largely a mystery. It is clear, however, that the medullary vasculature is very complex and that an efficient control of blood flow through this region is essential for the normal operation of the concentrating mechanism (Thurau and Levine, 1971).

According to Thurau (Thurau, 1964; Thurau and Levine, 1971) the pressure profile of the medullary capillaries is different from that of the cortical peritubular capillaries, and the hydrostatic pressure at the efferent arterioles may be as high as 50 mm Hg. Studies in golden hamsters suggested a substantial pressure drop along the descending limb of the vasa recta of about 6.5 mm Hg per millimeter of vessel length. Most of the pressure was dissipated along the descending limb because the residual capillary pressure in the vasa recta close to the papillary tip was about 8 mm Hg. Sanjana et al. (1975) reported values of 9.2 mm Hg for descending vasa recta and 7.8 mm Hg for ascending vasa recta in Munich–Wistar rats. According to these data the vascular resistance of the ascending vasa recta is much less than that of the descending vasa recta. This lower hydrostatic pressure in the ascending vasa recta is appropriate for a favorable environment for fluid entry from the tissue spaces into the vascular structures. Because there are more than twice as many ascending as descending vessels (Bottcher and Steinhausen, 1976) and the ascending vessels appear to have greater permeability than the descending vessels, it is reasonable that the greater bulk of the medullary fluid reabsorption occurs in the ascending vasa recta.

Results obtained by Gottschalk et al. (1962) and Sanjana et al. (1976) showed that the protein concentration and the colloid osmotic pressure (π) at both the base and the tip of the papillary vasa recta are higher than the systemic plasma protein concentration, indicating that the fluid reabsorption by the descending vasa recta is relatively low. In fact, π at the tip was slightly greater, suggesting a small loss of fluid between the base and the tip. However, there was a decrease in π from 26 to 18 mm Hg from the descending to the ascending vasa recta, indicating a substantial fluid flow into the ascending vasa recta (Sanjana et al., 1975, 1976). Thus, the fluid removal between the base and the tip of the descending vasa recta may be due to osmotic water abstraction, but the bulk of the water entry into the ascending vasa recta is due to a predominance of the colloid osmotic forces causing inward flow over the hydrostatic forces causing outward flow. The specific values for the effective reabsorption pressures cannot be established with certainty because neither the medullary interstitial hydrostatic pressures nor the interstitial colloid osmotic pressures are known. However, Sanjana et al. (1975) calculated that, if one assumed a lower boundary condition of 0 mm Hg for interstitial fluid pressure, then values for interstitial π as high as 12 mm Hg would still be compatible with a net inward driving force for fluid reabsorption by the vasa recta. Alternatively, if the interstitial fluid pressure were as high or higher than it is in the cortical spaces (Ott and Knox, 1976), the net hydrostatic pressure gradient could be rather small (3–5 mm Hg) and interstitial fluid colloid osmotic pressure could be even higher. It is apparent, however, that the exact quantification of transcapillary fluid dynamics of the medulla must await more exact knowledge regarding the actual values for interstitial hydrostatic and colloid osmotic forces, the reflection coefficient of the vasa recta capillaries to protein and perhaps to small solutes (Sanjana et al., 1976), and the actual volume of fluid reabsorbed by the medullary capillaries relative to the plasma flow.

The reflection coefficients of the medullary capillaries, in particular of the ascending vasa recta, remain a major unresolved issue. From the previous discussion it is apparent that the major force capable of reabsorbing fluid from the medullary interstitial spaces is the colloid osmotic pressure gradient. However, studies have generally demonstrated that these capillaries are quite permeable to large molecules (Shimamura and Morrison, 1973; Venkatachalam and Karnovsky, 1972) and that the medullary protein concentration is rather high (Williams et al., 1971). If this is the case, then the transcapillary colloid osmotic pressure gradient could be quite small, and the reflection coefficient might be much lower than that for peritubular capillaries in the cortex. This environment is less than ideal for the reabsorption of fluid from the tissue spaces back into the capillaries. Thus, it would seem that our understanding of fluid reabsorption by the medullary capillaries is not only quantitatively inadequate but also deficient in terms of basic qualitative information necessary to validate fundamental notions.

F. Regulation of Filtration and Reabsorption Dynamics

1. Effects of Singular Alterations in the Direct Determinants of Glomerular Filtration Rate and Peritubular Capillary Uptake

Because of the many factors that contribute to the overall levels of GFR and PCU, it is essential to place these in some type of quantitative framework in order to evaluate their relative significance. There have been many different mathematical models of glomerular function (Deen et al., 1972; Du Bois et al., 1975; Huss et al., 1975; Källskog et al., 1975a; Marshall and Trowbridge, 1974; Oken et al., 1981; Papenfuss and Gross, 1978; Riggs, 1970; Steven and Strobaek, 1974; White and Navar, 1975) and somewhat fewer evaluations of PCU dynamics (Blantz and Tucker, 1975;

Deen *et al.*, 1973a; Ott, 1981; White and Navar, 1975). Most of these have utilized basic data obtained from studies in the rat. Because there has been less consideration of the characteristics of glomerular and peritubular capillary function in the dog and because of direct experience with these species by the authors, the analysis presented in this section is based primarily on the report and model presented by White and Navar (1975) and applies specifically to the dog. The authors believe that the values and analysis presented correspond closely to glomerular and peritubular capillary dynamics in man.

One of the major problems to be considered is the changing concentration of the plasma proteins, and thus the colloid osmotic pressure, as fluid flows along the length of the capillaries (see Fig. 13). The relationship between the plasma protein concentration and the colloid osmotic pressure is nonlinear and depends on several factors, so that it varies among species (Navar and Navar, 1977). This has been taken into consideration in this model, presented in Fig. 15, which consists of two capillary systems in series. In essence, blood enters the glomerular unit across the afferent resistance and is continuously modified in composition as the filtrate is formed. As the fluid leaves the glomerulus there is an additional pressure drop due to the efferent resistance segment. Consequently, the net force is reversed, and the predominance of the colloid osmotic pressure leads to the reabsorption of fluid. Thus, the equations for both capillary systems are similar, and the specific system responses depend on the actual values involved. For the peritubular capillary model the factors involving interstitial fluid pressure and interstitial fluid colloid osmotic pressure had to be included (see Section III,D). As previously justified it was assumed that the reflection coefficient for protein was 1 and that the effective colloid osmotic pressure was equivalent to the maximum theoretical value.

This model has been utilized in two approaches. In the first approach certain desired values compatible with experimental data are used as base data, and the model parameters are then adjusted to provide derived data compatible with the base data. The base data are given in Table II and are based on numerous previous studies, some of which are listed. The pressure drop from the largest peritubular vessels to the smallest is not clearly established, but the data from the rat (Allison *et al.*, 1972) were used as a reference. These basic data were incorporated into the model, giving the profile shown in Fig. 16. These results are also shown in a schematic diagram in Fig. 17. In addition, values for the remaining dependent variables were derived and are shown in Table III. These provide values that can be considered representative for the dog.

The results of the analysis indicate that the dog glomerulus filters throughout the length of the glomerular capillary and that a small effective

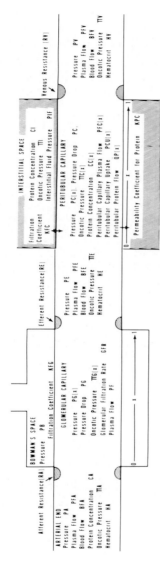

Fig. 15. Coupled model of glomerular and peritubular capillary dynamics (the symbols are identified in the model): (1) $dPF/dx = -KFG \, [PG(x) - PB - \pi G(x)]$; (2) $PG(x) = PG_0 - PG_1(x)$; (3) $\pi G(x) = [A \cdot C(x)]/[1 - B \cdot C(x)]$, where $A = 2.4$ and $B = 0.046$; (4) $C(x) = (CA \cdot PFA)/[PF(x)]$; (5) $GFR(x) = PFA - PF(x)$; (6) Total $GFR = PFA - PFE$; (7) $EFP(x) = PG(x) - PB - \pi G(x)$; (8) $PFA = (1 - HA)(PA - PG_0)/RA]$; (9) $PFE = (1 - HE)](PG_0 - PG_1 - PE)/RE]$; (10) $FF = GFR/PFA$; (11) $dPFC/dx = -KFC[PC(x) - PIF \times \pi I - \pi C(x)]$; (12) $PC(x) = PC_0 - PC_1(x)$; (13) $\pi C(x) = [A \cdot CC(x)]/[1 - B \cdot CC(x)]$; (14) $d\dot{Q}P/dx = -KPC[CC(x) - CI]$; (15) $QP(x) = PFC(x)CC(x)$; (16) $PCU(x) = PFC(x) - PFE$; (17) Total $PCU = PFV - PFE$; (18) $PFV = [(1 - HV)(PC_0 - PC_1 - PV)]/RV$. Equations (1)–(10) are related to glomerular dynamics, and Eqs. (11)–(18) are related to peritubular capillary dynamics. Some of the symbol notations in these equations differ slightly from those presented in earlier sections.

TABLE II

Base Data for Coupled Model of the Glomerular and Peritubular Capillaries

Parameter	Value	Reference
Arterial pressure (PA)	100 mm Hg[a]	—
Glomerular pressure (PG)	56–58 mm Hg	Thomas et al. (1979); Marchand and Mohrman (1980); Heller and Horacek (1980)
Glomerular pressure drop (PG$_1$)	1 mm Hg	Huss et al. (1975)
Bowman's space pressure (PB)	20 mm Hg	Knox et al. (1972b); Navar et al. (1977b)
Efferent arteriolar pressure (PC$_0$)	17 mm Hg	Allison et al. (1972)
Pressure drop of peritubular capillary (PC$_1$)	2–4 mm Hg	Allison et al. (1972)
Interstitial fluid pressure (PIF)	6 mm Hg	Ott et al. (1971, 1975)
Plasma protein concentration (CA)	5.6 g dl^{-1}	Navar and Navar (1977)
Interstitial protein concentration (CI)	2.8 g dl^{-1}	Knox et al. (1972b)
Plasma colloid osmotic pressure (πA)	18 mm Hg[b]	—
Interstitial colloid osmotic pressure (πI)	7.7 mm Hg[b]	—
Arterial blood hematocrit (HA)	0.40[a]	—
Efferent arteriolar hematocrit (HE)	0.49[c]	—
Single-nephron glomerular filtration rate (SNGFR)	45–50 nl min^{-1}	Navar et al. (1974, 1977b)
Peritubular capillary uptake (PCU)	46 nl min^{-1} [d]	—

[a] Initial condition.
[b] From protein concentration.
[c] From filtration fraction of 0.30.
[d] From SNGFR.

filtration pressure (4–8 mm Hg) remains at the efferent end. This is demonstrated in Fig. 16 by the separation of the lines showing the glomerular pressure and the sum of the proximal tubule pressure and πG. The filtration coefficient derived from this model is consistent with that obtained from experimental studies in several laboratories (Navar et al., 1977a; Ott and Marchand, 1976; Thomas et al., 1979). If the pressure drop (PG) was increased, then a greater value of glomerular filtration coefficient (KFG) was required to achieve the desired single-nephron GFR (SNGFR) and the probability of attaining filtration equilibrium was increased, as pointed out by DuBois et al. (1975).

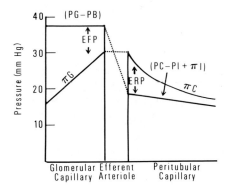

Fig. 16. Representative profiles of the changes in hydrostatic and plasma colloid osmotic pressures for glomerular and peritubular capillaries obtained from the model using base data from the dog. At the efferent arteriole there is a reversal of the predominance of forces such that the colloid osmotic pressure within the peritubular capillaries exceeds the sum of the forces responsible for fluid efflux. For abbreviations see Tables II and III.

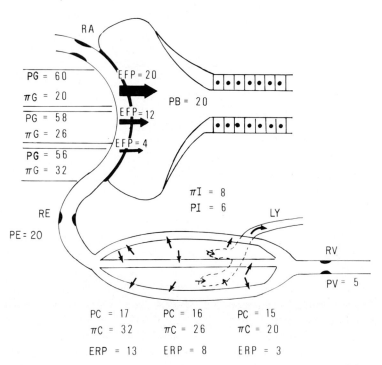

Fig. 17. Schematic of a nephrovascular unit depicting the hydraulic and colloid osmotic forces operating across the glomerular and peritubular capillaries. LY, Lymphatic vessels. For other abbreviations see Tables II and III.

TABLE III

Data Derived from Coupled Model of Glomerular and Peritubular
Capillaries Using Base Data Shown in Table II

Parameter	Value
Arterial blood flow (BFA)	262 nl min^{-1}
Arterial plasma flow (PFA)	157 nl min^{-1}
Efferent plasma flow (PFE)	110 nl min^{-1}
Efferent protein concentration (CE)	7.97 g 100 ml^{-1}
Efferent colloid osmotic pressure (πE)	30.2 mm Hg
Afferent arteriolar resistance (RA)	0.161 mm Hg nl^{-1} min
Efferent arteriolar resistance (RE)	0.187 mm Hg nl^{-1} min
Glomerular filtration coefficient (KFG)	3.51 nl min^{-1} (mm Hg)$^{-1}$
Peritubular filtration coefficient (KFC)	13 nl min^{-1} (mm Hg)$^{-1}$
Effective filtration pressure, glomerulus (EFP)	13.4 mm Hg
Effective reabsorption pressure (ERP)	3.5 mm Hg

For the peritubular capillary model the filtration coefficient (KFC) necessary to achieve a reabsorption of 46 nl min^{-1} was highly dependent on the values for interstitial fluid pressure and colloid osmotic pressure and also on the magnitude of the hydrostatic pressure drop in the peritubular capillaries. With the base data provided, a KFC of 13 nl min^{-1} (mm Hg)$^{-1}$ was necessary. With an increase in the pressure drop to 3–4 mm Hg, KFC could be reduced to 8–10 nl min^{-1} (mm Hg)$^{-1}$. As can be seen the profile is distinct from that obtained in the glomerular capillary because most of the uptake occurs early. This is compatible with the very high total surface area available for reabsorption. The derived values remain uncertain because they are highly dependent on the base values used. Ott (1981) obtained somewhat lower values for peritubular capillary pressures (11.3 mm Hg) and lower values for interstitial fluid pressures (5.7 mm Hg) and thus found a substantially greater net reabsorption pressure. The calculated KFC for his experiments (for the total reabsorbate) was about one-half of that derived using our base data. Ott observed that marked volume expansion with isotonic saline did not alter the KFC.

The first approach is particularly valuable in that it allows an assessment to be made of the influence of specific and singular perturbations on net fluid filtered or reabsorbed. These can be evaluated graphically or with the aid of sensitivity analysis (White and Navar, 1975). These evaluations have considered the effects of changes in plasma protein concentration, plasma flow, hydrostatic pressure gradient, and filtration coefficient on the net transcapillary fluid movement. The effects of changes in the net hydrostatic pressure gradient and in the initial plasma protein concentration on GFR and PCU are compared in Fig. 18. There is the generally well

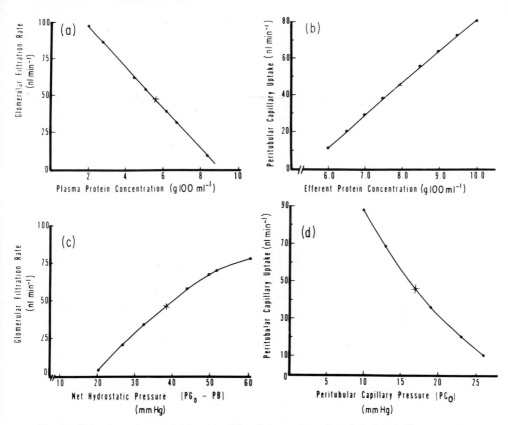

Fig. 18. Representative results from models of glomerular and peritubular capillary systems showing the effects of changes in initial plasma protein concentration (a and b) and hydrostatic pressure (c and d) on GFR (a and c) and PCU (b and d).

recognized effect of pressure, indicating a direct effect of pressure to increase GFR and decrease PCU. The marked sensitivity of PCU to the hydrostatic pressure seems worthy of emphasis. This relationship supports the suggestion that changes in peritubular capillary dynamics could exert substantial influences on net sodium reabsorption (Earley *et al.*, 1972). Also, the predicted influence of changes in plasma protein concentration are relatively linear. Both GFR and PCU show rather marked sensitivities to changes in plasma protein concentration. Because the concentration of protein entering the peritubular capillaries is influenced by the filtration fraction as well as the plasma protein concentration, the effects of filtration fraction changes on peritubular capillary uptake could be mediated through this mechanism (Brenner *et al.*, 1969).

The effects of changes in plasma flow in the absence of any other changes are shown in Fig. 19. In contrast to the reported studies based on rats that exhibit the characteristic of filtration equilibrium (Brenner *et al.*, 1972; Blantz *et al.*, 1974), the analysis based on dog studies indicates that changes in plasma flow per se have only modest effects on GFR and PCU. The GFR is much more sensitive to plasma flow at the lower values of plasma flow. In contrast to the effects of alterations in plasma protein concentration and hydrostatic pressure, plasma flow exerts balanced effects such that increases in plasma flow increase both GFR and PCU to approximately the same extent. Thus, specific changes in blood flow independent of other factors do not appear to cause an imbalance between filtration and reabsorption.

The effects of changes in the filtration coefficients on GFR or PCU are also depicted in Fig. 19. A similar relationship is apparent for each system such that changes in K_f are important at lower values for K_f and become less effective at the higher values. The major distinguishing feature is related to the physiologic operating range. For the glomerulus it appears that the normal K_f in the dog is in the range in which changes in either direction can cause profound changes in GFR. In contrast, this analysis indicates that K_f of the peritubular capillaries is sufficiently high that the effects of changes in this parameter on overall PCU are relatively modest. This interpretation agrees with the anatomic data indicating an immense peritubular capillary network surface area.

These results indicate that, in species not exhibiting the characteristics of filtration equilibrium, K_f may be of major physiologic significance in regulating filtration at the glomerulus and quantitatively may be of only minor importance in regulating PCU.

2. Integrated Responses to Alterations in the Vascular Resistance Elements

One useful advantage of the approach just explained is that it allows a theoretical evaluation to be made of the influence of specific perturbations independent of the changes in other associated variables. It is recognized, however, that this is not the physiologic manner in which the determinants of GFR and PCU are usually regulated. Under actual physiologic circumstances the vascular resistance elements constrict or dilate, resulting in coincident changes in the pressures and flows. Thus, a physiologically more realistic approach to the modeling of renal hemodynamics is to evaluate the effects of alterations in vascular resistance on the other system variables. In this type of model the resistances are changed, and new values for all affected variables are determined using iterative techniques.

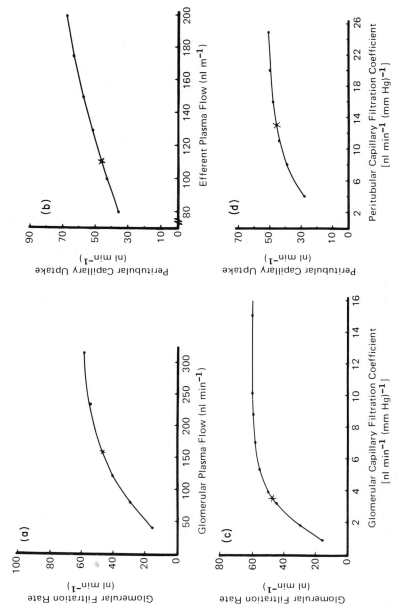

Fig. 19. Representative results from the glomerular and peritubular capillary models demonstrating the effects of variation in initial plasma flow (a and b) and the capillary filtration coefficient (c and d) on GFR (a and c) and PCU (b and d). The analysis was conducted using a data base representative for the dog, and thus the influence of plasma flow on GFR and PCU is modest.

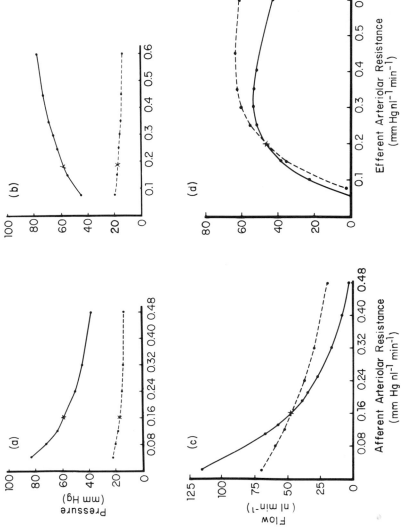

Fig. 20. Results from coupled model of glomerular and peritubular capillary dynamics showing the effects of variations in afferent arteriolar resistance (a and c) and efferent arteriolar resistance (b and d) on the intraluminal hydrostatic pressures (a and b; ——, glomerular capillary; ——, peritubular capillary) and transcapillary fluxes (c and d; ——, glomerular filtration rate; ——, peritubular capillary uptake) at the glomerular capillaries (——) and the peritubular capillaries (——).

The predicted effects of changes in afferent and efferent resistances above and below the normal values on glomerular pressure and peritubular capillary pressure are shown in Fig. 20. As afferent arteriolar resistance increases, there are decreases in both glomerular pressure and peritubular capillary pressure; however, the responsiveness of glomerular pressure is much greater. Accordingly, selective increases in afferent arteriolar resistance may exert greater effects on GFR than on PCU. These effects are shown in Fig. 20c. It should be emphasized, however, that these responses are only theoretical ones based on the maintenance of all extracapillary forces. In an actual physiologic setting these outside forces are also adjusted in order to maintain an overall balance between filtration and reabsorption. The predicted effects of selective changes in efferent arteriolar resistance are somewhat more complex because increases in efferent resistance lead to increases in glomerular pressure and decreases in peritubular capillary pressure. With small increases in efferent resistance, the effect of glomerular pressure in increasing GFR may predominate over the effects of an increased colloid osmotic pressure. With greater increases in efferent resistance, GFR is no longer affected because the protein concentration is sufficient to counteract the effects of increased glomerular pressure. The effects of increases in efferent resistance on peritubular uptake are not as marked. As efferent resistance increases, the filtration fraction rises and the efferent colloid osmotic pressure is increased to enhance the reabsorptive capability of the peritubular capillary network. The slight decrease in peritubular capillary pressure also contributes to this effect. This reaches a maximal level and remains stable with further increases in efferent resistance due to the reduction in PCU caused by the associated decreases in plasma flow.

These studies demonstrate that the effects of increases in the segmental vascular resistances can be quite complex and may not always be intuitively obvious. Perhaps the best demonstration of this point is the concept that interpretations of selective resistance adjustments can be made from changes in filtration fraction. This concept stems from the basic notion that selective increases in efferent arteriolar resistance do indeed cause increases in filtration fraction. However, increases in filtration fraction can also occur by other means, including combined changes in afferent and efferent resistance (Gomez, 1951; Smith, 1951). For example, if both afferent and efferent resistances increase to a proportional extent, the influence on GFR is much less than the effect on blood flow. Consequently, filtration fraction increases. Conversely, a vasodilator stimulus may reduce overall vascular resistance and decrease the filtration fraction to a variable extent depending on the relative effects on afferent and efferent resistances. A nonselective effect that leads to equivalent reductions in both afferent and efferent resistances would cause increases in renal blood flow (RBF) and associated GFR responses of lesser magnitude (assuming a system that is not in filtration equilibrium). This would lead to decreases in filtration fraction because RBF is increased to a greater extent. Therefore, it should be emphasized that it is not appropriate to draw conclusions regarding the segmental localization of renal vascular resistance changes based only on filtration fraction data.

IV. Distribution of Blood Flow within the Kidney

The intrarenal distribution of blood flow may be of importance in various experimental and clinical conditions. For example, the mechanisms involved in urine concentration depend, to a great extent, on the maintenance of an optimum medullary blood flow. It has also been suggested that the relative distribution of cortical blood flow among the outer superficial nephrons and the deeper nephrons participates in the regulation of sodium excretion (Barger, 1966). The relative hemodynamic effects of the intrarenal hormones such as angiotensin II or the prostaglandins may be exerted in such a manner that alterations in RBF distribution occur. It is evident, therefore, that without knowledge of the changes in intrarenal vascular resistance and flow distribution in different conditions it is not possible to understand the dynamics of the microcirculation in the kidney.

A. Methodologic Approaches to Regional Microcirculatory Studies

In the last decade much experimental work has been devoted to the measurement of intrarenal distribution of blood flow using different methods. Nevertheless, the effects of various neurogenic, humoral, and physical factors on different parts of the renal microcirculation have not yet been fully elucidated. This has been due in part to an inadequate evaluation of the methods used. Under normal conditions the mean values obtained by the various techniques used to measure intrarenal blood flow have shown reasonably good agreement. However, there is substantial variation with regard to the responses in intrarenal distribution estimated by various methods. Because these apparent discrepancies may result from errors inherent in the techniques, it seems relevant to mention briefly the theoretical and technical problems associated with the measurement of RBF distribution.

1. Microsphere Method

It has been extensively reported that the microsphere method is reliable for the estimation of cardiac output and RBF in various species (McNay and Abe, 1970a; Mendell and Hollenberg, 1971; Rudolph and Heymann, 1967; Stein et al., 1973). Most investigators use 15-μm carbonized radiolabeled microspheres with a specific gravity varying from 1.1 to 1.6. Labeled frog red blood cells, which have also been used, have an elliptical dimension of 18 $\times$ 10 μm and a density of 1.08 (Baehler et al., 1973). After the injection of particles into the left ventricle, which provides an adequate mixing of the spheres, the microspheres that flow into the kidney are trapped almost exclusively in the glomerular capillary bed (Katz et al., 1971; Stein et al., 1973). The side effects of increasing the number of microspheres injected during flow measurements have been studied by several investigators (Källskog et al., 1975d; Poujeol et al., 1975; Slotkoff et al., 1971). Although some slight effects have been noted, it is generally agreed that total RBF, GFR, and sodium excretion are not perceptibly altered if the cumulative dose is not larger than about 10^6 microspheres. The diameter of the afferent arterioles can be estimated from the spheres trapped in them or from the spheres that pass through the afferent arterioles and are trapped in the glomerular capillary network. Estimates based on such measurements indicate that the afferent arteriole in the dog kidney has a diameter of about 20 μm (Morkrid et al., 1978; Ofstad et al., 1975).

The major limitation of the microsphere method is due to possible rheologic differences between red blood cells and the rigid spheres. McNay and Abe (1970a) concluded that the microsphere distribution reflected accurately the distribution of intrarenal blood flow. However, subsequent observations by other investigators suggested that an axial distribution of 15-μm microspheres does occur and results in a lower microsphere concentration in the blood perfusing the deep glomeruli than in that flowing through the more superficial glomeruli (reviewed by Aukland, 1976, 1980, 1981). Studies using in vitro glass models have indicated that microspheres are separated to a much greater extent than erythrocytes by skimming (Palmer and Betts, 1975; Ofjord et al., 1981). This would lead to artifactually exaggerated flow values in the superficial glomeruli, not only because the relative microsphere concentration of the blood reaching the superficial glomeruli would be greater, but also because the average size of these microspheres would be larger and have a proportionally greater radioactivity than those in the inner cortex (Bankir et al., 1979). There is also the possibility that microspheres larger than 15–17 μm may have a lower probability of entering the afferent arterioles of the deep cortex in the dog due to steric restriction (Morkrid *et al.*, 1976). Furthermore, there is a thin cell-free and microsphere-free plasma film along the walls of the interlobular arteries. These factors collectively provide a lower probability of the microspheres entering the afferent arterioles, especially those of the deep cortex that are branched at right or recurrent angles.

Overall, the microsphere technique offers the advantage of convenience and, by the use of different radionuclides, measurements can be paired so that comparisons between control and experimental conditions can be obtained. The technique is considered to provide an accurate measurement of total glomerular blood flow. However, the absolute flow distribution obtained with different sizes of microspheres may not be quantitatively correct, although relative differences occurring in the same area during control and experimental conditions may be reasonably accurate.

2. Diffusible Tracers

a. Inert Gas Methods (*External Detection*). The inert gas (^{133}Xe, ^{85}Kr) washout method is based on the theory of Kety (1951) concerning the exchange of rapidly diffusible indicators between tissue and blood. The basic assumption is that the highly diffusible tracers dissolved in the blood entering the tissue will reach complete equilibrium with the total organ mass in one single passage; hence, it can be considered that the indicator activity in the venous blood is equal to that in the tissue. By compartmental analysis it is possible to examine the progressive loss of indicator from the kidney after the cessation of gas administration and arrive at several exponential relationships (three or more) that are consistent with the overall decay curve obtained. In some studies autoradiography has been employed in an effort to localize distinct regional components within the kidney that may be associated with the individual exponential relationships obtained (Jones and Herd, 1974; Thornburn *et al.*, 1963).

The exact meaning of the subdivisions of the washout curve into several exponential components has remained controversial. The division of the cortex into four zones is, of course, arbitrary, and the differences in the perfusion of adjacent thin layers of the cortical tissue must be small, although they differ significantly, as studies carried out with microspheres have shown. Accordingly, the first seemingly monoexponential component of the decay curve, which represents the cortical flow, is presumably a resultant of an infinite number of components with gradual transitions between high and low flow rates (Hársing *et al.*, 1975). Also, the relative volume of the tissue corresponding to the different slopes of the washout curve may change with increases or decreases in RBF (Rosivall *et al.*,

1979b). Consequently, the slopes of the decay curves do not represent the flow in well-defined and constant parts of the kidney. Furthermore, compartmental analysis is valid for a system having parallel compartments in which the disappearance of the indicator starts at the same time in all compartments, the flow within the compartments is homogenous and constant during the washout period, and there is no other flow that interferes with the washout. If blood flow is calculated per unit volume of tissue, it is also assumed that the tissue/blood partition coefficient is the same within the entire kidney. However, it has been shown that the postglomerular circulation comprises both parallel and serial coupled circuits (Rosivall *et al.*, 1979a,b), and the disappearance of the indicator does not start at the same time in the different compartments. It is also recognized that the inert gas flow is a considerable underestimation of the "medullary" flow because of recirculation of the indicator in this area. Furthermore, the flow of the third compartment may also be influenced by trapping of indicator in urine and lymph. The solubilities of Xe in blood, protein, lipid, and saline solution are different. Therefore, the tissue/blood partition coefficient may be different within the kidney and may change if the component of the tissue is not constant during the experiment (Szabó *et al.*, 1976).

Although this technique offers the advantages of being relatively noninvasive and easy to repeat, the results have always been difficult to interpret because of the many inherent assumptions and the complexity and dynamic nature of the renal microcirculation. Therefore, insights about the intrarenal blood flow distribution gained from the analysis of inert gas washout curves are not comparable with those obtained by other methods in which the regional perfusion is measured in an anatomically defined portion of the renal tissue. Passmore *et al.* (1977) developed a deep-freeze dissection technique to measure the washout of ^{85}Kr from outer cortex, inner cortex, and outer medulla separately. This technique allows only a single series of measurements to be made and relies on group comparisons. Such an approach makes it difficult to show small changes in the intrarenal flow distribution in response to specific manipulations.

b. Local Measurement of Diffusible Tracers: H_2, [^{125}I]Iodoantipyrine, Tritiated Water, and Sulfanilamide. Theoretically, local blood flow can be assessed by measuring the removal or uptake of a substance in a specific region of the kidney. For example, H_2 gas washout can be measured with platinum electrodes implanted into the tissue (Aukland *et al.*, 1964). During insertion of the electrodes some tissue trauma is unavoidable, but the data in the literature suggest that it does not impair the actual reactivity of the local resistance to blood flow (Aukland, 1980; Loyning, 1971). In addition to H_2 gas, [^{125}I]iodoantipyrine (Clausen *et al.*, 1979a; Hope *et al.*,

1976), tritiated water (Clausen *et al.*, 1979a), and, more recently, unlabeled sulfanilamide (Szabó *et al.*, 1980) have been used to determine intrarenal blood flow distribution using the measurement of local uptake of these inert diffusible tracers. The tracers leave the blood by glomerular filtration and by diffusion from the peritubular capillaries into the renal interstitium and tubular cells. Sulfanilamide is also taken up by the tubular cells and excreted into the urine (Szabó *et al.*, 1980). Techniques using most of these local tracers probably underestimate the medullary blood flow to an unknown extent due to the countercurrent diffusion between arterial and venous vasa recta, which slows down both the accumulation and washout of the tracer in the deep portions of the medulla.

The technical difficulties of determining local uptake rate are considerable because it is important to compare the arterial concentration curve of tracer with the kidney tracer content at the same time. Even small errors in the correction of catheter delay of arterial concentrations give rise to serious over- or underestimations of blood flow. The prolongation of the tracer infusion time causes a higher degree of saturation but also increases the error in calculated flow caused by an inappropriate tissue/blood partition coefficient and by inaccuracies in the measurements of tracer concentration in blood and tissue (Hope *et al.*, 1976). Nevertheless, long infusion times decrease the effect of timing error, minimizing the effect of the initial delay. Errors inherent in medullary countercurrent exchange of tracers remain (Clausen *et al.*, 1979a).

3. Rubidium-Uptake Method

The measurement of regional blood flow using ^{86}Rb is based on the finding that the behavior and distribution of ^{86}Rb are similar to those of potassium and that for a period of 10–120 sec following a bolus injection the fraction of Rb taken up by kidney is constant and is a function of the RBF fraction of cardiac output (Sapirstein, 1958; Steiner and King, 1970). This calculation of RBF is valid provided that the renal extraction of ^{86}Rb equals the total-body ^{86}Rb extraction ratio. Systemic and renal ^{86}Rb extraction ratios have been determined at different times after injection, and the results have shown that there is no significant difference between them 15–30 sec after ^{86}Rb injection (Rosivall *et al.*, 1981; Yarger *et al.*, 1978).

There are reports suggesting that ^{86}Rb extraction is inversely related to renal blood flow (Rosivall *et al.*, 1979b; Steiner and King, 1970), and this relationship has been demonstrated by direct measurements (Rosivall *et al.*, 1981). Such a relationship has also been observed in skeletal muscle (Sheehan and Renkin, 1972) and in heart muscle (Love and O'Meallie,

1963). Although it seems that there is slightly higher extraction of ^{86}Rb in rats than in dogs (Coelho, 1977; Steiner and King, 1970), there is a similar flow dependency (Rosivall et al., 1979b, 1981). Thus, it is possible that, during vasodilation, estimates of fractional flow distribution based on average extraction may not be representative of the true distribution. However, calculations show that the apparent error in fractional flow distribution is no more than 1.6% of total blood flow with a doubling of blood flow (Rosivall et al., 1981).

During the first minute after the ^{86}Rb bolus injection, the ^{86}Rb content of the kidney cortex is reasonably stable (Sapirstein, 1958; Yarger et al., 1978). There is, however, a possibility of redistribution between tissue regions having a different flow rate. After the first circulation, the ^{86}Rb ratio is higher in tissues having a high flow rate than in tissues having a low flow rate. Therefore, in the latter tissues, where the specific activity is low, the uptake of ^{86}Rb from the blood can continue, which might explain the dependency of the medullary ^{86}Rb content on the time elapsed since the indicator injection (Steiner and King, 1970; Yarger et al., 1978). Thus, estimations of medullary blood flow based on the ^{86}Rb method are generally higher than those obtained by other methods. However, the diffusibility of ^{86}Rb is substantially lower than that of the inert gases, and the ^{86}Rb is less likely to undergo as much countercurrent exchange. Also, during ^{86}Rb recirculation ^{86}Rb may be continuously taken up by the medulla and transported to the medulla by the tubular fluid.

Thus, ^{86}Rb uptake is a simple technique for the estimation of postglomerular blood flow clearly relating to a well-known anatomic area. It is possible to measure simultaneously the cortical and medullary blood flow as well, which is an advantage over previously discussed methods. However, the ^{86}Rb extraction depends on the flow in the medulla and is also time dependent. As with the local uptake techniques for [^{125}I]iodoantipyrine, tritiated water, and sulfanilamide, the major disadvantage is that the tissue must be excised in order to be measured, and all analysis and approaches must be based on the comparison of values from different groups of kidneys.

4. Medullary Blood Flow Measurements

The special anatomy of the medullary blood supply and the importance of medullary flow in renal function have resulted in several experimental approaches specifically directed toward measuring renal medullary blood flow. In one of the first methods (Kramer et al., 1960), Evan's blue was injected into the renal artery and detected by small photocells placed along the pelvic surface of medulla. The plasma flow was obtained by the transit time of the indicator. Lilienfield *et al.* (1961) used the accumulation rate of labeled albumin as an index of medullary blood flow. However, at that time the true shape of the medullary accumulation curve was assumed to be a straight line. More recently, it was demonstrated, using a step function input, that during early accumulation the shape is a curve rather than a straight line (Rasmussen, 1978).

Wolgast (1973) described a method for measuring the blood flow using ^{32}P-labeled red blood cells and small needle-shaped semiconductor detectors with which the mean transit time and the regional red blood cell volume could be determined. Although this technique has the potential problem of tissue damage caused by probe insertions, it yields consistent results and correlates well with results obtained by other methods. Other methods involve the transport of inert diffusible indicators such as ^{133}Xe, ^{86}Kr, H_2, tritiated water, sulfanilamide, and [^{125}I]iodoantipyrine or ^{86}Rb extraction. These techniques underestimate the medullary flow because they are influenced by the countercurrent system and the urine and lymph flows, and furthermore they are influenced by the reduced hematocrit values of blood perfusing the medulla. These low hematocrit values in the inner medulla are probably not the result of axial streaming because it has been shown that the inner medullary mean transit times of albumin and red blood cells are similar (Rasmussen, 1978).

5. General Considerations

From this brief review of the methods available for measuring intrarenal blood flow, it is evident that there is substantial uncertainty and confusion over the distribution of regional flow because of the errors inherent in all the techniques used. Thus, in studies using these approaches it is not possible to determine whether the alterations in measured flow truly reflect differences in blood flow distribution or are simply due to the specific method used. Certainly, one should be very cautious when comparing the data obtained in different species and with different techniques because of the uncertainty regarding the magnitude of the errors with the different methods.

In order to verify that changes in intrarenal blood flow are due to different experimental procedures, it is necessary to use a range of methods and to recognize their limitations. For example, microsphere measurements are often used as a reference base for intracortical zonal blood flow even though they only provide data regarding glomerular blood flow distribution. Also, the externally detected inert gas washout technique has been subjected to considerable criticism; however, it remains a valuable noninvasive method for studying renal hemodynamics and is one of the few method applicable to studies in human subjects.

B. Absolute and Relative Distribution of Glomerular, Peritubular, and Medullary Blood Flow

The average RBF is about $3-5$ ml min^{-1} g^{-1}, but there are great differences in the blood supply of different parts of the kidney. Under basal conditions the cortical blood flow ranges between 3.5 and 6.5 ml min^{-1} g^{-1}, and the medullary flow is in the range $1-3$ ml min^{-1} g^{-1}. Furthermore, the blood flow in the cortex and in the medulla is not homogenous. Disregarding the most superficial aglomerular layer of the kidney surface, there is a trend of decreasing flow from the surface of the kidney down to the tip of the papilla. This decrease in flow has been shown in both the preglomerular (Katz et al., 1971; McNay and Abe, 1970a) and postglomerular vessels (Coelho, 1977; Steiner and King, 1970; Yarger et al., 1978). The profile of the glomerular vessel density also shows a decrease from the superficial cortex to juxtamedullary cortex. After an aglomerular cortical layer, with just a few glomeruli, there is a peak in the second tissue layer and a tendency to decline toward the juxtamedullary cortex (Katz et al., 1971). The decrease in blood flow of the subsequent different cortical zones is apparently greater than the decrease in the number of glomeruli, and it has therefore been said that the blood flow per glomerulus in the outer cortex must be higher than that in the inner cortex. Using the microsphere method, the single-glomerular blood flow (SGBF) in the different cortical zones (Katz et al., 1971; McNay and Abe, 1970a) or in the different well-defined types of nephrons has been measured (Bankir et al., 1979; Källskog et al., 1975d; Mimran and Casellas, 1979; Sabto et al., 1978). In rats, values for the absolute flow in the superficial glomeruli have ranged from about 250 to 400 nl min^{-1} per glomerulus, whereas they have been about $100-300$ nl min^{-1} per glomerulus in the juxtamedullary glomeruli (Table IV). Bankir et al. (1979) determined a ratio of superficial to juxtamedullary glomerular blood flow of as high as 3, with 15-μm microspheres. However, this ratio measured in the same animal changed, from 1.74 to 0.98 (Mimran and Casellas, 1979) and from 2.3 to 1.18 (Yarger et al., 1978), when smaller microspheres were used. In the latter study the SNGFR was also obtained using Hanssen's technique, and a superficial/juxtamedullary ratio of 0.69 calculated. The single-nephron filtration fraction in superfical glomeruli calculated from the microsphere and Hanssens data in this study was only 0.19 using 15-μm microspheres and 0.25 using 9-μm microspheres. In dog, SGBF measured by Katz et al. (1971) was 544 nl min^{-1} for superficial glomeruli and 301 nl min^{-1} in the juxtamedullary glomeruli (Table IV).

As shown in Table V, the average outer cortical/inner cortical glomerular blood flow ratio for the rat kidney using the data from four authors is

TABLE IV

Glomerular Blood Flow Rates in Different Glomeruli Estimated by the Use of Microspheres in Dog and Rat[a]

Diameter of microspheres (μm)	Glomeruli			S/JM[b]	Animal	Ref.[c]
	Superficial	Midcortical	Juxtamedullary			
15	544	—	301	1.81	Dog	1
15	350	149	150	2.33	Rat	2–5
	(414–308)	(196–108)	(275–298)			
9	248	150	205	1.21	Rat	5
7–10	317	221	209	1.52	Rat	4

[a] Blood flow rates expressed as nanoliters per minute.
[b] Ratio of superficial to juxtamedullary glomerular blood flow.
[c] References: 1, Katz *et al.* (1971); 2, Bankir *et al.* (1979); 3, Källskog *et al.* (1975d); 4, Sabto *et al.* (1978); 5, Yarger *et al.* (1978).

2.10. In the dog (Table VI) the determined outer cortical/inner cortical glomerular flow ratio is lower and more consistent ranging from 1.38 (Passmore *et al.*, 1978) to 1.66 (Clausen *et al.*, 1979a). A ratio of 1.63 can be derived from the average of four authors' data (Table VI). This ratio depends not only on the SGBF but also on the glomerular density.

The SNGFR obtained by either micropuncture or Hanssen's technique in rats strongly suggests that the difference in the superficial and juxtamedullary glomerular blood flow is not as large as is reported. In particular, there remains the major discrepancy that GFR in deep nephrons is generally considered to be greater than that in superficial nephrons (Davis *et al.*, 1974; DeRouffignac *et al.*, 1970). This is opposite to that suggested for glomerular blood flow and suggests that there is a marked heterogeneity in the single-nephron filtration fractions, an explanation that is not generally accepted (Yarger *et al.*, 1978). Thus, it is likely that some major methodologic complication is contributing to the apparent values for SGBF of deep and superficial nephrons.

About 85% of the postglomerular blood flow is distributed to the cortical peritubular capillaries, and the remaining 15% goes to the medulla and renal papilla. Because of the small difference between preglomerular flow and postglomerular cortical outflow and because of methodologic variability, it is difficult to demonstrate real differences between the absolute preglomerular and postglomerular cortical flow calculated in milliliters per minute per gram. As shown in Tables V and VI, the outer cortical/inner cortical postglomerular flow ratio is similar to the preglomerular flow distribution ratios. However, the differences between the blood flows of the

TABLE V

Calculated Absolute Zonal Blood Flow[a] Measured by Different Techniques in Rat[b]

Technique	RBF	OC	IC	OM	IM	M	OC/IC	Ref.[c]
Microsphere (8.5–15 μm)	5.1 (4.5–6.1)	8.4 (5.6–9.8)	4.0 (3.0–4.7)	—	—	—	2.1	1–4
^{86}Rb	5.2 (4.5–6.1)	7.0 (5.3–8.7)	4.6 (4.0–5.1)	2.0 (1.5–2.4)	0.3	2.5 (1.4–3.3)	1.52	2–5
^{125}I-Ap	4.6	7.1	4.7	1.6	—	—	1.51	6
H$_2$	4.3	5.7	5.2	2.5	—	—	1.36	7
Sa	5.7 (5.2–6.1)	9.0 (8.9–9.1)	5.0 (4.2–5.8)	—	—	2.5 (2.3–2.7)	1.80	3
^{133}Xe	4.4 (3.4–5.4)	Comp. I 7.5 (4.6–10.4)	Comp. II 1.2	—	Comp. III 0.1	—	6.25	8,9

[a] Expressed as milliliters per minute per gram.

[b] Abbreviations: RBF, renal blood flow; OC, outer cortical; IC, inner cortical; OM, outer medullary; IM, inner medullary; M, medullary; ^{125}I-Ap, [^{125}I]iodoantipyrine; SA, sulfanilamide.

[c] References: 1, Mimran and Casellas (1979); 2, Rosivall et al. (1979a); 3, Szabó et al. (1980); 4, Yarger et al. (1978); 5, Coelho (1977); 6, Hope et al. (1976); 7, Parekh and Veith (1981); 8, Ayer et al. (1971); Källskog et al. (1975d).

TABLE VI

Calculated Absolute Zonal Blood Flow[a] Measured by Different Techniques in Dog[b]

Technique	RBF	OC	IC	OM	IM	OC/IC	Ref.[c]
Microsphere (10–15 μm)	3.2 (2.7–3.9)	5.2 (4.4–6.7)	3.2 (2.4–5.2)	— (0–0.5)	— (0–0.03)	1.63	1–3
^{86}Rb	3.6 (2.3–4.6)	7.4 (6.7–8.2)	4.8 (3.7–5.6)	2.5 (1.6–3.0)	1.5 (1.0–2.5)	1.54	4–7
^{125}I-AP	4.2 (3.9–4.5)	6.2 (5.7–6.6)	4.7 (4.4–5.0)	0.9 (0.8–0.9)	0.2	1.32	8
THO	3.8	5.4	4.4	1.0	—	1.23	8
H$_2$	3.6	3.3	3.5	0.8	—	0.94	9
^{133}Xe/^{85}Kr	4.0 (2.9–5.0)	Comp. I 5.3 (3.8–7.1)	Comp. II 1.6 (1.0–2.4)		Comp. III 0.4		3, 4, 7, 10
Deep-freeze dissection	—	7.6	4.4	2.6	—	1.73	3

[a] Expressed as milliliters per minute per gram.

[b] Abbreviations: RBF, renal blood flow; OC, outer cortical; IC, inner cortical; OM, outer medullary; IM, inner medullary; ^{125}I-AP, [^{125}I]iodoantipyrine; THO, tritiated water.

[c] References: 1, Clausen et al. (1979a,b); McNay and Abe (1970a); Passmore et al. (1978); 4, Härsing et al. (1975); 5, Rosivall et al. (1979b); 6, Steiner and King (1970); 7, Szabó et al. (1976); 8, Clausen et al. (1979a); 9, Loyning (1971); 10, Slotkoff et al. (1971).

two regions are less for the postglomerular pattern. This may be due to a real difference or, alternatively, may reflect a more realistic distribution of the diffusible indicators compared with that of the microspheres. The outer cortical/inner cortical postglomerular flow ratios in rats were 1.56 measured using [^{125}I]iodoantipyrine (Hope et al., 1976) and 1.22–1.27 measured using ^{86}Rb (Coelho, 1977; Yarger et al., 1978). In dogs a value of 1.31 was obtained by Clausen et al. (1979a) using [^{125}I]iodoantipyrine, and 1.29–1.69 was obtained using ^{86}Rb (Rosivall et al., 1979b; Steiner and King, 1970).

The medullary blood flow data strongly depend on the method used. In the rat there is a significant difference in the blood flow between the two parts of the outer medulla if flow is measured with [^{125}I]iodoantipyrine but only a slight difference when ^{86}Rb uptake is employed. Whereas there was practically no [^{125}I]iodoantipyrine activity in the inner medulla, the flow based on ^{86}Rb extraction is 1.26 ml min^{-1} g^{-1}. These data indicate that about 10% of the RBF supplies the outer medulla and 2.5% goes to the inner medulla (L. Rosivall, unpublished data). These results are in agreement with most of the medullary flow measurements indicating that there is a lower blood flow rate in the papilla (Coelho, 1977; Steiner and King, 1970).

It is generally accepted that the medulla is supplied by the efferent vessels of the juxtamedullary glomeruli. Thus, it might be expected that the glomerular blood flow of the innermost cortical zone (measured by the microsphere method) would be approximately equal to the combined postglomerular flow of the same cortical zone and of the medulla measured by diffusible indicators such as [^{125}I]iodoantipyrine, ^{86}Rb, and sulfanilamide. However, in both rats and dogs the deep cortical and medullary flow fraction measured by the microsphere method is lower than that obtained with diffusible indicators (Clausen et al., 1979a; Passmore et al., 1978; Rosivall et al., 1979a; Szabó et al., 1980). Figure 21 provides some comparisons made in the same experiments. This consistent difference indicates that there is a net inward postglomerular flow from the outer cortex to the inner cortex medulla. The blood supply to the medulla is provided not only by the efferent vessels of juxtamedullary glomeruli, but also by the vessels from midcortical glomeruli. This is consistent with morphologic observations that the postglomerular capillaries of the cortex and medulla form a continuous network (Beeuwkes, 1980; Fourman and Moffat, 1971) and that there are several "long" efferent arterioles, mainly in the middle cortex, which can reach the medulla (Beeuwkes, 1980). These considerations form the basis for the pre- and postglomerular flow patterns shown in Fig. 21.

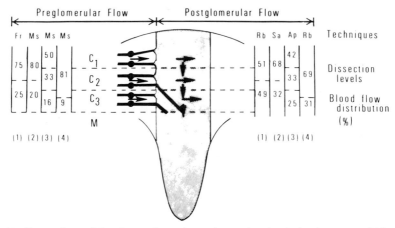

Fig. 21. Comparison of the glomerular and postglomerular circulation in outer, middle, and deep regions of the kidney. The numbers in the columns show the relative distribution of simultaneously measured preglomerular (left side) and postglomerular (right side) blood flow at different dissection levels obtained in different studies in (1) rat (Rosivall *et al.,* 1979a), (2) rat (Szabó *et al.,* 1980), (3) dog (Clausen *et al.,* 1979a), and (4) dog (Rosivall *et al.,* 1979b). In each case the innermost preglomerular flow fraction is lower than the corresponding postglomerular deep fraction (innermost zone and medulla). This means that the deep fraction of the peritubular capillary flow is not totally derived from the innermost cortical zone. On the basis of this and new morphologic data, we have constructed a schematic diagram of postglomerular blood flow. The arrows show the net blood flow direction within different zones. Fr, Frog erythrocytes; Ms, microspheres; Rb, rubidium; Sa, sulfanilamide; Ap, antipyrine; C_x, cortical zone; M, medulla.

V. Physiologic Control of the Renal Microcirculation

Although it is helpful to consider the specific effects of isolated changes in individual determinants of GFR and PCU, it should be recognized that the actual physiologic controlling elements usually alter several of the determinants concomitantly. In general, the physiologic regulation of GFR and PCU occurs as a consequence of changes in the preglomerular or postglomerular resistances, either selectively or combined. Alternatively, various factors may directly alter the filtration coefficients of the glomerular and peritubular capillary networks. These effects may be manifested on the total nephron population, or a heterogenous effect may occur, leading to regional redistribution of the intrarenal hemodynamic environment.

A. *Autoregulation and Intrinsic Control Mechanisms*

It is well recognized that most microcirculatory beds possess intrinsic autoregulatory mechanisms (Johnson, 1964), and the kidney is not an exception. In fact, the renal circulation has developed a highly efficient autoregulatory mechanism that can maintain total RBF and GFR essentially constant during variations in mean perfusion pressure from as low as 70–75 mm Hg to values substantially in excess of the normal physiologic range (Navar, 1978a; Selkurt *et al.*, 1949; Selkurt, 1963; Shipley and Study, 1951; Thurau and Kramer, 1959; Thurau, 1964). Studies have demonstrated that several different extrinsic manipulations, such as changes in arterial pressure and increases in venous pressure, ureteral pressure, or plasma colloid osmotic pressure, elicit intrinsic adjustments in renal vascular resistance in such a way that the direct effects of the extrinsic manipulation are partially counteracted (Navar, 1978a). Under some conditions, such as with changes in arterial or renal venous pressure, the autoregulatory adjustments in renal vascular resistance help to maintain both RBF and GFR (Guyton *et al.*, 1964). However, in other circumstances, such as with increases in plasma colloid osmotic pressure (Kállay and Debreczeni, 1970; Navar *et al.*, 1971) or increases in ureteral pressure (Nash and Selkurt, 1964), RBF may be increased above the control levels. Thus, the phenomenon of autoregulation can be regarded as the capacity of the renal vasculature to respond to extrinsic physical disturbances by intrinsic adjustments in renal vascular resistance in such a manner as to minimize the influence of the extrinsic manipulation on GFR (Navar *et al.*, 1981a,b). There are certainly several possible mechanisms that could be responsible for autoregulation. However, an impressive feature of this phenomenon is that the adjustments all seem to return GFR back toward the control level (Navar, 1978a; Navar *et al.*, 1980, 1981a,b). This is demonstrated in Table VII. For that reason it has been suggested that the mechanisms responsible do not have a primary function in maintaining RBF. Rather, the concept has emerged that the autoregulatory adjustments in resistance are the reflection of a negative feedback control system that responds to some function of altered filtered load and adjusts one or more determinants of glomerular function.

Under most conditions it has been determined that the vascular segment most consistently responsible for the autoregulatory adjustments in resistance is the afferent arteriolar segment (Navar, 1970; Robertson *et al.*, 1972; Thurau and Wober, 1962). This can be demonstrated readily by considering the alterations in intrarenal pressures during changes in arterial pressure. As shown in Fig. 22 both RBF and GFR demonstrate highly

TABLE VII
Intrinsic Responses of Renal Vasculature to Extrinsic Disturbances

Disturbance	Renal blood flow	Glomerular filtration rate	Renal vascular resistance
Changes in arterial blood pressure (70–180 mm Hg)	Remains constant (autoregulated)	Remains within 10% of control	Decreases as arterial pressure decreases
Increases in venous pressure (0–40 mm Hg)	Remains constant (autoregulated)	Remains constant or decreases slightly	Decreases as venous pressure increases
Increases in ureteral pressure (0–60 mm Hg)	Increases from 30 to 70%	Increases slightly, remains unchanged, or decreases slightly	Decreases as ureteral pressure increases
Increases in plasma colloid osmotic pressure	Increases from 30 to 100%	Remains within control range	Decreases as colloid osmotic pressure increases

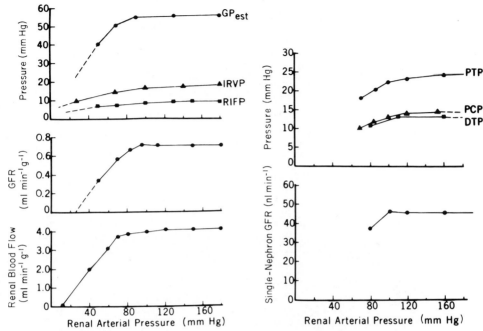

Fig. 22. Representative relationships between renal arterial pressure and various indices of renal function. Data were taken from studies in dogs (Baer and Navar, 1973; Navar *et al.*, 1977a; Ott et al., 1971). As demonstrated, glomerular pressure (GP_{est}), intrarenal venous pressure (IRVP), interstitial fluid pressure (RIFP), proximal tubule pressure (PTP), peritubular capillary pressure (PCP), and distal tubule pressure (DTP) all exhibit autoregulatory behavior. Single-nephron GFR data were calculated on the basis of distal tubular fluid collections (Navar *et al.*, 1977a). From Navar (1978a).

efficient autoregulation. In addition, glomerular pressure, proximal tubule pressure, distal tubule pressure, intrarenal venous pressure, and interstitial fluid pressure exhibit autoregulatory behavior over approximately the same pressure range. Thus, as shown in Fig. 23 the major site of the requisite resistance adjustments is proximal to the glomeruli, or at the level of the afferent arteriole. Under usual circumstances there are minimal changes in postglomerular resistance in direct response to changes in arterial pressure. However, it is possible that changes in intrarenal angiotensin II production may lead to increases in postglomerular resistance, especially when renal arterial pressure is maintained at lower levels conducive to high renin release rates (Fojas and Schmid, 1970). Similar assessments of the responses to changes in venous pressure, ureteral pressure, and plasma colloid osmotic pressure indicate that the afferent arteriolar

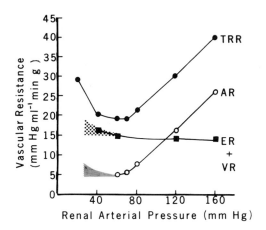

Fig. 23. Relationships between renal arterial pressure and total renal vascular resistance (TRR), preglomerular resistance (AR), and efferent plus venous resistance (ER + VR). Under most circumstances the autoregulatory adjustments in renal vascular resistance are due almost entirely to changes in afferent arteriolar resistance.

resistance is the dominant component responsible for the observed autoregulatory hemodynamic responses (Navar, 1978a).

It appears that all regions of the renal microcirculation exhibit autoregulatory behavior, but not to the same degree of efficiency. Studies in the dog (Navar *et al.,* 1977b) demonstrated that at higher arterial pressure there was coincident autoregulation of the total nephron population and the superficial nephrons. However, as arterial blood pressure was reduced, the superficial nephrons utilized all of their autoregulatory reserve at slightly higher arterial pressures. In contrast to earlier studies which had suggested that the juxtamedullary nephrons did not exhibit autoregulation (Thurau, 1964), the more recent data suggest that the deeper nephrons may have an even greater autoregulatory efficiency than the superficial nephrons. Studies using microspheres (Abe, 1971) and the ferrocyanide technique (Bonvalet *et al.,* 1972) have also demonstrated that the total nephron population can exhibit autoregulatory behavior; however, at the lower pressures, deep glomerular blood flow is preserved with greater efficiency than superficial glomerular blood flow (Clausen *et al.,* 1980; McNay and Abe, 1970a). Since the medullary circulation is essentially a postglomerular circuit, it might be expected that its response would be similar to those of the inner nephrons. This has been shown to be the case (Grangsjo and Wolgast, 1972; Loyning, 1971; Stern *et al.,* 1979), and autoregulation of medullary blood flow has been demonstrated. Hope *et al.* (1981) found that there was an unchanged zonal distribution of blood flow throughout the kidney, including the medulla, as perfusion pressure was varied. Thus, it would seem that the capacity for autoregulatory behavior is a general feature of all regions of the kidney. The slightly reduced autoregulatory capability of the superficial nephrons may simply be a reflection of the longer arterial path for blood flow to the outer cortical regions. This longer path may be of greater significance in the rat, which may have maximally dilated superficial nephron afferent arterioles at spontaneous arterial pressures (Källskog et al., 1975c). Because there is a measurable pressure drop of 20 mm Hg or more along the arteriolar tree of the rat (Boknam et al., 1981; Källskog et al., 1976), the preglomerular pressure to the superficial glomeruli of the rat may already be close to the lower limit of the autoregulatory range. The dog, however, seems to maintain its arterial pressure along the arterial pathway to the surface of the kidney (Navar et al., 1982a).

Although there is not complete agreement regarding the mechanism responsible for autoregulatory adjustments in resistance, most investigators now agree that the responses are the consequence of active adjustments in smooth muscle tone of the preglomerular arterioles. The myogenic hypothesis explains these adjustments as being the result of direct responses of the arteriolar muscle elements to a change in transmural pressure (Gilmore et al., 1980; Young and Marsh, 1981). Although it does appear that the arterioles can respond to sudden changes in pressure, there are several obstacles to the acceptance of the hypothesis of a major myogenic autoregulatory mechanism. At present, the nature of the receptor system capable of sensing transmural wall tension remains unknown. Also, it is difficult to determine how RBF per se could be the controlled entity during changes in arterial pressure but not be regulated during changes in ureteral pressure or venous pressure. In addition, the responses to increases in venous pressure seem to be opposite to those expected on the basis of the myogenic hypothesis. In some microcirculatory beds such as that of intestine, increases in venous pressure lead to increases, not decreases, in precapillary vascular resistance (Johnson, 1959). Whereas the results from the intestine are consistent with the predictions of the myogenic hypothesis, the renal responses to increases in venous pressure are not (Navar, 1978a). Thus, the basic myogenic hypothesis remains inadequate to explain the many different types of autoregulatory response, and there is no direct evidence supporting the concept that an intrinsic myogenic mechanism is the predominant mediator of sustained autoregulatory responses. Nevertheless, Aukland (1976) also assessed the available data and arrived at the opinion that some type of myogenic mechanism based on the Bayliss phenomenon (Bayliss, 1902) is an attractive possibility.

An alternative explanation for the mechanism of autoregulation is based on the well-known morphologic association between the macula densa segment of the distal nephron and the vascular elements of the same nephron (Fig. 5). As described in Section II,B, the juxtaglomerular complex seems particularly well suited to provide a means of communication between some aspect of distal tubular flow or composition and the vascular structures (Guyton *et al.*, 1964; Schloss, 1945–1946; Thurau, 1981). This idea has led to the *macula densa feedback hypothesis* as an explanation for the phenomenon of renal autoregulation. As previously mentioned one consistent feature of the autoregulatory responses is that GFR is returned toward normal following an extrinsic manipulation. The macula densa feedback hypothesis extends this basic view and predicts that disturbances leading to inappropriate increases in distal tubular flow would elicit afferent arteriolar vasoconstriction, whereas decreases in distal tubular flow would lead to afferent arteriolar vasodilation. According to this hypothesis, autoregulatory responses would be one manifestation of a mechanism serving an important homeostatic role by helping to maintain a balance between the filtered load to the tubules and the reabsorptive capabilities of the proximal tubule and loop of Henle (Navar *et al.*, 1981a,b; Thurau, 1981). Such a mechanism implies that the control of the renal microcirculation is linked closely to the functional status of the tubules and that autoregulation occurs at the level of each nephrovascular unit.

Although several other mechanisms have been postulated to explain renal autoregulation (Selkurt, 1963), only the myogenic and macula densa feedback theories are presently under major consideration. Since both theories utilize changes in smooth muscle activity as the final effector limb of the mechanism, it has been difficult to delineate specific experiments capable of ruling out the myogenic theory. However, the macula densa feedback hypothesis can be challenged directly, and numerous studies have been conducted to evaluate specific predictions of this theory (Navar, 1978a; Navar *et al.*, 1981a,b; Schnermann, 1981). One prediction of the macula densa feedback hypothesis is that experimental manipulations that decrease or lead to the cessation of distal tubular flow would elicit feedback-mediated afferent arteriolar vasodilation, utilize the preexisting autoregulatory reserve, and interfere with normal autoregulatory responses (Navar *et al.*, 1982a). The results of several previous studies are in accord with this prediction and can be summarized as follows:

1.   Acute elevations in intratubular pressures by ureteral obstruction or renal vein constriction result in afferent arteriolar vasodilation that helps to maintain GFR (Navar, 1978a).

2.   Increases in plasma colloid osmotic pressure that would be expected to decrease effective filtration pressure and reduce GFR lead to

decreases in renal vascular resistance such that RBF is increased and autoregulatory capability is diminished (Kállay and Debreczeni, 1970; Navar *et al.*, 1971).

3. The imposition of an ischemic episode (60–90 min) in the dog results in marked diminution of GFR even though RBF may be within the normal range (19,20). In this type of "nonfiltering kidney," RBF autoregulation is markedly compromised (Adams *et al.*, 1980; Williams *et al.*, 1981).

4. When arterial pressure is well above the lower level of the autoregulatory range, SNGFR measurements based on total collections from proximal tubules, which result in the cessation of normal flow to the distal tubule, are higher than SNGFR measurements based on techniques that do not interfere with normal distal tubular flow (Navar *et al.*, 1974; Ploth *et al.*, 1977; Schnermann *et al.*, 1971; Williams *et al.*, 1977). Figure 24 presents a composite graph of data from dogs comparing the estimates of SNGFR obtained in our laboratory using various methods.

5. In micropuncture studies an association of superficial SNGFR and whole-kidney GFR autoregulatory responses to decreases in renal arterial pressure is consistently observed only when SNGFR is measured by methods that do not interfere with distal volume delivery (Navar *et al.*, 1974; Moore *et al.*, 1979; Ploth *et al.*, 1977; Schnermann, 1981; Williams *et al.*, 1977). These results are internally consistent with other studies demonstrating that glomerular pressure, based on proximal stop-flow pressure measurements that result in the cessation of distal volume delivery, fails to exhibit autoregulatory behavior in response to reductions in renal arterial pressure within the autoregulatory range for superficial nephrons (Navar *et al.*, 1975).

Thus, a substantial body of evidence exists that is consistent with the fundamental premise of the macula densa feedback hypothesis that maintenance of flow to the distal nephron is essential for the integrity of the autoregulatory mechanism. Furthermore, studies by numerous laboratories have demonstrated that the requisite feedback mechanism exists and can elicit alterations in glomerular function in response to alterations in flow rate to the distal tubule (P. D. Bell *et al.*, 1978; Navar, 1978a; Navar *et al.*, 1980; Schnermann *et al.*, 1970; Wright and Briggs, 1977, 1979). These investigations have established the presence of a tubuloglomerular feedback mechanism capable of exerting relatively large decreases in SNGFR in response to increases in distal volume delivery, and such a mechanism could serve as the mediator of autoregulatory responses (Navar *et al.*, 1981b). The associated feedback-mediated decreases in stop-flow pressure in response to distal nephron perfusion are also quite substantial and sufficient to account for the SNGFR responses (P. D. Bell *et al.*, 1978;

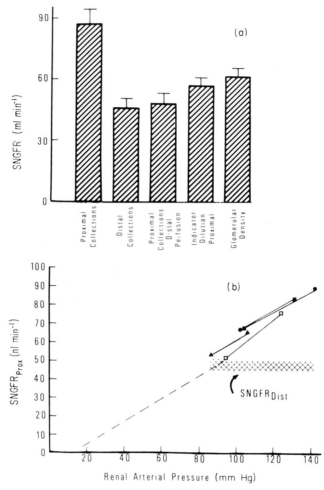

Fig. 24. Composite graph of SNGFR values obtained in dogs using different techniques at control arterial pressure (a) and in response to reductions in renal arterial pressure (b). Data in (a) demonstrate that SNGFR values measured during cessation of distal delivery (proximal collection) are higher than those obtained using means that do not interfere with distal flow rate (distal collections, proximal collections during distal tubule perfusions, and the indicator-dilution technique). The latter values agree with the SNGFR calculated on the basis of total GFR and glomerular density. Panel (b) shows the results from several studies demonstrating that SNGFR, measured during interruption of distal flow rate, does not exhibit autoregulation during reductions in renal arterial pressure. The hatched area represents SNGFR values obtained with techniques that do not interfere with distal volume delivery. Key: ●, Navar *et al.* (1974); □, Williams *et al.* (1977); ▲, Navar *et al.* (1977a); ■, Burke and Dachin (1979), control.

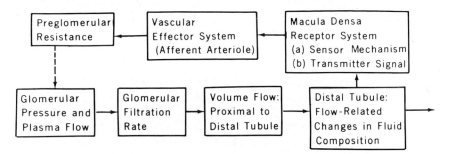

Fig. 25. Components of the feedback mechanism linking the glomerular vascular elements and the distal tubule. The solid arrows indicate direct effects (i.e., an increase in GFR causes an increase in tubular flow). The dashed arrow represents an inverse effect because an increase in resistance leads to decreases in plasma flow and glomerular pressure. From Navar *et al.* (1981b).

Bell and Navar, 1979; Schnermann *et al.*, 1973). These results have generally been interpreted as indicating that the changes in SNGFR occur as a consequence of changes in glomerular pressure caused by adjustments in the afferent arteriolar resistance (Navar 1978a; Navar *et al.*, 1980). More recent direct studies by Briggs and Wright (1979) have provided further support for this conclusion. Their results indicate that the resistance adjustments occurring during changes in flow rate to the distal tubule are localized at the afferent arteriolar segments and are consistent with the notion that the same mechanism is responsible for autoregulatory adjustments in vascular resistance and for feedback-mediated adjustments in the vascular resistance of single nephrons. Studies demonstrating that, during autoregulatory-induced reductions in whole-kidney vascular resistance, it is still possible to elicit feedback-mediated decreases in stop-flow pressure lend further support to this concept (Bell and Navar, 1979).

The literature related to the various aspects of the macula densa feedback hypothesis is vast and involves many controversies (Navar *et al.*, 1981b; Schnermann and Levine, 1975; Schnermann, 1981; Thurau, 1981; Wright and Briggs, 1979). However, the issue of critical importance here is that there is considerable evidence supporting the basic elements of the hypothesis that the major portion of renal autoregulatory adjustments in resistance are mediated by a feedback mechanism that responds to some compositional characteristic of distal tubular flow and transmits signals to the afferent arteriolar segment. The components involved in this feedback mechanism are illustrated in Fig. 25. The specific characteristics of the intraluminal and intracellular constituents involved in the mediation of the feedback signals remain under intensive investigation. More recent data suggest that macula densa cells sense flow-related changes in tubular

fluid osmolality that initiate the transmission of signals by activating a
cytosolic calcium system (Bell and Navar, 1982). It is now clear that
this basic feedback mechanism occurs at the single-nephron level and
is in a position to serve an important function regulating the renal microcirculatory environment. In addition to protecting the kidney from the effects of increases and decreases in arterial pressure, it provides an overall
stablization of hemodynamic inputs to the microcirculatory structures
and, in this manner, contributes to the optimum function of the kidney.
Furthermore, this intrinsic control mechanism interacts with several
other intrarenal and extrarenal systems to adjust the hemodynamic environment of the kidney.

B. *Influence of Renal Nerves and Catecholamines*

Although there is general agreement that the renal vasculature possesses a dense innervation consisting primarily of α adrenergic nerves
(Barajas, 1978) and is very responsive to infusions of epinephrine and norepinephrine (Kiil *et al.*, 1969), there is not a complete understanding of
the physiologic role exerted by the renal nerves in controling the renal microcirculation. Studies have indicated that the renal nerves can also influence tubular reabsorptive function directly (DiBona, 1978; Gottschalk, *et
al.*, 1981) and are an important mediator of renin release (Davis and
Freeman, 1976; LaGrange *et al.*, 1973). However, the major emphasis in
this section is on the effects of the nerves on renal microcirculatory dynamics, a topic that was also discussed in some detail by Aukland (1976).
Increases in renal nerve activity elicit renal vasoconstriction and variable changes in the distribution of RBF. Katz and Shear (1975) evaluated
the effects of direct nerve stimulation and the indirect neural effects mediated by carotid occlusion in dogs. A moderate degree of renal nerve
stimulation sufficient to decrease RBF by 20% failed to elicit changes in
GFR. Likewise, there was no major effect on the distribution of RBF.
When the renal nerves were activated by carotid occlusion, RBF again
decreased by about 20%; however, in this series GFR and sodium excretion decreased. The decrease in RBF appeared to be homogeneous
throughout the cortex, as assessed by microsphere distribution. It was
suggested that carotid occlusion and maintenance of systemic arterial
pressure exerted influences attributable to other factors in addition to the
renal nerves. These basic effects of renal nerve stimulation on RBF distribution were in contrast to those reported by Pomeranz *et al.* (1968), who
used the inert gas technique and reported that mild renal nerve stimulation led to preferential decreases in outer cortical perfusion. Banks
(1975) also reported that activation of the renal sympathetics by bilateral

carotid occlusion led to preferential decreases in the outer cortical flow. In contrast, Gotshall and Itskovitz (1977) suggested that reductions in RBF elicited by renal nerve stimulation were greater in the inner cortex than in the outer cortex. Nissen and Galskov (1972) observed that renal nerve stimulation caused a slightly greater reduction in deep blood flow than in subcapsular blood flow. Thus, there is no general agreement regarding those areas of the kidney that are most sensitive to increased renal nerve activity, although it is clear that all areas are quite responsive. It has also been shown that the medullary circulation, which was once thought to be protected from the effects of increased renal nerve activity (Trueta *et al.*, 1947), responds to increased nerve activity to about the same extent or perhaps slightly more (Aukland, 1968; Rosivall *et al.*, 1977).

In an attempt to evaluate the physiologic role of renal sympathetic tone in conscious animals, Gross and Kirchheim (1980) studied the effects of common carotid occlusion or a startling noise on RBF and renal nerve activity. Both stimuli increased nerve activity, but the effects of excitement were much greater. With carotid occlusion, RBF did not decrease significantly. With the startling noise, RBF decreased transiently by about 40%. In a study by Johns (1980) in cats, it was demonstrated that modest nerve stimulation decreased RBF but not GFR. Under these conditions, the RBF and GFR autoregulatory responses to decreases in renal perfusion pressure were not affected. Thus, the autoregulation mechanism can elicit decreases in renal vascular resistance even when renal nerve activity is exerting a vasoconstrictive influence.

In a study by Hermansson *et al.* (1981) the influence of renal nerve stimulation on glomerular filtration dynamics was evaluated using micropuncture techniques. Renal nerve stimulation elicited approximately equivalent effects on both afferent and efferent arteriolar conductances. Single-nephron plasma flow and GFR were reduced to about the same extent at both low levels (2 Hz) and higher levels (5 Hz) of renal nerve stimulation. At the higher level of stimulation, plasma flow and GFR were reduced to approximately 50% of control values, and both glomerular capillary pressure and peritubular capillary pressure were reduced. These studies again demonstrate the capacity of both afferent and efferent resistance vessels to respond to neural stimulation. At low levels of stimulation the increases in afferent and efferent resistance were similar; with higher levels of stimulation the responsiveness of the preglomerular resistance vessels was somewhat greater than that of the efferent arterioles. With very marked stimulation (10 Hz), glomerular ischemia resulted.

The effects of renal denervation on the renal microcirculation depend on the preexisting level of renal tone, which may be highly variable and dependent on the experimental preparation used. It has been reported that acute renal denervation in anesthetized dogs can result in denervation natriuresis without any evidence of significant changes in RBF, GFR, or intrarenal distribution of RBF as determined by the use of microspheres (Nomura et al., 1976). However, Bencsáth and Takács (1971) did observe an increase in medullary blood flow in hydropenic and normal anesthetized dogs following denervation. Thus, under conditions in which basal renal nerve activity is not excessively elevated, denervation appears to exert relatively modest effects on the overall renal circulation, although the effects on medullary blood flow may be of importance.

In general, the effects of norepinephrine and epinephrine infusions on renal hemodynamics resemble those exerted by renal nerve stimulation (Aukland, 1968), although it should be acknowledged that the vasoconstrictor effects are not directly comparable with the effects of endogenous release of amines because their intrarenal distribution is likely to be different. With moderate doses of epinephrine, the effects on RBF are somewhat greater than those observed for GFR and filtration fraction increases (Barclay et al., 1947; Smith, 1951). Smith and Gomez (Smith, 1951) concluded that these types of effects were best explained on the basis of approximately equivalent changes in afferent and efferent resistance. It was also suggested that the increased renal volume observed with low doses of epinephrine could be explained by constriction of the venules and increases in peritubular capillary pressure, leading to increases in interstitial fluid volume (Smith, 1951; Zimmerman et al., 1964).

Click et al. (1979) directly demonstrated the effects of norepinephrine and angiotensin on the afferent and efferent arterioles of kidney tissue grafted into the cheek pouch of hamsters. Both afferent and efferent arterioles responded to direct administration of norepinephrine, although the response of the efferent vessels was apparently less than that of the afferent arterioles. In micropuncture studies using the Munich–Wistar rat, Myers et al. (1975) administered norepinephrine systemically (2–4 μg min^{-1} kg^{-1}) and elicited decreases in glomerular blood flow without changes in GFR. Both glomerular pressure and peritubular capillary pressure increased. When arterial pressure was allowed to increase, afferent and efferent arteriolar resistance increased significantly. The increase in afferent resistance was markedly reduced when arterial pressure was maintained at control levels. Downstream venous resistance beyond the peritubular capillaries also increased slightly during both situations. Andreucci et al. (1976) observed that norepinephrine decreased glomerular pressure and efferent arteriolar pressure, indicating that this agent could increase preglomerular resistance to an extent greater than could be explained by an autoregulatory response to the elevated arterial pressure.

The infusion of epinephrine did not decrease the intrarenal pressure even though the increase in systemic arterial pressure was comparable, indicating that norepinephrine and epinephrine may have somewhat different quantitative effects on the pre- and postglomerular resistances.

The effects of epinephrine and norepinephrine on regional distribution of RBF have been studied using several techniques. The results from Xe washout studies suggested that the flow to the renal cortex was preferentially reduced by norepinephrine (Rentsch *et al.*, 1976). Gotshall and Itskovitz (1977) reported that the inner cortical vasculature was more responsive to norepinephrine than the outer cortex. The differences are rather small and not really at variance with the results of Tyssebotn and Kirkebo (1975), who observed proportional decreases in outer and inner cortical flows. Aukland (1968) also measured outer medullary hydrogen clearance and concluded that outer medullary blood flow decreased to about the same extent as total RBF in response to epinephrine, norepinephrine, angiotensin, and renal nerve stimulation. Interestingly, Grangsjo and Persson (1971) reported that sustained infusions of norepinephrine, but not epinephrine, could increase medullary blood flow even while cortical blood flow was decreased. This occurred only with low infusion rates ($0.2 \, \text{mg kg}^{-1} \, \text{min}^{-1}$), and higher infusions led to decreases in flow to all regions.

In summary, it can be concluded that neither renal nerve stimulation nor catecholamine infusions produce distinct or consistent differences in RBF distribution. It appears that all regions of the kidney are responsive to these effects. Some of the studies have hinted that there may be subtle differences in the medullary responses to epinephrine and norepinephrine, and this possibility deserves further investigation.

C. Contribution of the Renin–Angiotensin System

The literature related to the multiple effects of the renin–angiotensin system is voluminous, and no attempt has been made to provide a comprehensive review of the many findings. There are many sources that evaluate in detail the different components of the renin–angiotensin system (Oparil, 1976; Reid *et al.*, 1978), the mechanisms of renin release (Davis and Freeman, 1976), and the multiple actions of angiotensin (Levens *et al.*, 1981; Navar and Langford, 1974). From these studies there have emerged some basic concepts related to the influence of angiotensin II on renal hemodynamics and the microcirculatory environment. Since it is well recognized that angiotensin II can be formed both within the kidney and at extrarenal sites (Caldwell *et al.*, 1976; Erdos, 1977), this agent can serve as a circulating vasoactive substance or as an intrarenal hormone. The actions of angiotensin as a circulating hormone have been assessed by evaluating the responses to systemic or intraarterial infusions of angiotensin II. However, attempts to consider the role of angiotensin as an intrarenal hormone have involved more complicated approaches. Essentially, it has been suggested that angiotensin I is formed directly within the kidney as a consequence of changes in renin release (Thurau, 1974). The angiotensin I is then exposed to the influence of a converting enzyme present on the endothelial cells of the renal vessels and is converted to angiotensin II, which exerts a direct effect on responsive structures (Mendelsohn, 1979). Thus, endogenously formed angiotensin II may exert an influence on afferent arterioles if it is formed in the surrounding interstitial areas (Thurau, 1974) or could affect the efferent arterioles after its conversion in the glomerular capillaries (Hall et al., 1977a).

The effects of angiotensin on the renal circulation have been studied extensively (Navar and Langford, 1974), and it has generally been observed that angiotensin elicits dose-dependent decreases in RBF and proportionately smaller effects on GFR such that filtration fraction increases (Lohmeier and Cowley, 1979). At doses greater than 20 ng kg^{-1} min^{-1}, maximal sustained responses of approximately 50% decrease in RBF and 25% decrease in GFR have been obtained. Although higher doses can decrease RBF almost to zero, these effects are usually not sustained and the sustained RBF reductions may be less than at lower infusions. In addition it has been demonstrated that moderate infusions of angiotensin II or administration of angiotensin II antagonists do not prevent the normal autoregulatory decreases in vascular resistance following reductions in arterial pressure (Abe et al., 1976; Kiil et al., 1969; Fourcade et al., 1971; Gagnon et al., 1970).

Because angiotensin infusions usually result in greater reductions in RBF than in GFR, it has been suggested that the efferent arterioles have a greater sensitivity to angiotensin than the afferent arterioles; however, this is not necessarily the only explanation. Studies evaluating the effects of angiotensin II have demonstrated that both the afferent and efferent arteriolar resistances are increased by angiotensin II (Blantz et al., 1976; Myers et al., 1975). Myers et al. (1975) observed an increase in glomerular pressure and in the transglomerular hydrostatic pressure. When the increases in systemic arterial pressure were not transmitted to the kidney, the increases in afferent resistance were substantially less. In terms of peritubular capillary dynamics, proximal tubule fluid reabsorption was not significantly altered in spite of the marked increase in efferent colloid osmotic pressure. However, it was calculated that these were offset by the effects of changes in plasma flow and the small increases in capillary pressure. In the study by Blantz and Tucker (1975) similar effects were observed in plasma-volume-expanded rats. It was concluded that the increases in afferent resistance were greater than could be attributed specifically to autoregulatory increases in resistance. The SNGFR decreased significantly but not to the same extent as plasma flow, and K_f was reduced markedly by the infusions of angiotensin. It has been speculated that the contractile elements of the mesangial cells might be responsive to angiotensin and in some manner be responsible for the marked reductions in K_f (Blantz et al., 1976; Ichikawa et al., 1979).

Click et al. (1979) applied angiotensin II directly to the afferent and efferent arterioles of grafted renal tissue using a hamster cheek pouch preparation. Both afferent and efferent arterioles responded to angiotensin, and these responses were augmented in hypertensive (two-kidney Grollman procedure) hamsters. These data demonstrate that both afferent and efferent arterioles have the capacity to respond to angiotensin, and the apparent efferent preferential effect that is sometimes observed is not due to an insensitivity of the afferent vessel to this agent. In addition, direct morphologic investigations have demonstrated effects of angiotensin on the glomerular capillaries (Hornych and Richet, 1977). Following angiotensin II administrations, the glomerular capillaries were constricted and the cytoplasmic processes of the epithelial cells became irregular and fused. In micropuncture studies angiotensin II, infused directly into peritubular capillaries (Steven and Thorpe, 1977), caused an increase in peritubular and proximal tubule pressure. Angiotensin blockers led to a reduction in pressure of the peritubular capillaries, suggesting that angiotensin II could also influence peritubular capillary dynamics through a direct effect on the peritubular capillary structures or on venous resistance elements. Thus, angiotensin may have important regulatory influences on both glomerular and peritubular capillary dynamics. The exact manner in which these effects are manifested is not completely understood.

The effects of angiotensin on the regional distribution of RBF have also been studied extensively, but there is no clear agreement due to the different responses observed with different methods. Microsphere distribution studies have shown that angiotensin infusions produce greater decreases in the inner cortical fraction than in the outer regions (Britton, 1981; Itskovitz and McGiff, 1974). However, Rector et al. (1972) found essentially parallel decreases in every zone. Studies using the ^{85}Kr washout technique indicated that angiotensin infusions produced uniform decreases in the cortical blood flow (Carriere and Biron, 1970; Rentsch et al., 1976). Using autoradiograms, Carriere and Friborg (1969) observed that the subcapsular region of the cortex and the outer cortex were more sensitive to angiotensin than the inner cortex.

Although it is clear that intrarenal conversion of angiotensin I to angiotensin II occurs, the magnitude of the conversion has been variable, ranging from 1 to 20% (DiSalvo *et al.*, 1971; Franklin *et al.*, 1970; Oparil *et al.*, 1970). This degree of local renal conversion may be of sufficient magnitude to allow the renin–angiotensin system to participate in the local regulation of RBF and renal function (Britton, 1981; Hall *et al.*, 1977b; Mendelsohn, 1979; Ploth and Navar, 1979; Thurau, 1974). As a means of evaluating such possible intrarenal effects of angiotensin, pharmacologic inhibitors or antagonists that block the local formation or action of angiotensin II have been used (Hollenberg, 1979). The effects observed depend to a large extent on the preexisting level of activity of the renin–angiotensin system. Studies in animals having normal or enhanced renin levels have shown that angiotensin blockade increases RBF; however, the effects on GFR have been variable. Because of these variable effects on GFR and a general effect for filtration fraction to decrease upon administration of angiotensin blockers, it has been suggested that the influence of angiotensin is greater on the efferent arterioles than on the afferent arterioles (Freeman *et al.*, 1973; Hall *et al.*, 1977a). It has also been suggested that angiotensin formed intrarenally helps to maintain efferent arteriolar tone, particularly when renin secretory activity is enhanced, such as during sodium restriction or reduced renal perfusion pressure (Hall *et al.*, 1977b). This is based on the finding that GFR autoregulation is markedly attenuated in sodium-restricted dogs following angiotensin blockade or in renin-depleted dogs (Hall *et al.*, 1977a,b). There is disagreement, however, on this issue because other studies have failed to show a dissociation between RBF and GFR autoregulation during administration of angiotensin blockers (Gagnon *et al.*, 1974; Murray and Malvin, 1979; Navar *et al.*, 1982b).

In studies designed to investigate the effects of converting enzyme inhibition (CEI) on sodium-restricted dogs (Navar *et al.*, 1982b) attention was focused on the degree of association between RBF autoregulation and GFR autoregulation. As shown in Fig. 26, both RBF and GFR autoregulation were observed during control conditions and during infusion of SQ 14225. The specific effects of CEI on RBF, GFR, and filtration fraction are shown in Fig. 27. There were significant increases in RBF and GFR and a significant decrease in filtration fraction. By means of micropuncture techniques the effects of CEI on glomerular pressure and peritubular capillary pressure were also measured under conditions in which renal arterial pressure was maintained constant and the changes in segmental vascular resistance were calculated. These studies indicated that CEI induced approximately equivalent decreases in afferent and efferent arteriolar resistances. In other micropuncture experiments on sodium-re-

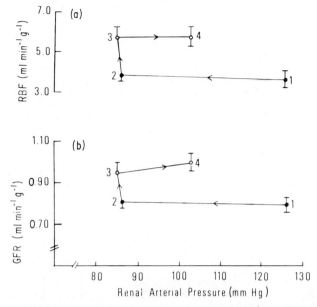

Fig. 26. Relationships between renal arterial pressure and RBF (a) or GFR (b) obtained in eight salt-restricted dogs before (points 1 and 2) and during the administration of the converting enzyme inhibitor SQ 14225 (points 3 and 4). 1, Control; 2, decrease in renal arterial pressure; 3, decrease in arterial pressure and converting enzyme inhibitor; 4, converting enzyme inhibitor.

stricted rats Steiner *et al.* (1979) observed that saralasin administration increased SNGFR and glomerular plasma flow and resulted in significant decreases in afferent resistance. Thus, the micropuncture experiments using angiotensin blockers do not support the hypothesis that angiotensin exerts a preferential effect on the efferent arterioles. Rather, they suggest that the increased activity of the renin–angiotensin system that occurs during sodium restriction exerts approximately equivalent vasoconstrictor influences on both preglomerular and postglomerular resistance elements.

Numerous discrepancies exist with regard to the overall contribution of the renin–angiotensin system to the control of renal hemodynamics. When the activity of the renin–angiotensin system is low, it appears that the angiotensin-dependent renal vascular tone is low (Fagard *et al.*, 1978). However, RBF and GFR values are similar to those occurring during high-renin states, when the angiotensin-dependent tone is accentuated (Navar *et al.*, 1982b). Presumably, another factor, such as the intrarenal prostaglandin system, is enhanced and counteracts the influence of the

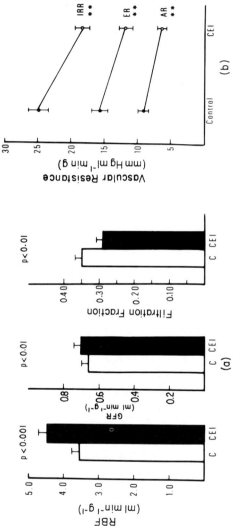

Fig. 27. Effects of converting enzyme inhibition (CEI) on (a) RBF, GFR, and filtration fraction and on (b) segmental vascular resistances ($n = 12$). For these experiments the renal arterial pressure was maintained at a constant value near the lower limit of the autoregulatory range. Resistances were calculated on the basis of whole-kidney hemodynamic data and superficial cortical measurements of glomerular pressure and peritubular capillary pressure. IRR, Intrarenal resistance; AR, afferent arteriole resistance; ER, efferent arteriole resistance. From Navar *et al.* (1982b), by permission of the American Heart Association, Inc.

angiotensin. This indicates that the role of the renin–angiotensin system as a regulator of the renal microcirculation may be quite complex and involve substantial interaction with other hormone systems (Brenner *et al.*, 1980; McGiff, 1980).

An alternative hypothesis that has been supported by Thurau and associates (Thurau, 1974, 1981; Thurau and Mason, 1974) is that the renin–angiotensin system is a major mediator of the distal tubuloglomerular feedback mechanism previously described. This feedback mechanism has been shown to regulate SNGFR in response to changes in distal flow rate or fluid composition at the level of the macula densa (Navar, 1978a; Schnermann, 1981; Wright and Briggs, 1979). Because it has been shown that angiotensin blockers lead to an attenuation of normal feedback responses (Ploth *et al.*, 1979; Stowe *et al.*, 1979), there is the possibility that angiotensin is involved, either directly or indirectly, in the tubuloglomerular feedback mechanism. The exact means by which this occurs remains uncertain, but it is possible that angiotensin is necessary for the full expression of tubuloglomerular feedback activity but does not serve as a direct mediator of the phenomenon (Ploth and Navar, 1979). It seems unlikely, however, that renin release from the juxtaglomerular cells directly into the lumen of the terminal portion of the afferent arterioles could exert a signifcant vasoconstrictor effect on afferent arterioles via the intrarenal formation of angiotensin. For this mechanism it would be more likely that the renin is released into the interstitial spaces of the kidney, and in this case the concentration of angiotensin could be high at both the afferent and efferent arterioles (Thurau, 1981).

D. Participation by Intrarenal Prostaglandins and Kinins

1. Prostaglandins

Cellular elements associated with the collecting tubules, the glomeruli, the medullary interstitium, and the blood vessels of the kidney have the capacity to form prostaglandins. There are several important prostaglandins; however, PGE_2 is the principal renal prostaglandin and is formed in the renal medulla (Baer and McGiff, 1980). In this region the degradative enzymes have low activity, and this may augment the local level of PGE_2 (McGiff, 1980). There is substantial evidence, however, that other prostaglandins, in particular PGI_2, are formed in the renal cortex also. The literature regarding prostaglandins and renal function is growing rapidly and is highly confusing. With regard to vascular effects there is the general consensus that the direct effect of the principal renal prostaglandins, PGI_2

and PGE$_2$, is vasodilation. However, there is also the possibility that prostaglandins can effect vasoconstriction, either directly or indirectly, under certain circumstances (Baer and McGiff, 1979). In addition, there is the general impression among workers in the field that there are significant interactions among the prostaglandin system, the kallikrein–kinin system, and the renin–angiotensin system (McGiff, 1980). Consequently, it is virtually impossible to provide a basic working hypothesis related to the singular role that prostaglandins may have in the regulation of renal hemodynamics. Only brief mention is made of some of the many possible interactions.

The possibility that prostaglandins could influence renal hemodynamics was established by experiments evaluating the effects of intraarterial infusions of various prostaglandins. Except for the paradoxical vasoconstrictor effects observed in the rat (Baer and McGiff, 1979), it has been generally observed that PGE$_2$, PGD$_2$, and PGI$_2$ all exert potent vasodilator effects (Baer and Navar, 1973; Lifschitz, 1981; Vander, 1968; Bolger *et al.*, 1977; Gerber *et al.*, 1978) when infused directly into the renal artery in dogs. In addition, the renal intraarterial infusion of arachidonic acid, precursor of the prostaglandins, can lead to increases in RBF, although a transient vasoconstriction is sometimes observed (Feigen *et al.*, 1977).

The effects of prostaglandins on intrarenal blood flow distribution have been studied in various laboratories. Using the ^{86}Rb technique, Bartha (1977) observed that PGE$_2$ proportionately increased both cortical and medullary blood flow. Chang *et al.* (1975b) and Larsson and Anggard (1974) found that, when endogenous prostaglandins were stimulated by infusion of sodium arachidonate, there was an increase in RBF to the inner cortical zones and in juxtamedullary blood flow but little change in the outer cortical areas. Likewise, Gerber *et al.* (1978) observed that PGI$_2$ infusion led to a preferential increase in RBF of the juxtamedullary cortical nephrons. In isolated perfused kidneys, PGE-like materials increased with time of perfusion, and these were associated with a redistribution of RBF so that the ratio of outer cortical/inner cortical blood flow diminished (Itskovitz *et al.*, 1974). It seems that most of the vasodilators have similar effects on the regional blood flow distribution (Carriere, 1975; Lameire *et al.*, 1977; Aukland, 1980; McNay and Abe, 1970b); that is, the relative increase in the inner cortical glomerular flow is greater than that of the outer glomerular cortical flow. These changes in the preglomerular flow, which do not always cause a demonstrable postglomerular blood flow redistribution, might be a consequence of a maximal vasodilation in the outer cortex during basal conditions or a consequence of the inherent errors existing in microsphere techniques, as discussed earlier.

In an analysis of intrarenal hemodynamics based on whole-kidney autoregulation experiments, it was observed that PGE_2 increased RBF but failed to alter GFR. Autoregulatory efficiency was reduced; however, the kidney still retained some capacity to alter renal vascular resistance in response to decreases in renal arterial pressure. Indirect calculations suggested that afferent resistance was reduced by about 50%, whereas efferent resistance was reduced by about 30%. There were apparent increases in glomerular and peritubular capillary pressures. It was suggested that GFR did not increase because the increase in proximal tubule pressure was sufficient to offset the increase in glomerular pressure and the transglomerular pressure remained unchanged (Baer and Navar, 1973). In micropuncture studies PGE_2 was infused systemically to Munich–Wistar rats (Baylis *et al.*, 1976), and it was noted that both afferent and efferent resistances decreased. In addition, the data indicated that PGE_2 could induce a substantial reduction in the filtration coefficient. Subsequent studies have established that the effects of prostaglandins on the filtration coefficient are not unique and that numerous humoral agents and vasodilators can elicit similar effects on the filtration coefficient in this strain of rats (Brenner *et al.*, 1980).

Another approach to evaluating the possible role of prostaglandins on renal hemodynamics has been the use of various inhibitors of prostaglandin synthesis. Many different nonsteroidal antiinflammatory agents have been used; however, the data must be interpreted with caution because of the many possible diverse actions of these drugs (Dunn and Hood, 1977). Nevertheless, it has been demonstrated that the administration of indomethacin or meclofenamate can induce reductions in RBF, and sometimes GFR, in anesthetized animals subjected to stressful surgery (McGiff, 1980; Lonigro *et al.*, 1973; Terragno *et al.*, 1977) and particularly in isolated perfused kidneys (Itskovitz *et al.*, 1974). It has also been observed that sodium-restricted dogs may exhibit marked decreases in renal plasma flow and GFR following treatment with indomethacin (DeForrest *et al.*, 1980). Thus, it has been suggested that activation of vasoconstrictor systems may also induce compensatory augmentation of renal synthesis of prostaglandins (Brody and Kadowitz, 1974; Dunn and Hood, 1977). In this manner intrarenal prostaglandins may serve a primary defensive role of sustaining renal function when other factors would reduce renal hemodynamic function (McGiff, 1980).

Aside from the stimulation of prostaglandins during specific stressful situations, it appears that this system does not participate to a major extent in the regulation of basal renal hemodynamics (Dunn and Hood, 1977). In spite of earlier work indicating that prostaglandins might participate in the mechanism of renal autoregulation (Herbaczynska-Cedro and Vane, 1970), subsequent studies demonstrated that whole-kidney autoregulatory responses were not impaired by inhibition of prostaglandin synthesis (Anderson et al., 1976; Finn and Arendshorst, 1976; Kaloyanides et al., 1976). However, studies by Schnermann and Briggs (1981) have indicated that cortical prostaglandins may be necessary to obtain maximum efficiency of superficial-nephron GFR and whole-kidney GFR autoregulation in the rat. In addition, the magnitude of the distal tubular feedback-mediated decrease in early proximal flow rate during increases in distal perfusion rate was diminished in the presence of prostaglandin synthase inhibitors. Feedback responsiveness was restored when exogenous PGI_2 was administered systemically. The mechanism of these effects remains difficult to decipher because the addition of the vasodilator PGI_2 restored the vasoconstrictor response occurring with increases in distal flow rate. It is clear that further work is needed in this area to resolve the many apparent roles that the intrarenal prostaglandins may have in the control of renal hemodynamics.

2. Kallikrein–Kinin System

Yet another intrarenal humoral system consists of kinin-generating enzymes that can release potent vasodepressor peptides into the circulation and tissues. However, it should be recognized that such systems are widespread throughout the body and probably are not involved in the specific regulation of the renal microcirculation (Carretero and Scicli, 1980, 1981). Over 90% of the renal kallikrein is in the cortex of the kidney, and there is abundant kallikrein in the urine that is secreted directly into the tubules. Since much of the renal kallikrein–kinin system is localized within the distal tubular network, the possible mechanism by which kinins influence renal hemodynamics remains unresolved (Carretero and Scicli, 1980; Levinsky, 1979; Kramer, 1979–1980). Nevertheless, it has been demonstrated that kinins, such as bradykinin, can increase RBF without increasing GFR and produce a natriuresis and diuresis (Willis et al., 1969). In general, bradykinin produces a greater increase in inner cortical flow than outer cortical flow when RBF distribution is assessed with microspheres (Stein et al., 1971).

Although it is recognized that the effects of arterial infusions of kinins probably do not mimic the effects of endogenous kinins, several studies have evaluated their effects on the renal microcirculation. Micropuncture studies in the rat by Baylis et al. (1976) demonstrated that bradykinin increased single-nephron plasma flow more than SNGFR and peritubular capillary pressure increased slightly. There were decreases in both afferent and efferent resistance, but the decrease in afferent resistance was

greater, presumably due to the concomitant autoregulatory-induced decrease induced by the reduction in systemic arterial pressure. As with
other vasodilators, bradykinin elicited a significant decrease in the glomerular filtration coefficient. Slight increases in peritubular capillary pressure along with decreases in the efferent arteriolar colloid osmotic pressure led to reductions in the net peritubular reabsorptive force. In the dog,
bradykinin also increased single-nephron plasma flow without increasing
SNGFR. There were approximately equivalent increases in glomerular
pressure and in proximal tubular pressure such that the net transglomerular capillary pressure did not change. In agreement with the studies in the
rat, bradykinin decreased afferent resistance more than efferent resistance. However, in contrast to the results from the rat, K_f was not significantly influenced by bradykinin in the dog (Thomas et al., 1982).

Studies related to inhibitors or blockers of the kallikrein–kinin system
have not been extensive. The angiotensin-converting enzyme and kini-
nase II are identical. However, this enzyme converts angiotensin I to the
active angiotensin II, whereas it deactivates bradykinin. The administration of CEI causes a combined effect of decreasing the activity of the angiotensin system and enhancing the activity of the kinin system (Erdos,
1977). Thus, many of the effects observed during the administration of
CEI could also be due to the accumulation of kinins. These effects are
reviewed in Section V,C. In another approach aprotinin was used to inhibit
kallikrein (Kramer et al., 1979). In non-volume-expanded rats, aprotinin
had no effects on GFR, plasma flow, or urine excretion rate. However,
aprotinin did reduce the responses to volume expansion, suggesting that
the increases in GFR and plasma flow that occur in the rat following volume expansion may be partially mediated by endogenous kinins.

It should be apparent that there is substantial uncertainty regarding the
influence of the intrarenal hormones on renal hemodynamics because of
the potential interaction among all the systems (Levinsky, 1979; Kramer,
1979–1980, McGiff, 1980; Nasjletti and Malik, 1981). Both the kallikrein–
kinin system and the renin–angiotensin system can stimulate the prostaglandin system. Likewise, prostaglandins have been shown to stimulate
renin release. In addition, prostaglandin inhibitors can augment the vasodilator response to bradykinin (Lonigro et al., 1978). The reason for the
enhanced activity is not clear, but the data indicate that an intact intrarenal prostaglandin system is not necessary for the mediation of bradykinin-induced vasodilation. It is interesting that prostaglandin inhibitors
have also been shown to augment the vasoconstrictor response to exogenous angiotensin (Baylis and Brenner, 1978). These results would suggest that endogenous prostaglandins are activated during conditions in
which tissue angiotensin levels are increased and that these tend to coun-

teract the vasoconstrictor effects of angiotensin. At present, this remains a fertile area for further studies aimed at assessing the quantitative roles of the various intrarenal hormonal systems in the regulation of the micro-circulation.

VI. Concluding Comments

During the preparation of this chapter it became apparent that, even with a presentation of this size, it would be impossible to provide a complete and comprehensive review of all the recent developments related to the renal microcirculation. The extreme complexity and degree of interaction among the various renal microcirculatory systems will continue to present exciting and challenging issues. Our knowledge concerning the inter-action among the various intrinsic, humoral, and neural mechanisms regu-lating renal microcirculatory dynamics remains incomplete. Furthermore, the quantitative contributions of these factors to the control of regional blood flow, and particularly medullary blood flow, have not been estab-lished. Greater work must be conducted on the specific permeability properties of the peritubular capillaries and the medullary capillaries; such studies will require close collaborative efforts between individuals skilled in morphologic approaches and those oriented predominantly toward functional measurements. Regulatory forces that influence perme-ability characteristics and operate at the level of individual capillary beds must be evaluated more extensively. These and many other issues will make this area of investigation a fruitful one for decades to come.

Acknowledgments

The experimental work conducted by the authors was supported by grants from the National Heart, Lung, and Blood Institute (HL 18426, HL 26371, and HL 25451). A. P. Evan's mor-phologic studies were supported by a grant from the National Institute of Arthritis and Meta-bolic Diseases.

The authors are grateful to Mrs. Cathy Dastmalchi and Mrs. Becky Smith for secretarial assistance and to Mrs. Ellen Bernstein for the illustration and photography.

László Rosivall was a Visiting Scientist at the University of Alabama in Birmingham, on leave from the Department of Pathophysiology of the Semmelweis University Medical School, Budapest, Hungary.

References

Abe, Y. (1971). *Jpn. Circ. J.* **35,** 1163–1173.

Abe, Y., Kishimoto, T., and Yamamoto, K. (1976). *Am. J. Physiol.* **231,** 1267–71.

Adams, P. L., Adams, F. F., Bell, P. D., and Navar, L. G. (1980). *Kidney Int.* **18,** 68–76.

Albertine, K. H., and O'Morchoe, C. C. C. (1979). *Kidney Int.* **16,** 470–480.

Allison, M. E., Lipsham, E. M., and Gottschalk, C. W. (1972). *Am. J. Physiol.* **223,** 975–983.

Anderson, R. J., Taher, M. S., Cronin, R. E., McDonald, K. M., and Schrier, R. W., (1976). *Am. J. Physiol.* **229,** 731–736.

Andreucci, U. E., Dal Canton, A., Corradi, A., Stanziale, R., and Migore, L. (1976). *Kidney Int.* **9,** 475–480.

Arendshorst, W. J., and Gottschalk, C. W. (1980). *Am. J. Physiol.* **239,** F171–F186.

Aukland, K. (1968). *Acta Physiol. Scand.* **72,** 498–509.

Aukland, K. (1976). *Int. Rev. Physiol.* **2,** 23–79.

Aukland, K. (1980). *Annu. Rev. Physiol.* **42,** 543–555.

Aukland, K. (1981). *In* "Advances in Physiological Sciences" (L. Takács, ed.), Vol. 2, pp. 191–198. Pergamon, Budapest.

Aukland, K., Bower, B. F., and Berliner, R. (1964). *Circ. Res.* **14,** 166–187.

Aukland, K., Heyeraas-Tonder, K., and Naess, G. (1977). *Acta Physiol. Scand.* **101,** 418–427.

Ausiello, D. A., Kreisberg, J. I., Roy, C., and Karnovsky, M. J. (1980). *J. Clin. Invest.* **65,** 754–760.

Ayer, G., Grandchamp, A., Wyler, T., and Turniger, B. (1971). *Circ. Res.* **29,** 128–135.

Baehler, R. W., Catanzaro, A. J., Stein, J. H., and Hunter, W. (1973). *Circ. Res.* **32,** 718–724.

Baer, P. G., and McGiff, J. C. (1979). *Eur. J. Pharmacol.* **54,** 359–363.

Baer, P. G., and McGiff, J. C. (1980). *Annu. Rev. Physiol.* **42,** 582–601.

Baer, P. G., and Navar, L. G. (1973). *Kidney Int.* **4,** 12–21.

Bankir, L., Trink Trang Tan, M. M., and Grunfeld, J. D. (1979). *Kidney Int.* **15,** 126–133.

Banks, R. D. (1975). *Proc. Soc. Exp. Biol. Med.* **150,** 327–330.

Barajas, L. (1970). *J. Ultrastruct. Res.* **33,** 116–147.

Barajas, L. (1978). *Fed. Proc. Fed. Am. Soc. Exp. Biol.* **37,** 1192–1201.

Barajas, L., and Muller, J. (1973). *J. Ultrastruct. Res.* **43,** 107–132.

Barclay, J., Cooke, W. T., and Kenney, R. A. (1947). *Am. J. Physiol.* **151,** 621–625.

Barger, A. C. (1966). *Ann. N.Y. Acad. Sci.* **139,** 276–284.

Barger, A. C., and Herd, J. A. (1973). *Handb. Physiol. Sect. 8 Renal Physiol.*

Bartha, J. (1977). *Acta Physiol. Acad. Sci. Hung.* **50,** 161–172.

Baylis, C., and Brenner, B. M. (1978). *Circ. Res.* **43,** 889–898.

Baylis, C., Deen, W. M., Myers, B. D., and Brenner, B. M. (1976). *Am. J. Physiol.* **230,** 1148–1158.

Bayliss, W. M. (1902). *J. Physiol. (London)* **28,** 220–231.

Beeuwkes, R., III (1971). *Am. J. Physiol.* **221,** 1361–1374.

Beeuwkes, R., III (1980). *Annu. Rev. Physiol.* **42,** 531–542.

Beeuwkes, R., III, and Bonventre, J. V. (1975). *Am. J. Physiol.* **229,** 695–713.

Bell, D. R., Pinter, G. G., and Wilson, P. D. (1978). *J. Physiol. (London)* **279,** 621–640.

Bell, P. D., and Navar, L. G. (1979). *Am. J. Physiol.* **237,** F204–F209.

Bell, P. D., and Navar, L. G. (1982). *Miner. Electrolyte Metab.* **8,** 61–77.

Bell, P. D., Thomas, C., Williams, R. H., and Navar, L. G. (1978). *Am. J. Physiol.* **234,** F154–F165.

Bell, R. D. (1971). *Lymphology* **4,** 74–78.

Bell, R. D., Sinclair, R. J., and Perry, W. L. (1974). *Lymphology* **3,** 143–148.

Bencsáth, P., and Takács, L. (1971). *J. Physiol. (London)* **212,** 629–640.

Blantz, R. C., and Tucker, B. J. (1975). *Am. J. Physiol.* **228,** 1927–1935.

Blantz, R. C., Rector, F. C., and Seldin, D. W. (1974). *Kidney Int.* **6,** 209–221.

Blantz, R. C., Konnen, K. S., and Tucker, B. J. (1976). *J. Clin. Invest.* **57,** 419–434.

Bohrer, M. P., Baylis, C., Humes, H. D., Glassock, R. J., Robertson, C. R., and Brenner, B. M. (1978). *J. Clin. Invest.* **61,** 72–78.

Bohrer, M. P., Deen, W. M., Robertson, C. R., Troy, J. L., and Brenner, B. M. (1979). *J. Gen. Physiol.* **74,** 583–593.

Boknam, L., Ericson, A. C., Aberg, B., and Ulfendahl, H. R. (1981). *Acta Physiol. Scand.* **111,** 159–163.

Bolger, P. M., Fisher, G. M., Shea, P. T., Ramwell, P. W., and Slotkoff, L. M. (1977). *Nature (London)* **267,** 628–630.

Bonvalet, J. P., Bencsáth, P., and DeRouffignac, C. (1972). *Am. J. Physiol.* **222,** 599–606.

Bottcher, W., and Steinhausen, M. (1976). *Kidney Int.* **10,** 574–580.

Brenner, B. M., Falchuk, K. H., Keimowitz, R. I., and Berliner, R. W. (1969). *J. Clin. Invest.* **48,** 1519–1531.

Brenner, B. M., Troy, J. L., and Daugharty, T. M. (1971). *J. Clin. Invest.* **50,** 1776–1780.

Brenner, B. M., Troy, J. L., Daugharty, T. M., and Deen, W. M. (1972). *Am. J. Physiol.* **223,** 1184–1190.

Brenner, B. M., Deen, W. M., and Robertson, C. R. (1974). *MTP Int. Rev. Sci. Physiol. Ser. One* **6,** 335–356.

Brenner, B. M., Badr, K. F., Schor, N., and Ichikawa, I. (1980). *Metabolism* **4,** 49–56.

Briggs, J. P., and Wright, F. S. (1979). *Am. J. Physiol.* **236,** F40–F47.

Britton, S. L. (1981). *Am. J. Physiol.* **240,** H914–H919.

Brody, M. J., and Kadowitz, P. J. (1974). *Fed. Proc. Fed. Am. Soc. Exp. Biol.* **33,** 48–60.

Burke, T. J., and Duchin, K. L. (1979). *Kidney Int.* **16,** 672–680.

Caldwell, P. R. B., Seegal, B. C., and Hsu, K. G. (1976). *Science (Washington, D.C.)* **191,** 1050–1051.

Carretero, O. A., and Scicli, A. G. (1980). *Am. J. Physiol.* **238,** F247–255.

Carretero, O. A., and Scicli, A. G. (1981). *Hypertension (Dallas)* **3** (Suppl. I), I-4–I-12.

Carriere, S., and Biron, P. (1970). *Am. J. Physiol.* **219,** 1642–1646.

Carriere, S. (1975). *Can. J. Physiol. Pharmacol.* **53,** 1–20.

Carriere, S., and Friborg, J. (1969). *Am. J. Physiol.* **217,** 1708–1715.

Casellas, D., and Mimran, A. (1981). *Anat. Rec.* **201,** 237–248.

Chang, R. L. S., Deen, W. M., Robertson, C. R., and Brenner, B. M. (1975). *Kidney Int.* **8,** 212–218.

Chang, L. C. T., Splawinski, J. A., Oates, J. A., and Nies, A. S. (1975). *Circ. Res.* **36,** 204–208.

Clausen, G., Hope, A., Kirkebo, A., Tyssebotn, A., and Aukland, I. (1979a). *Acta Physiol. Scand.* **107,** 69–81.

Clausen, G., Kirkebo, A., Tyssebotn, I., Ofjord, E. S., and Aukland, K. (1979b). *Acta Physiol. Scand.* **107,** 385–387.

Clausen, G., Hope, A., Kirkebo, A., Tyssebotn, I., and Aukland, K. (1980). *Acta Physiol. Scand.* **110,** 249–258.

Click, R. L., Joyner, W. L., and Gilmore, J. P. (1979). *Kidney Int.* **15,** 109–115.

Coelho, J. B. (1977). *Am. J. Physiol.* **233,** F333–F341.

Davis, J. O., and Freeman, R. H. (1976). *Physiol. Rev.* **56**, 1–56.
Davis, J. M., Brechtelsbauer, H., Prucksunand, P., Weigl, J., Schnermann, J., and Kramer, K. (1974). *Pfluegers Arch.* **350**, 259–272.
Deen, W. M., Robertson, C. R., and Brenner, B. M. (1972). *Am. J. Physiol.* **223**, 1178–1183.
Deen, W. M., Robertson, C. R., and Brenner, B. M. (1973a). *Biophys. J.* **13**, 340–358.
Deen, W. M., Robertson, C. R., and Brenner, B. M. (1973b). *Circ. Res.* **33**, 1–8.
Deen, W. M., Robertson, C. R., and Brenner, B. M. (1974). *Fed. Proc. Fed. Am. Soc. Exp. Biol.* **33**, 14–20.
Deen, W. M., Ueki, I. F., and Brenner, B. M. (1976). *Am. J. Physiol.* **231**, 283–291.
Deen, W. M., Satvat, B., and Jamieson, J. M. (1980). *Am. J. Physiol.* **238**, F126–F139.
DeForrest, J. M., Davis, J. O., Freeman, R. H., Seymour, A. A., Rowe, B. P., Williams, G. M., and Davis, T. P. (1980). *Circ. Res.* **47**, 99–107.
DeMuylder, C. G. (1952). "The Neurility of the Kidney." Thomas, Springfield, Illinois.
DeRouffignac, C., Deiss, S., Bonvalet, J. P. (1970). *Pfluegers Arch.* **315**, 273–290.
DiBona, G. (1978). *Fed. Proc. Fed. Am. Soc. Exp. Biol.* **37**, 1214–1217.
Dieterich, H. J. (1974). *Z. Anat. Entw. Ges.* **145**, 169–186.
Dinerstein, R. J., Vannici, J., Henderson, R. C., Roth, L. J., Goldberg, L. I., and Hoffman, P. C. (1979). *Science (Washington, D.C.)* **205**, 497–499.
Dirks, J. H., Clapp, J. R., and Berliner, R. W. (1966). *J. Clin. Invest.* **43**, 916–921.
DiSalvo, J., Peterson, A., Montefusco, C., and Menta, M. (1971). *Circ. Res.* **29**, 398–406.
DuBois, R., Decoodt, P., Gassee, J. P., Verniory, A., and Lambert, P. P. (1975). *Pfluegers Arch.* **356**, 299–316.
Dunn, M. J., and Hood, V. L. (1977). *Am. J. Physiol.* **233**, F169–F184.
Earley, L. E., Hymphreys, M. H., and Bartoli, E. (1972). *Circ. Res.* **31**, (Suppl. II), 1–18.
Edwards, J. G. (1956). *Anat. Rec.* **125**, 521–529.
Erdos, E. G. (1977). *Fed. Proc. Fed. Am. Soc. Exp. Biol.* **36**, 1760–1765.
Evan, A. P., and Dail, W. G. (1977). *Anat. Rec.* **187**, 135–145.
Evan, A. P., and Hay, D. A. (1981). *Anat. Rec.* **199**, 481.
Faarup, P., Saelan, H., and Ryo, G. (1971). *Acta Pathol. Microbiol. Scand. Sect.* **79**, 607–616.
Fagard, R. H., Amery, A. K., and Linjnen, P. J. (1978). *Pfluegers Arch.* **374**, 199–204.
Farquhar, M. G., and Kanwar, Y. S. (1980). *In* "Renal Pathophysiol" (A. Leaf, ed.), pp. 57–74. Raven, New York.
Feigen, L. P., Chapnich, B. M., Flemming, J. E., Flemming, J. M., and Kadowitz P. J. (1977). *Am. J. Physiol.* **233**, H573–H579.
Finn, W. F., and Arendshorst, W. J. (1976). *Am. J. Physiol.* **231**, 1541–1545.
Fojas, J. E., and Schmid, H. E. (1970). *Am. J. Physiol.* **219**, 464–468.
Fourcade, J. C., Navar, L. G., and Guyton, A. C. (1971). *Nephron* **8**, 1–16.
Fourman, J., and Moffat, D. B. (1971). "The Blood Vessels of the Kidney." Blackwell, Oxford.
Franklin, W. G., Peach, M. J., and Gilmore, J. P. (1970). *Circ. Res.* **27**, 321–324.
Freeman, R. H., Davis, J. O., Vitale, S. J., and Johnson, J. A. (1973). *Circ. Res.* **32**, 692–698.
Gagnon, J. A., Keller, H. I., Kokotis, W., and Schrier, R. W. (1970). *Am. J. Physiol.* **219**, 491–496.
Gagnon, J. A., Rice, M. K., and Flamenbaum, W. (1974). *Proc. Soc. Exp. Biol. Med.* **146**, 414–418.
Ganong, W. F. (1972). "Medizinesche Physiologie, Kurzgefaztes Lehrbeich der Physiologie des Menschem fur Studierende der Medizin and Arzte." Springer, Berlin.
Gartner, K., Banning, E., Vogel, G., and Ulbrich, M. (1973). *Pfluegers Arch.* **343**, 331–340.

Gassee, J. P., DuBois, R., Staroukine, M., and Lambert, P. P. (1976). *Pfluegers Arch.* **367,** 15–24.

Gerber, J. G., Nies, A. S., Friesinger, G. C., Gerkins, J. F., Branch, R. A., and Oates, J. A. (1978). *Prostaglandins* **16,** 519–528.

Gilmore, J. P., Cornish, K. G., Rogers, S. D., and Joyner, W. L. (1980). *Circ. Res.* **47,** 226–230.

Gomez, D. M. (1951). *J. Clin. Invest.* **30,** 1143–1155.

Gotshall, R. W., and Itskovitz, H. D. (1977). *Proc. Soc. Exp. Biol. Med.* **154,** 60–64.

Gottschalk, C. W. (1952). *Am. J. Physiol.* **169,** 180–187.

Gottschalk, C. W., Lassiter, W. E., and Mylle, M. (1962). *Excerpta Med. Sect.* **47,** 375–376.

Gottschalk, C. W., Colindres, R. E., Moss, N. G., Rogenes, P. R., and Szalay, L. (1981). *In* "Kidney and Body Fluids" (L. Takács, ed.), pp. 1–17. Pergamon, Budapest.

Grangsjo, G., and Persson, E. (1971). *Acta Anaesthesiol. Scand.* **15,** 71–95.

Grangsjo, G., and Wolgast, M. (1972). *Acta Physiol. Scand.* **85,** 228–236.

Graves, F. T. (1971). "The Arterial Anatomy of the Kidney" Williams & Wilkins, Baltimore, Maryland.

Gross, R., and Kirchheim, H. (1980). *Pfluegers Arch.* **383,** 233–239.

Guyton, A. C., Langston, J. B., and Navar, L. G. (1964). *Circ. Res.* **15** (Suppl. I), 187–196.

Hall, J. E., Guyton, A. G., and Cowley, A. W. (1977a). *Am. J. Physiol.* **232,** F215–F221.

Hall, J. E., Guyton, A. C., Jackson, T. E., Coleman, T. G., Lohmeier, T. E., and Trippodo, N. C. (1977b). *Am. J. Physiol.* **232,** F298–F306.

Hargens, A. R., Tucker, B. J., and Blantz, R. C. (1977). *Am. J. Physiol.* **233,** F269–F273.

Hársing, L., Pósch, E., Rosivall, L., and Szabó, G. (1975). *Acta Med. Acad. Sci. Hung.* **32,** 239–244.

Hatt. P. Y. (1967). *In* "Ultrastructure of the Kidney" (A. J. Dalton, and F. Haguenau, eds.), pp. 101–141. Academic Press, New York.

Heller, J., and Horacek, V. (1980). *Pfluegers Arch.* **385,** 253–258.

Heney, N. M., O'Morchoe, P. J., and O'Morchoe, C. C. (1971). *Urol.* **106,** 455–462.

Henry, L. P., Keyl, M. J., and Bell, R. D. (1969). *Am. J. Physiol.* **217,** 411–413.

Herbaczynska–Cedro, C. K., and Vane, J. R. (1970). *Circ. Res.* **27,** 571–587.

Hermansson, K., Larson, M., Kallskog, O., and Wolgast, M. (1981). *Pfluegers Arch.* **389,** 85–90.

Hollenberg, N. K. (1979). *Annu. Rev. Pharmacol. Toxicol.* **19,** 559–582.

Hope, A., Clausen, G., and Aukland, K. (1976). *Circ. Res.* **39,** 362–370.

Hope, A., Clausen, G., and Rosivall, L. (1981). *Acta Physiol. Scand* **113,** 455–463.

Hornych, H., and Richet, G. (1977). *Kidney Int.* **11,** 28–34.

Huber, G. C. (1907). *Am. J. Anat.* **6,** 391–406.

Huss, R. E., Marsh, D. J., and Kalaba, R. E. (1975). *Ann. Biomed. Eng.* **3,** 72–99.

Ichikawa, I., Miele, J. F., and Brenner, B. M. (1979). *Kidney Int.* **16,** 137–147.

Itskovitz, H. D., and McGiff, J. G. (1974). *Circ. Res.* **34–35** (Suppl. I), 65–73.

Itskovitz, H. D., Terragno, N. A., and McGiff, J. C. (1974). *Circ. Res.* **34,** 770–776.

Johns, E. J. (1980). *Br. J. Pharmacol.* **71,** 499–506.

Johnson, P. C. (1959). *Circ. Res.* **7,** 992–999.

Johnson, P. C. (1964). *Circ. Res.* **14–15** (Suppl. I), 2–9.

Jones, L. G., and Herd, J. A. (1974). *Am. J. Physiol.* **226,** 886–892.

Jorgensen, F., and Bentzon, M. W. (1968). *Lab. Invest.* **18,** 42–48.

Jorgensen, K. E., and Moller, J. V. (1979). *Am. J. Physiol.* **236,** F103–F111.

Kállay, K., and Debreczeni, L. A. (1970). *Acta Physiol. Acad. Sci. Hung.* **38,** 9–17.

Källskog, O., and Wolgast, M. (1975). *Acta Physiol. Scand.* **95,** 364–372.

Källskog, O., Lindbom, L. O., Ulfendahl, H. R., and Wolgast, M. (1975a). *Acta Physiol. Scand.* **95**, 191–200.
Källskog, O., Lindbom, L. O., Ulfendahl, H. R., and Wolgast, M. (1975b). *Acta Physiol. Scand.* **95**, 293–300.
Källskog, O., Lindbom, L. O., Ulfendahl, H. R., and Wolgast, M. (1975c). *Acta Physiol. Scand.* **94**, 289–300.
Källskog, O., Lindbom, L. O., Ulfendahl, H. R., and Wolgast, M. (1975d). *Acta Physiol. Scand.* **94**, 145–153.
Källskog, O., Lindbom, L. O., Ulfendahl, H. R., and Wolgast, M. (1976). *Pfluegers Arch.* **363**, 205–210.
Kaloyanides, G. J., Ahreno, R. E., Shepherd, J. A., and DiBona, G. F. (1976). *Circ. Res.* **38**, 67–73.
Kanwar, Y. S., and Farquhar, M. G. (1979). *Proc. Natl. Acad. Sci. USA* **76**, 1303–1307.
Katz, M. A., and Shear, L. (1975). *Nephron* **14**, 246–256.
Katz, M. A., Blantz, R. C., Rector, F. C., and Seldin, D. W. (1971). *Am. J. Physiol.* **220**, 1903–1913.
Kedem, O., and Katchalsky, A. (1958). *Biochim. Biophys. Acta* **27**, 229–246.
Kety, S. S. (1951). *Pharmacol. Rev.* **3**, 1–40.
Kiil, F., Kjekshus, J., and Loyning, E. (1969). *Acta Physiol. Scand.* **76**, 10–23.
Knox, F. G., Willis, L. R., Strandhoy, J. W., Schneider, E. G., Navar, L. G., and Ott, C. E. (1972a). *Am. J. Physiol.* **223**, 741–749.
Knox, F. G., Willis, L. R., Strandhoy, J. W., and Schneider, E. G. (1972b). *Kidney Int.* **2**, 11–16.
Koester, H. L., Locke, J. C., and Swann, H. G. (1955). *Tex. Rep. Biol. Med.* **13**, 251–271.
Kramer, H. J., (1979–1980). *Renal Physiol.* **2**, 107–121.
Kramer, H. J., Moch, T., Sichherer, L., and Dusing, R. (1979). *Clin. Sci.* **56**, 547–553.
Kramer, K., Thurau, K., and Deetjen, P. (1960). *Pfluegers Arch. Ges. Physiol.* **270**, 251–269.
Kriz, W. (1968). *In* "Urea and Kidney" (B. Schmidt, ed.), pp. 342–357. Neilsen, Amsterdam.
Kugelgen, A. V., and Braunger, B. (1962). *Z. Zellforsch. Mikrosk. Anat.* **57**, 766–808.
LaGrange, R. G., Sloop, C. H., and Schmid, H. E. (1973). *Circ. Res.* **33**, 704–712.
Lambert, P. P., DuBois, R., Decoodt, P., Gassee, J. P., and Verniory, A. (1975). *Pfluegers Arch.* **359**, 1–22.
Lameire, N. H., Lifschitz, M. D., and Stein, J. H. (1977). *Annu. Rev. Physiol.* **39**, 159–184.
Langer, K. H. (1975). *Cytobiologie* **10**, 161–184.
Larsson, C., and Anggard, E. (1974). *Eur. J. Pharmacol.* **25**, 327–334.
Latta, H. (1973). *Handb. Physiol. Sect.* 1–29.
LeBrie, S. J. (1967). *Am. J. Physiol.* **213**, 1225–1232.
Levens, N. R., Peach, M. J., and Carey, R. M. (1981). *Circ. Res.* **48**, 157–167.
Levinsky, N. G. (1979). *Circ. Res.* **44**, 441–451.
Lifschitz, M. D. (1981). *Kidney Int.* **19**, 781–785.
Lilienfield, L. S., Maganzine, H. C., and Bauer, M. H. (1961). *Circ. Res.* **9**, 614–617.
Ljungquist, A. (1963). *Acta Paediatr. Scand.* **52**, 443.
Ljungquist, A. (1975). *Kidney Int.* **8**, 239–244.
Lohmeier, T. E., and Cowley, A. W. (1979). *Circ. Res.* **44**, 154–160.
Lonigro, A. J., Itskovitz, H. D., Crowshaw, K., and McGiff, J. C. (1973). *Circ. Res.* **32**, 712–717.
Lonigro, A. J., Hagemann, M. H., Stephenson, A. H., and Fry, C. L. (1978). *Circ. Res.* **43**, 447–455.
Love, W. A., and O'Meallie, L. (1963). *Am. J. Physiol.* **205**, 382–384.

Loyning, E. W. (1971). *Acta Physiol. Scand.* **83,** 191–202.
MacCallum, D. B. (1939). *Am. J. Anat.* **65,** 69–103.
Marchand, G. R., and Mohrman, D. E. (1980). *Life. Sci.* **27,** 2571–2576.
Marsh, D. J., Huss, R. E., and Moore, L. C. (1974). *Proc. Summer Comput. Simul. Conf.* **1,** 720–731.
Marshall, E. A., and Trowbridge, E. A. (1974). *Theor. Biol.* **48,** 389–412.
McGiff, J. C. (1980). *Clin. Sci.* **59,** 1055–1165.
McIntosh, G. H., and Morris, B. (1971). *J. Physiol.* **214,** 365–376.
McNay, J. L., and Abe, Y. (1970a). *Circ. Res.* **27,** 571–587.
McNay, J. L., and Abe, Y. (1970b). *Circ. Res.* **27,** 1023–1032.
Mendell, P. L., and Hollenberg, N. K. (1971). *Am. J. Physiol.* **221,** 1617–1620.
Mendelsohn, F. A. O. (1979). *Clin. Sci.* **57,** 173–179.
Mimran, A., and Casellas, D. (1979). *Pfluegers Arch.* **382,** 233–240.
Mohos, S. C., and Skoza, L. (1970). *Exp. Mol. Pathol.* **12,** 316–323.
Moore, L. C., Schnermann, J., and Yarimizu, S. (1979). *Am. J. Physiol.* **237,** F63–F74.
Morkrid, L., Ofstad, Y., and Willasen, Y. (1976). *Circ. Res.* **39,** 608–615.
Morkrid, L., Ofstad, Y., and Willasen, Y. (1978). *Circ. Res.* **42,** 181–191.
Murray, R. D., and Malvin, R. L. (1979). *Am. J. Physiol.* **236,** F559–F566.
Myers, B. D., Deen, W. M., and Brenner, B. M. (1975). *Circ. Res.* **37,** 101–110.
Nash, F. D., and Selkurt, E. E. (1964). *Circ. Res.* **15,** (Suppl. 1), 142–147.
Nasjletti, A., and Malik, K. U. (1981). *Kidney Int.* **19,** 860–868.
Navar, L. G. (1970). *Am. J. Physiol.* **219,** 1658–1664.
Navar, L. G. (1978a). *Am. J. Physiol.* **234,** F357–F370.
Navar, L. G. (1978b). "Physiology of Membrane Disorders" (T. E. Andreoli, J. Hoffman, and D. Fanestil, eds.), pp. 593–626. Plenum, New York.
Navar, L. G., and Guyton, A. C. (1975). *In* "Circulatory Physiology: Dynamics and Control of the Body Fluids" (A. C. Guyton, A. E. Taylor, and H. J. Granger, eds.), Vol. 2, pp. 243–261. Saunders, Philadelphia, Pennsylvania.
Navar, L. G., and Langford, H. G. (1974). *Handb. Exp. Pharmacol.* **37,** 455–474.
Navar, L. G., Baer, P. G., Wallace, S. L., and McDaniel, J. K. (1971). *Am. J. Physiol.* **221,** 329–334.
Navar, L. G., Burke, T. J., Robinson, R. R., and Clapp, J. R. (1974). *J. Clin. Invest.* **53,** 516–525.
Navar, L. G., Chomdej, B., and Bell, P. D. (1975). *Am. J. Physiol.* **266,** 1596–1603.
Navar, L. G., Bell, P. D., White, R. W., Watts, R. L., and Williams, R. H. (1977a). *Kidney Int.* **12,** 137–149.
Navar, L. G., Bell, P. D., and Burke, T. J. (1977b). *Circ. Res.* **41,** 487–496.
Navar, L. G., Ploth, D. W., and Bell, P. D. (1980). *Annu. Rev. Physiol.* **42,** 557–571.
Navar, L. G., Bell, P. D., and Adams, P. L. (1981a). *In* "Advances in Physiological Sciences" (L. Takács, ed.), Vol. 2, pp. 205–215. Pergamon, Budapest.
Navar, L. G., Bell, P. D., and Ploth, D. W. (1981b). *Fed. Proc. Fed. Am. Soc. Exp. Biol.* **40,** 93–98.
Navar, L. G., Bell, P. D., and Burke, T. J. (1982a). *Kidney Int.* **22** (Suppl. 12), 5157–5164.
Navar, L. G., Jirakulsomchok, D., Bell, P. D., Thomas, C. E., and Huang, W. C. (1982b). *Hypertension (Dallas)* **4,** 58–68.
Navar, P. D., and Navar, L. G. (1977). *Am. J. Physiol.* **233,** H295–H298.
Nissen, O. I., and Galskov, A. (1972). *Circ. Res.* **30,** 82–96.
Nomura, G., Kibe, Y., Arai, S., Uno, D., and Takeuchi, J. (1976). *Nephron* **16,** 126–133.
Nordquist, R. E., Bell, R. D., Sinclair, R. J., and Keyl, M. J. (1973). *Lymphology* **6,** 13–19.

Oberling, C., and Hatt, P. Y. (1960). *Ann. Anat. Pathol.* **5**, 441–460.
Ofjord, E. S., Clausen, G., and Aukland, K. (1981). *Am. J. Physiol.* **241**, H342–H347.
Ofstad, J., Morkrid, L., and Williassen, Y. (1975). *Scand. J. Clin. Lab. Invest.* **35**, 767–774.
Oken, D. E., and Flamenbaum, W. (1971). *J. Clin. Invest.* **50**, 1498–1505.
Oken, D. E., Thomas, S. R., and Mikulecky, D. (1981). *Kidney Int.* **19**, 359–373.
O'Morchoe, C. C. C., Jarosz, H. M., Holmes, M. J., and O'Morchoe, P. J. (1977). *Lymphology* **10**, 204–208.
O'Morchoe, C. C. C., O'Morchoe, P. J., Holmes, M. J., and Jarosz, H. M. (1978). *Lymphology* **11**, 27–31.
Oparil, S. (1976). Annual Research Reviews: Renin (D. F. Horrobin, ed.). Eden, Montreal.
Oparil, S., Sanders, C. A. and Haber, E. (1970). *Circ. Res.* **26**, 591–599.
Ott, C. E. (1981). *Am. J. Physiol.* **240**, F106–F110.
Ott, C. E., and Knox, F. G. (1976). *Fed. Proc. Fed. Am. Soc. Exp. Biol.* **35**, 1872–1875.
Ott, C. E., Marchand, G. R., Diaz-Buro, J. A., and Knox, F. G. (1976). *Am. J. Physiol.* **231**, 235–239.
Ott, C. E., Navar, L. G., and Guyton, A. C. (1971). *Am. J. Physiol.* **221**, 394–400.
Ott, C. E., Cuche, J. L., and Knox, F. G. (1975). *J. Appl. Physiol.* **38**, 937–941.
Palmer, A. A., and Betts, W. H. (1975). *Biorheology* **12**, 283–292.
Papenfuss, H. D., and Gross, J. F. (1978). *Microvasc. Res.* **16**, 59–72.
Pappenheimer, J. R. (1955). *Klin. Wochenschr.* **33**, 362–365.
Pappenheimer, J. R., Renkin, E. M., and Borrero, L. M. (1951). *Am. J. Physiol.* **167**, 13–46.
Parekh, N., and Veith, U. (1981). *Kidney Int.* **19**, 306–316.
Parker, J. C., Parker, R. E., Granger, D. N., and Taylor, A. E. (1981). *Circ. Res.* **48**, 549–561.
Passmore, J. C., Neiberger, R. E., and Eden, S. W. (1977). *Am. J. Physiol.* **232**, H56–H58.
Passmore, J. C., Leffler, C. W., and Neiberger, R. E. (1978). *Circ. Shock* **5**, 327–338.
Pinter, G. G., and Wilson, P. D. (1981). *In* "Advances in Physiological Sciences" (L. Takács, ed.), Vol. 2, pp. 57–73. Pergamon, Budapest.
Ploth, D. W., and Navar, L. G. (1979). *Fed. Proc. Fed. Am. Soc. Exp. Biol.* **38**, 2280–2285.
Ploth, D. W., Schnermann, J., Dahlheim, H., Hermle, M., and Schmidmeier, E. (1977). *Kidney Int.* **12**, 253–267.
Ploth, D. W., Rudolph, J., LaGrange, R., and Navar, L. G. (1979). *J. Clin. Invest.* **64**, 1325–1335.
Pomeranz, B. H., Birtch, A. G., and Barger, A. C. (1968). *Am. J. Physiol.* **215**, 1067–1081.
Poujeol, P., Chabardes, D., Bonvalet, J. P., and DeRouffignac, C. (1975). *Pfluegers Arch.* **357**, 291–301.
Prong, L. A., Bjoraker, D. G., and Harvey, R. B. (1969). *Microvasc. Res.* **1**, 275–286.
Rasmussen, S. N. (1978). *Pfluegers Arch.* **373**, 153–159.
Rector, J. B., Stein, J. H., Bag, W. H., Osgood, R. W., and Ferris, T. F. (1972). *Am. J. Physiol.* **222**, 1125–1131.
Reid, I. A., Morris, B. J., and Ganong, W. F. (1978). *Annu. Rev. Physiol.* **40**, 377–410.
Renkin, E. M. (1977). *Circ. Res.* **41**, 735–743.
Renkin, E. M., and Gilmore, J. P. (1973). *Handb. Physiol. Sect. 8 Renal Physiol.* **8**, 185–248.
Rennke, H. G., and Venkatachalam, M. A. (1977). *Fed. Proc. Fed. Am. Soc. Exp. Biol.* **36**, 2619–2626.
Rennke, H. G., and Venkatachalam, M. A. (1979). *J. Clin. Invest.* **63**, 713–717.
Rennke, H. G., Patel, Y., and Venkatachalam, M. (1978). *Kidney Int.* **13**, 324–328.
Rentsch, H. P., Ayer, G., Valloton, M., Zeigler, W., and Trunager, B. (1976). *Eur. J. Clin. Invest.* **6**, 457–464.

Riggs, D. S. (1970). "Control Theory and Physiological Feedback Mechanisms," pp. 272–281. Williams & Wilkins, Baltimore, Maryland.

Robertson, C. R., Deen, W. M., Troy, J. L., and Brenner, B. M. (1972). *Am. J. Physiol.* **223**, 1191–1200.

Rojo-Ortega, J. M., Yeghiayan, E., and Genest, J. (1973). *Lab. Invest.* **29**, 336–341.

Rosivall, L., Walter, J., and Hársing, L. (1977). *Acta Physiol. Acad. Sci. Hung.* **50**, 409–416.

Rosivall, L., Pósch, E., Simmon, G., László, E., and Hársing, L. (1979a). *Acta Physiol. Acad. Sci. Hung.* **53**, 387–397.

Rosivall, L., Fazekas, A., Pósch, E., Szabó, G., and Hársing, L. (1979b). *Acta Physiol. Acad. Sci. Hung.* **53**, 399–408.

Rosivall, L., Hope, A., and Clausen, G. (1981). *Pfluegers Arch.* **390**, 216–218.

Rouiller, C., and Orci, L. (1971). *In* "The Kidney: Morphology, Biochemistry and Physiology" (C. Rouiller, and A. F. Muller, eds.) Vol. 4, pp. 1–80. Academic Press, New York.

Rudolph, A. M., and Heymann, M. A. (1967). *Circ. Res.* **21**, 163–184.

Sabto, J., Baukir, L., and Grunfeld, J. P. (1978). *Clin. Exp. Pharmacol. Physiol.* **5**, 559–565.

Sanjana, V. M., Johnston, P. A., Deen, W. M., Robertson, C. R., Brenner, B. M., and Jamison, R. L. (1975). *Am. J. Physiol.* **228**, 1921–1926.

Sanjana, V. M., Johnston, P. A., Robertson, C. R., and Jamison, R. L. (1976). *Am. J. Physiol.* **231**, 313–318.

Sapirstein, L. A. (1958). *Am. J. Physiol.* **00**, 161–168.

Schloss, G. (1945–1946). *Acta Anat.* **1**, 365–410.

Schnermann, J. (1981). *Fed. Proc. Fed. Am. Soc. Exp. Biol.* **40**, 109–115.

Schnermann, J., and Briggs, J. P. (1981). *Kidney Int.* **19**, 802–815.

Schnermann, J., and Levine, D. Z. (1975). *Can. J. Physiol. Pharmacol.* **53**, 325–329.

Schnermann, J., Wright, F. S., Davis, J. M., Stackelberg. W., and Grill, G. (1970). *Pfluegers Arch.* **318**, 147–175.

Schnermann, J., Davis, J. M., Wunderlich, P., Levine, D. Z., and Horster, M. (1971). *Pfluegers Arch.* **329**, 307–320.

Schnermann, J., Persson, E., Ulfendahl, H., Wolgast, M., and Wunderlich, P. (1972). *In* "Recent Advances in Renal Physiology" (H. Wirz and F. Spinell, eds.), pp. 43–50. Karger, Basel.

Schnermann, J., Persson, A. E. G., and Agerup, B. (1973). *J. Clin. Invest.* **52**, 862–869.

Schwartz, M. M., Karnovsky, M. J., and Venkatachalam, M. A. (1976). *Lab. Invest.* **35**, 161–170.

Selkurt, E. E. (1963). *Handb. Physiol. Sect. 2 Cardiovasc. Sys.* **2**, 1457–1516.

Selkurt, E. E., Hall, P. W., and Spencer, M. P. (1949). *Am. J. Physiol.* **159**, 369–378.

Shea, S. M., and Raskova, J. (1981). *Fed. Proc. Fed. Am. Soc. Exp. Biol.* **40**, 515.

Sheehan, R. M., and Renkin, E. M. (1972). *Circ. Res.* **30**, 588–607.

Shimamura, T., and Morrison, A. B. (1973). *Am. J. Pathol.* **71**, 155–166.

Shipley, R. E., and Study, R. S. (1951). *Am. J. Physiol.* **167**, 676–688.

Slotkoff, L. M., Logan, A., Jose, P., D'Avella, J., and Eisner, G. M. (1971). *Circ. Res.* **28**, 158–166.

Smith, H. W. (1951). *In* "The Kidney." Oxford Univ. Press, London and New York.

Stein, J. H., Ferris, T. F., Huprich, J. E., Smith, T. C., and Osgood, R. W. (1971). *J. Clin. Invest.* **50**, 1429–1438.

Stein, J. H., Boonjarern, S., Wilson, C. B., and Ferris, T. F. (1973). *Circ. Res.* **32**, 61–71.

Steiner, R. W., Tucker, B. J., and Blantz, R. C. (1979). *J. Clin. Invest.* **64**, 503–512.

Steiner, S. H., and King, R. D. (1970). *J. Surg. Res.* **10**, 133–146.

Stern, M. D., Bowen, P. D., Parma, R., Osgood, R. W., Bowman, R. L., and Stein, J. H. (1979). *Am. J. Physiol.* **236,** F80–F87.

Steven, K., and Strobaek, S. (1974). *Pfluegers Arch.* **348,** 317–331.

Steven, K., and Thorpe, D. H. (1977). *Acta Physiol. Scand.* **101,** 394–403.

Stowe, N. T., and Hook, J. B. (1976). *Arch. Int. Pharmacodyn. Ther.* **224,** 299–309.

Stowe, N., Schnermann, J., and Hermle, M. (1979). *Kidney Int.* **15,** 473–486.

Szabó, G., Pósch, E., Rosivall, L., Fazekas, A., and Hársing, L. (1976). *Pfluegers Arch.* **367,** 33–36.

Szabó, G., Fazekas, A., Rosivall, L., and Pósch, E. (1980). *Res. Exp. Med.* **177,** 23–32.

Taylor, A. E., and Granger, A. N. (1983). *Handb. Physiol. Sect. Microcirc.* (in press).

Terragno, N. A., Terragno, D. A., and McGiff, J. C. (1977). *Circ. Res.* **40,** 590–595.

Thomas, C. E., Bell, P. D., and Navar, L. G. (1979). *Kidney Int.* **15,** 502–512.

Thomas, C. E., Bell, P. D., and Navar, L. G. (1982). *Renal Physiol.* **5,** 197–205.

Thornburn, G. D., Kopald, H. H., Herd, J. A., Hollenberg, M., O'Morchoe, C. C. C., and Barger, A. C. (1963). *Circ. Res.* **13,** 290–307.

Thurau, K. (1964). *Am. J. Med.* **36,** 698–719.

Thurau, K. (1974). *Handb. Exp. Pharmacol.* **37,** 475–489.

Thurau, K. (1981). *In* "Advances in Physiology Sciences" (L. Takács, ed.), Vol. 2, pp. 75–82. Pergamon, Budapest.

Thurau, K., and Kramer, K. (1959). *Pfluegers Arch.* **269,** 77–93.

Thurau, K., and Levine, D. Z. (1971). *In* "The Kidney" (C. Rouiller, and A. F. Muller, eds.) Vol. 3, pp. 1–70. Academic Press, New York.

Thurau, K., and Mason, J. (1974). *MTP Int. Rev. Sci. Physiol. Ser. One* **6,** 357–389.

Thurau, K., and Wober, E. (1962). *Pfluegers Arch.* **274,** 553–566.

Tonder, K. J. H., and Aukland, K. (1979–1980). *Renal Physiol.* **2,** 214–221.

Trueta, J., Barclay, A. E., Daniel, P. M., Franklin, K. J., and Prichard, M. M. L. (1947). "Studies of the Renal Circulation." Blackwell, Oxford.

Tyssebotn, I., and Kirkebo, A. (1975). *Acta Physiol. Scand.* **95,** 318–328.

Vander, A. J. (1968). *Am. J. Physiol.* **214,** 218–221.

Vanrenterghem, Y., Vanholder, R., Lammens-Verslijpe, M., and Lambert, P. P. (1980). *Clin. Sci.* **58,** 65–75.

Venkatachalam, M. A., and Karnovsky, M. J. (1972). *Lab. Invest.* **27,** 435–444.

Virchow, R. (1857). *Anat. Physiol.* **12,** 310–325.

Von Baeyer, H., VanLiew, J. B., Klassen, J., and Boylan, J. W. (1976). *Kidney Int.* **10,** 425–437.

Weinstein, S. W., and Szyjewicz, J. (1978). *Am. J. Physiol.* **234,** F207–F214.

White, R. J., and Navar, L. G. (1975). *Proc. Summer Comput. Simul. Conf.* **2,** 878–888.

Williams, M. M. M., Moffat, D. B., and Creasey, M. (1971). *Q. J. Exp. Physiol.* **56,** 250–256.

Williams, R. H., Thomas, C., Bell, P. D., and Navar, L. G. (1977). *Am. J. Physiol.* **2,** F282–F289.

Williams, R. H., Thomas, C. E., Navar, L. G., and Evan, A. P. (1981). *Kidney Int.* **19,** 503–515.

Willis, L. R., Ludens, J. H., Hook, J. B., and Williamson, H. E. (1969). *Am. J. Physiol.* **217,** 1–5.

Wolgast, M. (1973). *Acta Physiol. Scand.* **88,** 215–225.

Wolgast, M., Persson, E., Schnermann, J., Ulfendahl, H., and Wunderlich, P. (1973). *Pfluegers Arch.* **340,** 123–131.

Wright, F. S., and Briggs, J. P. (1977). *Am. J. Physiol.* **233,** F1–F7.

Wright, F. S., and Briggs, J. P. (1979). *Physiol. Rev.* **59,** 958–1006.

Wunderlich, P., Persson, E., Schnermann, J., Ulfendahl, H. R., and Wolgast, M. (1971). *Pfluegers Arch.* **328,** 307–319.

Yarger, W. E., Boyd, M. A., and Schrader, N. W. (1978). *Am. J. Physiol.* **235,** H592–H600.

Young, D. K., and Marsh, D. J. (1981). *Am. J. Physiol.* **240,** F446–458.

Zimmerman, B. G., Abbound, F. M., and Eckstein, J. W. (1964). *Am. J. Physiol.* **206,** 701–706.

Index